# Oxford H
## of Perio

**Published and forthcoming Oxford Handbooks in Nursing**

OXFORD HANDBOOK OF

# Perioperative Practice

## SECOND EDITION

EDITED BY

**Suzanne J. Hughes**

Senior Lecturer in Adult Nursing
School of Healthcare Sciences
University of Cardiff
Cardiff, UK

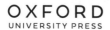

OXFORD
UNIVERSITY PRESS

# OXFORD
UNIVERSITY PRESS

Great Clarendon Street, Oxford, OX2 6DP,
United Kingdom

Oxford University Press is a department of the University of Oxford.
It furthers the University's objective of excellence in research, scholarship,
and education by publishing worldwide. Oxford is a registered trade mark of
Oxford University Press in the UK and in certain other countries

© Oxford University Press 2023

First Edition published in 2009
Second Edition published in 2023

Impression: 1

Published in the United States of America by Oxford University Press
198 Madison Avenue, New York, NY 10016, United States of America

British Library Cataloguing in Publication Data
Data available

Library of Congress Control Number: 2022930565

ISBN 978–0–19–878378–7

DOI: 10.1093/med/9780198783787.001.0001

Printed and bound in China by
C&C Offset Printing Co., Ltd.

**Tim Lewis**

Lecturer
Operating Department Practice
Retired
School of Healthcare Sciences
Cardiff University
Wales, UK

**Andy Mardell**

Practice Educator
Retired
Cardiff and Vale
University Health Board, Cardiff
University
Wales, UK

**Peter McNee**

Senior Lecturer
Children and Young People's
Nursing
School of Healthcare Sciences
Cardiff University
Wales, UK

**Sherran Milton**

National Training and
Guidance Lead
Public Health Wales: Health
Protection
Wales, UK

**Alun Morgan**

Lecturer
Operating Department Practice
Retired
School of Healthcare Sciences
Cardiff University
Wales, UK

**Tim Nagle**

Ward Manager
Cygnet Alders Clinic
Gloucester, UK

**Andy Parry**

Senior Lecturer
Adult Nursing
School of Healthcare Sciences
Cardiff University
Wales, UK

**Melda Price**

Lecturer
Children and Young People's
Nursing
Retired
School of Healthcare Sciences
Cardiff University
Wales, UK

**Anthony Pritchard**

Lecturer
Adult Nursing
School of Healthcare Sciences
Cardiff University
Wales, UK

**Natalea Purnell**

Staff Nurse
Department of Southmead
Emergency
North Bristol NHS Trust
Bristol, UK

**Melissa Rochon**

Quality & Safety Lead for
Surveillance
Royal Brompton and Harefield
Hospitals part of Guys and St
Thomas NHS Foundation Trust
Harefield, UK

**Andrew James Santos**

Lecturer
Adult Nursing
School of Healthcare Sciences
Cardiff University
Wales, UK

**Nelson RK Selvaraj**

Lecturer
Adult Nursing
School of Healthcare Sciences
Cardiff University
Wales, UK

**Hazel Smith**

Lecturer
Operating Department Practice
School of Healthcare Sciences
Cardiff University
Wales, UK

**Gemma Stacey-Emile**

Team Manager/Advanced Nurse
Practitioner
Memory Assessment Service
Hywel Dda University Health Board
Carmarthen, Wales, UK

**Ben Stanfield-Davies**

Head of Clinical Quality &
Professional Practice
Nuffield Health
London, UK

**Alicia Stringfellow**

Senior Lecturer
Mental Health Nursing
School of Healthcare Sciences
Cardiff University
Wales, UK

**Katie Summerhill**

Lecturer
Adult Nursing
School of Healthcare Sciences
Cardiff University
Wales, UK

**Neil Thomas**

Senior Lecturer
Adult Nursing
School of Healthcare Sciences
Cardiff University
Wales, UK

**Georgios Tsigkas**

Lecturer in Nursing
Queen Margaret University
Edinburgh, UK

**Susan Ward**

Senior Lecturer
Adult Nursing
School of Healthcare Sciences
Cardiff University
Wales, UK

**Gaynor Williams**

Senior Lecturer
Adult Nursing
School of Healthcare Sciences
Cardiff University
Wales, UK

**Afzal Zaidi**

Consultant Cardiothoracic Surgeon
Morriston Hospital
Swansea Bay University Health
Board, Swansea
Wales, UK

# Chapter 1

# Perioperative practice

# Team working

Surgery is a complex field that requires a coordinated, well-directed inter-disciplinary approach. There are three basic objectives of safe surgical patient care delivery and management and all team members play a vital role in achieving these objectives:

1. The delivery of a physiologically and psychologically prepared patient for the planned surgical journey.
2. The safe, efficient, and therapeutic alleviation of the patient's problem using sound evidence-based knowledge and a proficient technique.
3. The careful guidance of the patient's immediate postoperative care in order to minimize the possibility of complications.

Teams often work across functional divides in that they are drawn from many disciplines, with each member encompassing a distinct role, and failure to develop a collaborative approach will often result in a fragmented service for patients.

The understanding of each team member's role is an important aspect of ensuring a coordinated and collaborative approach. No individual alone can deliver a high-quality service; therefore, teamwork is vital in ensuring a first-class service.

Strategies pivotal to clinical governance include patient satisfaction, personal and professional growth, risk management, and team building. Effective teamwork can have a direct impact on the health and well-being of team members and the mortality and morbidity of patients.

There is also a need to recognize that if errors occur, they should be prevented from happening again by systematically learning from them, although they may not be completely eradicated. This would encourage individual practitioners to share experiences of both error prevention and actual errors with their team members without a fear of unfair treatment and to make error reduction possible in the future.

The focus of error prevention needs to be widened from individual to team responsibility and include the underlying organizational factors as well. Therefore, fostering shared responsibility to minimize error-making and learning from mistakes should be intimately connected.

All healthcare practitioners have a duty to use evidence-based practice which encompasses research utilization and highlights the impact that effective teamwork has on staff and patients.

Effective teams can ensure that staff feel a common purpose and work to promote the health and well-being of the patient through good communication, cooperation, and increased understanding of other professional roles.[1]

## Members of a high-performing and effective team

- Understand their own and other members' roles and responsibilities.
- Encourage contributions from other members and ensure that the views of new and junior members are acknowledged.
- Respect the role, expertise, competence, and contributions of allied disciplines and healthcare providers.
- Respect team leadership.
- Share a goal of high-quality care for the patient.
- Show commitment to team work in the best interest of the patient.
- Recognize they are important to the outcome of the task.
- Feel confident to speak up or intervene.

In the modern National Health Service (NHS), with medicine and healthcare increasing in complexity, high-quality care for patients will increasingly depend on high-quality teamwork, so the effectiveness of clinical teams is an important clinical governance issue.

## Reference

1. Roche F (2016). Human factors and non-technical skills: teamwork. Journal of Perioperative Practice, 26(12):285–288.

## Further reading

Catchpole K (2010). Errors in the operating theatre: how to spot and stop them. Journal of Health Services Research and Policy, 15(Suppl 1):48–51.

Kim FJ, da Silva RD, Gustafson D, et al. (2015). Current issues in patient safety in surgery: a review. Patient Safety in Surgery, 9:26.

Royal College of Anaesthetists (2020). Chapter 1: guidelines for the provision of anaesthetic services. London: Royal College of Anaesthetists.

Royal College of Surgeons (2014). The high performing surgical team: a guide to best practice. Available at: ⅋ https://www.rcseng.ac.uk/-/media/files/rcs/library-and-publications/non-journal-publications/rcs_gsp_teamworking_web.pdf

Wicker P, Dalby S (2016). Rapid perioperative care. Oxford: Wiley-Blackwell.

# Interprofessional team working

Defining the term '*interprofessional*' has proved problematic for almost a decade and there still doesn't appear to be a sound consensus of definition.

- The terms interprofessional, multiprofessional, multidisciplinary, and interdisciplinary are regularly used interchangeably without careful consideration of their underpinning meanings.
- Interprofessional working can be considered as interactions between team members; or a willingness to share and give up exclusive claims to specialized knowledge and authority if other professional groups can meet patient needs more efficiently and appropriately.
- Multiprofessional working comprises a group of people who come from different health and social care professions but who do not necessarily interact; or as a cooperative enterprise in which traditional forms and divisions of professional knowledge and authority are retained.
- Multidisciplinary working is often viewed as including practitioners who share the same professional background but who practise within different specialities.

The NHS promotes and emphasizes the importance of inter-professional teamwork as the way to providing seamless patient-centred care.

> Interprofessional teamwork and collaborative practice support healthcare practitioners' abilities to provide safe care and to perform as a cohesive team.[1]

Successful implementation of clinical governance within the NHS organization depends upon leaders who are able to inspire and motivate others. Leaders occur throughout an organization and are not necessarily the people at the top of the hierarchy or just managers. However, the running of the operating theatre should be undertaken by a theatre manager who is responsible for coordinating the operating lists and ensuring that effective communication systems are in place.

## The operating theatre team

The operating theatre team consists of a diverse range of healthcare professionals with different levels of training, experience, and responsibility.

*Consultant surgeons* hold the overall responsibility for managing patients' care and are assisted by a team of doctors and other healthcare professionals. Consultants usually specialize in one or two specific areas of surgery and are governed by the General Medical Council (GMC).[2]

*Associate specialist surgeons* carry out surgical procedures and work under the supervision of a consultant. They may run their own clinics, have personal waiting lists, and operate independently.

*Specialty/staff grade/career grade surgeons* will have had some experience as a registrar and have completed at least 2 years of surgical training after their foundation years. They may perform operations and outpatient consultations under the supervision of a consultant.

*Specialty surgical registrars* (StRs) spend up to 8 years gaining surgical experience. On successful completion of this training period, surgical StRs can apply for positions as consultants.

*Core surgical training* (CT1 and CT2) is when surgeons gain experience performing different surgical procedures following the completion of F2. Core training programmes will last up to 2 years (CT1 and CT2) depending on the grade and specialty.[3]

*Foundation doctors* (F1 and F2) are newly qualified doctors who spend 2 years in training in surgery and general medicine. Their role involves preparing patients for theatre and observing procedures conducted by the core training doctors (CT1 and CT2). They may assist in minor surgery under close supervision.

*Medical students* gain valuable experience and skills while observing and assisting in theatre. Despite them not being an essential part of the surgery itself, they gain great insight into surgery and anaesthetics as specialties. They will assist with many different tasks such as helping the nursing team with transporting the patient to scrubbing in and developing their suturing skills.

*Operating department practitioners* (ODPs) have an essential role within the operating theatre team and provide high standards of care to patients during the perioperative period. Their role is quite diverse in that on completion of a 3-year degree programme, they are qualified to act as anaesthetic assistants, scrub and circulating practitioners, and post-anaesthetic care practitioners.

*Theatre nurses* are qualified nurses who deliver high-quality nursing care to patients throughout the perioperative phase, including pre-assessment, anaesthetics, scrub, and recovery.

*Surgical care practitioners* are registered non-medical healthcare professionals, usually nurses and/or ODPs who have extended the scope of their practice by successfully completing an advanced practice programme. They work as members of the surgical team and perform surgical interventions and preoperative and postoperative care under the direct supervision of a senior surgeon. They are clinically responsible to the consultant surgeon and work within a specific speciality as a member of the extended surgical team.

*Surgical first assistants* are qualified theatre practitioners who provide assistance to the surgeon under direct supervision. They are registered nurses and/or ODPs but do not perform any surgical procedures.

*Scrub practitioners* are qualified nurses or ODPs and occasionally healthcare support workers. They are responsible for maintaining a safe operating room environment throughout the surgical procedure by ensuring essential checks of all instruments are performed and swabs, needles, blades, and sutures are correct and accounted for before, during, and following surgery (➜ see Chapter 16).

*Circulating practitioners* are qualified nurses, ODPs, and/or healthcare support workers who assist the scrub practitioner by preparing the operating theatre prior to surgery, ensuring all needed equipment is available. Intraoperatively, the circulating practitioner assists with patient transfer/positioning, manages surgical specimens and consumables, and completes perioperative documentation (➜ see Chapter 16).

*Anaesthetists* are specialist doctors responsible for providing anaesthesia and pain management to patients during the perioperative phase. Additional responsibilities include intensive care medicine, pain medicine, resuscitation and stabilization of patients within the emergency unit, obstetric anaesthesia and analgesia, and transport of acutely ill and injured patients.

*Anaesthesia associates* (AAs) are highly trained and skilled practitioners who work within an anaesthetic team under the direction and supervision of a consultant anaesthetist. They are fully trained professionals who have completed a 27-month postgraduate diploma and can play a role in pre-operative assessment, provision of sedation, cardiac arrest teams, and offer a range of other perioperative and non-perioperative support consistent with their scope of practice at qualification.[4] AAs cannot prescribe medication but can administer drugs on the prescription of the supervising consultant under patient-specific directives.

*Anaesthetic assistants* are qualified ODPs/nurses who provide continual assistance to the anaesthetist during the delivery, maintenance, and reversal of anaesthesia. They also assist anaesthetists outside of the operating theatre, for example, analgesia/anaesthesia in the obstetric department, emergency unit, and critical care environments. The Association of Anaesthetists of Great Britain and Ireland (AAGBI)[5] emphasizes that all anaesthetic assistants should follow a programme of professional development to anaesthetic care that meets the requirements of their regulatory body (Health and Care Professions Council (HCPC) and Nursing and Midwifery Council (NMC)) (➜ see Chapter 7).

*Post-anaesthetic care practitioners or recovery practitioners* provide care to patients in the immediate post-anaesthesia period. The provision of care by nurses/ODPs with expertise and experience in this environment is vital. They assist the patient through emergence from anaesthesia and the postoperative effects of surgery by continual assessment of their condition (➜ see Chapter 21).

*Operating theatre support staff* are essential to the running of surgical lists. Theatre porters and healthcare support workers are responsible for transporting patients to and from theatre, maintaining stock levels, cleaning theatres after use, ensuring adequate supplies of linen, and waste management. They are often the first person a patient sees on arrival in theatre so they provide a vital role in engaging with patients and family members and offering reassurance.

## References

1. Marrone SR (2018). Perioperative accountable care teams: improving surgical team efficiency and work satisfaction through interprofessional collaboration. Journal of Perioperative Practice, 28(9):223–230.
2. General Medical Council (2019). Good medical practice: working with doctors working for patients. London: General Medical Council.
3. Royal College of Surgeons (2020). Who's who in the surgical team. London: Royal College of Surgeons.
4. Royal College of Anaesthetists (2019). Anaesthesia associates. Available at: ℗ https://rcoa.ac.uk/training-careers/working-anaesthesia/anaesthesia-associates
5. Association of Anaesthetists of Great Britain and Ireland (2018). The anaesthesia team. Available at: ℗ http://dx.doi.org/10.21466/g.TAT.2018

*To Ollie*
*'Pedwerydd llawr i chi'*
*Love Mum x*

# Acknowledgements

The increasing scope and complexity of perioperative care makes it more challenging for a sole author to encompass. Therefore, this text adopts an inter-disciplinary and inter-professional approach, and I am very grateful to all the contributors from the original edition and the second edition for their commitment to this project.

Special thanks to Elizabeth Reeve, Senior Commissioning Editor at Oxford University Press, whose endless support, encouragement, and motivation has been very much appreciated; and has brought the project to fruition. Thanks also to Sylvia Warren, Senior Project Editor and Clement and Priya, Production Editors in India for their unwavering support and understanding. Also, a personal thanks to my previous co-editor, Andy Mardell for enabling me to build on our first edition.

I also wish to thank and formally acknowledge the following organisations for permission to reproduce some of their material in this book:
- Oxford University Press
- Difficult Airway Society
- Ethicon
- World Health Organisation
- Cardiff and Vale University Health Board
- Lippincott, Williams and Wilkins

To all current contributors, you made this possible and I cannot thank you enough for your patience. The last few years have not been easy for anyone, but your support and unwavering professionalism has inspired me to finish this text.

To my Mum and Dad, Anne and Brian Griffiths, who have been a consistent source of support and encouragement, throughout my life. My greatest role models, my inspiration, and my ardent supporters. There are not enough words I can say to describe just how important they have been to me, and what a powerful influence they continue to be. I love you both and miss you so much.

Finally, special thanks to my husband, Charlie, and my son, Oliver for their unconditional support and patience and frequent deliveries of food and champagne. I love you both.

# Preface

The subject of this book relates to practice within the perioperative environment. It addresses many key issues and outlines a thorough introduction to the principles and practice of anaesthetic practice, intraoperative care, post-anaesthesia practice and emergency care, including a comprehensive account of clinically focused aspects of this highly specialised discipline.

The aim of the *Oxford Handbook of Perioperative Practice second edition* is to further provide practical, easily accessible, concise and up-to-date evidence-based guidelines relating to all the essential elements of perioperative practice. This book has continued to take an inter-disciplinary and inter-professional approach to perioperative practice with contributors comprising of educationalists and clinicians from the fields of nursing, operating department practice and pharmacy throughout the United Kingdom.

This book is a sound introduction to perioperative practice for newly qualified practitioners, all those studying the subject or those who are considering embarking on a career in this highly specialised environment. It is also intended to provide relevant and useful information at the fingertips of practitioners faced with managing difficult patient cases.

It is by no means exhaustive of all arenas of perioperative practice but serves to assist perioperative practitioners to meet the needs of surgical patients to ensure safe and efficient care delivery and management of this clientele. I hope that you will find it useful and that it contributes to your transition from novice to advanced beginner perioperative practitioner.

Suzanne J. Hughes
Editor

# Contents

# Surgical terms

–ECTOMY: removal of an organ, for example, mastectomy, gastrectomy, orchidectomy, and colectomy.

–ITIS: inflammation of an organ or cavity, for example, appendicitis and peritonitis.

–ORRHAPHY: repair of tissues, for example, herniorrhaphy.

–OSCOPY: examination of a body cavity or deep structure using an instrument specifically designed for the purpose, for example, gastroscopy, laparoscopy, arthroscopy, and bronchoscopy.

–OSTOMY: fashioning of an artificial communication between a hollow viscus and the skin, for example, tracheostomy, colostomy, and ileostomy. The term may also apply to artificial openings between different viscera, for example, gastrojejunostomy and choledochoduodenostomy.

–OTOMY: cutting open, for example, laparotomy, arteriotomy, fasciotomy, and thoracotomy.

–PEXY: relocation and securing in position, for example, orchidopexy and rectopexy.

–PLASTY: reconstruction, for example, pyloroplasty, mammoplasty, and arthroplasty.

# Symbols and abbreviations

| | |
|---|---|
| ⮎ | cross reference |
| ✐ | website |
| ↓ | decreased |
| ↑ | increased |
| > | greater than |
| < | less than |
| AAA | abdominal aortic aneurysm |
| AAGBI | Association of Anaesthetists of Great Britain and Ireland |
| ABCDE | airway, breathing, circulation, disability, exposure |
| ABG | arterial blood gases |
| ACE | angiotensin-converting enzyme |
| ACh | acetylcholine |
| AChE | acetylcholinesterase |
| ACORN | Australian College of Operating Room Nurses |
| AF | atrial fibrillation |
| AfPP | Association for Perioperative Practice |
| AIDS | acquired immunodeficiency syndrome |
| AORN | Association of periOperative Registered Nurses |
| AP | anteroposterior |
| APL | adjustable pressure-limiting |
| ASA | American Society of Anesthesiologists |
| AV | atrioventricular |
| AVPU | Alert, Verbal, Pain, Unresponsive |
| BiPAP | biphasic positive airway pressure |
| BIS | bispectral index |
| BLS | basic life support |
| BME | black and minority ethnic |
| BMI | body mass index |
| BNF | *British National Formulary* |
| BP | blood pressure |
| bpm | beats per minute |
| BSE | bovine spongiform encephalopathy |
| BSL | British Sign Language |
| CABG | coronary artery bypass graft |

| | |
|---|---|
| CAD | coronary artery disease |
| CBT | cognitive behavioural therapy |
| CHG | chlorhexidine gluconate |
| CJD | Creutzfeldt–Jakob disease |
| CKD | chronic kidney disease |
| CNS | central nervous system |
| CO | cardiac output |
| $CO_2$ | carbon dioxide |
| COPD | chronic obstructive pulmonary disease |
| CPAP | continuous positive airway pressure |
| CPR | cardiopulmonary resuscitation |
| CRF | chronic renal failure |
| CRP | C-reactive protein |
| CSF | cerebrospinal fluid |
| CT | computed tomography |
| CVA | cardiovascular accident |
| CVP | central venous pressure |
| CWD | chronic wasting disease |
| DIC | disseminated intravascular coagulation |
| DLT | double-lumen tube |
| DM | diabetes mellitus |
| DMARD | disease modifying anti-rheumatoid drug |
| DNACPR | do not attempt cardiopulmonary resuscitation |
| DVT | deep venous thrombosis |
| ECF | extracellular fluid |
| ECG | electrocardiogram |
| ECT | electroconvulsive therapy |
| ED | emergency department |
| EEG | electroencephalogram |
| EMG | electromyogram/ electromyography |
| EMLA | eutectic mixture of local anaesthetic |
| ENT | ear, nose, and throat |
| ERAS | Enhanced Recovery after Surgery |
| ERCP | endoscopic retrograde cholangiopancreatography |

| | |
|---|---|
| ERPC | evacuation of retained products of conception |
| ETCO$_2$ | end-tidal carbon dioxide |
| ETT | endotracheal tube |
| FBC | full blood count |
| FEV$_1$ | forced expiratory volume in 1 second |
| FFP | fresh frozen plasma |
| FGM | female genital mutilation |
| FiO$_2$ | fraction of oxygen in inspired air |
| GA | general anaesthetic |
| GCS | Glasgow Coma Scale |
| GI | gastrointestinal |
| GMC | General Medical Council |
| GP | general practitioner |
| GTN | glyceryl trinitrate |
| HAART | highly active antiretroviral therapy |
| Hb | haemoglobin |
| HBV | hepatitis B virus |
| HCAI | healthcare-associated infection |
| HCPC | Health and Care Professions Council |
| HCV | hepatitis C virus |
| HDU | high dependency unit |
| HELLP | haemolysis, elevated liver enzymes, low platelets |
| HIV | human immunodeficiency virus |
| HME | heat and moisture exchange |
| HRA | Human Rights Act |
| HRT | hormone replacement therapy |
| ICD | intracardiac defibrillator |
| ICU | intensive care unit |
| ICP | intracranial pressure |
| ICS | intraoperative cell salvage |
| ID | internal diameter |
| ILMA | intubating laryngeal mask airway |
| IM | intramuscular |
| INR | international normalized ratio |
| IPPV | intermittent positive pressure ventilation |
| ITU | intensive therapy unit |
| IU | international units |
| IV | intravenous |
| IVC | inferior vena cava |
| L | litre(s) |
| LA | local anaesthetic |
| LFT | liver function test |
| LMA | laryngeal mask airway |
| LMP | last menstrual period |
| LMWH | low molecular weight heparin |
| LPA | lasting power of attorney |
| LSI | long-standing illness or disability |
| LV | left ventricle |
| MAC | minimum alveolar concentration |
| MAP | mean arterial pressure |
| mcg | microgram(s) |
| mg | milligram(s) |
| MH | malignant hyperthermia |
| MHRA | Medicines and Healthcare products Regulatory Agency |
| MI | myocardial infarction |
| mL | millilitre(s) |
| MLT | microlaryngoscopy tube |
| MRI | magnetic resonance imaging |
| MRSA | methicillin (or multiple)-resistant *Staphylococcus aureus* |
| MSSA | methicillin-sensitive *Staphylococcus aureus* |
| NBM | nil by mouth |
| NEWS | National Early Warning Score |
| NG | nasogastric |
| NHS | National Health Service |
| NIBP | non-invasive blood pressure |
| NICE | National Institute for Health and Care Excellence |
| NMC | Nursing and Midwifery Council |
| NMDA | N-methyl-D-aspartate |
| NSAID | non-steroidal anti-inflammatory drug |
| O$_2$ | oxygen |
| ODP | operating department practitioner |
| OIR | overnight intensive recovery |
| OTC | over the counter |
| PaCO$_2$ | arterial carbon dioxide tension |
| PACU | post-anaesthetic care unit |
| PaO$_2$ | arterial oxygen tension |
| PBM | patient blood management |
| PCA | patient-controlled analgesia |
| PCO$_2$ | partial pressure of carbon dioxide |
| PCS | postoperative cell salvage |
| PE | pulmonary embolism |
| PEA | pulseless electrical activity |

| | | | |
|---|---|---|---|
| pEEG | processed electroencephalography | SPC | summary of product characteristics |
| PEEP | positive end-expiratory pressure | SpO$_2$ | peripheral oxygen saturation |
| PEFR | peak expiratory flow rate | SSI | surgical site infection |
| PICU | paediatric intensive care unit | SSRI | selective serotonin reuptake inhibitor |
| PLMA | ProSeal™ laryngeal mask airway | TB | tuberculosis |
| PO | orally (*per os*) | TCA | target-controlled anaesthesia |
| PONV | postoperative nausea and vomiting | TCI | target-controlled infusion |
| PO$_2$ | partial pressure of oxygen | TENS | transcutaneous electric nerve stimulation |
| PPE | personal protective equipment | TIA | transient ischaemic attack |
| PR | *per rectum* | TIVA | total intravenous anaesthesia |
| RBC | red blood cell | TURP | transurethral resection of the prostate |
| RCN | Royal College of Nursing | U&Es | urea and electrolytes |
| RCoA | Royal College of Anaesthetists | UTI | urinary tract infection |
| RCOG | Royal College of Obstetricians and Gynaecologists | UV | ultraviolet |
| RCS | Royal College of Surgeons | VATS | video-assisted thoracoscopic surgery |
| RLMA | reinforced laryngeal mask airway | vCJD | variant Creutzfeldt–Jakob disease |
| RSI | rapid sequence induction | VF | ventricular fibrillation |
| SaO$_2$ | arterial oxygen saturation | VP | ventriculoperitoneal |
| SBAR | Situation, Background, Assessment, Recommendation | VT | ventricular tachycardia |
| SC | subcutaneous | VTE | venous thromboembolism |
| SIC | surgical intensive care | WCC | white cell count |
| SLE | systemic lupus erythematosus | WHO | World Health Organization |

# Contributors

**Sue Barker**
Psychologist
Retired
The British Psychological Society
Leicester, UK

**Geinor Bean**
Lecturer
Adult Nursing
School of Healthcare Sciences
Cardiff University
Wales, UK

**Nisha Bhudia**
Lead Pharmacist
Critical Care and Anaesthesia
Royal Brompton and Harefield
Hospitals Part of Guys and St
Thomas NHS Foundation Trust
Harefield, UK

**Sian Bill**
Lecturer
Children and Young People's
Nursing
School of Healthcare Sciences
Cardiff University
Wales, UK

**Alex Bradbury**
Lecturer
Operating Department Practice
School of Healthcare Sciences
Cardiff University
Wales, UK

**Rachel Brent**
Practice Educator
Cardiff and Vale
University Health Board
Wales, UK

**Jan Campsie**
Lecturer
Adult Nursing
School of Healthcare Sciences
Cardiff University
Wales, UK

**Felicia Cox**
Nurse Consultant
Pain Management
Royal Brompton and Harefield
Hospitals Part of Guys and St
Thomas NHS Foundation Trust
Harefield, UK

**Dawn Daniel**
Paediatric Practice
Development Nurse
Cwm Taf Morgannwg University
Health Board
Wales, UK

**Sandra Fender**
Lecturer
Adult Nursing
School of Healthcare Sciences
Cardiff University
Wales, UK

**Sarah Fry**
Senior Lecturer
Adult Nursing
School of Healthcare Sciences
Cardiff University
Wales, UK

**Hannah Grainger**
Senior Service Improvement Officer
Welsh Blood Service
Llantrisant
Wales, UK

**Nick Groves**
Consultant Anaesthetist
Nuffield Vale Hospital, Hensol
Wales, UK

**Gaynor Hamlington**
Senior Sister, Theatre
Wrexham Maelor Hospital
North Wales, UK

**Jayne Hancock**
Lecturer
Adult Nursing
School of Healthcare Sciences
Cardiff University
Wales, UK

**Alex Harmer**
Lecturer
Operating Department Practice
School of Healthcare Sciences
Cardiff University
Wales, UK

**Ricky Hellyar**
Senior Lecturer
Adult Nursing
School of Healthcare Sciences
Cardiff University
Wales, UK

**Paul Hennessy**
Lecturer
Operating Department Practice
School of Healthcare Sciences
Cardiff University
Wales, UK

**Charles Hughes**
Business Manager
ODP Retired
Cardiff, Wales, UK

**Suzanne Hughes**
Senior Lecturer
Adult Nursing
School of Healthcare Sciences
Cardiff University
Wales, UK

**Alison James**
Lecturer
Operating Department Practice
School of Healthcare Sciences
Cardiff University
Wales, UK

**Lindsey James-Lee**
Deputy Ward Manager
Cardiff and Vale
University Health Board
Wales, UK

**Claire Job**
Senior Lecturer
Adult Nursing
School of Healthcare Sciences
Cardiff University
Wales, UK

**Beverley Johnson**
Senior Lecturer
Adult Nursing
School of Healthcare Sciences
Cardiff University
Wales, UK

**Babs Jones**
Perioperative Education Lead
Cardiff and Vale
University Health Board, Cardiff
Wales, UK

**Gerwyn Jones**
Senior Lecturer
Mental Health Nursing
School of Healthcare Sciences
Cardiff University
Wales, UK

**Harri Jones**
Medical Student
School of Healthcare Sciences
Cardiff University
Wales, UK

**Kaye Jones-Mahoney**
Senior Lecturer
Adult Nursing
School of Medicine, Cardiff
University
Wales, UK

**Rhys Jones**
Pharmacy Student
School of Pharmacy and
Pharmaceutical Sciences, Cardiff
University
Wales, UK

**Moyra Journeaux**
Senior Lecturer
Harvey Besterman Education
Centre, Government of Jersey
Jersey, Channel Islands

# Further reading

Association for Perioperative Practice (2018). Theatre etiquette: a student's guide to theatres. Harrogate: Association for Perioperative Practice.

Forsyth C, Mason B (2017). Shared leadership and group identification in healthcare: the leadership beliefs of clinicians working in interprofessional teams. Journal of Interprofessional Care, 31(3):291–299.

Thomas J, Pollard KC, Sellman D (eds) (2014). Interprofessional working in health and social care (2nd ed). Hampshire: Palgrave.

# Theatre etiquette

The operating theatre has a unique atmosphere which can prove quite deceptive; however, there are certain conventions that the novice theatre practitioner ought to be aware of. These include:
- Minimizing distraction of the surgical team
- Noise levels
- Teamwork.

There should be no direct contact with the surgeons when they are operating. Any communication must go through the scrub practitioner who will pass on any message at a convenient moment or invite the circulating member of staff to speak to the surgeon.

Similarly, the noise levels in the operating theatre must be kept to a minimum while surgery is taking place. Care should be taken to keep the volume of conversations as low as possible.

## Movement (traffic)
- Staff wearing non-sterile theatre wear should keep their movements in and out of the operating theatre to a minimum.
- All operating theatre staff should enter and leave the operating theatre via a clearly identified door so as not to disturb airflow.
- Consideration should be given to the layout of the operating theatre to minimize flow of staff through the area as this can compromise the efficiency of ventilation systems.
- In addition to keeping clean and dirty areas separate, it is important to ensure that patient flow, from arrival to discharge, is orderly and logical.
- It is important to control traffic and activities in the operating theatre department as the number of people and the amount of activity influence the number of microorganisms that are present and therefore influence the risk of infection.

## Footwear
- Appropriate protective footwear with enclosed toes and heels should be worn and cleaned frequently.
- There is no evidence to suggest that the wearing of outside shoes in the operating theatre is a source of infection but they should be limited to use in contaminated cases only.
- The wearing of overshoes has been shown not only to be ineffective in reducing the bacterial load on the floor but also causes hands to become more easily contaminated when the overshoes are applied and removed.
- Local policy in respect of footwear should be adhered to.

## Surgical face masks
- Masks were originally worn to prevent patients from surgical site infections. They have been shown to be effective in reduction of contamination of the surgical field when worn by the surgical team but it is questionable whether they contribute to the overall reduction of wound infections.

- Surgical face masks should have a minimum of three layers in order to have >99% bacterial filtration efficacy.
- Respirator masks are recommended for protection during aerosol-generating procedures.
- Masks should never hang or dangle around the neck or be placed in a pocket for later use.
- If worn correctly, a surgical mask should help block large-particle droplets, splashes, sprays, or splatters that may contain viruses and bacteria, and keeping them from reaching the mouth and nose; it should also be worn with eye protection.
- Surgical face masks do not filter or block very small particles in the air that may be transmitted by coughs, sneezes, or certain medical procedures.
- If the mask cannot be easily readjusted or becomes wet, it should be replaced immediately as the filtration efficiency and its protective ability is compromised when the mask becomes wet, torn, or dislodged. Face masks should be discarded safely and replaced with a new one.
- To safely discard the mask, place it in a plastic bag and then place this in a clinical waste bag. It is recommended to handle only the tapes of the mask during disposal. Hands should be washed immediately after handling a used mask.
- There would appear to be little rationale for the wearing of masks by non-scrubbed staff (circulating and anaesthetic staff).
- Local policy in respect of surgical masks should be adhered to.

## Headwear and goggles

- The intention of covering the hair has been to reduce the risk of infection from bacteria that may be shed from the hair and skin of healthcare workers.
- Hats should be donned prior to theatre clothing to reduce the amount of shedding of particles from the head onto the suit.
- All hair must be covered and staff with long hair should wear a surgical hood or an elasticated hat.
- Men should wear a hood if they have facial hair.
- Most theatre departments purchase disposable hats which are discarded at the end of the working day.
- Cloth caps should be laundered daily at a temperature of at least 60°C and changed if they become soiled.
- Hands should be washed after the removal of hats.
- Hats, for example, turbans, kippot, veils, and headscarves, are permitted on religious grounds, provided that patient health and safety, infection control and security, and safety of staff are not compromised.
- Goggles or visors should be worn during aerosol-generating procedures and to protect against splashes.
- Visors should be worn when the risk of splattering or spray of bodily fluids is anticipated.
- Visors should be wrapped around the eye area to protect the side areas of the face.
- Local policy in respect of theatre hats should be adhered to.

## Theatre apparel

- Staff should be trained on donning and doffing personal protective equipment.
- All staff entering the operating theatre must wear a clean theatre suit.
- All staff should wear specific non-sterile theatre wear in all areas where operations are undertaken.
- Theatre scrubs should only be worn in dedicated areas and should never be worn for travelling to and from work.
- Consideration should also be given to the donning of a fresh suit prior to each operating session.
- Although 'bare below the elbow' is essential for hand hygiene during direct patient care delivery, local policy will advise on covering the forearm where necessary, for example, on religious grounds.

## Jewellery

- Local policy regarding jewellery should be adhered to.
- All jewellery should be removed prior to entering the operating theatre. Jewellery and watches can harbour microorganisms and make effective hand hygiene more difficult. Local policy may allow wedding rings and stud earrings.
- The operating team should remove artificial nails and nail polish before operations. False nails harbour microorganisms and make effective hand hygiene more difficult.

## Further reading

Association for Perioperative Practice (2018). Theatre etiquette: a guide to theatres. Harrogate: Association for Perioperative Practice.

Burden M (2019). The link between surgical site infection and traffic flow in the operating theatre. British Journal of Nursing, 28(1):18.

Datta R (2010). Use of surgical facemasks in the operation theatre: effective or habit? Medical Journal, Armed Forces India, 66(2):163–165.

Greenhalgh T, Chan XH, Khunti K, et al. (2020). What is the efficacy of standard face masks compared to respirator masks in preventing COVID-type respiratory illnesses in primary care staff? Oxford: Centre for Evidence Based Medicine.

Kelkar U, Gogate B, Kurpad S, et al. (2013). How effective are face masks in operation theatre? A time frame analysis and recommendations. International Journal of Infection Control, 9(1):1–6.

Loison G, Troughton R, Raymond F, et al. (2017). Compliance with clothing regulations and traffic flow in the operating room: a multi-centre study of staff discipline during surgical procedures. Journal of Hospital Infection, 96(3):281–285.

McKenna E (2019). Cloth hats: (w)hat's the issue. Journal of Perioperative Nursing, 32(4):21–25.

National Institute for Health and Care Excellence (2019). Surgical site infections: prevention and treatment. London: National Institute for Health and Care Excellence.

NHS England (2020). Uniforms and workwear: guidance for NHS employers. Available at: ℛ https://www.england.nhs.uk/wp-content/uploads/2020/04/Uniforms-and-Workwear-Guidance-2-April-2020.pdf

Roebuck A, Harrison EM (2017). Operating theatre etiquette, sterile technique and surgical site preparation. Surgery, 35(4):177–184.

# Clinical governance

The introduction of clinical governance in 1998 was designed to introduce a systematic approach to the delivery of high-quality healthcare. A duty of quality was placed on NHS organizations in the Health Act 1999.[1] This introduced corporate accountability for clinical quality and performance.

> In essence, clinical governance is a 'system through which NHS organisations are accountable for continuously improving the quality of their services and safeguarding high standards of care by creating an environment in which excellence in clinical care will flourish'.[2]

It is an umbrella term which emerged as a solution to address concerns raised following a series of incidents which drew attention to perceived falling standards in healthcare and provision of healthcare services in the early 1990s. The original vocabulary has since been developed and healthcare professionals will be familiar with current terms such as quality initiatives and patient safety.[3,4]

Clinical governance is a 'whole system' process which has a number of features:

• Patient-centred care should be at the core of every NHS organization. This means that patients should be kept well informed and be given the opportunity to participate in their care.
• Good information about the quality of services is available to those providing the services as well as to patients and the public.
• Good practice and research evidence is systematically adopted. As such, variations in the process, outcomes, and in access to healthcare can be greatly reduced.
• NHS organizations and their partners in social and private care should work together to provide quality assured services.
• Doctors, nurses, and allied health professionals must work in teams to a consistently high standard and identify ways to provide safe and improved care for their patients.
• Risks and hazards to patients are reduced to as low a level as possible, creating a safety culture throughout the NHS.

Overall responsibility for the provision of quality services and patient and staff safety lies with the chief executive. The arrangements for governance and the structures, systems, and processes organizations have in place differ according to where in the UK services are provided. However, the key principles remain the same (Fig. 1.1).

### How can healthcare professionals engage with the key principles?

*Leadership, strategy, and planning*

Clinical leaders are critical in ensuring that healthcare practice is safe, compassionate, and high quality. Developing a leadership capacity is a core feature of both the NMC Code[5] in relation to teamwork and empowerment of others by education and support.[6] The King's Fund review of the

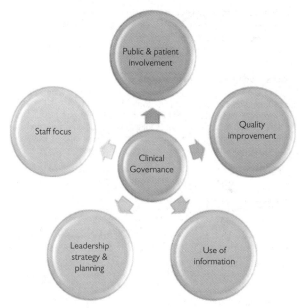

**Fig. 1.1** Main principles of clinical governance.

evidence base[7] consider the qualities and behaviours of leaders at all levels of the organization. Specifically, clinical leaders should be transformational, which suggests being participative and emotionally intelligent, being a role model for staff which aims to increase morale and motivation and ultimately influence quality outcomes in patient care.

### Staff focus

The type of leadership suggested by The King's Fund[7] aims to focus on the engagement and well-being of staff. A healthy workplace leads to a happy workplace[8] and positive working environments can influence positive patient outcomes. The management of stress, conflict, and an even work–life balance impacts performance and therefore good human resource management is essential.[9]

### Information focus

The use of information is critical to support all of the elements of governance. The use of developing technologies, for example, electronic patient records, smartphones, and related applications, influences how we engage with our patients, colleagues, and other agencies. This includes information provision in order to support practice, as well as data collected which evaluate performance. However, what is key for the healthcare professional is how they engage with technology, in terms of skills as well as motivation.

## Public and patient involvement

Engaging the public and patient in health provision requires facilitation of their contribution to service design and procedures as well as feedback on performance. This may be in the form of managing complaints to engaging the expert patient.

## Process for quality improvement

Healthcare professionals are encouraged to engage with a wide variety of quality improvement approaches and tools.[3,4]

Key to improving quality is to understand the underlying problem, utilizing the data collated by audit or other feedback and considering how these can be enhanced or simplified. Being able to utilize tools of change, leadership, and staff engagement is essential.

## References

1. Legislation.gov.uk (1999). Health Act 1999. Available at: ℜ https://www.legislation.gov.uk/ukpga/1999/8/contents
2. Scally G, Donaldson LJ (1998). Clinical governance and the drive for quality improvement in the new NHS in England. BMJ (Clinical Research Edition), 317(7150):61–65.
3. Healthcare Quality Improvement Partnership (2015). Guide to quality improvement methods. London: Healthcare Quality Improvement Partnership.
4. Public Health Wales. 1000 lives Improvement. Available at: ℜ http://www.1000livesplus.wales.nhs.uk/sitesplus/documents/1011/1000%20Lives%20Improvement%20Brochure%202018%20%28web%20version%29.pdf
5. Nursing and Midwifery Council (2018). The code: professional standards of practice and behaviour for nurses and midwives. London: Nursing and Midwifery Council.
6. Health and Care Professions Council (2016). Standards of conduct, performance and ethics. London: Health and Care Professions Council.
7. West M, Armit K, Loewenthal L, et al. (2015). Leadership and leadership development in health care: the evidence base. London: The King's Fund.
8. Royal College of Nursing (2015). Healthy workplace, healthy you. London: Royal College of Nursing.
9. Dawson J (2014). Staff experience and patient outcomes: what do we know? A report commissioned by NHS Employers on behalf of NHS England. London: NHS Employers.

# Applying principles of clinical governance to perioperative practice

The ethos of clinical governance is underpinned by strong leadership, positive teamwork, safe and effective practice, and, above all, a working environment that promotes, trust, candour, and collaboration for the benefit of the patient.

> The operating department team can reflect the clinical governance ethos, by endorsing the key principles of leadership, teamwork, and risk management.

## Leadership
- Leadership is important at all levels of the team, exercising it from the top requires vision and the ability to share that with others.
- Leadership is about personal self-awareness and also an understanding of the contribution made by all members of the team.

## Teamwork
- Everyone in the team should know and understand their own roles as well as others within the team.
- Staff appraisal is essential to help identify and address development and educational needs of both self and staff.
- Staff attitude and perceptions of teamwork are relative to the behaviour of the team and application to patient safety.

## Risk management
- Performing risk assessment and identifying risk profiles are essential to risk management.
- Departments will generate a risk profile that outlines the five or ten most common risks to the department and the actions that are taken to avoid these[1] (Fig. 1.2).
- Clinical incidents reporting will also ensure potential 'at-risk' situations are identified, and acted upon, before becoming a serious risk to patient/staff safety. Failure to acknowledge and address such situations reflects a breach of clinical governance principles.
- Formally reviewing service delivery by means of audit against recognized national standards will ensure evidence-based practice.
- Use of both this clinical incident and audit data enables the manager to detect trends and deal with these appropriately. It is important that actions taken as a result of an incident form are fed back to departmental staff.

## Patient safety
Patient safety is high in the agenda and there are several organizations that address it. NHS Improvement[2] supersedes the National Patient Safety Agency and has the responsibility for operating the National Reporting and Learning System (NRLS). Its patient safety collaborative aim is to 'support and encourage a culture of safety, continuous learning and improvement, across the health and care system'.

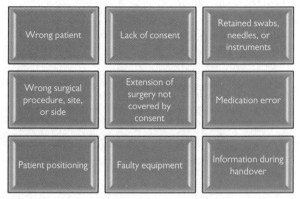

**Fig. 1.2** Areas of risk within the operating theatre.

Handover between sections within the operating department may result in the miscommunication or omission of important patient information, which can increase the risk of patient safety events. The use of the SBAR (situation, background, assessment, recommendation) technique provides a valuable tool for communicating critical information that requires attention and action and facilitates efficient handover between teams—thus contributing to effective escalation and increased patient safety.[3]

## References

1. NHS Improvement (2018). Never events. Available at: ☍ https://www.england.nhs.uk/publication/never-events/
2. NHS England and NHS Improvement (2021). Patient safety reports. Available at: ☍ https://www.england.nhs.uk/patient-safety/organisation-patient-safety-incident-reports/organisation-patient-safety-incident-reports-29-september-2021/
3. NHS Institute for Innovation and Improvement (2010). Safer care: SBAR. Available at: https://www.england.nhs.uk/improvement-hub/wp-content/uploads/sites/44/2017/11/SBAR-Implementation-and-Training-Guide.pdf

# Chapter 2

19

# Ethicolegal aspects of perioperative practice

# Accountability and responsibility

## Definitions

*Accountability*: someone who is accountable is completely responsible for what they do and must be able to give a satisfactory reason for it.[1]

*Responsibility*: to be responsible is to have control and authority over something or someone and the duty of taking care of it, him, or her.[2]

Although it would appear the two words have a similar meaning, there is a subtle difference. The perioperative healthcare professional would be both *responsible* and *accountable* for safe operative conditions whereas a healthcare support worker would only be responsible for tasks they have been delegated. Therefore, the main difference between *responsibility* and *accountability* is that *responsibility* can be shared whereas *accountability* cannot.

> If you are *accountable*, you are ultimately answerable for your actions and the actions of those you have delegated to.

Previous NMC (2008) and HCPC (2004) codes of conduct have explicitly provided explanations of these values. However, in the current NMC (2018) code[3] and HCPC (2016) standards[4] there is an emphasis on personal responsibility to patients, organization, and profession.

## When are perioperative practitioners accountable?

In their professional capacity, perioperative practitioners must comply with standards of conduct, performance, and ethics as stipulated by their professional regulatory body (HCPC or NMC). Each practitioner is accountable for his/her own:

- Actions
- Omissions.

A practitioner is therefore accountable for anything that he/she does, or fails to do, that does not meet the profession's required standard.

With the development of advanced practice,[5,6] practitioners who take on roles and tasks normally regulated by other professional standards (e.g. GMC) must ensure they take on that role/task to the same level as the other professional standard. Not to do so would be seen as negligent.[7]

## To whom are perioperative practitioners professionally accountable to?

It is recognized that practitioners are accountable to:

- The patient
- The public
- The employer
- The profession.

## Accountability to the patient

- Each patient has a right to receive the standard of care required of the perioperative practitioner by his/her profession.
- Where the actions (or omissions) of the practitioner are not of the required standard, the patient may seek redress.

- Where harm has been caused to the patient by the practitioner's action/omission, the patient may choose to sue the practitioner for his/her negligence in the civil courts (➔ see Negligence, p. XX).

## Accountability to the public

- All perioperative practitioners must act within the law.
- In extreme cases where the practitioner's actions/omissions have led to the death of a patient, a criminal charge of manslaughter or murder may be brought.

## Accountability to the employer

- Perioperative practitioners, by nature of their employment contracts, are required to undertake reasonable instructions of the employer.
- The employer may commence a disciplinary procedure against a practitioner whose actions/omissions are in breach of his/her employment contract (i.e. not the standard expected).
- Where the disciplinary procedure finds that the practitioner is in breach of contract, a range of sanctions, from a warning to dismissal, are available to the employer.

## Accountability to the profession

- Regulatory bodies (e.g. the HCPC and NMC) function to safeguard the health and well-being of the public.
- This function is discharged (in part) by considering any allegations of misconduct against registrants.
- Alleged misconduct is investigated in terms of the registrant's 'fitness to practise'.
- If the practitioner's actions/omissions are found to have affected his/her fitness to practise, the regulatory body has a range of sanctions it can apply.
- Sanctions include a caution, a Conditions of Practice Order, suspension, and, ultimately, removal of the registrant's name from the register.
- It should be noted that accountability to the patient, the public, or the employer may also result in the involvement of the regulatory body since any findings in any of these arenas may be reported to the regulatory body if 'fitness to practise' has been considered.

### An example

*A perioperative practitioner administers a massive overdose of a prescribed analgesic drug, without following the local policy of checking that drug dose, and the patient dies.*

Although there are many aspects of this scenario that would be considered, it is possible (as a worst-case scenario) that the patient's relatives sue for negligence (accountability to the patient), the practitioner is charged with manslaughter (accountability to the public), the employer commences disciplinary action (accountability to the employer), and the regulatory body reviews the practitioner's fitness to practise (accountability to the profession).

## References

1. Oxford English Dictionary. Accountable. Available at: &#x1F50D; https://www.oed.com/view/Entry/1198
2. Oxford English Dictionary. Responsible. Available at: &#x1F50D; https://www.oed.com/view/Entry/163863
3. Nursing and Midwifery Council (2018). The code: professional standards of practice and behaviour for nurses and midwives. London: Nursing and Midwifery Council.
4. Health and Care Professions Council (2016). Standards of conduct, performance and ethics. London: Health and Care Professions Council.
5. NHS England (2017). Multi-professional framework for advanced clinical practice in England. London: Department of Health.
6. National Leadership and Innovation Agency Healthcare (2010). Framework for advanced nursing, midwifery and allied health professional practice in Wales. Available at: &#x1F50D; https://www.wales.nhs.uk/sitesplus/documents/829/NLIAH%20Advanced%20Practice%20Framework.pdf
7. Wilsher v Essex Area Health Authority [1986] 3 All ER 801.

# Negligence

The tort of negligence is to ensure the public are able to seek redress where care has cause harm through poor practice or omission. In most legal cases of clinical negligence, a claim for compensation is heard in the civil court.

## The legal framework for clinical negligence claims

To succeed, the claimant must prove that:
- He/she was owed a legal duty of care by the defendant health carer (perioperative practitioner) and/or health provider (e.g. NHS trust/ health board).
- That the defendant was in breach of that duty of care (by failing to achieve the standard of care).
- The harm to the claimant (for which compensation is sought) was caused by, or materially contributed to, by the breach in the duty of care.

## Duty of care

- It is an accepted legal principle that a practitioner who takes on the responsibility of caring for a patient owes a duty of care to that patient.
- There is no legal duty, in the UK, to act as a 'Good Samaritan' (e.g.at the scene of an accident). However, if a practitioner does become involved, then a duty of care will exist.
- Applies equally to all health professionals and to support staff.
- The NHS trust/health board (or other healthcare provider) may also have a duty of care and either be liable in negligence claims for its own actions (primary liability) or be vicariously liable for negligence actions of its employees.
- Where an employee has breached the employer's policies and procedures, the employer might not have vicarious liability.
- The UK government has made professional indemnity arrangements a requirement for all healthcare professionals.
- In most clinical negligence claims the duty of care is not disputed by the defendant(s).

## Breach of duty

To identify whether a breach in duty occurred, a three-stage process is followed:
- Was the practitioner competent at undertaking the task?
- Was the practitioner undertaking the task using evidence-based practice (national and local policies)?
- If no policies exist, were they using appropriate evidence to guide their practice?

Case law provides guidance for practitioners on competence with Bolam v Friern Hospital Management Committee [1957][1] and Wilsher v Essex Area Health Authority [1986][2] offering what a competent practitioner should be expected to provide. Bolitho v City and Hackney Health Authority [1997][3] offers additional guidance on the use of evidence. Ultimately, if a practitioner is not competent, they should not undertake a task.

For example, if a practitioner is asked to take on a new, expanded, or advanced role, they must first undertake education, training, and supervised practice and be seen as competent before undertaking the role without supervision.

## Causation

Establishing that the breach of duty has caused the harm is notoriously difficult to prove in clinical negligence claims. There may be several reasons for the harm (that the patient claims) including pre-existing disease/trauma and recognized side effects of treatments. The following tests may be applied:

- The 'but for' test—used in straightforward cases. Would the harm have been caused but for the actions of the defendant? If not, the causal link is made.
- The 'chain of causation'—when there is an unbroken chain of events from the original act to the harm then the causal link is made.
- 'Reasonable foreseeability'—is the harm which was caused not too remote from the act or omission?

The onus is always on the claimant to prove that the cause of the harm was the action or omission of the defendant(s).

Where more than one possible cause may be presented, the decision by the court will be made using the civil standard of the 'balance of probabilities'—i.e. only if there is more than a 50% chance that the harm was caused by the negligence can the claim succeed.

## Gross negligence

On rare occasions where the negligence is considered to be extreme (e.g. when a patient dies), a claim of gross negligence may take the form of a charge of manslaughter. Gross negligence is therefore seen in a prosecution through the criminal courts.

## References

1. Bolam v Friern Hospital Management Committee [1957] 1 WLR 582.
2. Bolitho v City and Hackney Health Authority [1997]. House of Lords judgment. Available at: ℗ http://www.publications.parliament.uk/pa/ld199798/ldjudgmt/jd971113/boli01.htm
3. Wilsher v Essex Area Health Authority [1986] 3 All ER 801.

## Further reading

Brazier M, Cave E (2011). Medicine, patients and the law (5th ed). London: Penguin Books.
Gallagher A, Hodge S (2012). Ethics, law and professional issues? A practice-based approach for health professionals. Basingstoke: Palgrave Macmillan.

# Conscientious objection

Perioperative practitioners, as registered health professionals, are required by their respective regulatory bodies to provide care for patients without discrimination and with respect for the patient's rights. While few would disagree with these standards, difficulties do arise when practitioners find themselves in situations where participation in a patient's care is contrary to their own religious and personal beliefs.

This conscientious objection (to participation in care) can be considered in two ways:
• Legislation.
• Rights of the perioperative practitioner.

## Legislation

There are currently two Acts of Parliament that give health professionals the right to refuse to participate in procedures on the grounds of conscientious objection:
• Abortion Act 1967.
• Human Fertilisation and Embryology Act 1990.

*Requirements under the Acts*
• In the event of an emergency, the practitioner is required to participate in the patient's care (i.e. cannot claim conscientious objection).
• Practitioners will be responsible for proving their conscientious objection should it be required in legal proceedings.

It has been established, through the courts, that conscientious objection to participation in either an abortion or procedures for assisted conception (under these Acts) only applies to those directly involved in the technical procedure (i.e. conscientious objection may be claimed by a practitioner in the operating theatre during a termination but not by a practitioner checking the patient into the department).

## Rights of the perioperative practitioner

Where specific legislation does not address issues of conscientious objection, the position is less clear. Perioperative practitioners cannot simply be selective about patients in their care as the regulatory bodies require practitioners to practise in a non-discriminatory way. There are, however, some situations where a practitioner may have real concerns about specific practices. The Human Rights Act (HRA) 1998[1] identifies that:
• It is unlawful for any public authority (e.g. NHS trusts) to act in a way that is incompatible with the HRA
• Under Article 9, an individual (e.g. perioperative practitioner) has the right to freedom of thought, conscience, and religion, and the right to practise that religion
• Rights under Article 9 are not absolute—there are several limitations including public order and the protection of the rights and freedoms of others.

If a perioperative practitioner objects to undertaking a specific practice, because it is contrary to the practice of his/her religion, the NHS trust/health board will need to consider the objection.

This scenario has been tested in the Scottish courts.[2] Due to reconfiguration of services, two midwives took their employers to court for potential breech of their right to object to taking part in abortions. As labour ward coordinators, they felt they were taking part in the care of patients undergoing abortions. The court found that as they were not directly taking part in the treatment, they could not object to other aspects of their role including management of the labour ward.

Therefore, while the Scottish court agreed that the labour ward coordinators would not be expected to provide direct care, it is an important case for perioperative practitioners to be aware of and while making their objections known, ensure that they adhere to the current standards of performance, conduct, and ethics as stipulated by their professional body by:

- Considering not accepting employment where practices are contrary to their beliefs
- Informing the employer of the conscientious objection at the earliest opportunity—to allow other arrangements to be made to ensure that the patient's care does not suffer
- Acknowledging that each patient has the right to make his/her own care decisions
- Making no attempts to impose their beliefs on the patient
- Treating all patients with respect and dignity
- Accepting that in an emergency they cannot refuse to participate in the patient's care.

Considering the HRA 1998, it is evident that a balance between the rights of the patient to undergo a planned lawful surgical procedure and the rights of the practitioner to practise his/her religion has to be met.

## References

1. Legislation.gov.uk (1998). Human Rights Act 1998. Available at: https://www.legislation.gov.uk/ukpga/1998/42/schedule/1
2. Greater Glasgow Health Board (Appellant) v Doogan and another (Respondents) (Scotland) Michaelmas Term [2014] UKSC 68. On appeal from: [2013] CSIH 36.

# Informed consent

People are becoming more knowledgeable about their bodies, illnesses, and treatments and often feel the need to be more involved in the decisions made for their care. The law has always supported this through the law relating to consent to treatment.[1] The legal requirements for valid consent reflect the ethical ones: it must be given voluntarily by an appropriately informed patient, who has the capacity to exercise a choice—even if this choice appears irrational. Consent to treatment must be confirmed in writing. For consent to be valid,[2,3] it must be:

• Given by a person with the capacity to make the decision in question
• Given voluntarily
• Based on appropriate information (informed) and understood.

Anyone who is deemed mentally competent and aged >16 years can consent to treatment. Under Section 8 of the Family Law Reform Act (1969),[4] a minor of 16 or 17 can give valid consent but if a minor aged <16 years is mature and intelligent enough to understand the nature of the treatment, then they are lawfully able to give consent. This is termed as 'Gillick Competence'.[5] Issues of consent in the doctor–patient relationship arise in three main contexts:

• In the crime of battery.
• In the tort of battery.
• In the tort of negligence.

It is the surgeon's responsibility to assess the capacity of patients to make decisions about their care. In this assessment, surgeons must comply with the Mental Capacity Act 2005 (England and Wales),[6] the Adults with Incapacity (Scotland) Act 2000,[7] or the Mental Capacity Act (Northern Ireland) 2016,[8] including codes of practice and relevant regulatory guidance.[3]

The surgeon responsible for providing treatment remains responsible for making sure that the patient has been given enough time and appropriate information to make an informed decision and has given their consent before they start the treatment.[3]

There is a danger in the health professions to sideline the concept of consent as a concept affecting doctors only, but gaining consent also applies to all healthcare practitioners. Consent should be obtained for non-surgical treatment, such as taking blood, giving an injection, and providing fundamental care. Consent allied to the term informed means that patients should be given the amount of information needed to make an informed choice about a given treatment and can be written, oral or implied.[9]

> Act in the best interests of people at all times, gain consent before providing care and treatment, and respect a person's right to accept or refuse treatment.[10,11]

The issue is then raised about the amount of information that should be given. Considering the provision of information, the law was previously shown in the case of Sidaway v Governors of the Bethlem Royal Hospital & the Maudsley Hospital [1985][12] where the duty of care in the area of disclosure was decided on the basis of a responsible body of medical opinion.

More recently, the Montgomery v Lanarkshire Health Board case [2015][13] was a landmark for informed consent in the UK, which focused on consent and information disclosure in medical treatment and care. It signalled a move away from a 'doctor knows best' approach to one that focuses on disclosing information to which particular patients would attach significance. In other words, the Montgomery case closed the gap between regulatory guidance and case law by shifting the focus of consent towards the specific needs of the patient.[3]

The AAGBI[2] stipulates only three exceptions to this rule:
- The patient has expressed a fixed desire not to know the risks.
- Discussion of the risks would pose a serious threat to the patient, for example, suicide.
- In 'circumstances of necessity' where urgent treatment is needed but the patient lacks capacity, and where the treatment that is being delivered is in his/her best interests.

Although theoretically, a doctor who acts without obtaining a patient's consent may not only be exposed to liability in tort, but also runs the risk of facing a criminal prosecution for the crime of battery.

The Royal College of Surgeons highlights a ten-step process (Table 2.1) aimed at adult patients with capacity to optimize the time available for providing the required information and discussing options for treatment to facilitate patient decision-making.[3]

When caring for patients with mental health problems, it is essential to apply the legislation accurately and with due regard for such vulnerable patients.[14]

In an urgent or emergency situation where it is imperative to save life or prevent serious deterioration, the surgeon has to proceed with limited discussion or even without consent.[3]

## Consent for anaesthesia

Consent for anaesthesia has traditionally been considered as 'implied' once the patient consents to surgery, with the surgical consent stating that anaesthesia will be needed for the surgery and there are associated risks with anaesthesia. A separate consent form, signed by the patient, is not required for anaesthetic procedures that are done to facilitate another treatment, for example, surgery. Anaesthetists should record details of the discussion regarding anaesthesia in the patient record, noting the risks, benefits, and alternatives (including no treatment) that were explained.

The AAGBI outlines risks associated with the anaesthetic technique, specific risks relating to an anaesthesia procedure, common side effects of anaesthesia, and serious side effects (Box 2.1).[2] This information is seen as appropriate for patients during the consenting process.

## Exceptions to consent requirements

Medical emergencies, such as patients who are unconscious, will require decisions about patient care to be made urgently or immediate action to be taken to preserve life. In these cases, it will be inappropriate to delay treatment to try to facilitate the patient's autonomous decisions. Healthcare staff should act in the patient's best interests and attempt to communicate with them to keep them informed wherever possible.[3]

**Table 2.1** Ten-step process to consent

| | |
|---|---|
| **Step 1** | Explain the diagnosis to the patient in a language that is understood |
| **Step 2** | Explain the options for treatment including the risks and benefits and the option of no surgery |
| **Step 3** | Explain the consent and decision-making process so the patient understands what is expected of them |
| **Step 4** | Allow time for patients to deliberate on treatment options available including reading further information or accessing additional resources regarding their condition |
| **Step 5** | Discuss the patient's wishes, needs, views, and expectations regarding any treatment they might undertake. Ensure that the patient's views are respected |
| **Step 6** | Explain how different options will or will not achieve the patient's goals and any potential impact that the options taken will have |
| **Step 7** | Provide any relevant information not already covered, or any emerging information that may have altered the conditions surrounding the various options for treatment |
| **Step 8** | Is the person seeking consent satisfied that the patient understood the information provided? |
| **Step 9** | Respect the patient's decision |
| **Step 10** | The signing of the form and maintaining a decision-making record. Provide a copy of the consent form for the patient to review and retain |

Source: data from Royal College of Surgeons (2016). Consent: supported decision-making. London: Royal College of Surgeons.

---

**Box 2.1 Information for patients regarding anaesthesia during the consenting process**

*Common risk components of anaesthetic technique*
Fasting, effects of premedication, IV access, induction of anaesthesia (general, regional anaesthetic, local anaesthetic (LA)), non-invasive monitoring, intraoperative drugs/fluids, intraoperative discomfort/awareness of the procedure/surroundings if awake/sedated, postoperative analgesia/antiemetics/fluids, alternative techniques if one technique fails (e.g. general anaesthetic (GA) for caesarean section as an alternative to regional anaesthetic, or if the latter is inadequate).

*Specific risks related to procedure*
Invasive monitoring, recovery in a critical care environment; sedation; intubation/tracheotomy.

*Common side effects*
Nausea and vomiting; sore throat; suxamethonium pains, damage to teeth/lips; cognitive dysfunction; numbness/weakness/return of pain after LA techniques; postdural puncture headache.

Source: data from AAGBI (2017). Consent for anaesthesia. https://onlinelibrary.wiley.com/doi/full/10.1111/anae.13762

## Refusal/withdrawal of consent

Patients have a right to refuse treatment or withdraw their consent to treatment at any time, even if such treatment is considered life-threatening/limiting.

For an overview of the shared decision process of consent, see Fig. 2.1.

## References

1. Tingle J, Cribb A (eds) (2013). Nursing law and ethics (4th ed). London: Wiley-Blackwell.
2. Association of Anaesthetists of Great Britain and Ireland (2017). Consent for anaesthesia. Available at: ℰ https://onlinelibrary.wiley.com/doi/full/10.1111/anae.13762
3. Royal College of Surgeons (2016). Consent: supported decision-making. London: Royal College of Surgeons.
4. Legislation.gov.uk (1969). Family Law Reform Act 1969. Available at: ℰ https://www.legislation.gov.uk/ukpga/1969/46
5. Gillick v West Norfolk & Wisbeck Area Health Authority [1986] AC 112 House of Lords.
6. Legislation.gov.uk (2005). Mental Capacity Act 2005. Available at: ℰ https://www.legislation.gov.uk/ukpga/2005/9/contents
7. Legislation.gov.uk (2000). Adults with Incapacity (Scotland) Act 2000. Available at: ℰ https://www.legislation.gov.uk/asp/2000/4/contents
8. Department of Health (2016). Mental Capacity Act 2016 (Northern Ireland). Available at: ℰ https://www.health-ni.gov.uk/mca
9. Dowie I, Griffith R (2019). Dimond's legal aspects of nursing: a definitive guide to law for nurses (8th ed). Harlow: Pearson Education.
10. Nursing and Midwifery Council (2018). The code: professional standards of practice and behaviour for nurses and midwives. London: Nursing and Midwifery Council.
11. Health and Care Professions Council (2016). Standards of conduct, performance and ethics. London: Health and Care Professions Council.
12. Sidaway v Bethlem Royal Hospital Governors [1985] 1 All ER 643, [1985] 2 WLR 480, HL.
13. Montgomery v Lanarkshire Health Board [2015] UKSC 11.
14. Griffith R, Tengnah C (2020). Law and professional issues in nursing (5th ed). London: Learning Matters.

## Further reading

General Medical Council (2019). Good medical practice: working with doctors working for patients. London: General Medical Council.
Royal College of Anaesthetists (2021). Chapter 2: guidelines for the provision of anaesthesia services for the perioperative care of elective and urgent care patients. London: Royal College of Anaesthetists.

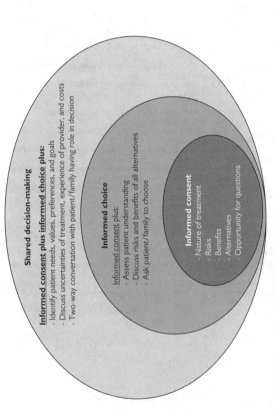

**Shared decision-making**

<u>Informed consent plus informed choice</u> plus:
- Identify patient needs, values, preferences, and goals
- Discuss uncertainties of treatment, experience of provider, and costs
- Two-way conversation with patient/family having role in decision

**Informed choice**

<u>Informed</u> consent plus:
- Assess patient understanding
- Discuss risks and benefits of all alternatives
- Ask patient/family to choose

**Informed consent**
- Nature of treatment
- Risks
- Benefits
- Alternatives
- Opportunity for questions

**Fig. 2.1** Overview of the shared decision process.

# Confidentiality

The NMC[1] and HCPC[2] state that all healthcare practitioners owe a duty of confidentiality to patients receiving care. This includes making sure that they are informed about their care and that information about them is shared appropriately. Patients have a right to privacy in all aspects of their care but necessary information with other healthcare professionals can only be shared when the interests of patient safety and public protection override the need for confidentiality.

Confidentiality is fraught with dilemmas and healthcare professionals have to accept accountability and take responsibility for their own actions. There is allowance for exceptional cases of disclosure where healthcare practitioners have a legal duty to report certain situations in which the safety of the patient and the welfare of the public is considered at risk, for example, suspected child/elder abuse, communicable diseases, dangerous patients, and any criminal activity. However as long as disclosure is reported in good faith and according to the law, most statutes provide immunity from civil and criminal liability.

A breach of confidentiality which cannot be justified may expose the practitioner to disciplinary proceedings with the possible consequence, if found guilty of professional misconduct, of being removed from the professional register.[1,2]

## References

1. Nursing and Midwifery Council (2018). The code: professional standards of practice and behaviour for nurses and midwives. London: Nursing and Midwifery Council.
2. Health and Care Professions Council (2016). Standards of conduct, performance and ethics. London: Health and Care Professions Council.

## Further reading

Buka P (2020). Essential law and ethics in nursing (3rd ed). Abingdon: Routledge.
Dowie I, Griffith R (2019). Dimond's legal aspects of nursing: a definitive guide to law for nurses (8th ed). Harlow: Pearson Education.

# Mental capacity

Making decisions about treatment and care for patients who lack capacity is governed in England and Wales by the Mental Capacity Act 2005,[1] and in Scotland by the Adults with Incapacity (Scotland) Act 2000.[2] In Northern Ireland, the Mental Capacity Act 2016 (Northern Ireland) 2016[3] protects those who lack capacity to consent to care or treatment and who need limits placed on their liberty to keep them safe. For the five key principles of the Mental Capacity Act 2005, see Table 2.2.

> Act in the best interests of patients at all times, adhere to all relevant laws about mental capacity, and make sure that the rights and best interests of those who lack capacity are at the centre of the decision-making process.[4,5]

- All Acts assume that patients have capacity to consent unless proved otherwise and to decide whether to agree to, or refuse, an examination, investigation, or treatment.
- A patient can only be suspected as lacking capacity if they cannot understand, retain, or use all information needed to make an informed decision.
- A patient cannot be assumed to lack mental capacity due to age, disability, appearance, behaviour, medical condition (including mental illness), their beliefs, their specious inability to communicate, or if they make an unwise decision.
- Mental capacity can fluctuate and a patient's capacity can temporarily be affected by pain, confusion, sepsis, or shock.
- The concept of incapacity can arise due to brain injury, dementia, mental illness, or learning disability.
- Any decision and/or intervention on behalf of a patient lacking capacity must be in his/her best interests. The intervention or decision made on behalf of a person lacking capacity must cause the least restriction of his/her rights and freedom of action to achieve the stated purpose.[6]

**Table 2.2** The five principles of the Mental Capacity Act 2005

| 1 | Presumption of capacity |
|---|---|
| 2 | Support to make a decision |
| 3 | Ability to make unwise decisions |
| 4 | Best interest |
| 5 | Least restrictive |

## Making decisions when a patient lacks mental capacity

- Consider whether the patient's lack of mental capacity is temporary or permanent.
- Consider evidence of the patient's previously expressed preferences, such as an advance directive, and the views of who has legal authority to make a decision on the patient's behalf (lasting power of attorney (LPA)).
- Adults may make an advance decision to refuse treatment or appoint a proxy to decide upon their behalf using a LPA. A valid and applicable advance decision or a decision of a validly appointed health and welfare LPA is legally binding, as is the decision of a court-appointed deputy with the appropriate powers.[7]
- In the absence of an LPA, consider the views of people close to the patient about the patient's preferences, feelings, beliefs, and values, and whether they consider the proposed treatment to be in the patient's best interests.

## References

1. Legislation.gov.uk (2005). Mental Capacity Act 2005. Available at: ℘ https://www.legislation.gov.uk/ukpga/2005/9/contents
2. Legislation.gov.uk (2000). Adults with Incapacity (Scotland) Act 2000. Available at: ℘ https://www.legislation.gov.uk/asp/2000/4/contents
3. Department of Health (2016). Mental Capacity Act 2016 (Northern Ireland). Available at: ℘ https://www.health-ni.gov.uk/mca
4. Nursing and Midwifery Council (2018). The code: professional standards of practice and behaviour for nurses and midwives. London: Nursing and Midwifery Council.
5. Health and Care Professions Council (2016). Standards of conduct, performance and ethics. London: Health and Care Professions Council.
6. General Medical Council (2019). Good medical practice: working with doctors working for patients. London: General Medical Council.
7. Association of Anaesthetists of Great Britain and Ireland (2017). Consent for anaesthesia. Available at: ℘ https://onlinelibrary.wiley.com/doi/full/10.1111/anae.13762

## Further reading

Legislation.gov.uk (1969). Family Law Reform Act 1969. Available at: ℘ https://www.legislation.gov.uk/ukpga/1969/46
Royal College of Anaesthetists (2021). Chapter 2: guidelines for the provision of anaesthesia services for the perioperative care of elective and urgent care patients. London: Royal College of Anaesthetists.
Royal College of Surgeons (2016). Consent: supported decision-making. London: Royal College of Surgeons.

# Lasting power of attorney

A LPA is a legal document that lets a person, known as the donor, to appoint one or more people, known as attorneys, to help that person make decisions or to make decisions on his/her behalf. This gives a person more control over what happens in the event of an accident or illness when the said person lacks mental capacity so cannot make their own decisions. There are two types of LPA as follows:
- LPA for health and welfare.
- LPA for property and financial affairs.

A person can choose to make one or both types of LPA, which must be registered with the Office of the Public Guardian before either can be used.

### Lasting power of attorney for health and welfare

This LPA can be used to give an attorney the power to make decisions when a donor is unable to make decisions regarding their own health and welfare. It can include:
- General daily living tasks (e.g. washing, dressing, eating)
- Medical and nursing care
- Social care and moving into a care home
- Life-sustaining treatment.

A LPA for health and welfare can only be used when a person (donor) is unable to make their own decisions.

### Lasting power of attorney for property and financial affairs

This LPA can be used to give an attorney the power to make decisions on behalf of the donor about money and property. This can include:
- Paying for private health and social care
- Managing a bank account
- Paying bills
- Collecting benefits or a pension
- Selling the donor's home.

A LPA for property and financial affairs can be used when registered with the donor's permission.

A donor can choose one or more people to be their attorney. If more than one attorney is appointed, then the donor decides if they will make decisions severally (separately) or jointly (together).
- Jointly: attorneys must always make decisions together.
- Jointly and severally: attorneys must make some decisions together and some individually.

An attorney must be someone who is aged 18 or over and has the mental capacity to make their own decisions:
- An attorney could be a husband, wife, partner, relative, friend, or professional (nurse, ODP, doctor) and trustworthy to make decisions in the donor's best interests.
- An attorney does not need to live in the UK or be a British citizen.

## Further reading

Association of Anaesthetists of Great Britain and Ireland (2017). Consent for anaesthesia. Available at: ✍ https://onlinelibrary.wiley.com/doi/full/10.1111/anae.13762

Department of Health (2016). Mental Capacity Act 2016 (Northern Ireland). Available at: ✍ https://www.health-ni.gov.uk/mca

Legislation.gov.uk (1969). Family Law Reform Act 1969. Available at: ✍ https://www.legislation.gov.uk/ukpga/1969/46

Legislation.gov.uk (2000). Adults with Incapacity (Scotland) Act 2000. Available at: ✍ https://www.legislation.gov.uk/asp/2000/4/contents

Legislation.gov.uk (2005). Mental Capacity Act 2005. Available at: ✍ https://www.legislation.gov.uk/ukpga/2005/9/contents

Royal College of Anaesthetists (2021). Chapter 2: guidelines for the provision of anaesthesia services for the perioperative care of elective and urgent care patients. London: Royal College of Anaesthetists.

Royal College of Surgeons (2016). Consent: supported decision-making. London: Royal College of Surgeons.

# Chapter 3

# Admission of surgical patients

# The admission process

Surgery consists of emergency or elective (planned) admissions and the admission process will vary to accommodate the needs of the individual.

The increase in emergency surgery in the UK to 40–50% of the workload[1] has led to a reconfiguration of services. The surgical journey for the patient while essentially remaining unchanged is now for a wide range of specialties and procedures facilitated through preadmission clinics, admission lounges, short stay surgery units, and generally much shorter lengths of stay for all.

In order to facilitate this process, Enhanced Recovery after Surgery (ERAS) initiatives highlight the need to improve preoperative care, to improve outcomes and thus speed up recovery.

The admission process is essential to quality care and communication within the surgical team. The surgical journey for patients who have a planned admission can be facilitated through:
• Preadmission programmes
• The provision of written and online information
• Preoperative assessment clinics
• Ward visits.

For urgent surgical admissions time is of the essence and preoperative care needs to be provided far more quickly to facilitate a comprehensive preoperative assessment and a safe patient journey. An essential element is effective communication between the patient and the team to ensure the patient is fully informed about the procedure, recovery, and discharge date.

## The patient's surgical journey

*Patient group directives*
See Fig. 3.1.
• Formerly known as group protocols.
• They provide a framework for the supply and administration of medications without an individualized prescription.
• Patient group directives allow identified, responsible, trained healthcare professionals to supply and administer medication to a group of patients who fit specific patient group directive criteria.
• Trust-wide policy.
• Underpinned by the best possible evidence base.
• Must be signed by a doctor, pharmacist, and organizing authority before it can be used.

*Integrated care pathways and care bundles*
• A multimodal care pathway to achieve optimal recovery which covers the whole of the patient's surgical journey for specific conditions (e.g. colorectal surgery, hip or knee surgery).
• A guide to good practice which ensures the patient is in the best possible condition for surgery.
• A multidisciplinary document that incorporates local and national policies/guidelines and best practice to plan safe/high-quality, personalized care.

- Forms all or part of the clinical record and details essential steps in the care of the patient with a specific surgical condition.
- Patient progress can be monitored and audited.
- Known to reduce postoperative morbidity.
- Maximizes interventions.
- Ensures optimal preparation of the patient.
- Keeps the patient fully informed.

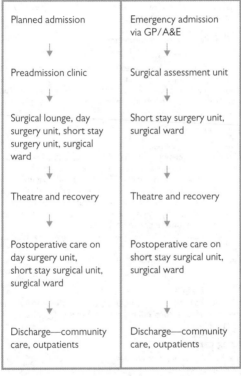

**Fig. 3.1** The surgical journey. A&E, accident and emergency; GP, general practitioner.

# Assessment of care

## Assessment

The aim of preoperative assessment, which ideally should take place 6 weeks before the elected date of surgery, is to:
- Maximize procedure-specific interventions
- Educate the patient to ensure they are fully informed
- Establish the level of risk and ensure the patient is aware of this
- Optimal preparation to ensure that the patient is prepared physically and psychologically for the procedure they are to undergo
- Identify the length of stay
- Plan multidisciplinary team interventions
- Discharge plan to a set/agreed discharge date.

Table 3.1 identifies some procedures to be undertaken during the assessment of surgical patients, although it should be noted that not all patients will require all investigations and National Institute for Health and Care Excellence (NICE) guidance[2] identifies recommended tests for minor, intermediate, major, and complex surgery.

## Planning care

The aim of planning care is to:
- Identify, reduce, or eliminate any individual risk factors that could potentially increase the risk to the patient during surgery
- Listen to the individual and establish their health beliefs and psychological/social/spiritual/financial issues to ensure the essential and fundamental needs of each client are identified and met
- Communicate effectively and provide individualized information based on the person's circumstances and experience
- Ensure that the needs of the client are met in line with the Equality Act 2010[3]
- To take into account individual language and cultural needs
- To ensure services are tailored to meet the needs of the individual.

## Implementing care

Table 3.2 identifies procedures to be undertaken in the preparation of surgical patients. Additional procedures can be found in ➔ Chapter 4 and in NICE guidance.[3]

## Evaluating care

- Completion of preoperative checklist.
- Patient is safely prepared and transferred to the operating theatre team.
- Sign in and commencement of the WHO surgical safety checklist.

**Table 3.1** Assessment of surgical patients

| | |
|---|---|
| Baseline observations | Electrocardiogram (ECG) |
| Chest X-ray | Pulmonary function tests |
| Past medical history | Allergies |
| Medication | Haematological investigations |
| Health education—smoking, obesity, alcohol consumption | Height, weight, body mass index (BMI) |
| Screening for infection control, e.g. methicillin-resistant *Staphylococcus aureus* (MRSA)—as per local policy | Complete local policy risk assessment tools, e.g. Waterlow |
| Latex screen | Manual handling |
| Nutrition | Autar deep venous thrombosis (DVT) scale |
| Record last menstrual period (LMP) | Glycated haemoglobin (HbA1c) |

**Table 3.2** Preparation of surgical patients

| | |
|---|---|
| Confirm biographical data | Informed consent |
| Correlate results of investigations, scans, radiographic images | Record baseline observations of temperature, pulse, and respiration (TPR), blood pressure (BP), oxygen saturation. |
| Urinalysis | 12-lead ECG |
| Anaesthetic assessment | Identify fasting regimen |
| Oral care | Hygiene needs |
| Identification of operation site | Record results of risk assessments |
| Document time premedication is given and ensure patient consent for rectal medication | Apply appropriate venous thromboembolism (VTE) prevention, as per local protocol |

## References

1. King's Fund (2014). Reconfiguring acute surgical services. Available at: ℘ https://www.kingsfund.org.uk/publications/reconfiguration-clinical-services/acute-surgical
2. National Institute for Health and Care Excellence (2016). Routine preoperative tests for elective surgery. NICE guideline [NG45]. Available at: ℘ https://www.nice.org.uk/guidance/ng45
3. Legislation.gov.uk (2010). Equality Act 2010. Available at: ℘ https://www.legislation.gov.uk/ukpga/2010/15/contents

# Patients with diverse healthcare needs

Patients with diverse health needs can present complexities for staff and require specialist knowledge and skills in order to effectively manage their care.

- Perioperative practitioners need a wide range of knowledge and skills to support the care of surgical patients with such healthcare needs.
- Patients with specific healthcare needs should be identified on the operating theatre list in order to ensure seamless care.
- By identifying and anticipating the needs of patients with complex problems, healthcare practitioners are able to quantify the nursing actions necessary to prevent problems occurring during the perioperative period.
- Diverse needs can be broadly categorized as physical disabilities, psychological disabilities, learning disabilities, and children and parents.

> Promoting diversity in healthcare can lead to the ability of healthcare providers to offer services that meet the unique social, cultural, and linguistic needs of their patients. In short, the better a patient is represented and understood, the better they can be treated.

## Physical disabilities

### Mobility

All patients with physical disabilities require care and consideration during the perioperative period.

- Patients with mobility difficulties caused by arthritis, or those with previous limb amputation, should be taken to theatre on a bed to avoid unnecessary transfers.
- Some procedures such as an epidural or spinal anaesthesia require positioning of the patient in the anaesthetic room.
- If a patient has restricted movement, the anaesthetic practitioner should identify:
  - How restricted is the movement?
  - Is the range of movement limited?
- Considerable care should also be taken when patients are anaesthetized in order to avoid nerve damage or excessive pressure on certain joints or limbs.

### Sensory impairment

Healthcare practitioners need a special understanding of patients with auditory, visual, speech, and cognitive impairment. Patients with these impairments are vulnerable and often feel quite anxious and isolated regarding their prospective surgical procedures. Assistance or specialist aids can be provided to patients with hearing, visual, or speech impairment, enabling them to receive and respond to information.

- Assistance or specialist aids are provided to patients with speaking, sight, or hearing difficulties, special needs, or learning disabilities, enabling them to receive and respond to information.

- If necessary, people are provided with access to a translator or a member of staff with appropriate language skills.
- Some people may have a limited capacity to understand, such as people with learning disabilities or mental illness. In such cases, every effort is made to help them comprehend what is being said and to involve them in the decision-making process with their carer or next of kin.

*Hearing impairment*
- Hearing aids and sound amplification technology can be of significant benefit to patients in the operating theatre.
- It is not necessary to remove a patient's hearing aid until he/she has been anaesthetized; it should then be replaced during reversal of anaesthesia.
- Ensure that any hearing aid is switched on and working and avoid the temptation to speak too loudly to the patient.
- Some patients can lip read so it is essential to face the patient and speak slowly and clearly.
- Some patients with a hearing impairment might prefer to communicate by writing; in this situation, handwriting should be clear, concise, and legible.
- British Sign Language (BSL) interpretation can be used for patients who request it, but adequate notice is generally required for interpreters— a family member can be involved with the patient's consent.

*Visual impairment*
- There are many conditions that can impair a patients' vision including cataract, glaucoma, diabetic retinopathy, age-related macular degeneration, acute closed-angle glaucoma, and primary open-angle glaucoma.
- In the perioperative environment, healthcare practitioners should stand or sit reasonably close to blind or partially sighted patients as they can often recognize outlines of individual faces.
- Sudden appearances at the theatre trolley or bedside should be avoided as this can startle patients.

*Speech impairment*
- Communication can be very difficult for patients, especially following a stroke; contact speech and language therapists for advice.

*Cognitive impairment*
- Some patients may have a limited capacity to understand (e.g. patients with mental illness or learning disabilities).
- Every effort must be made to help them comprehend what is being said and to involve them in the decision-making process with a family member, friend, carer, or next of kin.
- Information already given may need to be repeated.
- Written information can be left to remind the patient.

## Learning disabilities

*Autism*

- Autistic spectrum disorder refers to the whole range of 'autistic-style' symptoms with varying ranges of symptoms and degrees of severity.
- Autism is a subgroup of autistic spectrum disorder.
- Autism is a brain development disorder that affects communication and social interaction (Box 3.1).
- Problems with language and communication are common and speech usually develops later than usual.
- People with autism are more likely to have coexisting mental and physical disorders, and other developmental disorders.
- People with autism should have the opportunity to make informed decisions about their care, in partnership with their healthcare professionals.
- Care of young people in transition between paediatric services/child and adolescent mental health services (CAMHS) and adult services should be planned and managed according to the best practice guidance.
- No two autistic children are alike.
- There were approximately 17,970 new referrals for suspected autism in the first three-quarters of 2018–2019.
- Families, partners, and carers should have the opportunity to be involved in decisions about support and care if the patient with autism consents and has mental capacity to do so.

### Box 3.1 Problems that can be associated with autism

Patients with autism:

- May be unable to express themselves well
- May be unable to understand gestures, facial expressions, or tone of voice
- Can say odd things
- Make up their own words
- Express anger or aggression if routines are changed.
  Children with autism often hurt themselves when they are angry—they might bang their head or hit their face to get attention.

*In the perioperative environment*

- Changes in routine can be frightening and disorientating.
- A preoperative visit by the anaesthesia team is vital to ensure a smooth experience for everyone involved.
- Parents should be encouraged to discuss their child's particular needs, fears, communication level, and ability to cooperate and understand.
- Children should be prepared for theatre as they would for any unusual activity.
- Explain the sequence of events to the parents.
- Both parents/carers should be allowed in the anaesthetic room until anaesthesia has been induced.
- Preoperative sedation may assist to ease the transition from the parents to the anaesthetic room.

- It should not be used in place of preparing the child ahead of time and instead of talking to the child in the preoperative area.
- Just because a child with autism has communication difficulties, never assume that the child does not understand what is happening.
- Listen to the parents/carers as they know the child best.

*Down syndrome*

Down syndrome is a common genetic disorder characterized by intellectual disability, dysmorphic facial features, and a host of structural abnormalities. Individuals with Down syndrome tend to have a lower-than-average cognitive ability, often with mild-to-moderate learning disabilities. The life expectancy for people with Down syndrome is about 50–60 years. See Table 3.3 for associated medical conditions.

*In the perioperative environment*

- Patients may become belligerent when frightened.
- A preoperative visit by the anaesthesia team is vital to ensure a smooth experience for everyone involved.
- Encourage parents/carers to discuss the patient's particular needs, fears, communication level, and ability to cooperate and understand.
- Explain the sequence of events to the patient, parents, and/or carer.
- Parents/carers should be allowed in the anaesthetic room until anaesthesia has been induced.
- Never talk over the patient and never assume that the patient does not understand what is happening.

**Table 3.3** Medical conditions associated with Down syndrome

| | |
|---|---|
| **Cardiac** | Atrioventricular canal defects ventricular septal defect, tetralogy of Fallot |
| **Ear, nose, and throat (ENT)** | Conductive, sensorineural, mixed hearing loss, otitis media, sinusitis, pharyngitis, obstructive sleep apnoea |
| **Ophthalmic** | Cataracts, strabismus, nystagmus, congenital glaucoma, keratoconus |
| **Gastrointestinal** | Oesophageal atresia, duodenal atresia, pyloric stenosis, Meckel's diverticulum, Hirschsprung's disease, imperforate anus, gastro-oesophageal reflux |
| **Orthopaedic** | Hyperflexibility, scoliosis, hip dislocation, patellar subluxation/dislocation, foot deformity |
| **Neurological** | Intellectual disability, behavioural problems, Alzheimer's disease in older patients |
| **Haematological** | Risk of infections<br>Acute myeloblastic leukaemia, acute lymphoblastic leukaemia |
| **Endocrine** | Hypothyroidism |

## Further reading

Down's Syndrome Association. Homepage. Available at: ℜ http://www.downs-syndrome.org.uk

Mrdutt MM, Papaconstantinou HT, Robinson BD, et al. (2019). Preoperative frailty and surgical outcomes across diverse surgical subspecialties in a large health care system. Journal of the American College of Surgeons, 228(4):482–490.

National Autistic Society. Homepage. Available at: ℜ http://www.nas.org.uk

National Institute for Health and Care Excellence (2016). Autism spectrum disorder in adults: diagnosis and management. Clinical guideline [CG142]. Available at: ℜ https://www.nice.org.uk/guidance/cg142

National Institute for Health and Care Excellence (2017). Autism spectrum disorder in under 19s: recognition, referral and diagnosis. Clinical guideline [CG128]. Available at: ℜ https://www.nice.org.uk/guidance/cg128

National Institute for Health and Care Excellence (2018). Learning disabilities and behaviour that challenges: service design and delivery. Available at: ℜ https://www.nice.org.uk/guidance/ng93

NHS Digital. Homepage. Available at: ℜ https://digital.nhs.uk/

Peate I (ed) (2019). Alexander's nursing practice (5th ed). London: Elsevier.

Peate I, MacLeod J (eds) (2021). Pudner's nursing the surgical patient (4th ed). London: Elsevier.

Regulation and Quality Improvement Authority (2018). Guidelines on caring for people with a learning disability in general hospital settings. Belfast: Regulation and Quality Improvement Authority.

# Children, young people, and parents

The needs of children and young people must be considered during all stages of perioperative care, as they differ physiologically, emotionally, and socially from adults.

Operating theatres and operating lists specifically allocated for children are not always feasible. In these circumstances, children should be put to the start of the list with appropriately trained staff in the reception, anaesthetic room, theatre, and recovery areas.

A philosophy of family-centred care and partnership is advocated for children receiving perioperative care.[1] Parents and carers should be involved in partnership with all aspects of care and decision-making regarding the management of their children.[2]

- Communication must be at a level which is understandable and meets the cognitive and cultural needs of the child and family.
- Parents and children should be given the opportunity to ask questions during each stage of the perioperative journey.
- Provision should be made for parents to accompany children to the anaesthetic room.
- Provision should also be made for parents to stay in the anaesthetic room until the child has been anaesthetized; exceptions to this can include anticipated difficult intubation and rapid sequence intubation.
- When a parent accompanies a child into the anaesthetic room, a ward nurse or another suitable practitioner should also be present to escort the parent back to the ward.
- A registered children's nurse should be directly involved with children and young people within the perioperative environment.
- Healthcare practitioners caring for children and young people should be competent to practise advanced paediatric life support.
- Parents should be kept informed of their child's progress, especially if there is an unexpected delay in theatre.
- Many departments offer bleeps to parents so that they can be contacted in the event that anything needs to be discussed with them during surgery.

'Staff have a duty to understand and meet their legal responsibilities towards the children and young people they are caring for; including legal and ethical issues or potential conflicts between the interests of the child or young person and those of the parents.' Children's Act 2004

## Play and recreation

- Children in hospital, either as a day case or inpatient have a basic need for play and recreation; this should be met routinely in all hospital departments providing a service to children and young people.
- Play techniques should be encouraged across the interdisciplinary team, involving play-specialists, who can assist in the preparation for anaesthesia and surgery in children and young people.
- The team should be able to offer a variety of play interventions to support the child at each stage in his or her journey through the hospital system.

## References

1. Chorney JM, Kain ZN (2010). Family-centered paediatric perioperative care. Anaesthesiology, 112(3):751–755.
2. Zuo DZ, Houtrow AJ, Arango P, et al. (2012). Family-centred care: current applications and future directions in pediatric health care. Maternal Child Health Journal, 16(2):297–305.
3. Legislation.gov.uk (2004). Children Act 2004. Available at: ℛ https://www.legislation.gov.uk/ukpga/2004/31/contents

## Further reading

Health and Care Professions Council (2016). Standards of conduct, performance and ethics. London: Health and Care Professions Council.
Legislation.gov.uk (2004). Children Act 2004. Available at: ℛ https://www.legislation.gov.uk/ukpga/1989/41/contents
Nursing and Midwifery Council (2018). The code: professional standards of practice and behaviour for nurses and midwives. London: Nursing and Midwifery Council.
Royal College of Nursing (2011). Transferring children to and from theatre: RCN position statement and guideline for good practice. London: Royal College of Nursing.

# Communication and accessible information

Many people experience communication barriers across all care services, including language barriers, patients who are hard of hearing, people with sight loss, people with dual sensory loss (sight and hearing loss), and people with learning disabilities, learning difficulties or autism.[1] Standards to ensure accessible information are now in operation across the UK. They are in place to direct and define a consistent approach to identifying, recording, flagging, sharing, and meeting individuals' information and communication support needs by the NHS and social care service providers.[2]

The standard framework ensures that patients, carers, and parents who have information or communication needs relating to a disability, language barrier, impairment, or sensory loss receive both:

- Accessible information (information which is able to be read or received and understood by the individual or group for which it is intended)
- Communication support ('support which is needed to enable effective, accurate dialogue between a professional and a service user to take place').[2]

Where appropriate, staff should be trained in the use of different communication systems, for example, the use of text messaging, hearing induction loop systems, and basic BSL.[3]

> It is a legal requirement, under the Equality Act 2010, to ensure that reasonable adjustments are made to deliver equality of access to healthcare services for disabled people.[3]

### Language barriers

Healthcare practitioners will care for patients and relatives with language barriers at some point and standards of care delivery can become compromised if healthcare providers are unable to communicate with patients who do not speak the home language. A patient's language and communication needs should be routinely recorded by placing a flag or note that an interpreter is required on the person's case notes or electronic record.[2]

Language barriers between operating department staff and patients can severely undermine both effective communication and understanding of important healthcare information. For example, surgical patients may have a negative experience and are more at risk of delays in care provision and procedures, than fluent English/Welsh speakers. This may be due to difficulty understanding instructions or issues with informed consent.

Interpretation and translation services are available nationwide to allocate professional interpreters and translators for public sector use.[2] A professional interpreter will be registered on the National Register of Public Service which sets out a Code of Professional Conduct[4]; they can contribute to the provision of quality of care and promote patient safety by limiting the risk of adverse events. Interpreters should be used for all planned admissions, assessments, clinical consultations, informed consent, and discharge.

The role of the interpreter should be purely telling one person what another person is saying. If a translator is needed, they must be thoroughly briefed on the context of the information they convey and on the requirement for confidentiality.

## Language barriers in the perioperative environment

- Patients with language barriers within the perioperative environment are extremely vulnerable.
- When patients cannot communicate with health professionals, they can become distressed and this can make their treatment stressful and confusing.
- Every effort should be made to contact a translator. Lists of named interpreters should be available within all departments of the hospital.
- Friends and family members should not fulfil the role of a professional interpreter due to issues of confidentiality, impartiality, conflict of interest, and medical terminology. They should only be used as a temporary measure in cases such as emergency surgical treatment.
- Effective interpersonal skills are essential when caring for patients with language barriers. Attention should be paid to specific communication skills such as posture, eye contact, touch, and other non-verbal cues.

At no time should a child be expected to act as sole interpreter for another family member or patient.

## References

1. Wales Audit Office (2018). Speak my language: overcoming language and communication barriers in public services. Available at: ℘ http://www.audit.wales/system/files/publications/speak-my-language-2018-english.pdf
2. NHS England (2017). Accessible information standard. Available at: ℘ https://www.england.nhs.uk/publication/accessible-information-standard-overview-20172018/
3. NHS Wales (2014). All Wales standards for communication and information for people with sensory loss. Cardiff: Welsh Government.
4. National Register of Public Service Interpreters (2016). Code of professional conduct. Available at: ℘ http://www.nrpsi.org.uk/for-clients-of-interpreters/code-of-professional-conduct.html

# Anxiety and the influence of cognition

As has already been identified, one of the three basic objectives of safe, surgical, patient-care delivery and management is the delivery of a physiologically and psychologically prepared patient for the planned surgical journey. A key psychological issue faced by patients waiting for a surgical procedure is anxiety.

- Anxiety in itself is a standard response to a perceived or actual threat; it can become a problem for patients and impact the perioperative and postoperative phases of a patient's journey.
- Anxiety can result from a variety of factors and each individual's case is different. Factors may relate to gender, age, family dynamics, and educational level.
- To mitigate the effects of anxiety, the multidisciplinary team need to help the patient prepare for surgery by ensuring that they understand the rationale for surgery and the procedure up to and following surgery.
- It is imperative that the perceived threats or fears are identified during assessment:
  - These may include a fear of surgery, worries about the level and chronicity of pain they will experience postoperatively, or the impact that their health condition will have on their family, their employment, or their financial situation in the longer term. Equally, they may be concerned about being separated from family members for a period of time.
- Anxiety can be caused or maintained by the amount of stress a person experiences, together with their individual vulnerability to stress.
- One's personality plays a part, as does one's beliefs associated with the feared situation. Subsequently, to reduce levels of threat and stress, an individual will avoid the specific situations that cause them distress.
- Although this results in a reduction in anxiety in the short term, it only serves to maintain it in the longer term.

Here is an example of assessing a patient who has recently received assessments and diagnostic tests as a result of experiencing chest pain and breathlessness. They are scheduled to undergo an angiogram but are reticent about giving consent for the procedure due to their anxiety about their clinical condition and the procedure. A useful method of assessing an individual's anxiety involves exploring the patient's experience along four domains or systems (Fig. 3.2). This approach is typically used as part of cognitive behavioural therapy but it can be applied more broadly.

The initial aim is to identify the symptoms the patient experiences in each domain, then to help the patient understand how primarily our thoughts impact each domain in initiating and maintaining the anxiety. It also helps the patient to realize that although there are risks to any surgical procedure, some of their thoughts or cognitions may be exaggerated, thus exacerbating the perceived threat. In this example, the symptoms are shown in Fig. 3.3.

Having identified the key cognitions, the nurse needs to establish their strength of belief for each by asking 'On a scale of 0–100, zero being no belief and 100 being complete belief, how strongly do you believe each of these thoughts to be true?' Once the strength of belief has been established, this provides an opportunity for the nurse and patient to undertake

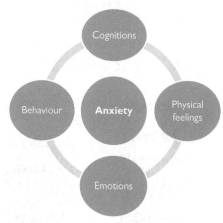

**Fig. 3.2** Effects of anxiety.

a guided discovery of the validity of the beliefs—with the nurse providing relevant education as required. Following the discussions and educational interventions, the patient's strength of belief is re-rated to establish the level of cognitive shift that has occurred as a result of the intervention. If a patient's anxiety is identified in advance of a planned procedure, this affords the opportunity to guide patients to self-help materials or to be referred for specific interventions for anxiety if necessary.

*Thoughts or cognitions*
- 'I am going to die.'
- 'I am going to have a heart attack in the operating theatre.'
- 'I am going to have a stroke.'
- 'I am not going to be able to stay still for the procedure and it will go wrong.'
- Racing thoughts.

*Physical feelings*
- Palpitations.
- Sweating.
- Dry mouth.
- Shaking.
- Feeling dizzy or lightheaded.
- Nausea.

*Emotions*
- Tearful.
- Nervous.
- Agitation.
- Fatigue.

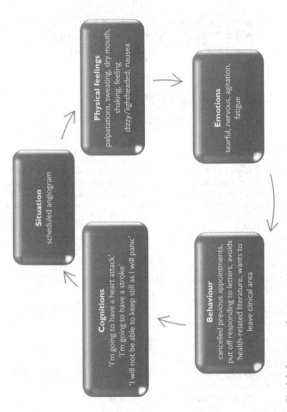

**Fig. 3.3** Symptoms of anxiety.

*Behaviour*
- Cancelled previous appointments.
- Has put off responding to letters from clinicians.
- Avoids reading any literature or watching television programmes relating to health issues.
- Attempted to leave the clinical area.

## Further reading

Alanazi AA (2014). Reducing anxiety in preoperative patients: a systematic review. British Journal of Nursing, 23(7):387–393.

Caumo W, Schmidt AP, Schneider CN, et al (2001). Risk factors for postoperative anxiety in adults. Anaesthesia, 56(8):720–728.

Dao TK, Youssef NA, Armsworth M, et al (2011). Randomized controlled trial of brief cognitive behavioural intervention for depression and anxiety symptoms preoperatively in patients undergoing coronary artery bypass graft surgery. Journal of Thoracic and Cardiovascular Surgery, 142(3):e109–e115.

Greenberger D, Padesky C (1995). Mind over mood: a cognitive therapy treatment manual for clients. New York: Guilford Press.

Mitchell M (2012). Anxiety management in minimal stay surgery. Nursing Times, 108(48):14–16.

Sigdel S (2015). Perioperative anxiety: a short review. Global Anaesthesia and Perioperative Medicine 1. Available at: ℘ http://www.oatext.com/Perioperative-anxiety-A-short-review.php#Article_Info

## Self-help materials

Getselfhelp.co.uk. Anxiety self-help. Available at: ℘ https://www.getselfhelp.co.uk/anxiety.htm

Northumberland, Tyne & Wear NHS Foundation Trust. Anxiety: An NHS Self Help Guide. Available at: ℘ https://web.ntw.nhs.uk/selfhelp/leaflets/Anxiety%20A4%202016%20FINAL.pdf

# Mental health

One in four people in the UK are affected by mental ill-health each year, more than those affected by cancer and heart disease.

- A range of conditions including depression, anxiety, psychosis, dementia, and personality disorders can impact a person's emotional well-being, physical health, relationships, and employment, and, depending on the severity of the illness, treatment may involve a complex mix of long-term psychosocial and pharmacological interventions (Box 3.2).
- Nonetheless, most people who experience mental ill-health will recover fully or be able to live well and manage their condition effectively.
- Despite this, there continues to be a significant amount of stigma and discrimination associated with mental illness that can leave the needs of those affected unmet or ignored.

Meeting the needs of those with mental ill-health in a fast-paced surgical environment can present some challenges to healthcare professionals. Taking time to talk and 'attend' to the patient using a range of interpersonal skills will help develop a trusting, therapeutic relationship that can promote a feeling of safety and aid recovery.

## Throughout the surgical journey

- Take time to establish a supportive relationship with those who have mental health conditions.
- Provide information that is clear and concise and establish the patient's level of understanding.
- Be prepared to offer support, repeated explanations, and reassurance.
- Liaise with mental health professionals for advice and support for both the patient and the surgical team.
- Recognize the importance of relatives and carers. With the patient's consent, they should be encouraged to stay with the patient for as long as possible and accompany the patient to theatre.
- Ascertain possible risk issues associated with the mental health condition.

## Communication

- It is important to communicate effectively with those who have mental health conditions and to demonstrate dignity and respect for the patient's rights.
- All information should be communicated clearly and concisely.
- Always establish the patient's level of understanding and be prepared to repeat information frequently.
- Allow time for the patient to ask questions.
- Work collaboratively with the patient and their relatives and carers and involve them in decision-making regarding their care and treatment.

## Box 3.2 Types of mental health conditions

- Depression.
- Anxiety.
- Obsessive–compulsive disorder.
- Post-traumatic stress disorder.
- Schizophrenia.
- Bipolar disorder.
- Dementia.
- Personality disorders.
- Eating disorders.

## Further reading

Bach S, Grant A (2015). Communication and interpersonal skills in nursing. London: Sage.

Legislation.gov.uk (2005). Mental Capacity Act 2005. Available at: ℜ https://www.legislation.gov.uk/ukpga/2005/9/contents

Legislation.gov.uk (2007). Mental Health Act 2007. Available at: ℜ https://www.legislation.gov.uk/ukpga/2007/12/contents

Moss B (2015). Communication skills for health and social care. London: Sage.

# Dementia

Delirium is described as an acute confusional state and dementia as a chronic confusional state but this differentiation is of limited guidance for healthcare staff.

The World Health Organization (WHO) defines dementia as a chronic and progressive disorder disturbing higher cortical functioning and personal activities of daily living.[1]

> Dementia is 'an umbrella term that describes a number of conditions of the brain: there is not just one condition called dementia. Dementia is a progressive and terminal condition. Each type of dementia affects the person in a different way.'[2]

Two people can have the same diagnosis for the same duration and their presentation is quite different. Therefore, how these disorders will be exhibited and the care required, in a surgical setting, will vary dramatically.

A full preoperative assessment should be undertaken which includes:
- Functional status, particularly activities of daily living
- Nutritional status including pressure sore risk
- Social issues such as support network.

A structured management plan including liaising with the ward or recovery area should be developed.

## Considerations prior to admission

The more 'knowledge' available about the person, the smoother the process should be for everyone. Some people have developed a 'This is me' document developed by the Alzheimer's Society. If they have, request to see it; if not, the following information will be useful:
- The name they like to be called.
- Brief details of their normal routines, including whether they need reminders or support with washing, dressing, eating and drinking, going to the toilet, or taking medication.
- Any difficulties the person may have with communication, and information on how best to communicate with them.
- Information about foods they particularly like or dislike, or any difficulties they have eating.
- Illness or pain that may bother them.
- Any cultural or religious needs.
- Information about sleeping patterns.
- Whether they like to be active or inactive—for example, if they walk about—and what can calm them when they are agitated.
- Whether they have an advance decision or a personal welfare LPA.[3]

## Communication

A person's ability to verbally communicate will deteriorate as the dementia progresses but the ability to communicate throughout the dementia journey is retained. It is therefore important to utilize all modes of communicating.

Some verbal and non-verbal suggestions to increase effective communication are[2]:

- Make eye contact
- Smile while speaking
- Use a friendly tone of voice
- Use short sentences
- Speak in the same language
- Do not be afraid of silence (it could be thinking time)
- Do not give too many messages at the same time
- Do not use defensive or aggressive body language
- Talk to someone at their eye level
- Make sure the room is quiet
- Do not speak to anyone at the same time
- Do not touch the person from behind.

## Carers

Carers are essential people to involve in perioperative care as they already have a close relationship with the person and can offer guidance and support. Being left alone or isolated can cause a deterioration of the dementia so having the carer as a member of the team is crucial. They can interpret communication and behaviour but also support in practical ways such as:

- Pain assessment
- Personal hygiene
- Mealtimes with eating and drinking
- Comfort and reassurance
- Ensuring sensory aids are available (glasses, hearing aids, etc.).

## Pain assessment and management

Special attention needs to be focused on pain and pain management as people with dementia are less likely to request pain relief.

In the early stages of dementia, the person could be asked about their pain with minimal choices such as 'Is your pain mild or severe?', but at later stages, an observational tool such as the Abbey Pain Scale is useful. Also consider if the person is able to move or cough. The Abbey pain scale involves assessment of:

- Vocalizations—such as crying
- Facial expression—such as grimacing
- Change of body language—such as holding parts of the body
- Behavioural change—such as refusing to eat
- Physiological change—such as BP
- Physical changes—such as skin tears.[4]

Opiates for pain management in patients with dementia should be minimized due to the risk of delirium; where they are required, it is recommended to take a 'start low and go slow' approach.

### Coexisting medical conditions

- A higher rate of medical conditions such as cardiovascular disease, chronic obstructive pulmonary disease, and renal impairment are found in people with dementia.
- Dementia is also linked with frailty. The more comorbidities, the greater postoperative risk.[5]

### Drug interactions

- Given the likelihood of comorbidities, there is also a high risk of polypharmacy and drug interactions.
- These will need careful consideration especially if delirium is to be minimized.
- There are specific drugs given to people with dementia and medical staff need to decide if they are to be reduced or stopped prior to surgery.
- Drugs used to reduce the cognitive symptoms of dementia:
  - N-methyl-D-aspartate (NMDA) receptor antagonists (such as memantine) enhance the side effects of anticholinergics and dopamine agonists.
  - Acetylcholine esterase inhibitors (such as donepezil) prolong the effect of depolarizing and decrease or reverse the effect of non-depolarizing neuromuscular blockers.[5]
  - Other drugs used to deal with emotional and behavioural symptoms related to dementia:
    - Specific serotonin reuptake inhibitors (SSRIs, such as citalopram) increase the risk of serotonin syndrome and enhance the effects of opiates and induction agents.
    - Atypical antipsychotics (such as risperidone) enhance the risk of vasodilation and hypotension with anaesthetics.[5]

### Sensitivity to anaesthetic agents

It is still unclear whether people with dementia have increased sensitivity to anaesthetic agents but given the higher number of older people with dementia, caution needs to be used.

### Consent issues

For all medical and nursing interventions, it is required that the person receiving treatment gives consent. There are exceptions to this regarding:
- A child
- An unconscious person
- A person on certain sections of the Mental Health Act 2007
- Those assessed not to have mental capacity.

Another person cannot give consent unless they have parental responsibility or have a LPA for welfare of the person. An adult should always be considered to have capacity to make their own decision unless they are assessed not to be able to. To assess mental capacity, the assessor should establish:
- If the person can understand what is being proposed
- If they can remember this information for as long as it takes to make the decision
- If they understand the implications or consequences of giving consent
- If they can communicate their decision.

The Mental Capacity Act 2005 makes provision for people to identify a person or people who they permit to make decisions for them if they lose capacity. A person with dementia is encouraged to do this before they lose capacity. The identified person or people are given LPA. If the person with dementia does not have the capacity to make the decision for the operation themselves, then the person with LPA for health and welfare must give consent for the operation to be carried out. If there is a disagreement between hospital professionals and the person/people with LPA then an application will need to be made through the courts to have the LPA status removed.[6]

## Postoperative complications—delirium

People with dementia are more likely to develop delirium after an anaesthetic which can lead to falls, pneumonia, and increased mortality.

Strategies to minimize risk:
- Avoid benzodiazepines and anticholinergics.
- Use prophylaxis with antipsychotic medication.
- Maximize early return home.
- Keep to patient routines as much as possible.
- Use bispectral index (BIS)-guided anaesthesia.
- Effective multimodal analgesia.
- Promotion of activities of daily living—sleep, mobility, hydration, elimination, vision, and hearing—along with reduction of disorientation through clear signage, use of lights, sounds etc.
- Maximize family support.[5]

## References

1. World Health Organization (2010). Mental and behavioural disorders (F00-F99). In: International Statistical Classification of Diseases and Related Health Problems 10th Revision (ICD-10). Version for 2010. Available at: ℜ http://apps.who.int/classifications/icd10/browse/2010/en#/F00-F09
2. Watchman K, Kerr D, Wilkinson H (2010). Supporting Derek, a practice development guide to support staff working with people who have a learning difficulty and dementia. York: Joseph Rowntree Foundation.
3. Alzheimer's Society (2018). Hospital care. Available at: ℜ https://www.alzheimers.org.uk/info/20046/help_with_dementia_care/40/hospital_care/2
4. Royal College of Physicians (2007). Clinical guidelines for the assessment of pain in older people. Available at: ℜ http://www.bgs.org.uk/Publications/Clinical%20Guidelines/pain%20concise%20guidelines%20WEB.pdf
5. Alcorn S, Foo I (2017). Perioperative management of patients with dementia. BJA Education, 17(3):94–98.
6. Legislation.gov.uk (2005). Mental Capacity Act 2005. Available at: ℜ https://www.legislation.gov.uk/ukpga/2005/9/contents

## Further reading

Legislation.gov.uk (2000). Adults with Incapacity (Scotland) Act 2000. Available at: ℜ https://www.legislation.gov.uk/asp/2000/4/contents
Department of Health (2016). Mental Capacity Act 2016 (Northern Ireland). Available at: ℜ https://www.health-ni.gov.uk/mca
Royal College of Anaesthetists (2019). Chapter 3: guidelines for the provision of anaesthesia services for intraoperative care. London: Royal College of Anaesthetists.
Royal College of Anaesthetists (2021). Chapter 2: guidelines for the provision of anaesthesia services for the perioperative care of elective and urgent care patients. London: Royal College of Anaesthetists.
Royal College of Surgeons (2016). Consent: supported decision-making. London: Royal College of Surgeons.

# Substance misuse

- Alcohol misuse.
- Drug misuse.
- Prescribed and non-prescribed medication.

Individuals use and misuse a range of legal and illegal substances, some are prescribed and bought over the counter (OTC) for pain relief. You will not always know whether individuals are involved with substance misuse treatment services and it is imperative that assumptions are not made regarding anyone's history or current use regarding substance misuse. The following list of substances identified is not exhaustive, but is provided as a baseline of knowledge and awareness.

## Substances that are misused

- Alcohol.
- Drugs:
  - Cannabis.
  - Amphetamine.
  - Cocaine.
  - Methamphetamine.
  - Mephedrone.
  - Synthetic cannabinoids (e.g. Spice).
  - Hallucinogens (e.g. LSD).
- Prescribed and non-prescribed medication:
  - Benzodiazepines (e.g. diazepam, lorazepam, temazepam).
  - Methadone.
  - Morphine.
  - Tramadol.
  - Co-codamol.
  - Codeine.
  - Fentanyl.
  - Dihydrocodeine.

### Alcohol misuse

- Each individual needs to be asked about their alcohol use as it is important not to make assumptions about people's consumption.
- Individuals may be physically dependant on alcohol; therefore, it is essential that they are observed for alcohol withdrawal symptoms.
- Individuals may not have informed the admissions team of their excessive alcohol use prior to admission and then feel very embarrassed disclosing this, especially if they begin to feel withdrawal symptoms of shaking begin.
- Ensure that you maintain an honest, open, and non-judgemental approach and do not make assumptions about how individuals may present regarding past and/or present alcohol use.

*Drug misuse*

- Each individual needs to be asked about their past and current drug use as it is important not to make assumptions about people's use.
- Individuals may be physically dependant on some drugs such as heroin and opiate-based medication such as tramadol, morphine, and fentanyl; therefore, it is essential that they are observed for opiate withdrawal symptoms.
- Individuals may not have informed the team of their drug use prior to admission and then feel very embarrassed disclosing this later in the admission.
- Ensure that you maintain an honest, open, and non-judgemental approach and do not make assumptions about how individuals may present regarding past and/or present drug use.
- If individuals disclose an opiate dependence, it is essential that their pain management is assessed and reviewed accordingly.
- Individuals who may have a history of planned abstinence from opiates may be upset, anxious, and concerned and even refuse opiate-based medication for pain as this may trigger past feelings.

*Prescribed and non-prescribed medication*

- Each individual needs to be asked about their past and current medication and whether they take it as prescribed, do not assume people take it as prescribed and seek clarification.
- Individuals may be physically dependant on some prescribed and non-prescribed medication such as cold remedies containing codeine which are bought OTC or diazepam and codeine which are prescribed by their GP.
- It is essential that all individuals are observed for opiate withdrawal symptoms.
- Individuals may not have informed the admissions team about how they are not taking medication as it is prescribed until they start to feel increased anxiety during the admission and then feel very embarrassed about disclosing this later in the admission.
- Ensure that you maintain an honest, open, and non-judgemental approach and do not make assumptions about how individuals may present during an admission regarding substance misuse.

# Further reading

Alcohol Change UK. Homepage. Available at: ℘ https://alcoholchange.org.uk/

Drug Wise (2017). Promoting evidence-based information on drugs, alcohol and tobacco. Available at: ℘ http://www.drugwise.org.uk

National Institute for Health and Care Excellence (2007). Drug misuse in over 16s: opioid detoxification. Clinical guideline [CG52]. Available at: ℘ https://www.nice.org.uk/guidance/cg52

National Institute for Health and Care Excellence (2016). Cirrhosis in over 16s: assessment and management. NICE guideline [NG50]. Available at: ℘ https://www.nice.org.uk/guidance/ng50

National Institute for Health and Care Excellence (2017). Alcohol-use disorders: diagnosis and management of physical complications. Clinical guideline [CG100]. Available at: ℘ https://www.nice.org.uk/guidance/cg100

National Institute for Health and Care Excellence (2020). Alcohol-use disorders overview. Available at: ℘ https://pathways.nice.org.uk/pathways/alcohol-use-disorders

National Institute for Health and Care Excellence (2020). Drug misuse prevention overview. Available at: ℘ https://pathways.nice.org.uk/pathways/drug-misuse-prevention

# Cultural competence

During the admission of a surgical patient, the nurse should make note of the patient's spiritual/cultural beliefs. These may be related to specific dietary needs, personal care needs such as washing and dressing, pain management, and medical interventions.

## Points to consider during admission

- Patients from black and minority ethnic (BME) backgrounds may prefer a family member with them during the admission process.
- For older BME patients this may be for a younger family member to act as a translator.
- The nurse should check if the patient is happy for intimate information to be shared, and the understanding of the family member to act as the translator.
- This practice may be discouraged in some hospitals but it is often the preferred choice of the BME patient.
- Muslim men and women prefer to be examined by a healthcare professional of the same sex, but the Islamic faith allows this to be relaxed in healthcare if no one of the same sex is available.
- Hindus place great value on washing under running water and it should be noted during their admission that this will be made available to them when dealing with personal hygiene.

---

- Hindu patients should not have their clothes and shoes stored in the same locker so as to keep the cleanest (the head) and dirtiest (the feet) parts of the body separate.

---

- The transgender patient should have their self-identified gender documented on admission.
- The transgender patient should be referred to as he or she according to their self-identified gender.
- If uncertain, healthcare professionals should not attempt to guess the self-identified gender of a transgender patient. The admission paperwork will give the nurse the opportunity to ask the patient if they have a preferred gender. This should not be ignored and should be acknowledged during the admission.
- The nurse does not have the right to share this personal information with colleagues unless the patient has agreed. It is important for the nurse to gain this consent during admission so that the transgender patient can be treated with dignity during their stay in hospital.

## Diet and culture

- Muslim men and women do not eat pork and prefer to eat halal meat. Jewish kosher food can be given as an alternative.
- Jewish patients should have kosher food made available.
- Hindu men and women usually follow a lacto-vegetarian diet (avoid meat and eggs). Fats derived from animals, e.g. dripping and lard are not permitted . Some may eat chicken, fish or lamb but beef is not eaten as it is considered a holy animal This should be documented on admission.

### Religion and culture (points to discuss on admission)

- Muslims are expected to pray five times each day: after dawn, at noon, mid-afternoon, early evening, and at night. If a patient is seriously ill, they can be exempt from prayers.
- Prayer is important to Christians and is particularly important at times of stress, such as illness. Christian patients should be offered the opportunity to see the hospital Chaplin and may especially like to pray with the Chaplin before surgery.
- The wearing of religious jewellery is important to Roman Catholics and the removal of this should be managed sensitively prior to surgery. Jewellery should only be removed with the patient's consent.

Worship is very important and is something many Hindus do every day to demonstrate their commitment to the faith. It is a way of showing love and devotion to their Hindu God Brahman. Hindus believe they have an atman, or piece of Brahman, within them. Hindu worshipping occurs at home or a temple to celebrate important festivals such as Diwali, the festival of lights.

Jews believe that there is a single God and that Judaism is a family faith that revolves around the home, e.g. the Sabbath meal, when families join together to welcome in the special day. Shabbat, the Jewish Sabbath, is a weekly holiday that celebrates creation and begins at sundown on Friday and ends with Havdalah—a short ceremony that separates Shabbat from the rest of the week, on a Saturday evening.

### Pain and culture

Cultural beliefs influence the experience and expression of pain.

- Some BME patients may be more expressive about their pain than other patients, and this cultural behaviour should not influence the way BME patients with pain are treated. The patient should be treated according to their expression of pain.
- Research has suggested that healthcare professionals may experience expressions of pain as follows:
  - Patients of African origin are highly expressive of pain-related symptoms.
  - Chinese patients have a low expression of pain-related symptoms.
  - South Asian patients are highly expressive of pain-related symptoms.

### Care of the transgender patient on the ward

The transgender patient should be accommodated according to their self-identified gender.

- This includes being placed in a male or female bay relating to their identified gender.
- This also applies to toilets facilities but exceptions are made if an open shower is used before surgery.
- When a transgender patient is too unwell to wash or dress themselves, staff should be aware of the patient's self-identified gender and treat them accordingly (e.g. if an individual identifies as a woman they should be given the choice to be washed by female staff).

## Further reading

Aziz S, Gatrad AR (2008). Caring for Muslim patients (2nd ed). London: Routledge.

Campbell CM, Edwards RR (2012). Ethnic differences in pain and pain management. Pain Management, 2(3):219–230.

Garneau AB, Pepin J (2015). Cultural competence: a constructivist definition. Journal of Transcultural Nursing, 26(1):9–15.

Gooren LJ (2011). Care of transsexual persons. New England Journal of Medicine, 354(13):1251–1257.

Holland K (2017). Cultural awareness in nursing and health care: an introductory text (3rd ed). Chicago, IL: Routledge Taylor & Francis Group.

McKennis AT (1999). Caring for the Islamic patient. AORN Journal, 69(6):1185–1196.

Monterrey SM, Jones AD, Perry N, et al. (2013). Cultural competence in nursing faculty: a journey, not a destination. Journal of Professional Nursing, 29(6):e51–e57.

Royal College of Nursing (2016). Caring for lesbian, gay, bisexual or trans clients or patients: guide for nurses and health care support workers on next of kin issues. London: Royal College of Nursing.

Smith FD (2016). Perioperative care of the transgender patient. AORN Journal, 103(2):152–160.

# Managing visitors in the perioperative environment

The continuing and often rapid development of products and techniques to provide improved treatment and more cost-effective practice, while maintaining the most beneficial outcomes for both patient and practitioner, realizes the need for programmes of hands-on training and education, provided by the healthcare industries that specialize in the relative areas.

- Historically, specialist representatives from industry, who have developed mutually beneficial partnerships with their colleagues within the critical care areas of the NHS, are often regarded as integral assets to the function of the department.
- Quite often, the specialist representative will have previously worked within the operating theatre department. This is, of course, dependent on the ability of the representative to forge a long-term relationship and acquire a considerable degree of trust, which does not happen overnight.

---

- The respect, well-being and integrity of the patient and their privacy are paramount; the visitor must be provided with boundaries that accentuate this.

---

With the appropriate training and guidelines, industry representatives have been welcomed into the operating theatres to provide support, education, and unbiased assessment of the needs and requirements of the department and its staff. This should, and no doubt will continue, with consideration to the following:

- Visitors should provide and constantly display, when practical, current identification relating to their role and their organization.
- The theatre management team must assess the risks of the visit and admission of the representative to the department as required by the Health and Safety at Work etc. Act 1974.
- The visit, involving entry into the clinical area, must be agreed and prearranged by the senior nursing and medical staff involved in the project or activity.
- It must be the equal responsibility of the representative and the operating theatre staff when confirming these arrangements to ensure that all parties have approved it and have communicated appropriately.
- Whether a former practitioner in the relative field or not, the representative should have successfully completed an accredited theatre access/operating theatre etiquette course that meets the requirements of the Life Science Industry Register for Tier 3—high-risk areas—and is valid for 2 years.
  - This provides the theatre staff with the assurance and confidence that the visitor has been educated appropriately in regard to behaviour and protocols.

---

- Medical representatives are merely promoting technology that the healthcare industry, through its need to provide better and more economical patient care, has demanded.

- It is necessary for the visitor to record their entry and exit times in the appropriate register and is prohibited from visiting areas of the department that are irrelevant to the procedures, without authorization.
- Medical representatives must be suitably attired in accordance with the local operating theatre recommendations and must not, at any time, engage in assisting with patient care.
- Representatives must be provided with all the health and safety information in relation to the specific department (e.g. fire exits, eye-wash and spill-stations), and the member of staff with first aid responsibilities.
- The patient must be consulted as to whether they wish to comply with the request that a representative be present during their procedure. This can be assisted in its presentation to the patient by the theatre staff member highlighting the relevant qualifications and experience of the visitor and the benefit that it will provide to the procedure being performed.
- Only with the consent of the medical staff can the representative assist in reassuring the patient directly of the relevance of their attendance during the procedure.
- When possible, demonstration and evaluation of the device in a non-clinical setting (i.e. a 'dry run') to the relevant nursing and medical staff is highly recommended, prior to the actual procedure itself.
- See Box 3.3.

---

**Box 3.3 Operating theatre protocols for visitors**

- Identify health and safety issues in the area relative to your own safety.
- Minimize risk to the patient.
- Protect the patient's anonymity and protect confidential information.
- Identify personal protective equipment specific to areas of the operating department.
- Abide by infection prevention and control policies in relation to operating room practice.
- Set up and manage capital equipment or medical disposables' trials effectively.

---

All operating theatres should have a detailed policy that applies to visitors in a high-risk environment.

---

### Further reading

Association of Perioperative Practice (2016). Standards and Recommendations for Safe Perioperative Practice. Harrogate: Association of Perioperative Practice.

Health and Safety Executive. Health and Safety at Work etc. Act 1974. Available at: ℜ http://www.hse.gov.uk/legislation/hswa.htm

Hughes CW (2003). A day in the life of a medical salesman. British Journal of Perioperative Nursing, 13(9):346–348.

Medical Industry Limited. E-learning and Life Science Industry National Credentialing Register. Available at: ℜ https://www.medicalindustry.co.uk/

# Prisoners attending for surgery

Prisons function to protect the public but, while people are detained, the prison also has a duty to protect those prisoners it holds. Her Majesty's Inspectorate of Prisons expects that prisoners are safe, treated with respect, have opportunities to engage in purposeful activities, are rehabilitated, and prepared for release.[1] Healthcare forms part of ensuring safety, showing respect and that prisoners are well for release. It is expected that prisoners have access to an equivalent level of healthcare in custody as they would receive in the community including access to specialist health services provided in hospital settings.

## General principles

The British Medical Association has previously claimed that prison staff often perceive hospitals and healthcare as the 'weak link' in keeping prisoners secure and that prisoners may exaggerate health complaints in order to seek escape.[2] However, prior to attending hospital for treatment the prisoner will have been assessed in prison by a medical professional such as a registered nurse, paramedic, or GP as requiring treatment. Prisoners attending hospital will be escorted by prison officers who remain accountable to the prison governor for the security of the prisoner. The prison service has clear processes in place to ensure the security and well-being of the prisoner and the safety of the public while the prisoner is receiving treatment in prison.[3]

- Prison healthcare teams may be able to offer minor surgery, X-rays, treatment of minor injuries, sexual health, and management of chronic conditions depending on facilities and staff skillset.
- Before attending hospital, the prisoner will have been assessed as requiring treatment that cannot be provided by the healthcare team working within the prison. A prisoner will only be sent to hospital if essential due to the security risks and the cost to the prison of providing escort staff.
- Prior to leaving the prison, a thorough risk assessment will be undertaken. The risk assessment will indicate any health reasons or restrictions on the use of restraints while the prisoner is outside of the prison. It also details the number of staff needed, the method of transportation used, and processes for visits while in hospital.
- Under normal circumstances, all prisoners will be handcuffed to officers at all times while outside of prison. Different methods of restraint are available and allow for the prisoner's confidentiality and dignity to be maintained while receiving healthcare.
- When attending surgery, restraints will normally be removed when the procedure is undertaken with officers remaining outside the surgical area. Prison officers are also instructed to remove restraints if they interfere with treatment or in a life-threatening situation.

Prison staff are accountable to the governor of their prison. They are responsible for protecting the public and the welfare of the prisoner. Healthcare professionals are accountable for the welfare of the patient and should deliver the same standard of care as to any other patient. This includes ensuring confidentiality, dignity, and respect and remaining non-judgemental. The presence of restraints and prison officers can make this challenging, but effective communication between healthcare staff and prison staff is key and will ensure safe care.

## Prisoners attending surgery

- Clinical areas should be advised in advance that they will be treating a prisoner by the prison healthcare team. This allows for the planning of how to ensure dignified, confidential, and safe care. Even in an emergency the prison healthcare team should be able to provide some advanced notice.
- Prisoners will always be escorted by at least two prison officers. Clinical staff should respect their role and communicate with the officers to ensure they understand what is required clinically so that security can be planned and organized appropriately.
- Prisoners will remain restrained until anaesthetized and unable to escape. Prison staff must dress appropriately in clinical areas but will not be present during surgical procedures.
- Prisoners will be restrained post surgery. It is important that escort staff are aware of any medical reasons why restraints should not be used or if specific wrists should not be handcuffed.
- Prisoners will be anxious about surgery in the same way as other patients but will not have access to support from family or friends unless visits have been authorized by the prison governor. Healthcare staff should reassure the prisoner patient and remain compassionate and empathetic as per governing body code of practice.

Clinical staff must communicate any life-threatening conditions or emergency treatment requirements to escorting staff. In these circumstances, restraints will be removed to allow treatment. Restraints must be removed if the use of a defibrillator is required.

## Key points

- Prisoners are entitled to the same level of healthcare as any other patient including being treated with respect, dignity, in confidence, and without judgement.
- The focus of the surgical staff should be the clinical needs of the patient and staff should not be perturbed in giving instruction to the escorting officers if their security focus is impeding care.
- Anxiety around attending for surgery may be increased for prisoner patients due to the presence of restraints, prison staff, and lack of family support through visits.
- Communication between prison healthcare, hospital staff, and prison staff should be clear and is vital to ensuring safe, effective care and to maintain security.

## References

1. Her Majesty's Inspectorate of Prisons (2017). Our expectations. Available at: ⅋ https://www.justiceinspectorates.gov.uk/hmiprisons/our-expectations/
2. British Medical Association (2009). The medical role in restraint and control: custodial settings. Guidance from the British Medical Association. Available at: ⅋ https://www.bma.org.uk/media/1860/bma-medical-role-in-restraint-2009.pdf
3. National Offender Management Service (2015). PSI33-2015 national security framework external escorts – external prisoner movement. Available at: ⅋ https://www.justice.gov.uk/downloads/offenders/psipso/psi-2015/psi-33-2015-external-prisoner-movement.pdf

## Further reading

National Institute for Health and Care Excellence (2016). Physical health of people in prison. NICE guideline [NG57]. Available at: ⅋ https://www.nice.org.uk/guidance/NG57
Royal College of Nursing (2017). Supporting nursing staff caring for patients from places of detention. London: Royal College of Nursing.

# Preadmission management

# Preoperative assessment

The primary aim of preoperative assessment is to identify the patient's health status and level of fitness and to optimize health in preparation for surgery and anaesthesia. It is also used to ascertain the functional ability/reserve of the patient and therefore quantify their operative risk.

## Key objectives

- To optimize pre-existing conditions and identify possible undiagnosed conditions.
- To identify and instigate relevant investigations according to predetermined protocols.
- To increase the patient's understanding of pre- and postoperative care.
- To provide information for the patient to decrease anxiety and fear.
- To establish that the patient is fully informed and wishes to undergo the planned procedure.
- To assess the patient's home situation, social circumstances, and availability of support.
- To reduce anaesthetic, surgical, and patient-specific risks of impending surgery.
- To discuss mode of anaesthesia prior to admission.
- To minimize the risk of late cancellations by ensuring that all essential resources and discharge requirements are identified.
- To provide an opportunity to discuss ways in which to improve their health and outcome of surgery such as weight loss and smoking cessation.
- To provide health education/promotion in order to reduce the potential for future comorbidities.

> A shared decision-making approach should take place as patients are likely to be less anxious if fully informed.

## Purpose of preoperative assessment

The overriding purpose of preoperative assessment is to obtain a comprehensive review of the patient's presenting condition and past medical history, ensuring that no aspect is overlooked. This includes:

- Comprehensive patient history taking
- Physical assessment
- Anaesthesia assessment, including airway assessment
- Risk assessment.

> All elective patients should be pre-assessed by a nurse/ODP/anaesthetic practitioner and anaesthetist prior to anaesthesia/sedation for surgery.

## History taking

- Introduce yourself to the patient and explain the purpose of the visit.
  - Patient preparedness requires knowledge-seeking and sense-making activities and usually this occurs in relation to healthcare professionals' intentions to support and involve patients in their care and decisions.
  - Different approaches to communication should be utilized in the consultations, for example, talking to the patient and talking with the patient.
  - Talking with the patient is essential for a successful preoperative assessment by listening to the patient, asking open questions, raising difficult topics, building on strengths and resources, and preparing for surgery.
- Confirm the patient's demographic details such as name, address, and date of birth.
- Confirm the surgeon's findings with the patient, that is, the presenting condition.
- Establish the patient's symptoms and question whether they have resolved or deteriorated; establish the site and side involved, if applicable, such as an arthroscopy.
- Enquire about past surgical and anaesthetic history and document any difficulties or cause for concern. This might include major cardiovascular or respiratory events, rare inherited disorders such as malignant hyperthermia (MH), and pseudocholinesterase deficiency.
- Establish any inherited blood disorders such as sickle cell disease and thalassaemia disorders.
- Ask questions about any allergies or sensitivities to medications, antibiotics, food, latex, or rubber; identify what reactions are experienced—these can include sneezing, wheezing, rash, nausea, vomiting, and diarrhoea.
- Record details of any triggers to allergies such as asthma or eczema.
- Identify VTE risk factors.
- Cardiopulmonary exercise testing may be necessary for some patients.

It is essential that patients provide a list of name(s) of current medication, dose, and quantity per day/week; this should also include any alternative or OTC medicines.

Additionally, it is important to establish the patient's cardiorespiratory status and identify any instances of breathlessness, chest pain, palpitations, fatigue, and claudication or sleep apnoea.

## Physical assessment

Preoperative assessment establishes if a patient is fit enough for anaesthesia, so the physical assessment and examination should focus primarily on the cardiorespiratory system. However, renal function, hepatobiliary system, and the endocrine system are examined in some patients. Additionally, the assessment should reveal any abnormalities, for example, obesity, scoliosis, or flexor contractions, to assess for potential positioning during anaesthesia. The systematic approach of inspection, palpation, percussion, and auscultation is recommended for a physical examination.

*Vital signs should be monitored and documented including*
- Non-invasive BP
- Pulse rate
- Oxygen saturation
- Height
- Weight
- BMI.

*Pre-assessment investigations are likely to include*
- MRSA screening
- Assessing the risk of VTE
- ECG if patient is >50 years; <50 years if indicated
- Urine analysis
- Pregnancy test if indicated
- Blood tests (full blood count (FBC), white cell count (WCC), C-reactive protein (CRP), platelets).

# Anaesthetic assessment

This should be undertaken by an anaesthetist; it is extremely important that a detailed medical, anaesthetic, and surgical history is taken and documented as this may indicate potential airway management difficulties.

- An airway assessment should always be undertaken following analysis of the medical history.
- Patients who have marked neck restrictions, anatomical abnormalities, a small mouth, or ill-fitting dentures could potentially be difficult to intubate.
- Congenital abnormalities such as Down syndrome, Marfan syndrome, and Treacher syndrome should be documented and brought to the attention of the anaesthetist.
- A history of snoring or obstructive sleep apnoea may be associated with airway difficulties and its presence should also be documented.

## Mallampati classification

The Mallampati classification is used to determine a potentially difficult airway. The patient is required to protrude the tongue as far as possible, while the anaesthetist inspects the pharyngeal structures from patient eye-level (➤ see Difficult airway assessment, p. 288).

## Patient information

On completion of the pre-assessment process, patients should be issued with advice to support the principles of ERAS. This should include both anaesthesia and surgical information (Table 4.1).

**Table 4.1** Patient information

| Anaesthesia | Surgery |
| --- | --- |
| • Reduced fasting guidelines | • Overview of surgical procedure |
| • Perioperative nutrition in order to optimize recovery and carbohydrate loading up to 2 hours prior to surgery if applicable | • Reasons for and benefits of surgery |
| | • Potential postoperative events/complications |
| • Types of anaesthesia | • Precautions post surgery |
| • Postoperative analgesia | • Showering/bathing |
| | • Wound care |

## Patient education

Patients should also be advised of attendance at education events that might prove informative and reduce anxiety. For example, many surgical specialities have developed short seminars that could assist in demystifying the surgical pathway. This could be led by the pre-assessment lead/team and consist of short talks focusing on the patient's journey by an anaesthetist, surgeon, anaesthetic, scrub and recovery staff, and surgical ward staff. Also included could be a discussion with a physiotherapist, occupational therapist, dietician, and pain teams.

This would be particularly beneficial for children. By including play specialists, children and their parents/guardian could visit the operating theatre (probably over a weekend) and dress up in theatre attire. They could also experience a three-lead ECG and engage in the use of a pulse oximeter.

# Short stay surgery

The AAGBI outlines the fundamental principles of day care:
- Patients should be selected according to their physiological status not their age (for normal exclusions see Table 4.2).
- Fitness for a procedure should relate to the patient's health as found at pre-assessment and not limited by American Society of Anesthesiologists (ASA) status.
- Obesity is not an absolute contraindication for day care in expert hands and with appropriate resources.
- Day surgery is particularly appropriate for children.

The medical criteria and patients who are excluded from short stay surgery differ according to locally agreed protocols.

Patient selection for short stay surgery will depend on:
- The procedure required
- The general health of the patient
- The patient's social circumstances.

In the interests of safety, pre-assessment should not be performed in the anaesthetic room if patients are admitted on the day of surgery.

## Medical criteria for short stay surgery

- Free from disease.
- Disease controlled.
- Asthma—not on steroids.
- Non-invasive blood pressure (NIBP) — on treatment.
- Diastolic BP <100 mmHg.
- Diabetes—diet controlled.
- No glycosuria.

## Social circumstances

- Patients should have adequate home circumstances with the presence of a responsible adult for 24 hours postoperatively.
- The patient's home situation should be compatible with postoperative care, with satisfactory standards of heating and lighting, together with adequate kitchen, bathroom, and toilet facilities.
- Patients should have telephone access.
- Patients should live within about 15 miles (24 kilometres)/1 hour from the hospital.
- Patients should have car transport home following surgery.
- If there is any doubt, medical referral is essential.

## Patient investigations

- BP/pulse.
- Blood tests—FBC/liver function tests (LFTs)/WCC/CRP.
- FBC—menstruating age.

**Box 4.1  Patient conditions normally excluded from short stay surgery**
- Chest disease.
- Renal failure.
- Uncontrolled hypertension.
- Symptomatic hiatus hernia.
- Severe psychiatric illness.
- Epilepsy.
- Type 1 diabetes.
- Severe rheumatoid arthritis.
- Chronic neurological disease.
- Previous adverse anaesthetic reactions (or relatives).
- BMI >40 kg/m$^2$—although some units will accept patients with a high BMI providing there is no other presenting comorbidity.

- Weight.
- ECG—patient older than 60 years.
- Assessed by anaesthetist.

## Benefits of anaesthetic assessment
- Identifies potential anaesthetic difficulties.
- Identifies medical conditions.
- Allows careful planning of care.
- Improves safety—minimizes risk.
- Provides preoperative information.
- Allays fear and anxiety.

## Pre-assessment of inpatients
- Vital part of anaesthetic care.
- Available for elective and emergency surgery.
- Usually includes assessment by anaesthetist who is responsible for their anaesthetic.
- Ensures continuity and rapport for anaesthetist and patient.

## Discharge criteria
See Box 4.2.

**Box 4.2  Patient discharge criteria for short stay surgery**
- Stable vital signs—1 hour.
- No sign of respiratory depression.
- Orientated to person, time, and place.
- Retain oral fluids.
- Dress and walk without assistance.
- No excessive pain, bleeding, or postoperative nausea or vomiting.
- Understands how to use oral analgesia supplied.
- Has a responsible adult to take them home.
- Has a carer at home for the next 24 hours.
- Written and verbal postoperative instructions have been received.
- Emergency contact number has been supplied.
- Void urine.

### Short stay surgery for children

The Royal College of Anaesthetists (RCoA)[1] and the AAGBI[2] specify that there should be a registered paediatric nurse present at all times when children are present on the short stay unit. They also state:

- Health and play specialists should play a key role within day surgery provision
- Children and adults should be managed separately on short stay units
- A nurse/ODP with an advanced paediatric life support qualification or an anaesthetist with paediatric competencies should be immediately available
- A preadmission programme for children should be considered, to decrease the impact and stress of admission to the day surgery unit on the day of surgery.

### Short stay surgery for urgent procedures

- Patients presenting with acute conditions requiring urgent surgery can be efficiently and effectively treated as day cases.
- After initial assessment, many patients can be discharged home and return for surgery at an appropriate time, either on a day-case list or as a scheduled patient on an operating list.
- Preoperative assessment should where possible be provided to the same standard as that used for elective day surgery.

### Advantages of short stay surgery

See Table 4.2.

**Table 4.2** Advantages of short stay surgery

| For the provider | For the patient |
| --- | --- |
| ↓ cost of treatment | Less time in hospital |
| ↓ recovery time | Fewer cancellations |
| ↓ waiting lists | ↓ infection |
| ↑ efficiency/£££ | ↓ anxiety |
| No emergencies | |
| Develop services | |

### References

1. Royal College of Anaesthetists (2021). Chapter 6: guidelines for the provision of anaesthesia services for day surgery. London: Royal College of Anaesthetists.
2. Bailey CR, Ahuja M, Bartholomew K, et al. (2019). Guidelines for day-case surgery 2019: guidelines from the Association of Anaesthetists and the British Association of Day Surgery. Anaesthesia, 74(6):778–792.

### Further reading

British Association of Day Surgery (2019). Spinal anaesthesia for day surgery patients: a practical guide (4th ed). London: British Association of Day Surgery.

Gray CE, Baruah-Young J, Payne CJ (2015). Preoperative assessment in patients presenting for elective surgery. Anaesthesia and Intensive Care Medicine, 16(9):425–430.

Hung OR, Murphy MF (2018). Hung's difficult and failed airway management. London: McGraw Hill.

Lake C (2015). Assessment of the emergency surgical patient. Anaesthesia and Intensive Care Medicine, 16(9):431–434.

McWhinnie D, Jackson I, Saha I, Thompson D, et al. (2020). Surgical same-day emergency care (2nd ed). London: British Association of Day Surgery.

National Institute for Health and Care Excellence (2016). Routine preoperative tests for elective surgery. NICE guideline [NG45]. Available at: https://www.nice.org.uk/guidance/NG45

National Institute for Health and Care Excellence (2018). Discharge planning. Emergency and acute medical care in over 16s: service delivery and organisation. Available at: https://www.nice.org.uk/guidance/ng94/evidence/35discharge-planning-pdf-172397464674

Pettersson ME, Öhlén J, Friberg F, et al. (2018). Prepared for surgery – communication in nurses' preoperative consultations with patients undergoing surgery for colorectal cancer after a person-centred intervention. Journal of Clinical Nursing, 27(13–14):2904–2916.

Royal College of Anaesthetists (2021). Chapter 2: guidelines for the provision of anaesthesia services for preoperative assessment and preparation. London: Royal College of Anaesthetists.

Wilkinson S (2018). Assessing the perioperative communication needs of a patient with learning disabilities: an holistic case study approach. Journal of Perioperative Practice, 28(10):278–282.

# Patients
# with comorbidities

# Chronic health

Patients with long-term and pre-existing conditions are increasing in the UK. In 2013, more than one in three adults (36%) reported having a long-standing illness or disability (LSI) and one in five (20%) reported having a limiting LSI. This has been attributed largely due to the increase in the ageing population.

- The likelihood of someone reporting having an LSI increases with age. In 2013, 69% of people aged 75 and over reported having an LSI. This compared with 15% of people aged 16–24. There are also some geographical differences, with people living in Wales (27%) more likely to report having a limiting LSI than those living in either England (19%) or Scotland (20%).[1]
- Patients with long-term or pre-existing conditions are likely to have more than one condition and have complex care requirements. Pre-existing long-term conditions can impact greatly upon the provision of nursing care during the perioperative phase and will potentially have an impact on the surgical outcome.

> Pre-existing conditions or comorbidities may be attributed to lifestyle or be inherited or acquired.

### Pre-existing conditions can include

- *Non-communicable diseases*: cardiovascular diseases, respiratory conditions, cancers, neurological diseases, and diabetes.[2]
- *Infectious diseases*: hepatitis, HIV/AIDS, tuberculosis (TB), and influenza.[3]
- *Musculoskeletal conditions*: rheumatoid arthritis, ankylosing spondylitis, fractures, and chronic pain.
- *Mental health disorders*: depression, dementia, schizophrenia, bipolar disorders, and developmental disorders including autism.

### Perioperative planning

- Use a validated risk stratification tool to supplement clinical assessment when planning surgery. Discuss the person's risks and surgical options with them to allow for informed shared decision-making.[4]
- The ASA physical status (PS) classification system is often used by UK anaesthetists to establish a person's functional capacity.[5]
- ASA grades are a simple scale describing a person's fitness to be given an anaesthetic for a procedure and can be used to appraise the urgency for surgical intervention.

### ASA grading of physical status

The ASA grading system:
- Serves as a tool from which anaesthetists can classify patients, avoid unnecessary surgical procedures, and manage risk effectively
- Aims to evaluate the severity of systemic diseases, physiological dysfunction, and anatomic abnormalities
- The tool is used to grade patient risk based on their medical history, appearance, and condition (Fig. 5.1).

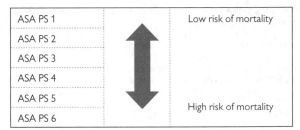

**Fig. 5.1** ASA PS grading risk of mortality.
Source: data from American Society of Anesthesiologists (2020). ASA Physical Status Classification System.

*ASA PS 1: a normal healthy patient*
- No physiological, psychological, psychiatric, biochemical, or organic disturbances.
- Healthy individual with good exercise tolerance.
- Excludes the elderly and neonates.

*ASA PS 2: patients with mild systemic disease*
- No functional limitations; has a well-controlled disease of one body system.
- Examples: controlled diabetes mellitus, hypertension, asthma, chronic bronchitis.
- Mild lifestyle issues—tobacco abuse, obesity.

*ASA PS 3: patients with severe systemic disease that is a threat to life*
- Some functional limitation; has a controlled disease of more than one body system or one major system.
- No immediate danger of death.
- Examples: stable angina, congestive cardiac failure, previous history of infarct, chronic renal failure (CRF).
- Lifestyle-affecting factors—morbid obesity.

*ASA PS 4: patients with severe systemic disease that is a constant threat to life*
- Has at least one severe disease that is poorly controlled or at end-stage.
- Possible risk of death as a result of disease.
- Examples: symptomatic chronic obstructive pulmonary disease (COPD), unstable angina, hepatorenal and/or endocrine failure.

*ASA PS 5: moribund patients who are not expected to survive 24 hours without the operation*
- Imminent risk of death.
- Surgery performed as a last resort or resuscitative effort.
- Multiorgan failure.
- Cerebral trauma.
- Examples: sepsis with haemodynamic instability, poorly controlled coagulopathy, ruptured aneurysm, large pulmonary embolism (PE).

*ASA PS 6: a declared brain-dead patient whose organs are being harvested for donor purposes*

- A specialist recovery area for people who have a high risk of complications or mortality, for example, because of previous surgical history or comorbidities is advocated by NICE.[4]
- NICE also advocates having a discussion about the options for postoperative pain management with patients before they have surgery. Comorbidities should be considered and a discussion had about the impact of the surgery on the patient's pre-existing condition and vice versa.

## References

1. Office for National Statistics (2015). Adult health in Great Britain, 2013. Available at: ℘ https://www.ons.gov.uk/peoplepopulationandcommunity/healthandsocialcare/health andlifeexpectancies/ compendium/ opinionsandlifestylesurvey/ 2015-03-19/ adulthealthingreatbritain2013
2. World Health Organization (2018). Non-communicable diseases. Available at: ℘ https://www.who.int/news-room/fact-sheets/detail/noncommunicable-diseases
3. World Health Organization (2020). Communicable diseases. Available at: ℘ https://www.euro.who.int/en/health-topics/communicable-diseases
4. National Institute for Health and Care Excellence (2020). Perioperative care in adults. NICE guideline [NG180]. Available at: ℘ https://www.nice.org.uk/guidance/ng180
5. American Society of Anaesthesiologists (2020). ASA physical status classification system. Available at: ℘ https://www.asahq.org/standards-and-guidelines/asa-physical-status-classification-system

## Further reading

Craig A, Hatfield A (2020). The complete recovery room book (6th ed). Oxford: Oxford University Press.

Department of Health (2004). Chronic disease management. London: Department of Health.

National Institute for Health and Care Excellence (2017). Nurse-led ASA grading in pre-operative assessment to guide investigations and risk scoring. Available at: ℘ https://www.nice.org.uk/sharedlearning/nurse-led-asa-grading-in-preoperative-assessment-to-guide-investigations-and-risk-scoring

Royal College of Anaesthetists (2021). Chapter 2: guidelines for the provision of anaesthesia services for preoperative assessment and preparation. London: Royal College of Anaesthetists.

World Health Organization (2021). Musculoskeletal diseases. Available at: ℘ https://www.who.int/news-room/fact-sheets/detail/musculoskeletal-conditions

# Lifestyle factors and induced disease

## Alcoholism

- Patients who are alcoholics and regular drinkers are tolerant to some sedatives (benzodiazepines) and anaesthetic agents (propofol) and will require higher dosages.
- Patients with alcoholism often emerge from anaesthesia in an aggressive and restless manner. They can thrash and move about in a semi-purposeful manner before they fully awake (e.g. they may try to sit up before rejecting their airway).
- They might appear dazed and will not respond to speech; this is a distinct feature.
- Thin/emaciated patients with alcoholism (usually in the latter stages of the disease) are prone to hypothermia.

## Drug addiction

- Patients who have substance misuse issues and also are without stable housing, as well as IV drug users, are often malnourished and in poor physical health.
- They are most likely to attend for emergency surgery.
- They have a very high risk of having blood-borne viruses and parasitic infections.

> *Always monitor blood glucose levels.*
> Some patients with alcoholism are susceptible to postoperative spontaneous hypoglycaemia.

### Amphetamines and cocaine

- These stimulate the activity of the sympathetic nervous system, causing a state of 'hyper-alertness'.
- They displace endogenous noradrenaline from nerve endings; addicts are prone to noradrenaline depletion particularly after drug use.
- Patients can become profoundly hypotensive postoperatively in recovery due to noradrenaline depletion. They may even require noradrenaline infusion to restore and maintain their arterial pressure.

### Opiate addiction

- Ideally, patients with opiate addiction will receive local/regional anaesthesia.
- Patients who are recovering from addiction may refuse opiates.
- In some cases, patients with drug addiction may overstate the intensity of their pain to obtain opiate analgesia.
- In general, patients with drug addiction will require higher doses than the average population due to opioid tolerance.
- Use caution if giving high doses and check the patient's drug history as he/she may be on a methadone regimen.

> *Do not withhold opiates.*
> If a patient is in pain, administer analgesia.

*Benzodiazepines*
- Many elderly patients or those with anxiety disorders might be considered as 'drug addicts' as they have been taking a benzodiazepine such as nitrazepam or diazepam for many years.
- Withdrawal of these drugs can cause acute agitation, aggression, violence, and even convulsions.
- If the patient is benzodiazepine dependent, administer their dose (if they have not already received it).

Caution is advised when caring for severely dependent patients who are experiencing withdrawal as they can become very violent.

## Obesity
- Obese patients will require higher oxygen ($O_2$) concentrations due to increased consumption as there is more tissue to be perfused.
- Positioning is very important; if possible, sit the patient up.
- BP readings cannot be relied on due to excess of body fat.
- If possible, monitor BP invasively via arterial access.
- IV access can be difficult to obtain due to body fat; this should therefore be well secured.

## Further reading

Craig A, Hatfield A (2020). The complete recovery room book (6th ed). Oxford: Oxford University Press.

Freedman R, Herbert L, O'Donnell A, et al. (eds) (2022). Oxford handbook of anaesthesia (5th ed). Oxford: Oxford University Press.

National Institute for Health and Care Excellence (2020). Perioperative care in adults. NICE guideline [180]. Available at: https://www.nice.org.uk/guidance/ng180

National Institute for Health and Care Excellence (2015). Obesity prevention. Clinical guideline [CG43]. Available at: https://www.nice.org.uk/guidance/cg43

Pollard B, Kitchen G (eds) (2017). Handbook of clinical anaesthesia (4th ed). London: CRC Press.

Royal College of Anaesthetists (2019). Chapter 3: guidelines for the provision of anaesthesia services for intraoperative care. London: Royal College of Anaesthetists.

Royal College of Anaesthetists (2019). Chapter 4: guidelines for the provision of postoperative care. London: Royal College of Anaesthetists.

Royal College of Anaesthetists (2021). Chapter 2: guidelines for the provision of anaesthesia services for preoperative assessment and preparation. London: Royal College of Anaesthetists.

Royal College of Anaesthetists (2021). Chapter 11: guidelines for the provision of anaesthesia services for inpatient pain management. London: Royal College of Anaesthetists.

# Obesity

Overweight and obesity are defined as abnormal or excessive fat accumulation that presents a risk to health.[1]

- Childhood obesity is one of the most serious public health challenges of the twenty-first century.
- Diabetes, ischaemic heart disease, and certain cancers are attributable to obesity.
- Weight loss management is now being prescribed.

BMI (Table 5.1) is used to classify overweight and obesity in adults and is defined as the weight in kilograms divided by the square of the height in metres ($kg/m^2$):

- Overweight = BMI $\geq 25$ $kg/m^2$.
- Obesity = BMI $\geq 30$ $kg/m^2$.

**Table 5.1** BMI classification (in $kg/m^2$)

| | |
|---|---|
| **Underweight** | <18.5 |
| **Normal range** | 18.5–24.9 |
| **Overweight** | $\geq 25$ |
| • Pre-obese | 25–29.9 |
| **Obese** | $\geq 30$ |
| • Obese class I | 30–34.9 |
| • Obese class II | 35–39.9 |
| • Obese class III | $\geq 40$ |

Associated obesity-related medical conditions include a diverse range of diseases (Box 5.1). Obesity also leads to an increased demand for healthcare services.

**Box 5.1 Associated obesity-related medical conditions**
- Hypertension.
- Coronary artery disease.
- Sudden (cardiac) death.
- Obstructive sleep apnoea.
- Restrictive lung disease.
- Diabetes.
- Degenerative joint disease.
- Gallstones.
- Cancer.
- Socioeconomic impairment.
- Psychosocial impairment.

## Preoperative assessment

- The preoperative assessment is crucial in identifying potential risk factors that might lead to perioperative adverse events.
- Bariatric surgery for adults with a BMI >50 kg/m$^2$ is recommended where surgery is considered appropriate and the patient is fit and meets the criteria for anaesthesia and surgery.
- The risk of perioperative pulmonary aspiration during subsequent procedures is increased after bariatric surgery and dramatic weight loss.
- Super morbidly obese patients (BMI >50 kg/m$^2$) should be assessed on an individual basis to ascertain whether additional equipment or staffing is required for their safe management.
- Obstructive sleep apnoea and the obesity hypoventilation syndrome are common in the bariatric surgical population, often occurring in 30–50% of patients.

> The Society for Obesity and Bariatric Anaesthesia outlines recommendations for screening and management of sleep disordered breathing in patients undergoing bariatric surgery.[2]

The hospital specialist and/or bariatric surgeon should discuss the following points with people who are severely obese if they are considering surgery to aid weight reduction:

- The potential benefits, longer-term implications of surgery-associated risks, complications, and perioperative mortality.
- The discussion should also include the person's family, where relevant.
- Choose the surgical intervention jointly with the person, taking into account the degree of obesity, comorbidities, the best available evidence on effectiveness and long-term effects, the facilities and equipment available, and the experience of the surgeon who would perform the operation.
- Carry out a comprehensive preoperative assessment of any psychological or clinical factors that may affect adherence to postoperative care requirements (such as changes to diet) before performing surgery.[3]
- Offer VTE prophylaxis to people undergoing bariatric surgery.[4]
- Mechanical VTE prophylaxis on admission for people undergoing bariatric surgery.
- Pharmacological VTE prophylaxis for a minimum of 7 days for people whose risk of VTE outweighs their risk of bleeding.

## Preoperative management

- One of the main problems for obese patients is respiratory compromise, which can be accentuated in the following positions:
  - Head-down.
  - Supine—aorto-caval compression may occur.
- Other problems that give rise for concern for both the anaesthetic and the surgical team can include:
  - Venous access
  - Airway management

- Regional anaesthesia—not usually recommended
- Hiatus hernia and the risk of aspiration
- BP monitoring—appropriate-sized cuff should be used
- Wound dehiscence.
- Prophylactic antiembolic therapy is advised with subcutaneous (SC) heparin and antiembolic stockings to reduce the risk of DVT and PE.
  - One dose of 5000 units to be taken 2 hours before surgery, then 5000 units every 8–12 hours.
- Premedication with medicines causing respiratory depression is not recommended.
- Antiemetic therapy and prophylactic antacids are advised before surgery to reduce the risk of acid aspiration.

## Anaesthetic management

- Airway management is often difficult in obese patients.
- Possible difficult airway should be assessed with consideration given to awake intubation.
- Rapid sequence induction with preoxygenation is required as obese patients are prone to gastric reflux.
- Antacids such as sodium citrate are advocated for use in the anaesthetic room prior to induction.
- Patients should be extubated awake in an upright position.

## Postoperative management

- Patients should be nursed in the upright position to aid respiratory function.
- Airway should be constantly monitored.
- Nasopharyngeal airway can aid breathing and reduce obstruction.
- Supplemental $O_2$ should be given as prescribed.
- Postoperative analgesia via IV route and/or patient-controlled analgesia (PCA) is recommended as intramuscular (IM) injection is often administered SC.
- Transport of patients may prove difficult so consideration should be given to transporting and transferring patients on a bed.
- Ensure there are enough staff for safe transfer and transport.
- Monitoring of vital signs including TPR, BP, and peripheral oxygen saturation ($SpO_2$).
- Invasive monitoring is recommended following major surgery.

## References

1. World Health Organization (2017). Obesity. Available at: ℅ https://www.who.int/health-topics/obesity#tab=tab_1
2. Society for Obesity and Bariatric Anaesthesia (2015). Guidelines for anaesthesia. Available at: ℅ https://www.sobauk.co.uk/guidelines-1
3. National Institute for Health and Care Excellence (2016). Surgery for obese adults. Available at: ℅ https://pathways.nice.org.uk/pathways/obesity
4. National Institute for Health and Care Excellence (2020). Venous thromboembolic diseases: diagnosis, management and thrombophilia testing. NICE guideline [NG158]. Available at: ℅ https://www.nice.org.uk/guidance/ng158

## Further reading

Al-Shaikh B, Stacey S (2018). Essentials of equipment in anaesthesia, critical care and perioperative medicine (5th ed). Edinburgh: Elsevier.

Bouch C, Cousins J (eds) (2018). Core topics in anaesthesia and perioperative care of the morbidly obese surgical patient. Cambridge: Cambridge University Press.

National Institute for Health and Care Excellence (2014). Obesity: identification, assessment and management. Clinical guideline [CG189]. Available at: ℅ https://www.nice.org.uk/guidance/cg189

National Institute for Health and Care Excellence (2015). Obesity prevention. Clinical guideline [CG43]. Available at: ℅ https://www.nice.org.uk/guidance/cg43

Royal College of Anaesthetists (2019). Chapter 3: guidelines for the provision of anaesthesia services for intraoperative care. London: Royal College of Anaesthetists.

Royal College of Anaesthetists (2019). Chapter 4: guidelines for the provision of postoperative care. London: Royal College of Anaesthetists.

Royal College of Anaesthetists (2020). Chapter 5: guidelines for the provision of emergency anaesthesia. London: Royal College of Anaesthetists.

Royal College of Anaesthetists (2021). Chapter 2: guidelines for the provision of anaesthesia services for preoperative assessment and preparation. London: Royal College of Anaesthetists.

Sinha A (ed) (2016). Morbid obesity: anaesthesia and perioperative management. Delhi: Byword Books.

# Respiratory disorders

For key definitions see Table 5.2.

## Asthma

- Asthma is defined as reversible airflow obstruction due to constriction of smooth muscles in the airways.
- Symptoms can include breathlessness, wheeze, cough, and sputum production.
- Poorly controlled asthma is a risk factor for the development of postoperative pulmonary complications but well-controlled asthma appears to confer little additional risk. The US National Asthma Education and Prevention Program consensus statement recommends that all patients with asthma undergo a preoperative evaluation to assess asthma control. Patients whose asthma is not well controlled should receive a step-up in asthma therapy; this may include a brief course of systemic glucocorticoids in patients whose forced expiratory volume in 1 second ($FEV_1$) or peak expiratory flow rate (PEFR) are below their predicted values or personal best.
- Patients with more severe asthma may also require additional medication and/or steroid therapy perioperatively if additional problems develop, such as chest infection.

## Chronic obstructive pulmonary disease

- COPD is a lung disease characterized by chronic obstruction of lung airflow that interferes with normal breathing and is not fully reversible.
- Known chronic obstructive lung disease is an important patient-related risk factor for postoperative pulmonary complications.
- COPD involves chronic bronchitis and emphysema and symptoms can include breathlessness, wheeze, cough, and sputum production.
- Nebulized bronchodilators are recommended prior to anaesthesia and surgery and continued for up to 48 hours.
- Intubation should generally be avoided but spontaneous breathing may be unsuitable for some patients.
- Patients should be monitored and observed closely perioperatively for potential pneumothorax.
- Deciding whether or not to proceed with surgery should rest with a consultant anaesthetist and consultant surgeon, taking account of the presence of comorbidities, the functional status of the patient, and the necessity of the surgery.
- The medical management of the patient should be optimized prior to surgery and might involve pulmonary rehabilitation.

### Preoperative assessment

Patients with respiratory disease are at risk of developing problems postoperatively, therefore it is advisable that elective surgery occurs only when respiratory function is optimal.

- For patients with suspected or known pulmonary diseases, a meticulous preoperative evaluation is needed because regional anaesthetic or GA can precipitate several unwanted physiological events caused by positive pressure ventilation, patient positioning, and drugs used during GA.

- Preoperative assessment of patients with respiratory disease requiring surgery should include the following:
  - Assessment of exercise tolerance: enquire about the functional aspects of daily life on breathlessness such as climbing stairs, walking outside, and sleeping (how many pillows?). If a patient has difficulty in climbing one flight of stairs, has a $SpO_2$ of <95% on air, or appears cyanosed then consider checking arterial blood gases (ABG).
  - Smoking history should also be assessed and the patient advised to stop smoking prior to surgery.
  - A thorough review of the patient's medications should be undertaken including regular and OTC drugs.
  - In patients where there is a reversible airflow obstruction, make sure they are optimally treated before surgery; this could be a consideration of a trial of oral prednisolone and medical review, or a change to nebulized bronchodilators prior to surgery.
  - Routine baseline blood tests such as FBC to identify anaemia or polycythaemia would be advised in line with the surgery type (minor, intermediate, major) and the ASA classification system (➔ Chronic health, p. 80).

If it is identified that the patient has a poor exercise tolerance (less than one flight of stairs) and is due to undergo surgery or an investigation that may impact breathing or make breathing painful postoperatively, then discuss with the anaesthetist whether the high dependency unit (HDU)/intensive therapy unit (ITU) would be more appropriate postoperatively.

Some patients may also benefit from preoperative chest physiotherapy.

A number of factors have been identified that greatly increase the risk of pulmonary complications during surgery, these include:
- Upper abdominal, thoracic (open), aortic, head and neck, neurosurgical, and abdominal aortic aneurysm surgery
- Emergency surgery
- Age >65 years
- Surgery lasting >3 hours
- Poor general health status as defined by ASA class >2
- Heart failure
- Serum albumin <3 g/dL
- Chronic obstructive lung disease
- Intraoperative long-acting neuromuscular blockade
- Functional dependence.

Further identification of patients at risk following surgery may be identified using a risk stratification tool such as the ASA PS or the Surgical Outcomes Risk Tool (SORT).

## Anaesthesia management

- Regional anaesthesia (e.g. epidural) may be beneficial for patients with severe pulmonary impairment and prevents the need for postoperative opioids.

**Table 5.2** Respiratory definitions

| | |
|---|---|
| **Tidal volume** | The amount of air that is moved in and out of the lungs during each breath |
| **Minute volume** | The volume of air that is moved in and out of the lungs in 1 minute |
| **Hypercarbia** | Excess carbon dioxide ($CO_2$) in the body |
| **Hypoxia** | Lack of $O_2$ that affects the normal function of cells |
| **Hypoxaemia** | $PaO_2$ is <60 mmHg |
| **Hypoventilation** | Failure of the lungs to eliminate $CO_2$ and measured by a rise in the partial pressure of $CO_2$ in arterial blood |

*Source:* data from Craig A, Hatfield A (2020). The Complete Recovery Room Book (6th ed). Oxford: Oxford University Press.

## Postoperative management

- Ensure patient is sitting in a supine/upright position where possible.
- Chest physiotherapy in recovery and on the ward as prescribed to aid in sputum clearance and prevent atelectasis.
- Early mobilization whenever possible.
- Bronchodilator therapy as prescribed: nebulized until fully mobile—change back to inhalers at least 24 hours before discharge.
- Effective analgesia to aid respiratory function—consider regular and simple analgesia such as paracetamol, or non-steroidal anti-inflammatory drugs (NSAIDs) (cautious/observe for bronchospasm). Opioids could be used but be careful as patients with respiratory conditions could be very sensitive to respiratory depression from opioids.
- If the patient is showing signs of infective exacerbation of their condition (pyrexia, increased amounts of purulent sputum), consider sending sputum sample for cultures and commence antibiotic as per protocol. If the patient is very unwell, consider the possibility of postoperative pneumonia.
- Accurate monitoring of fluid balance as patients with respiratory disease are at increased risk of pulmonary oedema.

## Further reading

Agostini P, Cieslik H, Rathinam S, et al. (2010). Postoperative pulmonary complications following thoracic surgery: are there any modifiable risk factors? Thorax, 65(9):815–818.

Craig A, Hatfield A (2020). The complete recovery room book (6th ed). Oxford: Oxford University Press.

Diaz-Fuentes G, Hashmi HR, Venkatram S (2016). Perioperative evaluation of patients with pulmonary conditions undergoing non-cardiothoracic surgery. Health Services Insights 2016:9(Suppl 1) 9–23.

National Heart, Lung, and Blood Institute (2007). Expert Panel Report 3: guidelines for the Diagnosis and Management of Asthma.

National Institute for Health and Care Excellence (2016). Routine preoperative tests for elective surgery. Available at: ℘ https://www.nice.org.uk/guidance/ng45

National Institute for Health and Care Excellence (2018). Chronic obstructive pulmonary disease in over 16s: diagnosis and management. NICE guideline [NG115]. Available at: ℘ https://www.nice.org.uk/guidance/ng115

National Institute for Health and Care Excellence (2020). Asthma: diagnosis, management and chronic asthma management. NICE guideline [NG80]. Available at: ℘ https://www.nice.org.uk/guidance/ng80

National Institute of Health Research (2018). A reminder that too much oxygen increases mortality in acutely ill adults. Available at: ℘ https://evidence.nihr.ac.uk/alert/a-reminder-that-too-much-oxygen-increases-mortality-in-acutely-ill-adults/

Protopapa K, Simpson J, Smith N, et al. (2014). Development and validation of the Surgical Outcome Risk Tool (SORT). British Journal of Surgery, 101(13):1774–1783.

Sheldon C, Wilson I (2000). Respiratory disorders. In: Nicholls A, Wilson I (eds) Perioperative medicine: managing surgical patients with medical problems. Oxford: Oxford University Press.

Smetana G, Lawrence V, Cornell J (2006). Preoperative pulmonary risk stratification for noncardiothoracic surgery: systematic review for the American College of Physicians. Annals of Internal Medicine, 2006;144(8):581–595.

Woods B, Sladen R (2009). Perioperative considerations for the patient with asthma and bronchospasm. British Journal of Anaesthesia, 103(Suppl):i57–i65.

# Cardiac disorders

### Cardiac risk

- Cardiac disease is one of the commonest causes of morbidity and mortality in surgical patients.
- Up to 20% of patients undergoing surgery have preoperative evidence of myocardial ischaemia.

### Predictors of perioperative risk

*Major risk*

- Recent myocardial infarction (MI) <1 month prior to surgery.
- Unstable angina.
- Decompensated heart failure.
- Significant arrhythmia.
- Severe valvular heart disease.
- Previous cardiac surgery.
- Previous percutaneous coronary angioplasty with stent.
- Congenital heart disease.

*Intermediate risk*

- History of cardiac ischaemia.
- A degree of heart failure.
- History of cerebrovascular disease.
- Abnormal renal function.
- Diabetes.

*Minor risk*

- Advanced age.
- Abnormal ECG.
- Some arrythmia.
- Low exercise tolerance.
- Uncontrolled systemic hypertension.

### Preoperative management

Comprehensive pre-assessment by a consultant anaesthetist and pre-assessment nurse should include:

- Past medical history including cardiac events
- Comprehensive cardiorespiratory physical assessment
- Airway, breathing, circulation, disability, exposure (ABCDE) assessment
- 12-lead ECG
- Cardiopulmonary exercise testing.

Pharmacological stress testing and magnetic resonance stress perfusion imaging may be required for some patients.

- Elective surgery should be postponed for up to 6 months following recent MI—refer to cardiologist if necessary.
- Assessment of renal function.
- Patients with pacemakers should have these identified and checked to ensure correct functionality. This should include a 12-lead ECG.
- Liaison with pacemaker clinics is sometimes necessary for cardiovascular evaluation for non-cardiac surgery.
- Continuation and optimization of pharmacological therapy for the cardiovascular disorders.

## Anaesthesia management

- Anaesthetizing patients with cardiovascular disease is one of the greatest challenges facing anaesthesiologists.
- Different cardiac disorders will require slightly different anaesthetic management.
- Close patient monitoring during the perioperative period and throughout procedure.
- Invasive monitoring including arterial BP, and central venous pressure (CVP) ± cardiac output if necessary for high- to intermediate-risk patients undergoing major surgery.
- ECG monitoring should use five-lead placement.
- Avoid hypotension and hypertension.
- Consider availability of high dependency or intensive care bed for close observation, again depending on predictive risk and type of surgery.
- Short bursts of bipolar diathermy are recommended as electrocautery for patients with pacemakers.
- Regional analgesia is effective in reducing the risk of tachycardia.

## Postoperative management

- Accurate fluid balance should be monitored frequently with recordings of hourly urine output.
- Monitoring of vital signs including TPR, BP, and $SpO_2$. An ABCDE systematic approach should be applied.
- Invasive monitoring including arterial BP, CVP ± cardiac output may be required following emergency surgery, and for those high- to intermediate-risk patients who have undergone major surgery.
- Following major surgery all patients should have supplemental $O_2$ for 3–4 days and this must be prescribed.
- Optimal analgesia prescribed to reduce the risk of tachycardia.
- Monitor haemoglobin (Hb) levels.

## Further reading

Alyesh D, Eagle K (2017). Peroperative evaluation for non-cardiac surgery. In: Fuster V, Harrington R, Narula J, et al. (eds) Hurst's the heart (14th ed). New York: McGraw Hill.

Byrne K, Goldstone K, Simmons P (2022). Cardiac anaesthesia. In: Freedman R, Herbert L, O'Donnell A, et al. (eds) Oxford handbook of anaesthesia (5th ed). Oxford: Oxford University Press.

Fleisher LA, Fleischmann KE, Auerbach AD, et al. (2014). 2014 ACC/ACH guideline on perioperative cardiovascular evaluation and management of patients undergoing non-cardiac surgery: a report of the American College of Cardiology/American Heart Association Task Force on Practice Guidelines. Circulation, 130(24):e278–e333.

Pardo M, Miller R (eds) (2018). Basics of anesthesia (7th ed). Philadelphia, PA: Elsevier.

Payne S (2022). Cardiovascular disease. In: Freedman R, Herbert L, O'Donnell A, et al. (eds) Oxford handbook of anaesthesia (5th ed). Oxford: Oxford University Press.

Rafiq A, Sklyar E, Bella J (2017). Cardiac evaluation and monitoring of patients undergoing noncardiac surgery. Health Services Insights, 9:1178632916686074.

Reich D, Mittnacht A, Kaplan J (2017). Anesthesia and the patient with cardiovascular disease. In: Fuster V, Harrington R, Narula J, et al. (eds) Hurst's the heart (14th ed). New York: McGraw Hill.

Wallace A (2018). Cardiovascular disease. In: Pardo M, Miller R (eds) Basics of anesthesia (7th ed). Philadelphia, PA: Elsevier.

# Haematology disorders

Haematology disorders can include anaemia, sickle cell disease, coagulation disorders, thrombocytopenia, haemophilia, and porphyria.

## Anaemia

- Anaemia can be defined as a reduction in red cell mass leading to decreased Hb and haematocrit levels in the blood.
- The most common form of anaemia is iron deficiency anaemia (Box 5.2) and this occurs when the Hb concentrations fall below the following levels:
  - Females: <12 g/dL.
  - Males: <13 g/dL.
- The most common symptoms associated with iron deficiency anaemia include:
  - Tiredness
  - Lethargy
  - Dyspnoea
  - Palpitations.
- Changes in physical appearance can also occur including dry, flaking nails, spoon-shaped nails, pale complexion, abnormally smooth tongue, and painful ulcers on the corners of the mouth.
- One of the commonest causes of anaemia is gastrointestinal (GI) blood loss and this can occur with stomach ulcers, cancer, menstruation, pregnancy, diet, and NSAIDs.

> **Box 5.2 Symptoms of iron deficiency anaemia**
> - Tiredness and lack of energy.
> - Shortness of breath.
> - Noticeable heartbeats (heart palpitations).
> - Pale skin.
>
> *Less common symptoms of iron deficiency anaemia*
> - Hair loss.
> - Spoon-shaped nails.
> - Headaches.
> - Tinnitus.
> - Food tasting strange.
> - Feeling itchy.
> - Sore tongue.
> - Dysphagia.
> - Mouth ulcers.
> - Restless legs syndrome.

*Perioperative considerations*
- Pre-assessment prior to surgery to include FBC and anaemia corrected by oral iron or vitamin $B_{12}$ injections if necessary.
- Blood transfusion is only recommended if Hb concentration is <7 g/dL.

- Transfusing a patient with pernicious anaemia may increase the risk of heart failure.
- Adequate patient monitoring is essential and should include:
  - $SpO_2$
  - TPR
  - BP.

## Sickle cell disease

- Sickle cell anaemia is one of the most common genetic diseases in the UK and affects the ability to carry $O_2$ around the body.
- The shape and texture of blood cells change, becoming hard and sticky and shaped like sickles. These cells then die prematurely, leading to a shortage of red blood cells.
- Sickle cell anaemia is more prevalent in Afro-Caribbean, black African, and black British people.
- The only cure for sickle cell anaemia is a bone marrow transplant.
- The symptoms of sickle cell anaemia usually commence from 3 months of age and can include:
  - Anaemia
  - Hand–foot syndrome
  - Jaundice
  - Frequent infections.

*Perioperative considerations*
- Preoperative assessment should include antibody screening.
- Consideration should be given to the possibility of dehydration, hypoxia, infection, and pain and be avoided.
- The operating theatre should be warmed to avoid patient hypothermia.
- Adequate patient monitoring is essential and should include:
  - $SpO_2$
  - TPR
  - BP.
- Consider perioperative fluid regimen.
- Postoperative $O_2$ therapy as prescribed.

## Further reading

Freedman R, Herbert L, O'Donnell A, et al. (eds) (2022). Oxford handbook of anaesthesia (5th ed). Oxford: Oxford University Press.
National Institute for Health and Care Excellence (2015). Blood transfusion: evidence. NICE guideline [NG24]. Available at: ℘ https://www.nice.org.uk/Guidance/NG24/Evidence
Pollard B, Kitchen G (eds) (2017). Handbook of clinical anaesthesia (4th ed). London: CRC Press.

# Gastrointestinal disorders

GI disorders encompass a wide range of diseases including liver disease, obstructive jaundice, inflammatory bowel disease, and gastric ulceration.

## Gastro-oesophageal reflux

- Caused by abnormal oesophageal motility and increased gastric pressure.
- Could also be caused by an incompetent lower oesophageal sphincter.
- Patients with oesophageal reflux are at risk of acid aspiration during GA.
- An antacid prophylactic regimen is usually administered to patients a few days prior to surgery.
- Sodium citrate can be administered orally immediately prior to induction of anaesthesia.
- Consider rapid sequence induction for GA.
- Extubate head-down in left lateral position.

## Liver disease

- Causes of liver disease in adults can include alcohol, cirrhosis, and hepatitis B or hepatitis C infection.
- Causes of liver disease in children can include congenital, biliary atresia, and viral hepatitis.
- Risks associated with liver disease include bleeding, acute kidney injury, and decompensation of chronic liver disease.
- Complications of liver disease can include bleeding, hypoglycaemia, ascites, renal failure, infection, and encephalopathy.
- See Table 5.3 for a list of safe anaesthetic drugs for use in liver failure.

## Pancreatitis

- Pancreatic proteases are secreted in inactive forms which are not activated until they reach the intestines.
- If the enzymes are activated while in the pancreas, the result is pancreatitis.
- Severe form causes necrosis and haemorrhage.
- Do not assume acute pancreatitis is alcohol related, it could also be caused by gallstones, metabolic causes such as hyper- or hypolipidaemia, prescription drugs, and hereditary causes.
- Consider surgery as first-line treatment in adults with painful chronic pancreatitis that is causing obstruction of the main pancreatic duct.
- Surgery is, however, often of high risk due to the acutely ill patient and is dependent on the functional and anatomic abnormalities of the pancreas.
- Most surgery will therefore be endoscopic or laparoscopic procedures.

## Gallstones (cholelithiasis)

- Usually formed in the gall bladder and made of cholesterol but can also be caused by bilirubin which is a waste product formed in the gall bladder.
- Pregnancy is associated with an increased risk of gallstone formation, which in turn is an important cause of pancreatitis in pregnancy.
- Complications can include acute inflammation of the bile duct and pancreas.

**Table 5.3** Safe anaesthetic drugs in liver failure

| | |
|---|---|
| **Premedication drugs** | Lorazepam |
| **Induction agents** | Propofol, thiopental, etomidate |
| **Inhalational agents** | Isoflurane, sevoflurane, desflurane |
| **Muscle relaxants** | Atracurium, cisatracurium |
| **Opiate drugs** | Remifentanil |
| **Analgesic drugs** | Paracetamol |

- Jaundice can occur with obstruction of the bile duct.
- If surgery is recommended, a laparoscopic cholecystectomy will be performed to remove the gall bladder.

## Coeliac disease

- Gluten reacts with the lining of the small bowel and triggers an immune response.
- The villi are attacked by the immune system and destroyed.
- Results in lack of absorption of nutrients—leads to vitamin and mineral deficiencies.
- Consider serological testing to determine diagnosis of coeliac disease.
- Advice regarding a gluten-free diet should be provided by a healthcare professional.

## Crohn's disease

- Chronic inflammatory bowel disease can affect any part of the GI tract but often affects the ileum and/or ascending colon.
- Affects *all* layers of the intestinal wall and age of onset most commonly 20–30 years.
- Unknown cause, but runs in families.
- Inflammation process begins in the submucosa and works inwards and outwards, abscesses and fistulas can form due to the deep ulcerations in the intestinal wall.
- The lumen of the intestine can therefore become narrowed and obstructed.

## Ulcerative colitis

- Chronic inflammatory bowel disease that begins in the rectum and sigmoid colon but may spread to entire colon.
- Involves only the inner mucosa.
- Unknown cause, although genetic links identified; usually begins between ages of 15 and 40 years.
- Involves intermittent periods of remission and relapse causing acute abdominal pain and diarrhoea.
- Complications include perforation of the colon, toxic megacolon, haemorrhage, and long-term risk of bowel cancer.
- See Table 5.4.

**Table 5.4** Overview of ulcerative colitis and Crohn's disease

|  | **Ulcerative colitis** | **Crohn's disease** |
| --- | --- | --- |
| **Incidence** | Usually between 15 and 40 years of age | Usually between 20 and 30 years of age |
| **Cause** | Unknown, genetic links, ?autoimmune | Unknown, genetic links, ?autoimmune |
| **Area of bowel affected** | Rectum always involved with variable spread along colon | Any part of GI tract, most common in terminal ileum |
| **Depth of involvement** | Mucosa and submucosa | All layers of wall |
| **Appearance of mucosa** | Continuous lesions, mucosa is red and inflamed | 'Skip' lesions, areas of normal tissue surrounded by ulceration |

## Diverticulitis

- Diverticula are small pouches of mucosa that protrude through the muscular wall of the large bowel.
- Occurs mainly in the descending and sigmoid colon due to increased pressure in weak areas of the colon.
- Diverticula occurs when faeces impact the pouches and cause inflammation.
- Diet low in fibre leads to a low volume of colonic content and a reduction in diameter of colon.
- Diagnosis often made through barium enema or colonoscopy.
- In complications such as obstruction, perforation, or haemorrhage, immediate surgical intervention may be required.

## Perioperative considerations

- Pre-assessment of the patient is essential prior to anaesthesia and surgery.
- Avoid use of halothane due to the possibility of postoperative liver dysfunction.
- Inform appropriate healthcare professionals if a patient has positive hepatitis viral serology.
- Postoperative monitoring of renal function is required.
- Assess levels of consciousness.
- Monitor blood glucose levels.
- Monitor the patient's vital signs.
- $O_2$ therapy as prescribed.
- Effective postoperative analgesia should be prescribed.
- DVT prophylaxis as per policy.
- Accurate fluid balance should be monitored.
- Monitor wounds and drains for output.
- Do not offer prophylactic antimicrobials to people with acute pancreatitis.

- Offer people with acute pancreatitis an endoscopic approach for managing infected or suspected infected pancreatic necrosis when anatomically possible.
- Therapeutic management for patients with Crohn's disease and ulcerative colitis involves corticosteroids to prevent inflammation.
- Caution must be taken prescribing laxatives for inflammatory disorders of the bowel.

## Further reading

Freedman R, Herbert L, O'Donnell A, et al. (eds) (2022). Oxford handbook of anaesthesia (5th ed). Oxford: Oxford University Press.

National Institute for Health and Care Excellence (2015). Coeliac disease: recognition, assessment and management. NICE guideline [NG20]. Available at: ℘ https://www.nice.org.uk/guidance/ng20

National Institute for Health and Care Excellence (2019). Crohn's disease: management. NICE guideline [NG129]. Available at: ℘ https://www.nice.org.uk/guidance/ng129

National Institute for Health and Care Excellence (2020). Colorectal cancer. Quality standard [QS20]. Available at: ℘ https://www.nice.org.uk/guidance/qs20

Pollard B, Kitchen G (eds) (2017). Handbook of clinical anaesthesia (4th ed). London: CRC Press.

Royal College of Anaesthetists (2019). Chapter 3: guidelines for the provision of anaesthesia services for intraoperative care. London: Royal College of Anaesthetists.

Royal College of Anaesthetists (2019). Chapter 4: guidelines for the provision of postoperative care. London: Royal College of Anaesthetists.

Royal College of Anaesthetists (2021). Chapter 2: guidelines for the provision of anaesthesia services for preoperative assessment and preparation. London: Royal College of Anaesthetists.

Royal College of Anaesthetists (2021). Chapter 11: guidelines for the provision of anaesthesia services for inpatient pain management. London: Royal College of Anaesthetists.

# Renal disorders

- Chronic kidney disease (CKD) can be defined as a gradual and eventual permanent loss of kidney function over time.
- CKD has been identified as a condition that is often under-diagnosed with no obvious symptoms.
- Common causes include hypertension, diabetes, and familial, and the damage usually occurs very gradually over years.
- Patients with kidney problems tend to be susceptible to heart attacks and strokes.
- Afro-Caribbean and South Asian patients are at significantly greater risk of renal failure than people from white ethnic backgrounds.
- For patients in established renal failure, the optimal choice is renal transplantation.
- It is recommended that the use of NICE guidance on preoperative testing should be followed in all surgical units.

## Preoperative management

- Pre-assessment should include drug history and drug allergies.
- Regular monitoring of vital signs.
- Consider anaemia or cardiovascular problems if reduced exercise tolerance is identified.
- An intensive care bed should be available for major surgical procedures.

## Anaesthesia management

- The use of NIBP and cannulation should be avoided in an arm with an atrioventricular (AV) fistula.
- Cannulation of the dorsum of the dorsum of the hand is recommended.
- Cannulation of the forearm and antecubital fossa should be avoided.
- The majority of drugs used in anaesthesia can reduce glomerular filtration rate, urine output, and blood flow (Table 5.5).

## Postoperative management

- Accurate fluid balance should be monitored frequently with recordings of hourly urine output.
- Avoid dehydration.
- NSAIDs should be avoided.

## Renal failure

Renal failure can occur perioperatively when oliguria and an increasing serum creatinine level develop. Patients at risk of acute kidney injury include those with the following conditions:

- Septic shock.
- Fluid depletion.
- Heart failure, hypertension, vascular disease.
- CRF.
- Elderly patients with hypertension and diabetes.
- Patients taking NSAIDs, angiotensin-converting enzyme (ACE) inhibitors, diuretics, and chemotherapy.

**Table 5.5** Safe anaesthetic drugs in chronic renal failure

| | |
|---|---|
| **Premedication drugs** | Midazolam, temazepam |
| **Induction agents** | Propofol, thiopental, etomidate |
| **Inhalational agents** | Isoflurane, halothane, desflurane |
| **Muscle relaxants** | Suxamethonium, atracurium, cisatracurium |
| **Opiate drugs** | Remifentanil, alfentanil |
| **Local anaesthetic drugs** | Lidocaine, bupivacaine |
| **Analgesic drugs** | Paracetamol |

## Further reading

Freedman R, Herbert L, O'Donnell A, et al. (eds) (2022). Oxford handbook of anaesthesia (5th ed). Oxford: Oxford University Press.

National Institute for Health and Care Excellence (2020). Acute kidney injury: prevention, detection and management. NICE guideline [NG148]. Available at: ℘ https://www.nice.org.uk/guidance/ng148

National Institute for Health and Care Excellence (2020). Intravenous fluid therapy in children and young people in hospital. NICE guideline [NG29]. Available at: ℘ https://www.nice.org.uk/guidance/ng29

National Institute for Health and Care Excellence (2020). Perioperative care in adults. NICE guideline [NG180]. Available at: ℘ https://www.nice.org.uk/guidance/ng180

National Institute for Health and Care Excellence (2020). Sepsis. Quality standard [QS161]. Available at: ℘ https://www.nice.org.uk/guidance/qs161

National Institute for Health and Care Excellence (2020). COVID-19 rapid guideline: chronic kidney disease. NICE guideline [NG176]. Available at: ℘ https://www.nice.org.uk/guidance/ng176

Pollard B, Kitchen G (eds) (2017). Handbook of clinical anaesthesia (4th ed). London: CRC Press.

Royal College of Anaesthetists (2019). Chapter 3: guidelines for the provision of anaesthesia services for intraoperative care. London: Royal College of Anaesthetists.

Royal College of Anaesthetists (2019). Chapter 4: guidelines for the provision of postoperative care. London: Royal College of Anaesthetists.

Royal College of Anaesthetists (2021). Chapter 2: guidelines for the provision of anaesthesia services for preoperative assessment and preparation. London: Royal College of Anaesthetists.

Royal College of Anaesthetists (2021). Chapter 11: guidelines for the provision of anaesthesia services for inpatient pain management. London: Royal College of Anaesthetists.

# Bone and joint disorders

## Rheumatology

- Rheumatoid arthritis is defined as a chronic, disabling autoimmune disease characterized by inflammation of the synovial tissue of the peripheral joints and is more prevalent in women than in men.
- Symptoms can include stiffness, swelling, pain, and progressive joint destruction.
- An interdisciplinary approach to managing musculoskeletal conditions is recommended usually involving the following health disciplines:
  - Rheumatologists, orthopaedic surgeons, nursing, physiotherapy, and occupational therapy.
  - Orthotics, prosthetics, podiatry, and dietetics usually support the above disciplines.
- Rheumatology services provide specialist advice, treatment, pharmacological management, and support for considerable numbers of people affected by rheumatological conditions (Table 5.6).

## Preoperative management

Pre-assessment by members of the nursing, anaesthetic, and medical team is essential and should include the following investigations:
- Full history and physical examination.
- Chest X-ray, 12-lead ECG, FBC, and urea and electrolytes (U&Es).
- Neck X-ray for cervical instability.
- Pulmonary function tests.
- Airway assessment to assess intubation risk.
- Assessment may also be undertaken by occupational therapists and physiotherapists to discuss the home environment and postoperative exercise regimens.
- Ensure VTE policy is initiated.
- Steroid cover should be implemented perioperatively and reduced to maintenance level postoperatively.

## Anaesthetic management

- Airway management with sedation can be problematic as patients are often in the supine position for orthopaedic surgery.
- A protective neck collar is recommended prior to induction of anaesthesia for patients with cervical instability.
- The use of spinal and epidural anaesthesia may prove difficult in some patients with joint deformities.
- Tracheal intubation might be problematic in patients with scoliosis and spondyloarthropathies.
- Care should be taken when moving, handling, and transferring patients with bone and joint disorders.
- Patients should be positioned carefully with appropriate protection and padding of pressure areas.
- Patients should be actively warmed intraoperatively.
- GA ± epidural is recommended for major orthopaedic procedures.

## Postoperative management

- All patients with bone and joint disorders should be transferred onto beds following surgery.
- Monitor patient's vital signs.
- $O_2$ therapy as prescribed.
- Effective postoperative analgesia should be prescribed.
- DVT prophylaxis as per policy.
- Accurate fluid balance should be monitored.
- For patients with rheumatoid disease, disease-modifying anti-rheumatoid drugs (DMARDs) should be resumed as soon as possible following surgery.
- Monitor wounds and drains for output.
- Care of the immobile patient.

**Table 5.6** Rheumatology conditions

| Inflammatory diseases | Ankylosing spondylitis<br>Psoriatic arthritis<br>Reactive arthritis |
|---|---|
| Autoimmune rheumatic diseases | Rheumatoid arthritis<br>Systemic lupus erythematosus (SLE)<br>Scleroderma<br>Myositis<br>Sjogren's syndrome<br>Systemic vasculitis |
| Soft tissue/regional pain disorders | Generalized and non-articular pain syndromes<br>Tendonitis<br>Bursitis |
| Bone diseases | Osteoporosis<br>Paget's disease |
| Osteoarthritis | |
| Back pain | |

## Further reading

Axford J (2018). Pre-operative evaluation and perioperative management of patients with rheumatic disease. Available at: ℬ https://www.uptodate.com/contents/preoperative-evaluation-and-perioperative-management-of-patients-with-rheumatic-diseases

Department of Health (2006). Musculoskeletal services framework. A joint responsibility: doing it differently. London: The Stationery Office.

Griffiths R, Brooks D (2022). Orthopaedic surgery. In: Freedman R, Herbert L, O'Donnell A, et al. (eds) Oxford handbook of anaesthesia (5th ed). Oxford: Oxford University Press.

Howell D (2022). Bone, joint, and connective tissue disorders. In: Freedman R, Herbert L, O'Donnell A, et al. (eds) Oxford handbook of anaesthesia (5th ed). Oxford: Oxford University Press.

Marshall P (2000). Bone and joint disorders. In: Nicholls A, Wilson I (eds) Perioperative medicine: managing surgical patients with medical problems. Oxford: Oxford University Press.

National Institute of Health and Care Excellence. (2018). Musculoskeletal conditions. https://www.nice.org.uk/guidance/conditions-and-diseases/musculoskeletal-conditions

National Institute for Health and Care Excellence (2020). Joint replacement (primary): hip, knee and shoulder. NICE guideline [NG157]. Available at: ℬ https://www.nice.org.uk/guidance/ng157

National Institute for Health and Care Excellence (2020). Perioperative care in adults. NICE guideline [NG180]. Available at: 🔗 https://www.nice.org.uk/guidance/ng180

National Institute for Health and Care Excellence (2020). Rheumatoid arthritis in over 16s. Quality standard [QS33]. Available at: 🔗 https://www.nice.org.uk/guidance/qs33

National Institute for Health and Care Excellence (2020). Venous thromboembolic diseases: diagnosis, management and thrombophilia testing. NICE guideline [NG158]. Available at: 🔗 https://www.nice.org.uk/guidance/ng158

Royal College of Anaesthetists (2020). Chapter 16: guidelines for the provision of anaesthesia services for trauma and orthopaedic surgery London: Royal College of Anaesthetists.

# Neurological and muscular disorders: overview and multiple sclerosis

- Patients with neurological and muscular disorders (Box 5.3) should be cared for by practitioners with the appropriate neurological and resuscitation skills and facilities.
- An interdisciplinary approach to care delivery and management is essential to maximize the patient experience.
- Treatment must comply with national and local standards and guidelines.

---

**Box 5.3 Examples of neurological and muscular disorders**
- Myasthenia gravis.
- Multiple sclerosis (MS).
- Stroke—ischaemic, haemorrhagic, and transient ischaemic attack (TIA).
- Parkinson's disease.
- Muscular dystrophy.
- Motor neurone disease.
- Epilepsy.
- Headache.
- Dementia.
- Guillain–Barré syndrome.
- Head injury.

---

### Multiple sclerosis

- MS is a common disabling neurological disease and autoimmune condition, resulting from damage to the myelin sheath which interferes with transmission of messages between the central nervous system (CNS) and other parts of the body.
- Treatment can involve disease-modifying drugs which include long-term immunotherapy and immunosuppressants, short-term high-dose corticosteroids, and medication for symptom management. Patients may also use unproven complementary and alternative therapies to manage symptoms.

*Problems associated with MS can vary from mild to severe and can include*
- Fatigue
- Altered sensation
- Neuropathic pain
- Altered balance
- Muscle weakness and reduced mobility
- Dysphagia
- Cognitive difficulties and memory problems
- Mood changes
- Tremor
- Bladder and bowel changes including commonly urinary urgency and constipation
- Dysphasia

- Muscle pain, spasms, and stiffness
- Sexual dysfunction
- Visual disturbances.

*Preoperative management*
- Detailed neurological assessment—essential to obtain a baseline assessment of function.
- Assessment of respiratory function.
- Antiembolic stockings should be applied to reduce the risk of DVT and PE.
- Consider positioning and safe management of airway in patients with disabling MS.

*Anaesthesia management*
- GA, epidural, and LA are not contraindicated as they do not alter the course of MS. Epidural blocks may cause exacerbation of underlying symptoms, but these effects are lessened where minimal concentrations of opioid and LA are used in combination.
- Discussion around the comparative risks of regional nerve or plexus blocks are prudent, however, if anaesthetic is to be used in a limb where other limbs are already weakened by a neurological problem.
- Caution should be applied to the use of non-depolarizing drugs in patients with high levels of disability. Suxamethonium should be avoided in this group of patients as it is associated with a large efflux of $K^+$ in debilitated patients.
- Cardiovascular monitoring is essential.

*Postoperative management*
- Monitor all vital signs—hypotension may result from autonomic instability and temperature fluctuations can result in delayed recovery or exacerbation of underlying symptoms.
- Patients with severe or advanced MS, who are more likely to have respiratory problems or are seriously weakened will be at greater risk of developing post-anaesthetic complications.
- Patients may have trouble coughing up sputum, increasing the risk of chest infection; sputum clearance is essential to reduce the risk of respiratory compromise.
- Exacerbation of pre-existing symptoms may be noted following anaesthetic but will usually recover to baseline with appropriate multidisciplinary team input.

## Further reading

Chikwe J, Walther A, Jones P (2009). Perioperative medicine: managing surgical patients with medical problems (2nd ed). Oxford: Oxford University Press.

Drake E, Drake M, Bird J, et al. (2006). Obstetric regional blocks for women with multiple sclerosis: a survey of UK experience. International Journal of Obstetric Anaesthetics, 15(2):115–123.

Multiple Sclerosis Society. Homepage. Available at: http://www.mssociety.org.uk

Multiple Sclerosis Trust. Homepage. Available at: http://www.mstrust.org.uk

National Institute for Health and Care Excellence (2014). Multiple sclerosis in adults: management. Clinical guideline [CG186]. Available at: https://www.nice.org.uk/guidance/cg186

Royal College of Anaesthetists (2020). Chapter 14: guidelines for the provision of neuro-anaesthetic services. London: Royal College of Anaesthetists.

Stuart M, Bergstrom L (2011). Pregnancy and multiple sclerosis Journal of Midwifery and Womens Health, 56(1):41–47.

Young A, Selin Kabadayi S, et al. (2022). Neurological and muscular disorders. In: Freedman R, Herbert L, O'Donnell A, et al. (eds) Oxford handbook of anaesthesia (5th ed). Oxford: Oxford University Press.

# Stroke

## Definition

- A stroke or a cerebrovascular accident (CVA) is a life-threatening condition, also known as a 'brain attack' where the blood supply to the brain is partially or completely cut off.
- The effect of the stroke therefore depends on the location and size of the artery affected.
- Stroke is a medical emergency and there is a significant beneficial effect on the patient's chances of recovery the sooner the stroke is diagnosed.

## Epidemiology

- Each year approximately 130,000 people in the UK have a first or recurrent stroke.
- Stroke can lead to major disability and is the third-most common cause of death in the Western world.
- It is estimated that up to 70% of all strokes could be avoided if the risk factors were treated and people adopted healthier lifestyles.

## Symptoms

The main symptoms of a stroke can be remembered with the acronym FAST; however, the onset of a haemorrhagic stroke can be sudden, causing a severe headache and/or unconsciousness.

- Face—the patient's face may have dropped to one side.
- Arms—the patient may have weakness in one or both arms.
- Speech—their speech may be slurred, illegible, or they may seem to be confused.
- Time—test the three symptoms, time to call 999.

## Types of stroke

There are three major categories of stroke:

### Ischaemic stroke

Ischaemic stroke is caused by a blockage cutting off blood supply to the brain.

- This is the most common type of stroke accounting for almost 85% of patients affected.
- Risk factors include atherosclerosis, atrial fibrillation, and small blood vessel disease.
- Can be caused by a thrombus which is a blood clot that forms in a blood vessel, a lacunar infarct that affects very small blood vessels deep in the brain, or an embolism which is a clot that travels around the body potentially lodging in the blood vessels supplying oxygenated blood to the brain.
- An ischaemic stroke can be classified using the Bamford classification which categorizes the stoke based on initial presentation of clinical signs and symptoms:
  - TACS—total anterior circulation stroke.
  - PACS—partial anterior circulation stroke.
  - LACS—lacunar syndrome.
  - POCS—posterior circulation syndrome.

- Treatment can include clot-busting medication or thrombolysis (tissue plasminogen activator) if the stroke is caused by a blood clot, however, there are many risk factors and caution should be used.
- An ischaemic stroke needs to be accurately diagnosed as giving thrombolysis to a patient with a haemorrhagic stroke would be catastrophic.
- Thrombolysis should be used within hours of onset of symptoms.
- Contraindications include subarachnoid haemorrhage, history of GI bleeding, pregnancy, and pancreatitis.
- BP monitoring is also extremely important.
- A thrombectomy could also be performed where the blood clot is mechanically removed.
- Long-term treatment will include anticoagulants.

*Haemorrhagic stroke*

Haemorrhagic strokes are caused by bleeding in or around the brain.
- Classified as an intracerebral haemorrhage (within the brain) or a subarachnoid haemorrhage (in the fluid-filled spaces around the blood vessels outside the brain).
- Risk factors include high BP and an aneurysm caused by rupture of a blood vessel.
- Diagnosis of a subarachnoid haemorrhage may include performing a lumbar puncture to explore if any blood has leaked into the patient's cerebral spinal fluid.
- Treatment is focused on restoring intracranial haemodynamics.
- Surgery may include a craniotomy allowing the drainage of bleeding, removal of clots, or blood vessel repair.
- If the patient has hydrocephalus (increased build-up of fluid around the brain), surgery to remove the fluid may need to be performed.

*Transient ischaemic attack*

A TIA, often referred to as a mini stroke, happens when the blood supply to part of the brain is interrupted for a very short time.

## Preoperative management

Pre-assessment is essential by members of the nursing, anaesthetic, and medical team and should include the following investigations:
- Full history and physical examination.
- Chest X-ray, 12-lead ECG, FBC, and U&Es.
- Pulmonary function tests.
- Airway assessment to assess intubation risk. Patient may have lost swallow reflex so may be at risk of aspiration.
- Ensure VTE policy is initiated.
- Close monitoring of BP ensuring adequate perfusion.
- $O_2$ therapy as required.
- Monitoring of blood glucose levels.

## Postoperative management

- Monitor patient's vital signs.
- $O_2$ therapy as prescribed.
- Effective positioning of patient.
- Be aware of dysphagia.

- Effective postoperative analgesia should be prescribed.
- DVT prophylaxis as per policy.
- Accurate fluid and electrolyte management.
- Monitor wounds and drains for output.
- Care of the immobile patient.

## Further reading

Barrett KM, Meschia JF (2013). Stroke. London: John Wiley and Sons.

Freedman R, Herbert L, O'Donnell A, et al. (eds) (2022). Oxford handbook of anaesthesia (5th ed). Oxford: Oxford University Press.

Lindley RI (2017). Stroke. Oxford: Oxford University Press.

Stroke Association. Homepage. Available at: ℘ https://www.stroke.org.uk/

Nathanson MH, Andrzejowski J, Dinsmore J, et al. (2020). Guidelines for safe transfer of the brain-injured patient: trauma and stroke, 2019: guidelines from the Association of Anaesthetists and the Neuro Anaesthesia and Critical Care Society. Anaesthesia, 75(2):234–246.

National Institute for Health and Care Excellence (2003). Stroke rehabilitation in adults. Clinical guideline [CG162]. Available at: ℘ https://www.nice.org.uk/guidance/cg162/

National Institute for Health and Care Excellence (2019). Hypertension in adults: diagnosis and management. NICE guideline [NG136]. Available at: ℘ https://www.nice.org.uk/guidance/NG136

National Institute for Health and Care Excellence (2019). Stroke and transient ischaemic attacks in over 16s: diagnosis and initial management. NICE guideline [NG128]. Available at: ℘ https://www.nice.org.uk/guidance/NG128

Pollard B, Kitchen G (eds) (2017). Handbook of clinical anaesthesia (4th ed). London: CRC Press.

Royal College of Anaesthetists (2021). Chapter 14: guidelines for the provision of neuroanaesthetic services. London: Royal College of Anaesthetists.

# Epilepsy

A seizure can be described as a sudden surge of electrical activity in the brain.[1]

A convulsion is a sudden, violent, irregular movement of the body, caused by involuntary contraction of muscles and associated especially with brain disorders such as epilepsy.

Seizures can occur as a result of epilepsy or as a result of an underlying pathology such as a CNS imbalance.

Irrespective of their cause, seizures should be managed similarly, with maintaining the airway taking precedence.

### Types of seizures

There are several types of seizure that a patient can endure. These can be broadly categorized as generalized, partial, and complex partial seizures (Table 5.7).

**Table 5.7** Types of seizures

| | |
| --- | --- |
| **Generalized seizures** | Summarize the traditional 'fit'. These describe tonic/clonic (grand mal) convulsions, myoclonic (brief arm contractions), and clonic seizures (rhythmic symmetrical movements of the arms, neck, and face) |
| **Partial seizures (also known as focal seizures)** | Usually non-motor and involve sensory, autonomic, and/or higher conscious impairment |
| **Complex partial seizures** | Involve loss of consciousness, spatial awareness, and memory. Seizures can progress from one type to another. For example, complex partial seizures commonly develop into generalized seizures |

### Causes

These are the predominant causes of seizures in the recovery room:
- An epileptic who has not taken his/her medication or is undiagnosed.
- Alcohol or drug withdrawal.
- Adverse reaction to anaesthetic agents.
- Neurosurgery (e.g. brain tumour or brain infection).

*More common causes might include*
- Hyperpyrexia and sepsis
- Hypoglycaemia
- Hypoxia
- Fluid overload
- Hypocalcaemia
- Norpethidine toxicity (pethidine overdose).

*Least common causes might include*
- Adverse reaction to anaesthetic agents. With the exception of epilepsy, this is one of the most common reasons for postoperative seizures

- Methohexitone, propofol, enflurane, and LAs are agents, which can directly stimulate convulsions
- The only visible symptom of epilepsy is seizures or fits
- It may be hard to tell if someone is having a seizure, as some seizures only cause a person to have vacant episodes, which may go unnoticed. Specific symptoms depend on which part of the brain is involved and often occur suddenly (Box 5.4).

> **Box 5.4  Seizure symptoms**
> - Brief blackout followed by a period of confusion (the person cannot remember for a short time).
> - Changes in behaviour, such as picking at one's clothing.
> - Drooling or frothing at the mouth.
> - Eye movements.
> - Grunting and snorting.
> - Loss of bladder or bowel control.
> - Mood changes, such as sudden anger, unexplainable fear, panic, joy, or laughter.
> - Shaking of the entire body.
> - Sudden falling.
> - Tasting a bitter or metallic flavour.
> - Teeth clenching.
> - Temporary stop in breathing.
> - Uncontrollable muscle spasms with twitching and jerking limbs.

Symptoms may stop after a few seconds or minutes, or continue for up to 15 minutes. They rarely continue longer. The person may have warning symptoms before the attack, such as:
- Fear or anxiety
- Nausea
- Vertigo (feeling as if you are spinning or moving)
- Visual symptoms (such as flashing bright lights, spots, or wavy lines before the eyes).

> Refractory convulsive status epilepticus can be treated with midazolam, propofol, or thiopentone.[1]

## Preoperative management
- A comprehensive care pathway utilizing an interdisciplinary approach to care delivery and management is essential.
- Epilepsy nurse specialists should be an integral part of the care of patients with epilepsy.
- Short stay surgery and anaesthesia is suitable for patients with well-controlled disease.
- Comprehensive pre-assessment of patient to include drug history and frequency of seizures.
- Antiepileptic therapy should be continued until the time of surgery.

## Anaesthesia management

- Premedication can include the use of diazepam or lorazepam.
- Thiopental is the drug of choice for induction of GA, due to its anticonvulsant properties.
- Atracurium or cisatracurium is recommended for muscle relaxation.
- Suxamethonium and vecuronium can increase the risk of dystonias.

## Postoperative management

- All neurosurgical patients are at an increased risk of postoperative seizure, this may be attributed to the surgery or the patient's medical history (which indicates the need for surgery).
- Epilepsy drugs should be recommenced as soon as possible postoperatively.
- Ensure IV access.
- Ensure availability of ventilatory support if required.
- Monitoring of vital signs including TPR, BP, and $SpO_2$.
- Antiemetic therapy should include ondansetron or cyclizine to reduce the risk of dystonias.
- Monitor for postoperative convulsions.

If seizure occurs, call for anaesthetist and:
- Maintain airway
- Administer $O_2$
- Assess cardiorespiratory function
- Ensure safety of patient but do not restrain
- Constant reassurance is necessary as the patient may be confused and not fully aware of surroundings
- Monitor length of seizure
- Patients may feel tired and need to sleep following a seizure.

## Reference

1. National Institute for Health and Care Excellence (2020). Epilepsies: diagnosis and management. Clinical guideline [CG137]. Available at: ᗺ https://www.nice.org.uk/guidance/cg137

## Further reading

Craig A, Hatfield A (2020). The complete recovery room book (6th ed). Oxford: Oxford University Press.

Denison D (2007). Degenerative neurological dysfunction: nursing management. In: Daniels R, Nosek L, Nicoll LH (eds) Contemporary medical-surgical nursing. New York: Thomson Delmar Learning.

Epilepsy Action. Homepage. Available at: ᗺ https://www.epilepsy.org.uk/

Freedman R, Herbert L, O'Donnell A, et al. (eds) (2022). Oxford handbook of anaesthesia (5th ed). Oxford: Oxford University Press.

Nathanson MH, Andrzejowski J, Dinsmore J, et al. (2020). Guidelines for safe transfer of the brain-injured patient: trauma and stroke, 2019: guidelines from the Association of Anaesthetists and the Neuro Anaesthesia and Critical Care Society. Anaesthesia, 75(2):234–246.

National Institute for Health and Care Excellence (2018). Brain tumours (primary) and brain metastases in adults. NICE guideline [NG99]. Available at: ᗺ https://www.nice.org.uk/guidance/ng99

National Institute for Health and Care Excellence (2019). Suspected neurological conditions: recognition and referral. NICE guideline [NG127]. Available at: ᗺ https://www.nice.org.uk/guidance/ng127

Royal College of Anaesthetists (2021). Chapter 14: guidelines for the provision of neuro-anaesthetic services. London: Royal College of Anaesthetists.

# Myasthenia gravis

- An autoimmune disease characterized by fluctuating muscle weakness that can sometimes be fatal (Box 5.5).
- Myasthenia gravis is a long-term condition that typically has phases when it improves and phases when it gets worse.
- It usually affects most of the body, spreading from the eyes and face to other areas over weeks, months, or years.
- The immune system damages the communication system between the nerves and muscles, making the muscles weak and easily fatigued.
- Treatment involves the use of anticholinesterase drugs such as neostigmine and atropine to counteract the muscarinic side effects that can include abdominal cramps and bradycardia.
- Myasthenic crisis causes paralysis of the respiratory muscles necessitating ventilation.

---

**Box 5.5 Symptoms of myasthenia gravis**

- Droopy eyelids/bulbar palsy.
- Diplopia.
- Facial weakness.
- Slurred speech.
- Weakness in limbs.
- Ptosis.
- Shortness of breath/respiratory insufficiency.
- Problems with chewing and swallowing.
- Symptoms have a tendency to worsen with fatigue.

---

### Preoperative management

- Patients with stable disease can usually present for most surgical procedures.
- Postoperatively, patients with myasthenia gravis are at risk of respiratory difficulties because of an inadequate cough reflex to clear their mucous owing to intrinsic muscle weakness.
- Sputum can then block the bronchi causing collapse of the lung.
- Comprehensive pre-assessment of the patient to include assessment of neurological and respiratory function.
- Anticholinesterase therapy should be continued until induction of anaesthesia.
- Pre-medication is not recommended.
- Assessment by the speech and language team is advised.

### Anaesthesia management

- Regional anaesthesia should be considered to avoid the use of opiate drugs and the possibility of respiratory depression.
- Rapid sequence induction may be employed with GA utilizing a minimal dose of suxamethonium.
- Neuromuscular blockade should be avoided as intubation and ventilation are achievable in the absence of muscle-relaxing drugs.

- If non-depolarizing muscle relaxants are used, the drugs of choice
  include atracurium, vecuronium, or mivacurium.
- Reversal agents are not recommended due to risk of overdose—if
  necessary, one dose of neostigmine is advocated.
- Nerve stimulators should be used to assess neuromuscular function
  prior to extubation.

## Postoperative management

- Delayed emergence from anaesthesia may occur.
- Ventilatory support should be available postoperatively.
- Transfer to ITU for postoperative management may be necessary.
- Full patient monitoring—TPR, BP, ECG, $SpO_2$, level of consciousness,
  and urinary output.
- Drug therapy should be recommenced immediately; enteral
  administration of medicines via a nasogastric tube may be necessary.
- Postoperative analgesia—epidural or PCA.
- Respiratory problems may occur, for example, infection, sputum
  retention, and respiratory failure.
- Intensive physiotherapy may be required pre- and postoperatively.

## Further reading

Craig A, Hatfield A (2020). The complete recovery room book (6th ed). Oxford: Oxford University Press.

Freedman R, Herbert L, O'Donnell A, et al. (eds) (2022). Oxford handbook of anaesthesia (5th ed). Oxford: Oxford University Press.

Nathanson MH, Andrzejowski J, Dinsmore J, et al. (2020). Guidelines for safe transfer of the brain-injured patient: trauma and stroke, 2019: guidelines from the Association of Anaesthetists and the Neuro Anaesthesia and Critical Care Society. Anaesthesia, 75(2):234–246.

National Institute for Health and Care Excellence (2018). Brain tumours (primary) and brain metastases in adults. NICE guideline [NG99]. Available at: ⌖ https://www.nice.org.uk/guidance/ng99

National Institute for Health and Care Excellence (2019). Suspected neurological conditions: recognition and referral. NICE guideline [NG127]. Available at: ⌖ https://www.nice.org.uk/guidance/ng127

Royal College of Anaesthetists (2021). Chapter 14: guidelines for the provision of neuro-anaesthetic services. London: Royal College of Anaesthetists.

# Cancer

The numbers of people living with and beyond cancer is increasing. By 2030, it is estimated that there will be 4 million people living with a diagnosis of cancer in the UK. Surgery remains the primary treatment modality for people with cancer, but also as cancer survivorship grows, further surgical intervention in the person's lifetime is a likely event. People living with cancer will often have other comorbidities which can add to the complexity of the care needed to optimize surgical outcome and recovery. The perioperative period of any person can cause anxiety; evidence indicates this is particularly true for people with cancer. The key to recovery and a positive postsurgical outcome for people affected by cancer is the application of the clinical concept of 'prehabilitation'.

## Preoperative management

- Many patients with cancer will require anaesthesia/surgery either for primary debulking tumour removal or to treat an adverse consequence of the malignant process or its treatment. Perioperative healthcare providers will be challenged to manage cancer patients not only for their primary intervention, but also through their complex journeys following surgical intervention.
- Cancer and its therapy can adversely affect every major organ system with profound implications for perioperative management.
- Cancer surgery is usually not elective, and therefore the amount of time available to medically optimize a patient may be limited.
- Preoperative assessment and care of people affected by cancer is crucial to the postoperative outcome of any surgical intervention.
- Holistic assessment is essential; evidence suggests that often complex physical, psychological, social, and emotional issues, such as anxiety, can be present prior to surgery, and these impact postoperative recovery.
- The clinical concept of 'prehabilitation' aims to coordinate the surgical multiprofessional team in interventions to maximize health and well-being prior to surgery in order to boost the person's recovery potential (Table 5.8).
- Aim to increase the mobility and exercise level of the person in the period leading up to surgery. Improvement in exercise level has been shown to benefit postoperative outcomes. Exercise can be safe and achievable for even frail older adults. Any improvement above baseline can be beneficial. The patient can monitor their own exercise using a simple pedometer or pedometer application.
- Preoperative assessment of comorbid conditions is essential when considering mobility and the return to preoperative ambulation, including conditions such as rheumatoid arthritis and osteoarthritis.
- Aim to optimize nutrition and hydration in the preoperative period, a high-protein diet has been positively correlated with reduced postoperative complications.
- Psychological prehabilitation is important for people affected by cancer when offered ahead of their surgery. Practically, consider signposting to self-help groups, third-sector helplines, or obtain further advice from the patient's cancer specialist nurse.

**Table 5.8** Summary of prehabilitation advice and management

| Maximize mobility | Support nutrition | Remember psychological health |
|---|---|---|
| Aim for an increase from baseline | Optimize hydration preoperatively | Positive psychological effect of 'prehabilitation engagement' |
| Recommend patient self-management using a pedometer or mobile app | Avoid bowel preparation if not surgically appropriate to minimize dehydration | Signpost to self-help, third-sector support mechanisms |
| Early mobilization postoperatively | A high-protein diet | Consider appropriate pharmacological management of anxiety if indicated |

### Anaesthesia and surgical management

- The optimal goal should be one of fluid management; Hartmann's solution is recommended unless there is a specific indication for normal saline. It is good practice to only use IV fluids for as short a period as possible and only while monitoring the patient both clinically and biochemically.
- Patient positioning during surgery and in recovery is important in the prevention of secondary complications such as a neuropathic or muscular injury. Minimize this by ensuring proper alignment of injured or arthritic joints.
- Cancer patients with tumour involving head, neck, and mediastinum may present with established or potential airway compromise. Assessment of the airway by physical examination and appropriate imaging is of paramount importance. Awake fibreoptic intubations should be considered for large head and neck tumours where there is a risk of airway compromise on induction of GA. Where fibreoptic intubation is deemed hazardous or impossible, elective tracheostomy should be considered. Continuing postoperative endotracheal intubation is often prudent until airway patency is assured.

### Postoperative management

- Use a multidisciplinary team approach to individualized person-centred interventions and care.
- Ensure the patient has appropriate analgesia prescribed on a regular basis and available as required for breakthrough pain. Maximize opioid-sparing analgesia to support pain control. Patients with cancer may be receiving long-acting forms of opioids and may require conversion to short-acting forms of analgesia in the perioperative period. Assess pain regularly, adjusting analgesia as needed.
- Ensure close monitoring of the person clinically and biochemically; optimizing fluid balance, to make the best use of individualized care planning and enhance recovery.

- Aim where possible to optimize gut function and consider early oral enteral feeding within 12 hours of the postoperative period.
- Aim where possible for the person to mobilize early in in the postoperative period; within 6 hours (if practical). Use postoperative mobility scoring daily to monitor and encourage mobilization.

## Further reading

Arain MR, Buggy DJ (2007). Anaesthesia for cancer patients. Current Opinion in Anaesthesiology, 20(3):247–253.

Freedman R, Herbert L, O'Donnell A, et al. (eds) (2022). Oxford handbook of anaesthesia (5th ed). Oxford: Oxford University Press.

Gudaitytė J, Dvylys D, Šimeliūnaitė I (2017). Anaesthetic challenges in cancer patients: current therapies and pain management. Acta Medica Lituanica, 24(2):121–127.

Henke Yarbro C. Wujcik D, Holmes Gobel B (2018). Cancer nursing: principles and practice (8th ed). Burlington MA: Jones and Bartlett Learning.

Kabata P, Jastrzebski T, Kakol M, et al. (2015). Preoperative nutritional support in cancer patients with no clinical signs of malnutrition-prospective randomized controlled trial. Supportive Care in Cancer, 23(2):365–370.

Maddams J, Utley M, Moller H (2012). Projections of cancer prevalence in the United Kingdom, 2010–2040. British Journal of Cancer, 107(7):1195–1202.

Riedel B, MacCallum P, Wigmore T, et al. (2013). Cancer anaesthesia. Best Practice and Research Clinical Anaesthesiology, 27(4):397–398.

Royal College of Anaesthetists (2019–2021). Guidelines for the provision of anaesthetic services. London: Royal College of Anaesthetists.

Tsimopoulou I, Pasquali S, Howard R, et al. (2015). Psychological prehabilitation before cancer surgery: a systematic review. Annals of Surgical Oncology, 22(13):4117–4123.

Valkenet K, Van deport IG, Dronkers JJ, et al. (2011). The effects of perioperative exercise therapy on postoperative outcome. Clinical Rehabilitation, 25(2):99–111.

# Patients with HIV

- Human immunodeficiency virus (HIV) is a virus that belongs to a specific type of viruses called retroviruses.
- HIV can be transmitted through sexual intercourse without the use of condoms, sharing infected needles between users of illegal IV drugs, from mother to child through breastfeeding, and less commonly through transfusion of infected blood.
- HIV destroys the CD4+ or T cells of the human immune system making it weaker and more susceptible to infections.[1]
- The normal range of CD4+ cells in a human body is around 1200 CD4+ cells/mL.
- CD4+ cell reduction to <200 cells/mL may lead to a syndrome that is called acquired immune deficiency syndrome (AIDS) where the immune system is no longer able to defend the antigens and the pathogen microorganisms, which enhances a person's morbidity. This is also now referred to as uncontrolled HIV.
- However, HIV will not necessarily always progress to AIDS as there are a variety of drugs available which slow and sometimes impede the progression of the infection.
- Highly active antiretroviral therapy (HAART) is an advanced combination treatment regimen of two or more antiretroviral drugs and since 1996 it has managed to transform HIV from a death sentence to a long-term condition.
- HAART can reduce the HIV viral load in the blood thus protecting the CD4+ cells and hindering the progression to uncontrolled HIV.

> Neither HIV viral load nor CD4+ cell count in blood plasma should be determinants of the elective and/or emergency surgery for patients with HIV/AIDS.[2,3]

## Preoperative management

- Newly diagnosed patients have almost the same morbidity risk after surgery than everyone else.
- Therefore, the preoperative management of patients with HIV/AIDS should be similar to patients who do not have HIV/AIDS.
- An explicit health history should be taken before any minor or major surgery, including history of substance use, in order to try to predict the outcome of the surgery and the morbidity.[4]
- Evidence shows that factors such as overall health, nutritional status, and single organ or multiple organ failure, are more reliable predictors than the CD4+ cell count and the viral load in the blood plasma.
- Take the weight and height of the patient in order to calculate the BMI and determine the nutritional status.
- A number of tests should be done, such as FBC, renal function, as well as a urine sample for toxicology if there is clinician concern about drug use.[5]
- History of previous infection and colonization with MRSA and especially in men who have sex with men.

- It is recommended that patients with a history of MRSA receive vancomycin if it is required.
- Provide patient with reassurance throughout the surgical journal and provide appropriate information and person-centred care.

## Anaesthesia management

- GA is generally well tolerated by patients with HIV/AIDS.
- However, patients with HIV/AIDS should be assessed for hepatic dysfunction before the administration of any medication, as it may affect the dosage of a variety of anaesthetics and antibiotics.
- Renal dysfunction is common among patients with HIV/AIDS, so renal function should be assessed prior to the administration of any anaesthetic or antibiotic.
- Sufficient monitoring should be taking place during the surgery including TPR, BP, and $SpO_2$.

## Perioperative management

- HAART administration during the perioperative management period should be interrupted as little as possible.
- Drug interaction resources, such as the *British National Formulary* (*BNF*), should be consulted prior to the administration of any medication to check potential interactions with any drug used in HAART.

## Postoperative management

- Keep monitoring the vital signs.
- Monitor any signs of infection as patients with HIV/AIDS are more susceptible to infection because of their weakened immune system, including TPR, BP, FBC, and CRP.
- Preferably, transfer the patient into a side room to prevent the transmission of hospital infections from other patients.
- It is essential that the antiretroviral drugs are given consistently postoperatively.
- Liaise with the multidisciplinary team in order to implement an individual care plan for the patient including a dietician and a mental health nurse.
- Universal pain control algorithms should be followed postoperatively regardless of any substance misuse by the patient.
- It is essential that patients with HIV/AIDS are mobilized as soon as possible after the surgery as they are more susceptible to thromboembolic complications.[6]

## References

1. Naif HM (2013). Pathogenesis of HIV infection. Infectious Disease Reports, 5(Suppl 1):26–30.
2. Madiba TE, Muckart DJJ, Thomson SR (2009). Human immunodeficiency disease: how should it affect surgical decision-making? World Journal of Surgery, 33(5):899–909.
3. Yang D, Zhao H, Gao G, et al. (2014). Relationship between CD4(+) T lymphocyte cell count and the prognosis (including the healing of the incision wound) of HIV/AIDS patients who had undergone surgical operation. Chinese Medical Association Publishing, 35(12):1333–1336.
4. Durvasula R, Miller T (2014). Substance abuse treatment in persons with HIV/AIDS: challenges in managing triple diagnosis. Behavioral Medicine, 40(2):43–52.
5. Naicker S, Rahmania S, Kopp J (2015). HIV and chronic kidney disease. Clinical Nephrology, 83(7, Suppl 1):32–38.
6. Bibas M, Biava G, Antinori A (2011). HIV-associated venous thromboembolism. Mediterranean Journal of Hematology and Infectious Diseases, 3(1):e2011030.

## Further reading

Baid H, Creed F, Hargreaves J (2016). Oxford handbook of critical care nursing (2nd ed). Oxford: Oxford University Press.

McCormack B, McCance T (2017). Person-centred practice in nursing and health care: theory and practice (2nd ed). Chichester: Wiley Blackwell.

National Institute for Health and Care Excellence (2016). HIV testing: increasing uptake among people who may have undiagnosed HIV. NICE guideline [NG60]. Available at: ℘ https://www.nice.org.uk/guidance/ng60

National Institute for Health and Care Excellence (2018). Venous thromboembolism in over 16s: reducing the risk of hospital-acquired deep vein thrombosis or pulmonary embolism. NICE guideline [NG89]. Available at: ℘ https://www.nice.org.uk/guidance/ng89

# Endocrine and metabolic disorders

Examples of endocrine and metabolic disorders include:
- Acromegaly
- Diabetes mellitus
- Hyperkalaemia
- Hypokalaemia
- Hypernatraemia
- Hyponatraemia
- Parathyroid disease
- Cushing's syndrome
- Obesity
- Thyroid disease.

## Diabetes

There are two main types of diabetes:
- *Type 1 diabetes*: occurs when the body is unable to produce insulin; onset is usually before the age of 40 and is the least common of the two types.
- *Type 2 diabetes*: is the most common of the two types and develops when the body doesn't make enough insulin; onset is usually after the age of 40 and is linked to obesity.

The main problem experienced by diabetic patients is blood glucose control. Complications of this are listed in Box 5.6.

---

**Box 5.6 Complications of poor blood glucose control**
- Ischaemic heart disease.
- Retinopathy.
- Peripheral vascular disease.
- Cerebrovascular disease.
- Neuropathy.
- Nephropathy.
- Hypoglycaemia:
  - Blood glucose <3.5 mmol/L.
  - Symptoms include sweating, tachycardia, confusion, unconsciousness, convulsions.
- Hyperglycaemia:
  - Blood glucose up to 20–25 mmol/L.
  - Symptoms include thirst, dehydration.

---

*Preoperative management*
- Diabetes is the most common endocrine disease encountered before surgery.
- Fasting times, the surgical stress response, and inactivity can all have a negative impact on blood sugar control.
- Preoperative fasting times for patients with diabetes should be minimal.
- Diabetic patients should be first on the operating theatre list.
- Short stay surgery and anaesthesia is suitable for patients with well-controlled disease.

- Comprehensive pre-assessment of patient to include monitoring of blood glucose levels, urine analysis, creatinine and electrolytes, and ECG if the patient is >30 years old.
- Regular monitoring of blood sugar levels is essential.
- Locally agreed regimens for blood sugar control of diabetic patients should be in place.
- Risks associated with complications of diabetes should be minimized.

*Anaesthetic management*
- If blood glucose level >10 mmol/L, consider insulin/glucose regimen.
- Rapid sequence induction of GA may be required as diabetic patients are prone to gastric reflux.
- Hypoglycaemia may not be evident during anaesthesia so blood glucose levels should be monitored regularly.
- Regional anaesthesia should be considered for surgery to the extremities.

*Postoperative management*
- Monitoring of blood glucose levels.
- Monitoring of vital signs including TPR, BP, and $SpO_2$.
- Self-managing patients should return to controlling their blood sugars as soon as deemed appropriate.
- Medical staff should inform the patient's GP of their recent admission and procedure to ensure a seamless transition of care and so an appropriate follow-up in primary care can take place.

## Further reading

Levy D (2018). Practical diabetes care (4th ed). Oxford: Wiley-Blackwell.

National Institute for Health and Care Excellence (2017). Type 2 diabetes: prevention in people at high risk. Public health guideline [PH38]. Available at: ℳ https://www.nice.org.uk/guidance/ph38

National Institute for Health and Care Excellence (2020). Diabetes (type 1 and type 2) in children and young people: diagnosis and management. NICE guideline [NG18]. Available at: ℳ https://www.nice.org.uk/guidance/ng18

National Institute for Health and Care Excellence (2020). Type 1 diabetes in adults: diagnosis and management. NICE guideline [NG17]. Available at: ℳ https://www.nice.org.uk/guidance/ng17

National Institute for Health and Care Excellence (2020). Type 2 diabetes in adults: management. NICE guideline [NG28]. Available at: ℳ https://www.nice.org.uk/guidance/ng28

Rodriguez-Saldana J (ed) (2019). The diabetes textbook: clinical principles, patient management and public health issues. New York: Springer.

## Hyponatraemia

- Hyponatraemia is a common electrolyte imbalance that is seen in many different patient cases across the hospital.
- Hyponatraemia is considered when the serum sodium level is below the normal range (normal range is 135–145 mEq/L).
- Complications from hyponatraemia could range from subtle to life-threatening.
- Most patients are asymptomatic.
- A patient who develops hyponatraemia is susceptible to increased mortality, increased morbidity, and it can increase their hospital stay, causing further complications (Box 5.7).

> **Box 5.7 Signs and symptoms of hyponatraemia**
> - Nausea and vomiting.
> - Headache.
> - Seizures.
> - Confusion.
> - Loss of energy, drowsiness, and fatigue.
> - Restlessness and irritability.
> - Muscle weakness, spasms, or cramps.
> - Seizures and coma if severe.

*Preoperative management*
- Locally agreed guidelines should be looked at for guidance.
- Sodium replacement regimens should be followed, as too rapid correction of low sodium levels could be neurologically damaging.
- Diuretics and laxatives should be stopped.
- If a patient has diarrhoea, then this could also be a cause of the decrease in sodium levels, so loperamide should be prescribe to try and manage the diarrhoea.
- If the hyponatraemia is severe or not correcting itself as anticipated, an endocrinologist should be contacted for advice and support.

Preoperative hyponatraemia is an independent risk factor for postoperative mortality in adults.[1]

*Anaesthetic management*
- Standard monitoring equipment: ECG, NIBP, $SpO_2$.
- Propofol and sufentanil.
- Monitor fluid intake and output.

*Postoperative management*
- Monitor sodium levels, as you would monitor all blood levels.
- Fluid replacement should be closely monitored as a patient could become overloaded and find it hard to manage the extra fluid.
- An endocrinologist should be contacted to gain advice on how to manage hyponatraemia and postoperative management.

## Reference

1. Benzon HA, Bobrowski A, Suresh S, et al. (2019). Impact of preoperative hyponatraemia on paediatric perioperative mortality. British Journal of Anaesthesia, *123*(5):618–626.

## Further reading

Hirst C, Allahabadia A, Cosgrove J (2015). The adult patient with hyponatraemia. British Journal of Anaesthesia, *15*(5):248–252.

National Institute for Health and Care Excellence (2020). Hyponatraemia. Available at: ℘ https://cks.nice.org.uk/topics/hyponatraemia/

National Institute for Health and Care Excellence (2020). Intravenous fluid therapy in adults in hospital. Clinical guideline [CG174]. Available at: ℘ https://www.nice.org.uk/guidance/cg174

National Institute for Health and Care Excellence (2020). Perioperative care in adults. NICE guideline [NG180]. Available at: ℘ https://www.nice.org.uk/guidance/ng180

Teran FJ, Simon EE (2006). Epidemiology and significance of hyponatraemia. In: Simon EE (ed) Hyponatraemia: evaluation and treatment (2nd ed). London: Springer.

Spasovski G, Vanholder R, Allolio B, et al. (2014). Clinical practice guideline on diagnosis and treatment of hyponatraemia. Nephrology Dialysis Transplantation, 29(2):i1–i39.

Woodcock T, Barker P, Daniel S, et al. (2020). Guidelines for the management of glucocorticoids during the peri-operative period for patients with adrenal insufficiency: Guidelines from the Association of Anaesthetists, the Royal College of Physicians and the Society for Endocrinology UK. Anaesthesia, 75(5):654–663.

## Hypernatraemia

- Hypernatraemia occurs when the sodium levels are too high in the blood with the levels exceeding 145 mEq/L.
- This could be caused from overuse of normal saline to replace lost fluids which can cause the sodium in people's blood to increase to dangerous levels; to combat this, using alternative solutions to replace lost fluid is advised (e.g. Hartmann's solution) or follow your local guidelines and policies.
- Quick diagnosis can be lifesaving (Box 5.8).
- If not diagnosed quickly, the patient may require intensive care to reverse hypernatraemia.

### Box 5.8 Signs and symptoms of hypernatraemia

Initial signs are:
- Irritability, restlessness, weakness.

Followed by:
- Vomiting, muscular twitching, fever, high-pitched crying and tachypnoea in infants.

Severe signs (develop with acute rise of sodium >160 mmol/L):
- Altered mental status.
- Lethargy.
- Seizures.
- Hyperreflexia.
- Coma.

*Preoperative management*
- Diuretics and laxatives should be stopped.
- If isotonic replacement is not working to reduce the hypernatraemia then dextrose should be used to offload the fluid.
- If there is a history of renal failure or poor renal function then haemodialysis or filtration should be considered.
- If the patient is also hypovolaemic, then monitor urinary output and renal function.

*Anaesthetic management*
- Standard monitoring equipment: ECG, NIBP, $SpO_2$.
- Propofol and sufentanil.
- Monitor fluid intake and output.

*Postoperative management*
- Monitoring sodium levels, as you would monitor all blood levels.
- Fluid replacement should be closely monitored as a patient could become overloaded and find it hard to manage the extra fluid.
- There should be a clearly documented plan for patient care for the next 24 hours and ensure there is a clear monitoring plan for the next doctors to continue and for the nurses to follow.
- The plan should be communicated to look out for early warning signs of what should be looked for, for example, an acceptable heart rate, BP, what National Early Warning Score (NEWS) is acceptable, and when it is appropriate to contact others for further advice.

## Further reading

National Institute for Health and Care Excellence (2017). Intravenous fluid therapy in adults in hospital. Clinical guideline [CG174]. Available at: ℬ https://www.nice.org.uk/guidance/cg174

National Institute for Health and Care Excellence (2020). Hypernatraemia. Available at: ℬ https://cks.nice.org.uk/topics/hypernatraemia/

Woodcock T, Barker P, Daniel S, et al. (2020). Guidelines for the management of glucocorticoids during the peri-operative period for patients with adrenal insufficiency: Guidelines from the Association of Anaesthetists, the Royal College of Physicians and the Society for Endocrinology UK. Anaesthesia, 75(5):654–663.

## Hyperkalaemia

Hyperkalaemia occurs when potassium is above the normal range in a person's blood, this is typically diagnosed when the potassium is ≥5.5 mmol/L.

> Patiromer is a treatment for people with hyperkalaemia and can be used for adults with CKD or heart failure.[1]

*Preoperative management*
- It is important to know the function of the person's kidneys through their estimated glomerular filtration rate.
- It is also good practice to get an ECG to see if there are any abnormalities; this can be made easier if you have a pre-hyperkalaemia ECG to compare it to.
- Insulin-glucose infusions are proven to be the most effective way to lower potassium levels, you need to ensure you do not do this too quickly as this can cause ECG changes.
- Regular monitoring of the patient's ECG, BP, and heart rate should be completed.
- Advice from senior doctors should be sought if you have any questions or doubts about treating hyperkalaemia.
- Low-potassium diet.

*Anaesthetic management*
- Standard monitoring equipment: ECG, NIBP, $SpO_2$.
- Avoid propofol—contraindicated in hyperkalaemia.
- Avoid suxamethonium.
- Monitor fluid intake and output.
- Hyperventilation can decrease serum potassium as it clears acidosis.

- Blood transfusion must be minimal.
- Intraoperative blood loss should be replaced by normal saline 0.9%.
- Intraoperative monitoring of serum potassium, ECG change, capillary glucose level, and urine output will improve patient outcome.[2]

*Postoperative management*

- Postoperative patients are best managed in ITU or HDU settings as they may show signs of acidosis and/or have an electrolyte shift that requires the skills of the doctors and nurses in these areas. These areas will also have local policies that will help manage a patient's conditions after surgery.
- Monitor ECG, respiratory rate, and blood glucose levels.
- Avoid NSAIDs.

## References

1. National Institute for Health and Care Excellence (2020). Patiromer for treating hyperkalaemia. Technology appraisal guidance [TA623]. Available at: ℘ https://www.nice.org.uk/guidance/ta623
2. Lema GF, Tesema HG, Fentie DY, et al. (2019). Evidence-based perioperative management of patients with high serum potassium level in resource-limited areas: a systematic review. International Journal of Surgery Open, 21:21–29.

## Further reading

Alfonzo A, Harrison A, Baines R, et al. (2020). Clinical practice guidelines treatment of acute hyperkalaemia in adults. The Renal Association. Available at: ℘ https://ukkidney.org/sites/renal.org/files/RENAL%20ASSOCIATION%20HYPERKALAEMIA%20GUIDELINE%202020.pdf

National Institute for Health and Care Excellence (2017). Intravenous fluid therapy in adults in hospital. Clinical guideline [CG174]. Available at: ℘ https://www.nice.org.uk/guidance/cg174

National Institute for Health and Care Excellence (2020). Intravenous fluid therapy in children and young people in hospital. NICE guideline [NG29]. Available at: ℘ https://www.nice.org.uk/guidance/ng29

National Institute for Health and Care Excellence (2020). Perioperative care in adults. NICE guideline [NG180]. Available at: ℘ https://www.nice.org.uk/guidance/ng180

Woodcock T, Barker P, Daniel S, et al. (2020). Guidelines for the management of glucocorticoids during the peri-operative period for patients with adrenal insufficiency: Guidelines from the Association of Anaesthetists, the Royal College of Physicians and the Society for Endocrinology UK. Anaesthesia, 75(5):654–663.

# Chapter 6

# Patient safety

# Preoperative preparation for surgery

A preoperative checklist (Table 6.1) must be completed prior to any surgical intervention and it is the responsibility of all surgical and perioperative practitioners to undertake this task. The ward nurse/nurse in charge must ensure that the patient is fully prepared for theatre. Patients should be assessed to ensure adequate preoperative education has been received and that they understand the nature and potential outcome of the surgery. The preoperative checklist should be checked prior to induction of anaesthesia on at least four or five occasions:

- At ward level when the patient is being prepared for surgery.
- Prior to the patient leaving the ward for the operating theatre.
- When the patient arrives at the operating theatre reception.
- When the patient arrives in the anaesthetic room and or operating theatre.

## Patient safety

- Ensure the patient is scheduled for surgery as per theatre list although some variance may occur between elective and emergency procedures.
- Identification band on wrist and ankle.
- Identification band has correct information.
- Preoperative optimization clinic for older people.[1]

## Patient wristbands

Standardizing the design of patient wristbands, the information on them, and the processes used to produce and check them will improve patient safety. Patients' ID wristbands must meet the National Patient Safety Agency design requirements. Clear guidelines from NICE[2] outline how wristbands should be produced, applied, and checked as follows:

- Wristbands should be white with black text and applied to the dominant hand.
- They should be generated and printed from hospital information systems and must include surname, first name, address, date of birth, and ID/NHS number.
- A red wristband should be worn by patients with allergies/reaction and by those who do not wish to receive blood.

## Informed consent

- Must be written, verbal, or implied as all are equally valid in law.
- Consent in writing is infinitely superior as a form of evidence.
- Patients should receive an explanation of the surgery and anaesthetic and the risks involved in both.
- If the patient has any doubt, call the surgical team back.
- Refer to ➲ Chapter 2, for further information.

## Allergy status

- Hypersensitivity—refers to a drug-induced antigen–antibody reaction.
  - Type I—anaphylactic reaction.
  - Type IV—delayed reaction.
- This must be identified to theatre staff by use of a prominent red band.
- Such allergies and reactions include medicines (antibiotics), latex, tape (sticky plasters) food (particularly eggs due to propofol administration), and skin preparation (iodine).

**Table 6.1** Preoperative checklist

| Ward: Name: Address: | ID No.: | Contact No.: |
|---|---|---|
| Consultant: | Age: | |
| | DOB: | |
| **Allergies/reactions**<br>Drug/food/tape/latex/skin prep/other | Weight:<br>Height:<br>Urinalysis:<br>Blood glucose: | NIBP:<br>Pulse:<br>RR:<br>$SpO_2$: |
| Preferred name:<br>Preferred language:<br>Interpreter required: Yes/no<br>Communication barriers: Yes/no<br>State: | ASA score:<br>NEWS score:<br>Covid-19 status:<br>Frailty score:<br>Sensory impairment: Yes/no | State of consciousness:<br>Alert/drowsy/confused<br>Agitated/unconscious |

| *To be completed at ward level and prior to leaving; on arrival at theatre reception; in the anaesthetic room and/or operating theatre; and prior to premedication if applicable* | **Ward nurse**<br>**Initials**<br>**Yes/No/NA** | **Theatre reception**<br>**Initials**<br>**Yes/No/NA** | **Anaesthetic room**<br>**Initials**<br>**Yes/No/NA** | **Operating theatre**<br>**Initials**<br>**Yes/No/NA** |
|---|---|---|---|---|
| Correct patient for surgery; ID bands ×2 checked | | | | |
| Surgical consent form: completed, correct, signed | | | | |
| Anaesthetic consent form: completed, correct, signed | | | | |

(continued)

**Table 6.1 (Contd.)**

| | |
|---|---|
| Surgical site prepped, marked, and correct | |
| Surgical site shaved if applicable | |
| Fasting status: last time food eaten | |
| Fasting status: last time fluids taken | |
| Urine voided (time): or urinary catheter *in situ* | |
| Bowel preparation: type/time | |
| Teeth: own/loose/caps/crowns/bridge | |
| Dentures: top/bottom/both/loose | |
| Hearing aid: with patient/left on ward | |
| Spectacles: with patient/left on ward | |
| Contact lenses: removed | |
| Jewellery/body piercings: taped/removed | |
| Cosmetics/nail polish/acrylic nails: removed | |
| Prosthesis/implant: type and location | |
| VTE prophylaxis: type and location | |
| Preoperative shower | |
| Medication chart | |
| Medical and nursing records | |

IV fluid therapy chart

X-rays/scans (to accompany patient)

Pregnancy status

Blood results, group and save/cross-match/INR

Identify relevant surgical issues to consider:

**Print name, designation, and time of check**

**Ward nurse:**

**Theatre reception:**

**Anaesthetic assistant:**

**Theatre nurse/ODP:**

### Teeth and dentures

- Dental crowns, caps, bridges, and loose teeth must be identified and recorded as these may be damaged, dislodged, or inhaled during intubation.
- Some anaesthetists allow dentures that are securely fitted to remain *in situ* as this can improve the structure of the airway.
- Problems can occur with an oropharyngeal airway and this may need to be replaced with a nasal airway.

### Patient's weight

- The patient's weight must be documented on the prescription chart.
- The weight of paediatric and elderly patients must be recorded— anaesthetic drugs are calculated according to the weight of these patients.

### References

1. Royal College of Anaesthetists (2020). Chapter 10: guidelines for the provision of paediatric anaesthesia services. London: Royal College of Anaesthetists.
2. National Institute for Health and Care Excellence (2020). Perioperative care in adults. NICE guideline [NG180]. Available at: ℛ https://www.nice.org.uk/guidance/ng180

### Further reading

Yentis SM, Hartle AJ, Barker IR, et al. (2017). AAGBI: consent for anaesthesia 2017: Association of Anaesthetists of Great Britain and Ireland. Anaesthesia, 72(1):93–105.

# Jewellery and body piercing

All jewellery should be removed and kept on the ward or given to relatives, although wedding rings can remain but should be securely taped. Jewellery has the potential to transmit bacteria and fungi to an open wound.

- All metal jewellery carries electrical conduction risks (e.g. electrosurgical cautery).
- Care should be taken if a patient wishes to keep jewellery on for religious reasons; these should be securely taped to avoid injury to the patient and/or perioperative personnel.
- Swelling is common postoperatively, so rings, where possible, should be removed.

Nursing and medical staff are constantly faced with various types of body piercing. Although each health board/NHS trust usually has its own set of guidelines, each case should be addressed individually and sensitively according to the type of anaesthesia or surgical procedure. There are a number of types of jewellery used for body piercing as follows:

- *Labret stud*—a straight bar with a fixed flat end and an unscrewable ball on the other end.
- *Barbell*—a straight, curved, or circular bar with an unscrewable ball at one end.
- *Captive ring*—an open ring in which a ball with two small dimples is inserted and the ball is clicked into position and held in place.
- *Flesh tunnel*—a ring inserted through a hole, usually the ear, to enlarge the hole in the skin.

A general guide for body piercing is that if it is not in the way, and does not interfere with anaesthesia or the surgical site/procedure, leave it alone. However, it is important to ensure that piercings are secure and documented. If body jewellery is to be removed, the best person to undertake this task is the patient.

### Risk assessment

- Body piercings have the potential to be caught and/or ripped by ECG leads, drapes, surgical clips, or instruments.
- There is an increased risk of pressure to chin/lip causing soft tissue damage from anaesthetic masks or nipple-piercing pressure if the patient is to lie prone.
- This should be assessed and documented by the anaesthetic practitioner prior to commencement of anaesthesia.

### Surgical procedures

- Body piercings should generally be removed if they are in close proximity to the surgical site or any other associated procedure (Table 6.2).
- However, this is ultimately the decision of the anaesthetist and/or surgeon.

*Tongue and lip piercing*
- All tongue and lip jewellery should be removed before a GA but advice should be sought from the anaesthetist.
- Barbells may cause obstruction to the airway during anaesthesia.
- Tongue labrets can contain a gemstone which is at risk of falling out and entering the airway as they are only glued in.

*Nasal and naval piercing*
- Nasal septum, nose, or ear piercing should be removed if the patient is to have ENT surgery.
- Naval and breast piercing should be removed for laparoscopic or breast surgery.

*Male genital piercing*
- Penile piercing can be pulled to one side if the patient requires a urinary catheter.
- For urological surgery it should be removed.

*Female genital piercing*
- The site of piercing should be assessed for surgical access.
- It should be removed if it is likely to hinder the type of surgery to be performed.
- It does not have to be removed if the surgical procedure is elsewhere on the body.

If there are signs of infection around the piercing site, it must be removed. Treatment for the infection may precede the surgery.

**Table 6.2** Examples of body piercing positions

| Body part | Position |
| --- | --- |
| Ear | Lobes, tragus, helix, conch, orbital, industrial, daith, rook |
| Nose | Septum, septril, nostril, bridge, nasallang, rhino |
| Tongue | Inch from tip in centre, uvula, tongue web |
| Lip | Bottom or top—labret, medusa, cyber bite |
| Face | Chin, eyebrow, cheek |
| Navel | Round, vertical, light bulb |
| Female nipple | Base of nipple |
| Male nipple | Placed well into areola |
| Female genitals | Labia majora, labia minora, clitoris, horizontal and vertical hood |
| Male genitals | Foreskin, frenum, lorum |

*If the body piercing remains for the surgical procedure*
- The site and type of piercing should be documented on the preoperative checklist.
- A check should be made in the postoperative period to ensure it is still *in situ*, which should also be documented.

In the event that a patient decides not to remove piercings, jewellery or acrylic nails, then a consent form should be signed by the patient stating that all associated risks are accepted and the health board/NHS trust would not be liable for any injuries caused.

## Further reading

Delaisse J, Varada S, Au SC, et al. (2014). Perioperative management of the patient with body piercings. Journal of Dermatology and Clinical Research, 2(1):1–4.

Holbrook J, Minocha J, Laumann A (2012). Body piercing: complications and prevention of health risks. American Journal of Clinical Dermatology 13(1):1–17.

Marenzi B (2004). Body piercing: a patient safety issue. Journal of Perianaesthesia Nursing, 19(1):4–10.

Mercier FJ, Bonnett MP (2009). Tattooing and various piercing: anaesthetic considerations. Current Opinion in Anaesthesiology, 22(3):436–441.

Meyer D (2000). Body piercing: old traditions creating new challenges. Journal of Emergency Nursing, 26(6):612–614.

National Institute for Health and Care Excellence (2020). Perioperative care in adults. NICE guideline [NG180]. Available at: ℘ https://www.nice.org.uk/guidance/ng180

Royal College of Anaesthetists (2020). Chapter 10: guidelines for the provision of paediatric anaesthesia services. London: Royal College of Anaesthetists.

Yentis SM, Hartle AJ, Barker IR, et al. (2017). AAGBI: consent for anaesthesia 2017: Association of Anaesthetists of Great Britain and Ireland. Anaesthesia, 72(1):93–105.

# Cosmetics, nail polish, and other considerations

## Cosmetics

Foundation and lipstick may disguise changes in the patient's colour (e.g. cyanosis). Coloured and clear nail vanish can distort or disguise changes in the patient's peripheral colour.

## Nail polish

- Nail polish is routinely removed prior to surgery but the research is inconsistent regarding the reason for this.
- Previously it was suggested that nail polish affected the efficacy of pulse oximeters in that they distorted the actual reading.

---

- Pulse oximeters work based on different absorption of red light by oxygenated and non-oxygenated Hb.

---

- Previous research suggested nail polish can reduce pulse oximeter reading by 2–6%; blue and brown polish caused the largest variances but no colours had variances >1%, within 2% clinical threshold.[1]
- Hinkelbein et al.[2] found that nail polish did not alter pulse oximetry readings in mechanically ventilated patients to a clinically relevant extent although they did advise it might be appropriate in some cases to decrease potential error of measurement.
- More recently, it has been found that fingernail polish does not cause a clinically significant change in pulse oximeter readings in healthy people.[3]
- A study by Yeganehkhah et al.[4] investigated the effect of different colours of glittered nail polishes on $SpO_2$ measurements. Although glitter particles in nail polish could affect the light absorption of haemoglobin, the authors concluded that different colours of glittered nail polishes did not affect pulse oximetry measurements in healthy subjects; therefore, they argued that it is not necessary to remove the glittered nail polish routinely in clinical, surgical, and emergency settings.

## Acrylic nails

- Artificial acrylic nails remain fashionable and are used to strengthen and lengthen nails.
- Acrylic nails are an extension on the natural nail and are a combination of a liquid monomer and a powder polymer. They create a hard protective layer over natural nails.
- Back in 1997, Peters[5] investigated the effects of unpolished acrylic nails on $SpO_2$ measurement using a sample of 30 women, aged 18–61 years and found no statistical difference existed between readings.
- A recent study revealed that nail treatments do not affect readings of patients' oxygen levels. Of the treatments examined (nail polish and acrylic nails), neither caused >1% variation in $SpO_2$ readings. Additionally, neither nail polish nor acrylic nails resulted in an $SpO_2$ of <95%, at which intervention with oxygen therapy is recommended.[3]

Recent study results contradict the view widely held by many medical personnel that nail polish and artificial nails must be removed to obtain an accurate measurement of oxygen saturation.[3]

## Gel nails

- Gel-based manicures have gained popularity in recent years due to their attractiveness and longevity.
- They are not an extension of natural nails but a polish that can last for up to 2 weeks and is cured under an ultraviolet (UV) light.
- Gel polish can be difficult to remove, and the process involves soaking nails in acetone and buffing off the polish.
- A study by Yek et al.[6] evaluated the effect of gel-based nails with two oximeters, using different technology and wavelength combinations.
- Gel-based manicures can result in overestimations of actual readings, delaying detection of hypoxaemia. The authors advise that gel nail polish should be routinely removed prior to surgery or an alternative monitoring technique sought.

## Polygel nails

- Polygel can be applied as an overlay on natural nails, or as a nail enhancement.
- It is cured under a UV light, but it is a lot lighter than both gel and acrylic nails.
- To remove polygel nails, the polish is buffed off rather than soaked off.
- There is no research regarding polygel nails and oxygen levels at the time of writing.

## Prosthetic devices

- Some prosthesis should normally be removed for safe keeping and retained on the ward.
- The removal of devices such as wigs, false eyes, glasses, contact lenses, and artificial limbs can cause distress to patients and it is not always necessary to remove these.
- Maintaining patients' dignity is essential so the necessity for removal should be discussed with the anaesthesia and/or surgical team and the patient; if removal is necessary, a prosthesis can be removed immediately prior to anaesthesia and replaced in the recovery room.
- It is often practical to allow patients to retain hearing aids for induction, reversal, and post-anaesthetic care.
- Some prosthetic devices such as orthopaedic implants should be documented appropriately and brought to the attention of perioperative personnel.

## Surgical site marking

- Wrong-site surgery is a never event and a serious, preventable patient safety incident.[7]
- Although surgery performed at an incorrect site is rare, when it happens it can be devastating for patients and their families.
- The NHS Improvement and the Royal College of Surgeons (RCS) developed national guidelines for implementation across the NHS, which are shown in Table 6.3.[8]

**Table 6.3** RCS guidelines for surgical site marking

| How to mark | Indelible marker pen |
| --- | --- |
| Where to mark | Mark at or near intended incision |
| Who marks | Operating surgeon/other present |
| With whom | Patient/carer involvement |
| Time and place | Mark on day of surgery |
| Verify | Documented by surgeon, check by nurse |

## Surgical skin preparation

- Shower or bath to prepare skin.
- Operation site marked correctly.
- Hair removal at the operative site is mostly carried out according to surgeon's preference.
- Research shows it is preferable to remove hair as near as possible to the time of surgery.
- ➲ See Chapter 13 for additional information.

## Shaving

- Close skin shaving can cause soft tissue abrasions and cuts which can encourage growth of bacteria.
- Depilatory creams are not widely used due to localized skin reactions.
- Electric shavers are preferred as they cause less trauma to skin.
- Razors can increase the risk of infection.
- ➲ See Chapter 13 for additional information.

## Premedication

Due to the difficulty of timing premedication to optimize effectiveness, there is a tendency to use them less frequently. However, they may be prescribed for the following reasons:

- Prophylactic antibiotic therapy.
- Prophylactic antiemetic therapy.
- Postoperative analgesia (e.g. diclofenac *per rectum* (PR)).
- Sedative agents to reduce patient anxiety.

## References

1. Rodden AM, Spicer L, Diaz VA, et al. (2007). Does fingernail polish affect pulse oximeter readings? Intensive and Critical Care Nursing, 23(1):51–55.
2. Hinkelbein J, Genzwuerker HV, Sogl R, et al. (2007). Effect of nail polish on oxygen saturation determined by pulse oximetry in critically ill patients. Resuscitation, 72(1):82–91.
3. Purcell J, Mannion S (2018). Medical fashion victims? Do nail polishes and acrylic nails affect digital pulse oximetry and patient management in the clinical setting? European Journal of Anaesthesiology, 35(e-Suppl 56):01AP05-1.
4. Yeganehkhah M, Dadkhahtehrani T, Bagheri A, et al. (2019). Effect of glittered nail polish on pulse oximetry measurements in healthy subjects. Iranian Journal of Nursing and Midwifery Research, 24(1):25–29.
5. Peters SM (1997). The effect of acrylic nails on the measurement of oxygen saturation as determined by pulse oximetry. American Association of Nurse Anaesthetists Journal 65(4):361–363.

6. Yek JLJ, Abdullah HR, Goh JPS, et al. (2019). The effects of gel-based manicure on pulse oximetry. Singapore Medical Journal 60(8):432–435.
7. Bathla S, Chadwick M, Nevins EJ, et al. (2017). Preoperative site marking: are we adhering to good surgical practice? Journal of Patient Safety, 17(6):e503–e508.
8. Royal College of Surgeons (2013). Good surgical practice: a guide to good practice. Available at: ℜ https://www.rcseng.ac.uk/standards-and-research/gsp/

## Further reading

Boyd-Carson H, Gana T, Lockwood S, et al. (2020). A review of surgical and peri-operative factors to consider in emergency laparotomy care. Anaesthesia, 2020;75(Suppl 1):e75–e82.
National Institute for Health and Care Excellence (2020). Perioperative care in adults. NICE guideline [NG180]. Available at: ℜ https://www.nice.org.uk/guidance/ng180
Royal College of Anaesthetists (2020). Chapter 10: guidelines for the provision of paediatric anaesthesia services. London: Royal College of Anaesthetists.
Yentis SM, Hartle AJ, Barker IR, et al. (2017). AAGBI: consent for anaesthesia 2017: Association of Anaesthetists of Great Britain and Ireland. Anaesthesia, 72(1):93–105.

# Preoperative fasting

The purpose of fasting patients preoperatively is to minimize the volume of gastric contents and reduce the risk of regurgitation and aspiration during anaesthesia. Fasting guidelines from NICE[1] are:

- Solid food (milk and milky drinks)—6 hours
- Breastfed infants—4 hours
- Clear fluids (water, black tea, and black coffee):
  - 2 hours for adults
  - 1 hour for children.

> It is widely recognized that prolonged fasting for elective surgery in both children and adults can be detrimental and can adversely affects patient well-being.[2]

- The chewing of gum is controversial but the pragmatic approach is to treat it as if it were an oral fluid and prohibit for 2 hours preoperatively.
- Many studies have emphasized the harmful effects of prolonged fasting but patients continue to be deprived of food and drink for excessively long periods (Table 6.4). This has led to much deviation from clinical practice guidelines.

Hewson and Moppett[3] outline potential reasons for disparity between guidelines and clinical reality in preoperative eating and drinking:

- Risk aversion on the part of staff and patients that pulmonary aspiration may occur despite following guidance.
- Poor professional and organizational incentivization to implement and disseminate best practice.
- Deficits in knowledge among staff and patients.

They also point out that the decision-making of multiple staff can lead to further prolongation of fasting times.

Morrison et al.[4] discussed how the 2-hour fasting time for clear fluids can translate into a considerably longer fasting time in reality. They discuss how:

- Prolonged fasting of clear fluids is unnecessary, and results in patient dissatisfaction and discomfort, and potentially causes harm
- Prolonged fasting does not reliably result in an empty stomach; having a drink of water may reduce residual gastric volumes and increase pH a short time later
- If regurgitation and aspiration of clear fluid occurs, it is unlikely to result in morbidity.

There is evidence to suggest that patients who fast for long periods during the preoperative phase often recover slowly postoperatively:

- Prolonged fasting can have both physical and psychological implications postoperatively and is particularly harmful in small children and elderly, infirm patients.
- Altered digestion can occur with pain, injury, and opiate analgesia.

The benefits of implementing evidence-based preoperative fasting times are outlined below and include a decreased incidence of:

- Dehydration
- Headache
- Postoperative nausea and vomiting
- Hunger and thirst
- Anxiety and discomfort.

**Table 6.4** Implications of prolonged fasting

| Physical | Psychological |
|----------|---------------|
| Dehydration | Anxiety |
| Catabolism | Discomfort |
| Nausea | Irritability |
| Vomiting | Electrolyte imbalance |
| Hypoglycaemia | Ketosis |

## Dehydration

- Dehydration is an excessive loss of fluid and minerals from the body and it can be described as mild, moderate, or severe. Nurses/ODPs must be cognisant of the risk of fluid imbalance and patients should be monitored for signs of dehydration.
- Postoperative fluid replacement is often prescribed to counteract fasting and blood loss.
- Patients who remain fasted following surgery will often be administered IV fluid to avoid dehydration.
- Water, as a means of hydration, can reduce confusion and headache so it is therefore essential that patients are not fasted longer than the recommended timescale.

*Stages and symptoms of dehydration*
- Mild—headache, lack of energy, tiredness.
- Moderate—dry mouth, decreased alertness, sunken eyes, muscle cramps.
- Severe—confusion, disorientated, tachycardia, tachypnoea.

## Nausea and vomiting

- Prolonged fasting preoperatively can cause nausea and vomiting in the postoperative period, and reintroducing oral fluid postoperatively can sometimes be equally problematic.
- If patients are nauseous on induction of anaesthesia, this is likely to persist into the postoperative period.
- The Royal College of Nursing (RCN) recommends that postoperative patients should be encouraged to drink when they are ready, providing there are no medical or surgical contraindications.

## Headache

- Preoperative fasting can be associated with postoperative headache and the interruption of daily caffeine consumption can cause caffeine withdrawal headache.

- Dehydration, prolonged preoperative fasting, and caffeine withdrawal can cause headaches during the perioperative period.
- Caffeine normally induces vasoconstriction; acute withdrawal in those with a high daily intake will cause rebound vasodilatation and headache.
- Prophylactic administration of caffeine tablets might be considered for surgical patients who are accustomed to a high daily intake of caffeine.

## Hypoglycaemia

Hypoglycaemia occurs when the blood glucose decreases to 2.7–3.3 mmol/L and can be caused by too much insulin, excessive physical activity, or too little food.

- The clinical manifestations of mild-to-moderate hypoglycaemia can include sweating, tachycardia, nervousness, hunger, headache, confusion, light-headedness, and drowsiness.
- Elderly patients are at an increased risk of dehydration.
- Patients who are prescribed insulin or insulin secretion-stimulating medication may experience hypoglycaemia as a result of perioperative fasting.

## References

1. National Institute for Health and Care Excellence (2020). Perioperative care in adults – evidence review for pre-operative fasting. NICE guideline [NG180]. Available at: ℘ https://www.nice.org.uk/guidance/ng180
2. Fawcett WJ, Thomas M (2019). Pre-operative fasting in adults and children: clinical practice and guidelines. Anaesthesia, 74(1):83–88.
3. Hewson DW, Moppett I (2020). Preoperative fasting and prevention of pulmonary aspiration in adults: research feast, quality improvement famine. British Journal of Anaesthesia, 124(4):361–363.
4. Morrison CE, Ritchie-McLean S, Jha A, et al. (2020). Two hours too long: time to review fasting guidelines for clear fluids. British Journal of Anaesthesia, 124(4):363–366.

## Further reading

Craig A, Hatfield A (2020). The complete recovery room book (6th ed). Oxford: Oxford University Press.

Freedman R, Herbert L, O'Donnell A, et al. (eds) (2022). Oxford handbook of anaesthesia (5th ed). Oxford: Oxford University Press.

Gan TJ, Belani KG, Bergese S, et al. (2019). Fourth consensus guidelines for the management of postoperative nausea and vomiting. Anesthesia and Analgesia, 131(2):411–448.

Hampl KF, Schneider MC, Ruttimann U, et al. (1995). Perioperative administration of caffeine tablets for prevention of postoperative headaches. Canadian Journal of Anesthesia, 42(9):789–792.

Longchamp A, Harputlugil E, Corpataux JM, et al. (2017). Is overnight fasting before surgery too much or not enough? How basic aging research can guide preoperative nutritional recommendations to improve surgical outcomes: a mini-review. Gerontology, 63(3):228–237.

Matsota PK, Christodoulopoulou TC, Batistaki CZ, et al. (2017). Factors associated with the presence of postoperative headache in elective surgery patients: a prospective single center cohort study. Journal of Anesthesia, 31(2):225–236.

National Institute for Health and Care Excellence (2020). Intravenous fluid therapy in children and young people in hospital. NICE guideline [NG29]. Available at: ℘ https://www.nice.org.uk/guidance/ng29

Royal College of Anaesthetists (2021). Chapter 2: guidelines for the provision of anaesthesia services for preoperative assessment and preparation. London: Royal College of Anaesthetists.

Royal College of Nursing (2005). Perioperative fasting in adults and children: an RCN guideline for the multidisciplinary team. London: Royal College of Nursing.

Smith I, Kranke P, Murat I, et al. (2011). Perioperative fasting in adults and children: guidelines from the European Society of Anaesthesiology. European Journal of Anaesthesiology, 28(8):556–569.

# Patient safety: surgical safety checklist

In 2008, the WHO launched its campaign 'Safe Surgery Saves Lives' to reduce the number of errors occurring in surgery.

- The focus of the campaign, which remains in operation was the surgical
  safety checklist.[1]
- During each phase, the WHO emphasized that a checklist coordinator
  must confirm that the surgical team has completed the listed tasks
  before proceeding with the procedure.
- The checklists must be conducted by teams of healthcare professionals
  who have trained together and who have received appropriate
  education in the human factors that underpin safe teamwork.[2]

---

- Safety is of paramount importance in surgery. Effective team working
  is an essential component in maximizing safety and avoiding adverse
  incidents.[3]

---

- The checklist has been shown to improve outcomes in surgery by
  standardizing care and reinforcing safety processes but it is only a device
  to promote systemic change and prompt safer behaviour.
- Like all tools, its effectiveness depends on skilful use.[2]
- It must be used prior to all surgical procedures, including dental
  procedures.[4]
- The checklist has been expanded to comprise five steps (Table 6.5) of a
  surgical procedure.[3]
- NICE[4] recommends adding further steps to the WHO surgical safety
  checklist as necessary to eliminate preventable events.
- All surgeons should lead on the implementation of the 'five steps'
  within their teams in order to ensure safety, improve efficiency of the
  operating list, enrich the trainee experience, and build team morale.[3]

## References

1. World Health Organization (2009). WHO guidelines for safe surgery. Geneva: World Health
   Organization.
2. NHS England (2019). National safety standards for invasive procedures (NatSSIPs).
   London: Department of Health and Social Care.
3. Royal College of Surgeons (2014). Ensuring consistency in patient safety. London: Royal College
   of Surgeons.
4. National Institute for Health and Care Excellence (2020). Perioperative care in adults – evidence
   review for pre-operative fasting. NICE guideline [NG180]. Available at: ℘ https://www.nice.org.
   uk/guidance/ng180

**Table 6.5** Five steps of patient safety

| | |
|---|---|
| **Team briefing** | All members of the surgical team should attend the team briefing at the beginning of the list to ensure a shared understanding of the requirements of that list, identify skill levels, staffing, and equipment requirements, and prepare for anticipated problems |
| **Sign in** | Used prior to induction of anaesthesia and allows the team to ensure that the patient's known allergies have been checked and that the surgical site on the patient's body has been properly marked and will be visible in the operative field after draping |
| **Time out** | Used prior to skin incision and enables members of the wider theatre team to introduce themselves and identify any concerns at this stage |
| **Sign out** | Used prior to the patient leaving the operating theatre and ensures that instruments, sponges, and needles have been counted to ensure that none have been left behind in the patient's body |
| **Debriefing** | All members of the surgical team should participate in a discussion at the end of the operating list, or at the end of the session, to consider good points of the operating process and teamwork, review any issues that occurred, answer concerns that the team may have, and identify areas for improvement |

## Further reading

Freedman R, Herbert L, O'Donnell A, et al. (eds) (2022). Oxford handbook of anaesthesia (5th ed). Oxford: Oxford University Press.

Jain D, Sharma R, Reddy S (2018). WHO safe surgery checklist: barriers to universal acceptance. Journal of Anaesthesiology, Clinical Pharmacology, 34(1):7–10.

Royal College of Nursing (2005). Perioperative fasting in adults and children: an RCN guideline for the multidisciplinary team. London: Royal College of Nursing.

Royal College of Anaesthetists (2021). Chapter 2: guidelines for the provision of anaesthesia services for preoperative assessment and preparation. London: Royal College of Anaesthetists.

# Venous thromboembolism

Venous thromboembolism (VTE) is the formation of a blood clot in a vein which, on occasion, may dislodge and give rise to an embolism.

- A pulmonary embolus (PE) is the result of the deep vein thrombosis (DVT) breaking off and travelling through the right side of the heart into the pulmonary circulation, leading to an infarct within the lung tissue.
- A DVT is a clot that forms mostly in the deep veins of the legs or pelvis.

The deep veins in the leg that are likely to be affected include:
- Great saphenous vein
- Femoral vein
- Popliteal vein
- Deep veins of the knee.

If a VTE occurs, it is usually diagnosed 3–14 days postoperatively.
- There is an increased risk of developing VTE with middle-aged and elderly patients, patients on prolonged bed rest, and following major surgery of the lower abdomen pelvis or hip joints (Box 6.1).
- All patients should be individually assessed at pre-assessment clinic and on admission to hospital to identify the risk of developing a VTE.[1]
- They should also be provided with written and oral information on the signs and symptoms of VTE.

---

**Box 6.1  Patient risk factors for VTE**

- Cancer treatment.
- Cardiac/respiratory failure.
- Acute medical illness.
- Burn patients.
- Age >60 years.
- Immobility.
- Obesity—BMI >30 kg/m².
- Pregnancy.
- Familial.
- Smoking.
- Use of oral contraceptives/ hormone replacement therapy (HRT).
- Varicose veins.
- Previous VTE.
- Severe infection.
- Continuous travel of >3 hours 4 weeks pre/post surgery.
- Confined to bed.
- Dehydration.

---

## Signs and symptoms of DVT

- Leg or arm swelling that comes on without warning.
- Pain or soreness when you stand or walk.
- Warmth in the area that hurts.
- Enlarged veins.
- Skin that looks red or blue.

## Signs and symptoms of PE

- Shortness of breath.
- Chest pain that worsens on inspiration.
- Coughing up blood.
- Higher heart rate.

## Prophylactic treatment of VTE

For indications see Box 6.2.

---

**Box 6.2 Indications for VTE prophylaxis**

- Bariatric surgery.
- Surgery in older people.
- Critical care patients.
- Cardiac/vascular surgery.
- Thoracic surgery.
- Spinal surgery.
- Neurosurgery:
  - Craniotomy.
- Non-obstetric surgery:
  - Caesarean section in high-risk patients.
- High-risk patients in trauma and orthopaedic surgery:
- Total knee replacement, total hip replacement, hip fracture surgery.

---

There are two main forms of prophylactic treatment to reduce the risk of VTE:

*Mechanical treatment*
- Intermittent pneumatic compression.
- Antiembolism compression stockings, which work by promoting venous flow and reducing stasis. They should not be prescribed to patients with:
  - Suspected or proven peripheral arterial disease
  - Severe leg oedema
  - Dermatitis, gangrene, or recent skin graft peripheral arterial bypass grafting
  - Peripheral neuropathy or other causes of sensory impairment
  - Fragile 'tissue paper' skin
  - Major limb deformity or unusual leg size or shape preventing correct fit.[1]

*Pharmacological treatment*
- Anticoagulant therapy with low-molecular-weight heparin (LMWH) for immediate effect, followed by warfarin in the long term to reduce the risk of recurrence.
- Antiplatelet drugs will decrease platelet aggregation and inhibit thrombus formation; they are usually effective in the arterial circulation, where anticoagulants have little effect.
- Aspirin, an antiplatelet drug, provides some protection against VTE but is considered less effective than other pharmacological methods.

'Mechanical methods of VTE prophylaxis, including graduated compression stockings, intermittent pneumatic compression devices, and venous foot pumps, should be available for any procedure that lasts more than one hour, and for all patients receiving general anaesthesia.'[2]

NICE recommends that both methods of treatment (mechanical and pharmacological) should be considered for all patients to reduce the incidence of VTE.

Early ambulation should be encouraged following surgery. Adequate analgesia postoperatively will encourage early mobilization and will also decrease the risk of VTE.

Patients should be encouraged to continue the use of compression stockings until normal mobility has been restored.

## Anaesthesia and VTE

- In the perioperative environment, the immobility of the patient during anaesthesia can deprive the deep veins in the legs of the pumping action of the calf muscles, causing pooling of venous blood and venous dilation that can predispose the patient to thrombosis formation.
- Regional anaesthesia can further reduce the risk of VTE in comparison to GA.

## References

1. National Institute for Health and Care Excellence (2019). Venous thromboembolism in over 16s: reducing the risk of hospital-acquired deep vein thrombosis or pulmonary embolism. NICE guideline [NG89]. Available at: ℘ https://www.nice.org.uk/guidance/ng89
2. Royal College of Anaesthetists (2020). Chapter 17: guidelines for the provision of anaesthesia services for burn and plastics surgery. London: Royal College of Anaesthetists.

## Further reading

Afshari A, Ageno W, Ahmed A, et al. (2018). European Guidelines on perioperative venous thromboembolism prophylaxis. European Journal of Anaesthesiology, 35(2):77–83.

Craig A, Hatfield A (2020). The complete recovery room book (6th ed). Oxford: Oxford University Press.

Freedman R, Herbert L, O'Donnell A, et al. (eds) (2022). Oxford handbook of anaesthesia (5th ed). Oxford: Oxford University Press.

Harrison R, Daly L (2006). Acute medical emergencies: a nursing guide (2nd ed). London: Churchill Livingstone.

Illingworth C, Timmons S (2007). An audit of intermittent pneumatic compression (IPC) in the prophylaxis of asymptomatic deep vein thrombosis (DVT). Journal of Perioperative Practice, 17(11):522–528.

Joint Formulary Committee (2021). British national formulary. Available at: ℘ https://bnf.nice.org.uk/

National Institute for Health and Care Excellence (2020). Perioperative care in adults. NICE guideline [NG180]. Available at: ℘ https://www.nice.org.uk/guidance/ng180

National Institute for Health and Care Excellence (2020). Venous thromboembolic diseases: diagnosis, management and thrombophilia testing. NICE guideline [NG158]. Available at: ℘ https://www.nice.org.uk/guidance/ng158

Royal College of Anaesthetists (2019). Chapter 3: guidelines for the provision of anaesthesia services for intraoperative care. London: Royal College of Anaesthetists.

Royal College of Anaesthetists (2019). Chapter 4: guidelines for the provision of postoperative care. London: Royal College of Anaesthetists.

# Enhanced Recovery After Surgery (ERAS)

- ERAS is an evidenced-based, multimodal, patient-centred pathway aiming to optimize the surgical outcome of patients undergoing major surgery by improving both patient experience and clinical outcomes.[1-3]
- It consists of a selected number of individual interventions which demonstrate an improvement in patient outcomes when implemented together, rather than when implemented as isolated interventions.[2,4-6]
- ERAS can therefore be classified as a multimodal, evidence 'care bundle' approach, which is defined by the Institute of Healthcare Improvement as:
  - 'A small set of evidence-based interventions for a defined patient segment/population and care setting that, when implemented together, will result in significantly better outcomes than when implemented individually'.[7]

## Care bundles

- Care bundles are a group of key drivers or interventions that are evidence based and considered to have the highest impact on patient outcomes following surgery.[3]
- To comply with a specific pathway, all the interventions within the pathway must be performed together.
- Each care bundle/pathway typically includes 15–20 elements or components combined to form a multimodal pathway/guideline.
- These elements span through the continuum of the preoperative, intraoperative, and postoperative periods.
- When used together in a complementary fashion they can decrease postoperative stress responses, thereby reducing duration of postoperative ileus, surgical complications, incisional pain, recovery time, and length of hospital stay.[8,9]
- Studies have revealed that ERAS care pathways can reduce surgical stress, maintain postoperative physiological function, and enhance mobilization after surgery.
- Evidence suggests that utilizing ERAS pathways has resulted in reduced rates of morbidity, faster recovery, and shorter length of stay in hospital which can ultimately lead to an improved outcome for the patient.[3,10-13]
- The use of an ERAS pathway[14,15] has been shown to:
  - Reduce care time by >30%
  - Reduce postoperative complications by up to 50%.

> The ERAS Society has developed and published guidelines which have been tailored to specific surgical fields. These can be found at: ℘ http://erassociety.org/guidelines/list-of-guidelines/

ERAS covers all aspects of the patient's journey. The main principles include[16]:

- *Preoperative strategies*: preoperative strategies of ERAS protocols involve medical risk evaluation and patient education.
- *Intraoperative strategies*: intraoperative strategies in ERAS protocols include selection of anaesthetic agents and techniques, lung-protective ventilation, fluid management, temperature regulation, and choice of the surgical approach.

- *Postoperative strategies*: postoperative goals in ERAS protocols include prevention and relief of pain or nausea and vomiting, and facilitation of early nutrition and mobilization.

Some of the main factors that keep patients in the hospital after surgery include the need for parenteral analgesia, the need for IV fluids secondary to gut dysfunction, bed rest, and poor nutrition.[3]

- The key elements of the ERAS pathway address these factors, helping to highlight how they interact to enhance the patient's recovery.
- While all the factors may have a positive impact on the patient's care, to achieve maximum benefit, all of these components—that is, a curtailed preoperative fasting, with carbohydrate loading, pre-emptive analgesia, early postoperative mobilization, timely nutrition, and fluids postoperatively—should be combined and delivered to all patients.
- Additionally, the ERAS pathway provides guidance to all involved in the perioperative care of the patient, thus enabling them to work as a well-coordinated team to provide the best care.[3]
- See Box 6.3.

---

**Box 6.3  Benefits of ERAS**

*For patients*

- It helps people to recover sooner so that life can return to normal as quickly as possible.
- It gives people a better overall experience due to higher-quality care and services.
- It lets people choose what's best for them throughout the course of their treatment with help from their GP and the wider healthcare team ('No decision about me without me').
- Many people who have experienced enhanced recovery say that it makes a hospital stay much less stressful.

*For providers*

- It gives patients a better overall experience through higher-quality care and services.
- It introduces innovative best practices that empower and motivate staff.
- It accelerates the clinical decision-making process by empowering multidisciplinary teams.
- It does not increase multidisciplinary team workload.
- It ensures the most efficient use of healthcare resources.

*For primary care*

- It gives patients a better overall experience through higher-quality care and services.
- Within England, it puts GPs in control of commissioning the right pathways for their patients.
- Earlier patient discharge doesn't create an extra workload for primary or social care services.
- It improves efficiency and productivity while improving quality.
- GPs and patients work in partnership through informed decision-making and greater choice.
- It is a clinically proven approach to faster patient recovery.

## References

1. Kehlet H (1997). Multimodal approach to control postoperative pathophysiology and rehabilitation. British Journal of Anaesthesia, 78(5):606–617.
2. Gustafsson UO, Scott MJ, Schwenk W, et al. (2013). Guidelines for perioperative care in elective colonic surgery: Enhanced Recovery After Surgery (ERAS) Society recommendations. World Journal of Surgery, 37(2):259–284.
3. Barlow R, Fairlie S (2013). The all Wales Enhanced Recovery after Surgery Collaborative. Final combined report. 1000 lives plus. Available at: ℘ http://www.1000livesplus.wales.nhs.uk/sitesplus/documents/1011/ERAS%20Programme%20Final%20Combined%20Report.pdf
4. Department of Health (2010). Delivering enhanced recovery: helping patients to get better sooner after surgery. London: Department of Health.
5. Kehlet H, Wilmore DW (2008). Evidence-based surgical care and the evolution of fast-track surgery. Annals of Surgery, 248(2):189–198.
6. NHS Wales (2010). Enhanced recovery after surgery. Cardiff: NHS Wales.
7. NHS Wales (2011). Enhanced recovery after surgery (hip and knee joint arthroplasty). Cardiff: NHS Wales.
8. Resar R, Griffin FA, Haraden C, et al. (2012). Using care bundles to improve health care quality. IHI Innovation Series white paper. Cambridge, MA: Institute for Healthcare Improvement.
9. Ljungqvist O, Scott M, Fearon KC (2017). Enhanced recovery after surgery: a review. JAMA Surgery, 152(3):292–298.
10. Wind J, Hofland J, Preckel B, et al. (2006). Perioperative strategy in colonic surgery: laparoscopy and/or FAst track multimodal management versus standard care (LAFA trial). BMC Surgery, 6:16.
11. Khoo CK, Vickery CJ, Forsyth N, et al. (2007). A prospective randomized controlled trial of multimodal perioperative management protocol in patients undergoing elective colorectal resection for cancer. Annals of Surgery, 245(6):867–872.
12. Lv L, Shao YF, Zhou YB (2012). The enhanced recovery after surgery (ERAS) pathway for patients undergoing colorectal surgery: an update of meta-analysis of randomised controlled trials. International Journal of Colorectal Disease, 27(12):1549–1554.
13. Shao YF, Zhou YB (2012). The enhanced recovery after surgery (ERAS) pathway for patients undergoing colorectal surgery: a meta-analysis of randomised controlled trials. International Journal of Colorectal Disease, 27(12):1549–1554.
14. Fearon KC, Ljungqvist O, Von Meyenfeldt M, et al. (2005). Enhanced recovery after surgery: a consensus review of clinical care for patients undergoing colonic resection. Clinical Nutrition, 24(3):466–477.
15. Varandhan KK, Neal KR, Dejong CH, et al. (2010). The enhanced recover after surgery (ERAS) pathway for patients undergoing major elective open colorectal surgery: a meta-analysis of randomized trials. Clinical Nutrition, 29(4):434–440.
16. Ricciardi R, MacKay G, Joshi GP (2017). Enhanced recovery after colorectal surgery. Available at: ℘ http://www.uptodate.com/contents/enhanced-recovery-after-colorectal-surgery

## Further reading

Greenshields N, Mythen M (2020). Enhanced recovery after surgery. Current Anesthesiology Reports, 10:49–55.
Royal College of Anaesthetists (2019). Chapter 3: guidelines for the provision of anaesthesia services for intraoperative care. London: Royal College of Anaesthetists.
Royal College of Anaesthetists (2019). Chapter 4: guidelines for the provision of postoperative care. London: Royal College of Anaesthetists.
Royal College of Anaesthetists (2021). Chapter 2: guidelines for the provision of anaesthesia services for preoperative assessment and preparation. London: Royal College of Anaesthetists.

# Communication

- Patients who are undergoing surgery may be anxious and feeling vulnerable.
- This can be the case if they are undergoing elective surgery, where the final outcome is unknown, such as surgery for cancer where the prognosis is not clear, or in an emergency when events may unfold very quickly and there is an equal amount of uncertainty as to what is going to happen.
- For most practitioners, their interaction with patients will be prior to their anaesthetic and then in the recovery room.
- As the practitioner and patient are unlikely to have met previously, there is little time to establish a relationship in a manner that other professionals might.
- It is vital therefore that the perioperative practitioner is able to gain the trust of the patient and the family, should they be present.
- This is a skill that most practitioners will grow more confident in with more experience.

## Surgery under local anaesthetic

- It is good practice to have a member of staff attend to the patient while the patient is undergoing the procedure.
- The member of staff should provide the information and reassurance as required.
- The member of staff should let the patient know what is going to happen and what is happening while it occurs.

## Non-verbal communication

This is a large part of communication. Types include:
- Eye contact and gaze
- Facial expression
- Proximity
- Touch
- Paralanguage.

## Patients who do not speak English

Under these circumstances, an independent interpreter may need to accompany the patient into the anaesthetic room and be present in the recovery room to ensure that the patient can understand instructions and advice.

### Use of family members

- It is considered poor practice to utilize a member of the patient's family. However, in urgent or emergency circumstances when it is not possible to use an official interpreter, it may prove necessary.
- Where possible, use an official interpreter. These are often available through the hospital or organization's advocacy arrangements and need to be arranged prior to the patient's arrival at the theatre doors.

## Other communication difficulties

*Patients with hearing difficulties*

- Patients who have regional anaesthetic/LA should keep their hearing aids in throughout the surgical procedure.
- Patients with hearing difficulties who normally wear hearing aids should be allowed to wear these until the last possible moment, which is usually when the GA has been commenced; in some instances, a hearing aid can just be 'turned off' and 'turned on' again in the recovery room.
- If a hearing aid is removed, it should be safely stored until it can be repositioned to aid communication in the recovery period.
- The hearing aid can be repositioned as soon as a patient emerges from anaesthesia, either before the patient leaves theatre or as soon as the patient enters the recovery room.

*With patients that are hard of hearing*

- Position yourself so that they can see you talking.
- Ensure that speech is clear and at an appropriate volume.
- Use touch where appropriate.

*Patients with visual impairment*

- Introduce yourself to the patient in the normal way by telling them your name and who you are so that they become familiar with your voice.
- Touch may be useful where appropriate.
- Allow spectacles to be worn until the last possible moment (usually when the GA has been commenced) and allow them to be put on as soon as possible in the recovery stage.
- Children with visual impairment are generally accompanied to theatre with their parents or guardians and it is often best to be guided as to what works with the child by utilizing the parents in the pre- and postoperative phases.
- ➲ See Chapter 3 for further information.

# Dignity, anxiety, and promoting equality when preparing the patient for theatre

## Dignity

Vulnerable perioperative patients have the right to be treated in a dignified manner whether conscious or anaesthetized. Practitioners should consider the way that they would want themselves or family members treated while undergoing perioperative care.

### Introduction

- Greet the patient in a professional manner. Introduce yourself by name and a simple explanation of your title. Remember that members of the general public are unlikely to understand specialist titles.
- For example, 'Hello Mr/Mrs/Ms/Miss [name] my name is [your name] and I am one of the team looking after you today'.
- Refer to patients by their title and last name unless invited to do otherwise. This is particularly true of older patients who may feel uncomfortable being called by their first name by a younger person.

### Exposure

- When the patient is being prepared for anaesthetic or surgery and access is required to their body, such as when skin preparation is being applied, the minimal area should be exposed and only when it is necessary to do so.

### Postoperative phase

- During this phase, the practitioner should, when appropriate, introduce themselves (this may be required more than once) and inform the patient what they do and what they will be doing.
- Care should be taken when looking under the patient's bedclothes for drains by explaining to the patient that this is being done and why, since the patient may be drifting off to sleep and be startled by such an intervention.

## Anxiety

- Patients undergoing a surgical intervention are likely to have some anxiety even if they have undergone a procedure in the past.
- Anxiety may manifest itself in several different ways. Some people will want to talk or be spoken to, while others may be quiet.
- Some patients will want to know everything, while others may be so frightened that they would prefer to know nothing and simply place their trust in the healthcare professional looking after them.
- This is a professional call made by the staff member.
- Each patient should be treated in appropriate manner that is right for them.

### Ways to reduce anxiety

- Providing information helps reduce anxiety and pain.
- Explanations should be given to the patient (and their carer or family member if present) as to what will be happening to them.

- Information should be given in a suitable way so that the patient understands.
- Patients should be given the opportunity to ask questions.

## Promoting equality

- All staff are required to treat patients without favour or discrimination.
- All patients are equal in terms of the care that is delivered, no matter how difficult a member of staff feels that a person or a group may be.
- This is enshrined in both the NMC's 'Code'[1] and the HCPC's 'Standards of conduct, performance and ethics'[2].

## References

1. Nursing and Midwifery Council (2018). The code: professional standards of practice and behaviour for nurses and midwives. London: Nursing and Midwifery Council.
2. Health and Care Professions Council (2016). Standards of conduct, performance and ethics. London: Health and Care Professions Council.

# Children, parents, and carers

It is now accepted practice to allow one or both parents of a baby or child into the anaesthetic room. This serves two main purposes:
• To help minimize the trauma to the child.
• To help the parents to be included in the child's care.

### Parental involvement in the preoperative stage
• The child is accompanied to the theatre department by the parent(s).
• After the final preoperative checks are made, the receiving theatre practitioner should accompany the child and parent(s) to the anaesthetic room. Since the parent(s) will remain until the child is anaesthetized another member of staff will be required to escort them from the anaesthetic room.
• Where appropriate, the parent(s) may be able to distract the child so the anaesthetist can undertake the IV cannulation.
• Once the child is anaesthetized, the parent(s) can be escorted from the anaesthetic room and then the department.
• Before the parent(s) leave, the practitioner should explain to them what the arrangements are for meeting up with their child in the recovery room following the operation.
• This can be an emotional time and parents may need a few moments to compose themselves.

### Parental involvement in the postoperative stage
• Usually, the parent(s) come into the recovery room as the child is awakening from the anaesthetic.
• It is advisable to have a short conversation with the parent(s) before they come into the recovery room to explain to them what to expect in the way of the child's condition, drains, drips, and items of monitoring equipment.
• The parent(s) should be involved with as much of the child's care as possible as this can be of comfort to the child and parent(s).
• Throughout this process, appropriate explanations should be provided about interventions such as the administration of medication.
• At the appropriate time, the child will be allowed to leave the recovery room and to return to the ward area. The practitioner should accompany the child and parent(s) from the unit.

Children should be managed in a paediatric recovery unit in the period immediately after anaesthesia. The staff in this area should have paediatric experience and current paediatric competencies, including resuscitation.[1]

### Communication
Careful and appropriate explanations of what is to happen will be required for the parent(s) and the child.

The age of the child will determine the manner and terms used to speak to them.

## Parental anxiety

Having a child who needs surgery can cause considerable anxiety for parents and it is important that this is recognized. Parents who are anxious may demonstrate a range of emotions from being tearful to being angry and it is important that parents:

- Are provided with clear, concise, and up-to-date information on a regular basis
- Have their fears and anxieties recognized and are given time to discuss these if required
- Are provided with reassurance and support.

## Reference

1. Royal College of Anaesthetists (2020). Chapter 10: guidelines for the provision of paediatric anaesthesia services. London: Royal College of Anaesthetists.

## Further reading

Chorney JM, Kain ZN (2010). Family-centered paediatric perioperative care. Anaesthesiology, 112(3):751–755.

Freedman R, Herbert L, O'Donnell A, et al. (eds) (2022). Oxford handbook of anaesthesia (5th ed). Oxford: Oxford University Press.

Health and Care Professions Council (2016). Standards of conduct, performance and ethics. London: Health and Care Professions Council.

Nursing and Midwifery Council 2018 The code: professional standards of practice and behaviour for nurses and midwives London: Nursing and Midwifery Council.

Royal College of Nursing (2011). Transferring children to and from theatre: RCN position statement and guideline for good practice. London: Royal College of Nursing.

# Caring for the adolescent child

## Adolescence

Adolescent development is generally divided into three phases:
- Early (11–14 years).
- Middle (14–17 years).
- Late (17–24 years).

A number of terms are used to describe adolescence including teenager (13–19 years) and young people (10–24 years). There are approximately 11.7 million young people aged 10–24 years living within the UK and although the majority of these are healthy individuals, some will be admitted into hospital for a surgical procedure. Adolescents who are admitted into hospital need to:
- Be managed in an age-appropriate way
- Have their wishes taken into account.

## Managing young people: general principles

- Young people are very conscious of their bodies and body image and it is important to maintain their dignity at all times. This is particularly important for young girls who may be menstruating when they are taken to theatre.
- The emotions of young people can fluctuate rapidly during adolescence and any situations out of the ordinary such as a hospital admission can cause them to become stressed and anxious. Young people will respond differently to stress, but it is not unusual for young males to become angry and defensive. It is important that any situation such as this should be deescalated and the adolescent should be managed with patience and understanding.
- Depending on their age and stage of development, some young people may want to be involved in the decision-making process.

*The preoperative stage*
- In some trusts/health boards, young people can give their own consent from the age of 15 years. Even where the parents still provide legal consent, the young person must assent to treatment.
- Some young people could have body piercings so in addition to the usual preoperative checks, you will need to check if the young person has piercings. Depending on local policy, these may need to be removed before surgery.
- Where appropriate, young people may want to use headphones to listen to music as a form of distraction when they are in the anaesthetic room.

*The postoperative stage*

Depending on their stage of development, young people may still want their parents to accompany them to the anaesthetic room.

- Young people may request that their parents meet them in the recovery room and that decision should be respected.

- Throughout this process, appropriate explanations should be provided of interventions such as the administration of medication.
- At the appropriate time, the young person will be allowed to leave the recovery room and to return to the ward area. The practitioner should accompany them from the unit.

*Communication*
- Even where parents are present, careful and appropriate explanations of what is to happen should also be provided to the young person.
- The developmental stage of the young person will determine the manner and terms used to speak to them. However, short and simple sentences should be used and jargon should be avoided at all times.

## Further reading

Bill S, Knight Y (2007). Adolescence: In: Valentine F, Lowes L (eds) Care of children with chronic illness. Oxford: Blackwell Publishing.

Dolgin KG (2010). The adolescent: development, relationships, and culture. (13th ed). Boston, MA: Pearson.

Hagel A, Coleman C, Brooks F (2015). Key data on adolescence. London: Association for Young People's Health.

Royal College of Anaesthetists (2020). Chapter 10: guidelines for the provision of paediatric anaesthesia services. London: Royal College of Anaesthetists.

Royal College of Nursing (2017). Getting it right for young people in your practice (3rd ed). London: Royal College of Nursing.

World Health Organization (2014). Health for the world's adolescents: a second chance in the second decade. Geneva: World Health Organization.

# Safeguarding children and young people

Safeguarding children and young people is every professional's responsibility.
- All healthcare staff who come into contact with children and young people carry a responsibility to safeguard and promote their welfare and should know the process to follow should they have safeguarding concerns including child protection.[1]
- All healthcare organizations have a duty to safeguard and protect children, promote their welfare, and fully cooperate with statutory agencies when safeguarding concerns are raised—this requirement is enshrined in law: in England and Wales, Children Act 2004; Northern Ireland, Children (Northern Ireland) Order 1995; and Scotland Children (Scotland) Act 1995.

## Definitions

In the UK, children are legally defined as individuals below the age of 18 years. This is consistent across UK safeguarding policy, guidance, and legislation. NICE clinical guidelines on child maltreatment[2] offer the following distinctions:
- Infant: <1 year.
- Child: 1 year to <13 years.
- Young person: 13–17 years.

Safeguarding and child protection are often seen as interchangeable terms; however, they are different. Safeguarding encompasses child protection but also the wider well-being of the child. This includes:
- Protecting children from maltreatment
- Preventing impairment of the child's health and development
- Ensuring that children are growing up in circumstances consistent with the provision of safe and effective care
- The taking of actions to ensure that children have the best life chances in order to enter adulthood successfully.[3]

Child protection is part of safeguarding practice and is the process of protecting individual children who may be suffering or be likely to suffer significant harm as a result of abuse or neglect.

Child abuse is a form of maltreatment of a child and describes the infliction of harm or failing to prevent harm in a child or young person. There are four categories of child maltreatment:
- Physical abuse.
- Sexual abuse.
- Emotional abuse.
- Neglect.

## Categories

*Physical abuse*

A form of abuse, which may involve hitting, shaking, throwing, poisoning, burning or scalding, drowning, suffocating, or otherwise causing physical harm to a child. Physical harm may also be caused when a parent or carer fabricates the symptoms of, or deliberately induces, illness in a child.[3]

*Sexual abuse*

Involves forcing or enticing a child or young person to take part in sexual activities, not necessarily involving a high level of violence, whether or not the child is aware of what is happening.

The activities may involve physical contact, including assault by penetration (e.g. rape or oral sex) or non-penetrative acts such as masturbation, kissing, rubbing, and touching outside of clothing. They may also include non-contact activities, such as involving children in looking at, or in the production of, sexual images, watching sexual activities, encouraging children to behave in sexually inappropriate ways, or grooming a child in preparation for abuse (including via the internet).

Sexual abuse is not solely perpetrated by adult males. Women can also commit acts of sexual abuse, as can other children.[3]

*Emotional abuse*

The persistent emotional maltreatment of a child such as to cause severe and persistent adverse effects on the child's emotional development.

It may involve conveying to a child that they are worthless or unloved, inadequate, or valued only insofar as they meet the needs of another person. It may include not giving the child opportunities to express their views, deliberately silencing them or 'making fun' of what they say or how they communicate.

It may feature age or developmentally inappropriate expectations being imposed on children. These may include interactions that are beyond a child's developmental capability, as well as overprotection and limitation of exploration and learning, or preventing the child participating in normal social interaction.

It may involve seeing or hearing the ill-treatment of another. It may involve serious bullying (including cyberbullying), causing children frequently to feel frightened or in danger, or the exploitation or corruption of children. Some level of emotional abuse is involved in all types of maltreatment of a child, though it may occur alone.[3]

*Neglect*

The persistent failure to meet a child's basic physical and/or psychological needs, likely to result in the serious impairment of the child's health or development. Neglect may occur during pregnancy as a result of maternal substance abuse. Once a child is born, neglect may involve a parent or carer failing to:

- Provide adequate food, clothing, and shelter (including exclusion from home or abandonment)
- Protect a child from physical and emotional harm or danger
- Ensure adequate supervision (including the use of inadequate care-givers)
- Ensure access to appropriate medical care or treatment.

It may also include neglect of, or unresponsiveness to, a child's basic emotional needs.[3]

## Female genital mutilation

Female genital mutilation (FGM) is an illegal practice within the UK. The practice impacts both the child's physical and emotional health. FGM is a physical abuse and is defined as all procedures which involve the partial or total removal of the external genitalia or other injury to female genital organs for non-medical reasons.[4,5] The WHO identifies four types of FGM[6]:

- *Type 1*: often referred to as *clitoridectomy*, this is the partial or total removal of the clitoris (a small, sensitive, and erectile part of the female genitals), and in very rare cases, only the prepuce (the fold of skin surrounding the clitoris).
- *Type 2*: often referred to as *excision*, this is the partial or total removal of the clitoris and the labia minora (the inner folds of the vulva), with or without excision of the labia majora (the outer folds of skin of the vulva).
- *Type 3*: often referred to as *infibulation*, this is the narrowing of the vaginal opening through the creation of a covering seal. The seal is formed by cutting and repositioning the labia minora, or labia majora, sometimes through stitching, with or without removal of the clitoris (clitoridectomy).
- *Type 4*: this includes all other harmful procedures to the female genitalia for non-medical purposes, such as pricking, piercing, incising, scraping, and cauterizing the genital area.

## Reporting safeguarding concerns

It is important to always raise any safeguarding concerns within your own organization. Across the UK, specialist safeguarding designated professionals are in post to support staff in the referral process. In England, Wales, and Northern Ireland, named doctors, nurses, and midwifes fulfil this role. In Scotland, nurse consultants, child protection advisors, and lead clinicians would fulfil these specialist roles. All healthcare organizations will have an established referral process in order to raise concerns; the starting point is always to discuss your concerns with your safeguarding leads.

## References

1. Royal College of Paediatrics and Child Health (2019). Safeguarding children and young people: roles and competencies for healthcare staff. Available at: ℘ https://www.rcn.org.uk/professional-development/publications/pub-007366
2. National Institute for Health and Care Excellence (2009). Child maltreatment: when to suspect child maltreatment. Clinical guideline [CG89]. Available at: ℘ https://www.nice.org.uk/guidance/cg89
3. HM Government (2015). Working together to safeguard children: a guide to inter-agency working to safeguard and promote the welfare of children. London: Department for Education.
4. Department of Health (2016). Female genital mutilation risk and safeguarding; guidance for professionals. London: Department of Health.
5. Royal College of Midwives, Royal College of Nursing, Royal College of Obstetricians and Gynaecologists, et al. (2013). Tackling FGM in the UK: intercollegiate recommendations for identifying, recording and reporting. London: Royal College of Midwives.
6. World Health Organization (WHO) (2022). Female genital mutilation: fact sheet. Available at: ℘ https://www.who.int/en/news-room/fact-sheets/detail/female-genital-mutilation

## Further reading

Dean E (2014). The hidden toll of FGM. Nursing Standard, 28(36):20–22.

Griffith R, Tegnah C (2017). Law and professional issues in nursing (4th ed). Exeter: Learning Matters Ltd.

Legislation.gov.uk (1989). Children Act 1989. Available at: ℜ https://www.legislation.gov.uk/ukpga/1989/41/contents

Legislation.gov.uk (2004). Children Act 2004. Available at: ℜ https://www.legislation.gov.uk/ukpga/2004/31/contents

NHS, The Children's Society (2017). Seen and Heard e-learning course. [The Seen and Heard course is narrated by young people, sharing real experiences about what it's like to be an abused or exploited child with 'something to tell'.] Available at: ℜ https://learning.seenandheard.org.uk/

Powell C (2016). Safeguarding and child protection for nurses, midwives and health visitors: a practical guide. Berkshire: Open University Press.

# Adults at risk

All healthcare professionals have a duty to safeguard patients with a particular responsibility to protect those who cannot protect themselves. A key principle of practice is the professional duty to empower patients to make autonomous decisions to manage their care and treatment. This approach is fundamental within healthcare regulation but also underpinned by legislation:
- Human Rights Act 1998.
- Mental Capacity Act 2005.
- Equality Act 2010.
- Care Act 2014.

## Definitions

The Care Act (2014) statutory guidance 14.2 describes a vulnerable adult as someone who:
- Has needs for care and support regardless of whether or not those needs are currently being met
- Is experiencing or is at risk of experiencing abuse and neglect
- As a result of care and support needs are unable to protect themselves from either the risk or experience of abuse or neglect (Fig. 6.1).

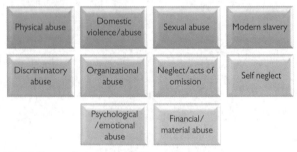

| Physical abuse | Domestic violence/abuse | Sexual abuse | Modern slavery |
| Discriminatory abuse | Organizational abuse | Neglect/acts of omission | Self neglect |
| | Psychological /emotional abuse | Financial/ material abuse | |

**Fig. 6.1** Common forms of abuse in adults.

## Who abuses and neglects adults?

- Spouses/partners/other family members.
- Neighbours.
- Friends.
- Acquaintances.
- Local residents.
- People who deliberately exploit adults they perceive as vulnerable to abuse.
- Paid staff or professionals and volunteers.
- Strangers.

## Principles of safeguarding

- Empowerment: there should be a presumption that decisions around care and consent should be led by the individual patient unless they lack capacity.
- Protection: those in greatest need should be provided with support and representation.
- Prevention: demonstrates the need to be proactive and act before harm occurs.
- Proportionality: where a risk is presented, the most proportionate and least intrusive response should be made.
- Partnerships: local solutions should be established through services working with their communities.
- Accountability: there should be accountability and transparency in delivering safeguarding to ensure that healthcare professionals know what is expected of them and others and are prepared to act on concerns.[2]

## Reporting safeguarding concerns

NHS England[3] has produced guidance on the approach that professionals should take when they have a safeguarding concern:

- Assess the situation, that is, are emergency services required?
- Ensure the safety and well-being of the individual.
- Establish what the individual's views and wishes are about the safeguarding issue and procedure.
- Maintain any evidence.
- Follow local procedures for reporting incidents/risks.
- Remain calm and try not to show any shock or disbelief.
- Listen carefully and demonstrate understanding by acknowledging regret and concern that this has happened.
- Inform the person that you are required to share the information, explaining what information will be shared and why.
- Make a written record of what the person has told you, using their words, what you have seen, and your actions.

All reasonable steps must be taken to safeguard the patient by sharing concerns with relevant agencies such as social services in line with regulatory guidance, policy, and legislation on disclosure. In the first instance, local procedures should be followed with concerns raised with the health organizations designated or named professionals for safeguarding adults. As healthcare professionals, it is important to ensure that any safeguarding concerns are raised if a patient is identified as vulnerable, or is at risk and in need of extra support and protection.

## References

1. Legislation.gov.uk (2014). Care Act 2014. Available at: ℘ http://www.legislation.gov.uk/ukpga/2014/23/contents
2. Department of Health (2011). Safeguarding adults: the role of health service practitioners. London: The Stationery Office.
3. NHS England (2014). Safeguarding adults. Available at: ℘ https://www.england.nhs.uk/wp-content/uploads/2017/02/adult-pocket-guide.pdf

## Further reading

Betts V, Marks-Maran D, Morris-Thompson T (2014). Safeguarding vulnerable adults. Nursing Standard, 28(38):37–41.

Dalphinis J (2016). Safeguarding adults: an update on legal principles. Practice Nurse, 46(9):12–16.

Department of Health and Social Care (2018). Care and support statutory guidance. Available at: ℘ https://www.gov.uk/government/publications/care-act-statutory-guidance/care-and-support-statutory-guidance

Francis R (2013). Report of the Mid Staffordshire NHS Foundation Trust Public Inquiry: Final Report. The Stationery Office: London.

Griffith R, Tegnah C (2017). Law and professional issues in nursing (4th ed). Exeter: Learning Matters Ltd.

NHS England (2016). Safeguarding adults: roles and competencies for healthcare staff. London: NHS England.

Nursing and Midwifery Council (2015). The code: professional standards of practice and behaviour for nurses and midwives. London: Nursing and Midwifery Council.

Welsh Government (2014). Social Services and Well Being (Wales) Act. Available at: ℘ https://www.legislation.gov.uk/anaw/2014/4/section/1

# Principles of anaesthesia

# Role of the anaesthetic practitioner

An anaesthetic practitioner is a qualified ODP or nurse who provides continual assistance to the anaesthetist during the delivery, maintenance, and reversal of anaesthesia.

In order to maintain safe levels of patient care throughout any surgical or anaesthetic procedure, the anaesthetic practitioner must be clinically competent and have a current and sound knowledge base of:
- Relevant anatomy and physiology
- The principles and practice of elective and emergency anaesthesia
- Airway management and difficult airway management
- Pharmacodynamics and pharmacokinetics of anaesthetic pharmacology
- Principles and practice of resuscitation.

## Priorities for the anaesthetic practitioner include
- Ensuring best practice and the patient's best interests at all times in accordance with local, national, and legal frameworks
- Contributing to all aspects of patient care, which includes the provision of emotional and physical support of the patient throughout the perioperative phase
- Anticipating the patient's and anaesthetist's requirements
- Patient management options
- Airway management and difficult airway management protocols including procedures for difficult and failed intubation
- Monitoring of the patient during anaesthesia
- Monitoring of the patient during in hospital or out of hospital transfer, ensuring that the patient's needs are met until handover to another healthcare professional.

Ensuring compliance with professional and mandatory training at all times, the anaesthetic practitioner must also engage with professional and educational development in the specialist area of perioperative care within regulatory requirements. Additionally, practitioners must contribute to the training and development of students and non-regulated personnel. See Box 7.1.

**Box 7.1 Additional aspects of the anaesthetic practitioner role**

*Duties*
- Excellent interpersonal skills including verbal and non-verbal communication skills.
- Preparation and checking of the anaesthetic room and operating theatre environment and equipment.
- Checking and stocking of all anaesthetic equipment to be used including any emergency equipment that may be required.
- Participating, if required, with the emergency response team to provide clinical assistance to all environments within the hospital (e.g. cardiac arrest calls).
- Care of catheters, drains, CVP lines, epidural catheters, arterial lines, and peripheral lines.
- Caring for ventilated patients.
- Perioperative teaching and information giving.
- Ensuring and adhering to handling and moving policies when transferring patients to trolleys and beds; ensuring safe and correct positioning of patients.

*Knowledge*
- Principles and practice of cross-infection.
- Evidence-based practice and national guidelines.
- Risk management strategies in the clinical area.
- Post-anaesthetic care in a range of surgical specialties.

## Further reading

Association of Anaesthetists of Great Britain and Ireland (2018). The anaesthesia team. Available at: ℳ http://dx.doi.org/10.21466/g.TAT.2018

College of Operating Department Practitioners (2011). Bachelor of Science (Hons) in Operating Department Practice – England, Northern Ireland and Wales, Bachelor of Science in Operating Department Practice – Scotland Curriculum Document. London: College of Operating Department Practitioners.

Difficult Airway Society. Homepage. Available at: ℳ http://www.das.uk.com

Freedman R, Herbert L, O'Donnell A, et al. (eds) (2022). Oxford handbook of anaesthesia (5th ed). Oxford: Oxford University Press.

Health and Care Professions Council (2016). Standards of conduct, performance and ethics London: Health and Care Professions Council.

Nursing and Midwifery Council (2018). The code: professional standards of practice and behaviour for nurses and midwives. London: Nursing and Midwifery Council.

NHS Scotland (2012). Portfolio of core competencies for anaesthetic assistants. Edinburgh: NHS Education for Scotland.

Perioperative Care Collaborative (2017). National core curriculum for perioperative nursing. London: Perioperative Care Collaborative.

Royal College of Anaesthetists (2019–2021). Guidelines for the provision of anaesthetic services. Available at: ℳ https://www.rcoa.ac.uk/gpas

# Anaesthesia

The term 'anaesthesia' is derived from two Greek words, which together mean 'loss of feeling or sensation'. Today the term reflects modern-day anaesthetic techniques and can also mean 'relaxation and pain relief for surgery'. Anaesthesia is one of the most significant developments of modern medicine as it allows once-unbearable surgical procedures to be performed while the patient is unconscious, pain free, and relaxed. There are predominantly four types of anaesthesia:

- General anaesthesia (GA).
- Local anaesthesia (LA).
- Regional anaesthesia.
- Combination of these three.

### General anaesthesia

GA is defined as:

- A state of total unconsciousness resulting from anaesthetic drugs within a controlled environment
- The administration of an agent or agents to render the patient unconscious and insensitive to pain and non-reactive to any form of surgical stimulation
- Induction of anaesthesia is achieved by IV (a combination of several drugs) or inhalational methods with the use of volatile agents
- Volatile agents, which are inhaled, are also utilized for maintenance of anaesthesia.

The development of new technology and safer anaesthetic pharmacology means that modern anaesthesia is now relatively safe. GA is usually used for all surgical procedures that cannot be performed under a LA or regional anaesthetic. GA is characterized by multiple aspects, such as unconsciousness, amnesia, depression of motor reflexes, and the lack of pain sensation. There is much debate around the actual mechanisms of action for GA; however, there is consensus that the predominate mode of action is within the CNS[2].

### IV induction

- Suitable for routine and emergency surgical procedures.
- On induction, patients are preoxygenated with 100% $O_2$ using a face mask. The duration of oxygenation is dependent on whether the procedure is an emergency or routine and could last anything from 3 minutes to three large breaths dependent on the patient's condition.
- All anaesthetic drugs necessary for the procedure should be prepared and appropriately labelled.
- The AAGBI recommend that all patients should be monitored in the anaesthetic room prior to induction of anaesthesia.[1] This should include:
  - Capnography
  - ECG
  - NIBP
  - Respiratory rate
  - $SpO_2$.

- The following must also be available:
  - A nerve stimulator whenever a muscle relaxant is used.
  - A means of measuring the patient's temperature.
- Anaesthesia induction agents include:
  - Propofol
  - Thiopental
  - Etomidate
  - Ketamine.

## Complications of IV induction

- Cardiovascular and respiratory depression.
- Arterial injection.
- Injection into SC tissue.
- Drug reaction.

## References

1. Association of Anaesthetists of Great Britain and Ireland (2019). Checklist for draw-over anaesthetic equipment. Available at: &#x1F50D; http://dx.doi.org/10.21466/g.CFDAE2.2019
2. Antkowiak B (2001). How do general anaesthetics work? The Science of Nature, 88(5):201–213.

## Further reading

Freedman R, Herbert L, O'Donnell A, et al. (eds) (2022). Oxford handbook of anaesthesia (5th ed). Oxford: Oxford University Press.
Royal College of Anaesthetists (2019–2021). Guidelines for the provision of anaesthetic services. London: Royal College of Anaesthetists.
Royal College of Anaesthetists (2021). Chapter 2: guidelines for the provision of anaesthesia services for preoperative assessment and preparation. London: Royal College of Anaesthetists.
Simpson PJ, Popat M (2002). Understanding anaesthesia (4th ed). Oxford: Butterworth-Heinemann.

# Triad of anaesthesia

The triad of anaesthesia was developed to describe the three basic requirements of an anaesthetic that must be achieved to ensure a successful outcome. The triad is associated with all anaesthetic techniques and these requirements provide a balanced combination of anaesthetic drugs and other agents that induce:
- Narcosis
- Analgesia
- Relaxation.

## Narcosis

Narcosis means that the patient is rendered unconscious/unaware following the administration of:
- Narcotic drugs
- Sedative drugs
- IV anaesthetic induction agents
- Inhalational gas induction agents.

## Analgesia

- Analgesia means lack of pain and suppresses physiological reflexes that occur following surgical stimulation and is often achieved by powerful narcotics, local block, or local infiltration.
- A surgical incision induces a complex series of physiological responses if made in a conscious patient[1] and can cause:
  - Tachycardia
  - Hypertension
  - Hyperventilation
  - Sweating
  - Vomiting.
- The administration of narcotic analgesic drugs limits such physiological responses to surgical stimulation.

## Relaxation

- Relaxation refers to the reduction or absence of muscle tone which can be retained even when the patient is deeply unconscious, and is achieved by the use of muscle-relaxing drugs and local blockade.
- Following the administration of relaxation drugs, patients will then require assisted or controlled ventilation until the drug has been reversed.
- Patient relaxation is important for endotracheal intubation, and abdominal and laparoscopic surgery.

Maintenance of anaesthesia can then be provided with $O_2$, nitrous oxide ($N_2O$), and either a volatile agent or total intravenous anaesthesia (TIVA), with additional increments of muscle relaxant as required. Modern anaesthetic agents allow the proportions of the three components of the triad to be more easily adjusted according to patients' individual requirements.

## Reference

1. Whelan E, Davies H (2010). The pharmacology of drugs used in general anaesthesia. In: Davey A, Ince C (eds) Fundamentals of operating department practice. Cambridge: Cambridge University Press.

## Further reading

Association of Anaesthetists of Great Britain and Ireland (2019). Controlled drugs in peri-operative care. Available at: ℞ http://dx.doi.org/10.21466/g.CDIPC.2006

Freedman R, Herbert L, O'Donnell A, et al. (eds) (2022). Oxford handbook of anaesthesia (5th ed). Oxford: Oxford University Press.

Pollard B, Kitchen G (eds) (2017). Handbook of clinical anaesthesia (4th ed). London: CRC Press.

Royal College of Anaesthetists (2019–2021). Guidelines for the provision of anaesthetic services. London: Royal College of Anaesthetists.

Scarth E, Smith S (2016). Drugs in anaesthesia and intensive care (5th ed). Oxford: Oxford University Press.

Simpson PJ, Popat M (2002). Understanding anaesthesia (4th ed). Oxford: Butterworth-Heinemann.

# Inhalational anaesthesia

Inhalational anaesthesia is the delivery of a volatile agent from a vaporizer through a breathing circuit to a patient. Inhalational anaesthesia can be sub-divided into:
- Induction
- Maintenance.

## Induction

The potency of an inhaled anaesthetic is quantified by its minimum alveolar concentration (MAC). The alveolus is the area of the lung in which gas leaves the lung and enters the bloodstream. MAC is defined as the amount of gas in the lungs required to prevent 50% of humans from moving when given a painful stimulus such as a surgical incision. IV medications can be characterized as to their 'equivalent MAC' so that their potencies can be compared to the inhaled medications.

During respiration, the patient inhales the volatile agent, the concentration of which builds in the alveoli which diffuses across the alveoli capillary membrane into the bloodstream, resulting in the gradual loss of consciousness.

*Indications for use*
- To avoid IV induction with children or patients with needle phobia.
- To maintain spontaneous respiration where difficult intubation is expected (e.g. acute epiglottitis or anatomical anomalies).
- Bronchopleural fistula.
- Inhaled foreign body.

*Management*
- Explanation and emotional support for patients.
- Close-fitting facemask.
- Preparation for immediate IV access.
- Availability of full-range airway management equipment.

*Complications*
- Delay in induction due to breath holding or obstruction.
- Difficulties with cannulation.
- Staff exposure to the inhalational agent.

Unconsciousness in most cases may be reversed promptly by the withdrawal of the inhalational agent. The use of volatile agents is contraindicated for use in patients with any history or familial association with MH.

## Maintenance

Volatile agents are the choice for maintenance of anaesthesia, in conjunction with $O_2$, analgesia, and muscle relaxants. These agents include:
- Isoflurane
- Sevoflurane
- Desflurane.

*Management*
- Monitoring and maintaining the level of volatile agent within the vaporizer.
- Ensuring patency of breathing circuits.

- Minimize the risk of environmental pollution with the use of active scavenging.
- Ensure availability and use of a vapour analyser.
- Circle breathing systems with vapour and $CO_2$ analysers are indicated for use with volatile agents to minimize cost and environmental pollution.

*Complications*
- Disconnection of breathing circuits.
- Delayed recovery.

## Stages of anaesthesia

All anaesthetic drugs produce anaesthesia by their effect on the CNS. Anaesthetic gases are inhaled and are then transferred from the lungs to the circulation and finally to the CNS to be effective. By administering an anaesthetic gas alone, the progress of each patient towards deep anaesthesia is divided into four stages (Table 7.1).

**Table 7.1** Stages of anaesthesia

| Stage | Progress of anaesthetic gas induction |
|---|---|
| 1 | The stage of analgesia; lasts from the beginning of administration of the gas until consciousness is lost |
| 2 | Refers to the stage of excitement, which lasts from loss of consciousness until regular breathing begins and settles. During this stage patients have been known to hold their breath, struggle, cough, or even vomit |
| 3 | Indicates that surgical anaesthesia has been achieved; once the patient's breathing has settled the procedure may begin |
| 4 | If additional anaesthetic is administered, the patient reaches the fourth stage, otherwise referred to as 'overdose' and breathing and circulation will cease |

Reproduced from Morton NS (1997). Assisting the anaesthetist. Oxford: Oxford University Press, with permission from Oxford University Press.

## Further reading

Al-Shaikh B, Stacey S (2018). Essentials of equipment in anaesthesia, critical care and perioperative medicine (5th ed). Edinburgh: Elsevier.

Aston D, Rivers A, Dharmadasa A (2014). Equipment in anaesthesia and critical care: a complete guide for the FRCA. Banbury: Scion.

Davey A, Ince CS (2010). Fundamentals of operating department practice. Cambridge: Cambridge University Press.

Freedman R, Herbert L, O'Donnell A, et al. (eds) (2022). Oxford handbook of anaesthesia (5th ed). Oxford: Oxford University Press.

Middleton B, Phillips J, Stacey S (2021). Physics in anaesthesia: for FRCA candidates, ODPs and nurse anaesthetists (2nd ed). Banbury: Scion.

Pollard B, Kitchen G (eds) (2017). Handbook of clinical anaesthesia (4th ed). London: CRC Press.

Royal College of Anaesthetists (2019–2021). Guidelines for the provision of anaesthetic services. London: Royal College of Anaesthetists.

Scarth E, Smith S (2016). Drugs in anaesthesia and intensive care (5th ed). Oxford: Oxford University Press.

Thompson J, Moppett I, Wiles M (eds) (2019). Smith and Aitkenhead's textbook of anaesthesia (7th ed). Edinburgh: Elsevier.

# Total intravenous anaesthesia

TIVA is the delivery of anaesthesia with no inhalational agents. Delivery is via a microprocessor-controlled syringe pump which delivers a prescribed target dose of an anaesthetic agent which is calculated on the basis of weight, age, and sex. TIVA may also be called target-controlled anaesthesia (TCA) or target-controlled infusion (TCI).

### Indications for use

- MH risk.
- Long QT syndrome (QTc ≥500 ms).
- History of severe postoperative nausea and vomiting (PONV).
- 'Tubeless' ENT and thoracic surgery.
- Patients with anticipated difficult intubation/extubation.
- Neurosurgery—to limit intracranial volume.
- Surgery requiring neurophysiological monitoring.
- Myasthenia gravis/neuromuscular disorders, and situations where neuromuscular blockers are of disadvantage.
- Anaesthesia in non-theatre environments.
- Transfer of an anaesthetized patient between environments.
- Day-case surgery.
- Patient choice.

### Advantages

- Rapid induction of GA.
- Rapid recovery with minimal 'hangover' effect.
- Can be used for sedation or as an adjunct to regional anaesthesia.
- Reduced PONV.
- Laryngoscopy/bronchoscope where inhalational agents may cause airway irritation.
- Safe for use with patients with MH.
- Predictability for bariatric patients.
- Suitable for high-risk patients, for example, the elderly and patients with relevant pre-existing disease (➜ see Chapter 5 for further details).
- Gentle gradual approach.
- Control over depth of anaesthesia.

### Disadvantages

- Pain on induction.
- Contraindicated for patients with hypolipidaemia for long-term use (i.e. ITU).
- Propofol TCI is not licensed for paediatric use.
- Potential interruption to delivery.

### Clinical management

- IV access must be protected, visible, and accessible at all times. If the IV access becomes dislodged or detached this will interrupt delivery and therefore predispose the patient to awareness. This is an added concern with patients who are paralysed as part of their management.

- IV delivery systems must include an antireflux valve at the access site to ensure antisiphon and prevent reflux. It is suggested that if TIVA is used in conjunction with IV fluids, it should have a separate and dedicated IV access point.
- Accurate assessment of depth of anaesthesia is difficult during TIVA, so care in preventing awareness is essential, especially if muscle relaxants are used.

## Further reading

Al-Rifai Z, Mulvey D (2016). Principles of total intravenous anaesthesia: practical aspects of using total intravenous anaesthesia. British Journal of Anaesthesia Education, 16(8):276–280.

Al-Shaikh B, Stacey S (2018). Essentials of equipment in anaesthesia, critical care and perioperative medicine (5th ed). Edinburgh: Elsevier.

Antkowiak B (2001). How do general anaesthetics work? The Science of Nature, 88(5):201–213.

Aston D, Rivers A, Dharmadasa A (2014). Equipment in anaesthesia and critical care: a complete guide for the FRCA. Banbury: Scion.

Davey A, Ince CS (2010). Fundamentals of operating department practice. Cambridge: Cambridge University Press.

Freedman R, Herbert L, O'Donnell A, et al. (eds) (2022). Oxford handbook of anaesthesia (5th ed). Oxford: Oxford University Press.

Middleton B, Phillips J, Stacey S (2021). Physics in anaesthesia: for FRCA candidates, ODPs and nurse anaesthetists (2nd ed). Banbury: Scion.

Pollard B, Kitchen G (eds) (2017). Handbook of clinical anaesthesia (4th ed). London: CRC Press.

Royal College of Anaesthetists (2019–2021). Guidelines for the provision of anaesthetic services. London: Royal College of Anaesthetists.

Scarth E, Smith S (2016). Drugs in anaesthesia and intensive care (5th ed). Oxford: Oxford University Press.

Thompson J, Moppett I, Wiles M (eds) (2019). Smith and Aitkenhead's textbook of anaesthesia (7th ed). Edinburgh: Elsevier.

Virtual Anaesthesia Textbook (2017). Intravenous agents, TCI and TIVA. Available at: ℗ http://www.virtual-anesthesia-textbook.com/vat/iva.htm

## Local anaesthesia

LAs are drugs that reversibly block the conduction of nerve impulses along nerve axons. Occasionally, patients can be sedated throughout the LA procedure if they are particularly anxious. There are many ways in which the LA can be used; this will depend on potency, toxicity, duration of action, stability, solubility in water, and the ability to penetrate mucous membranes by the drug. Other variations which will determine the LA which is used will be the type of procedure and the mode of delivery for the LA.[1]

### Administration

When administering LAs, care should be taken in calculating safe drug dosage. Take account of:
- Patient's age
- Weight
- Physique and health.

Other factors include:
- Absorption
- Excretion
- Potency of the drug
- Vascularity of the area in which the LA is to be applied when injecting.[1]

LAs will also cause some degree of vasodilatation; consequently, quite often vasoconstrictors will be added to the LA which increase its potency and duration of action by ensuring the drug is localized in the tissue. The vasoconstrictors also increase the safety by decreasing the rate of absorption. Adrenaline-containing solutions should never be used for infiltration around end-arteries, for example, penis, ring block of fingers, or other areas with a terminal vascular supply, as the intense vasoconstriction may lead to severe ischaemia and necrosis.[2]

LA often does not work when injected in and around infected tissue. This is due to the infected tissue having a more acidic environment, therefore delaying the action and reducing the effect of the LA. Infected tissue often has an increased blood supply therefore the anaesthetic is removed from the injection area before it can affect the nerve axon and neuron.[3] LA can be administered in several ways:
- Topical: topical anaesthetics are normally applied to both the skin or mucus membrane and its onset of action can range from 5 to 60 minutes. Topical anaesthetics are used typically prior to injection or cannulation and cutaneous contact (usually under an occlusive dressing) should be maintained for the maximum period directed by the drug data sheet prior to venepuncture to ensure maximum effect.[2]
- Local infiltration: this technique is normally used for minor procedures such as dental extractions and suturing of skin wounds.
- Regional (conductional anaesthesia): this can be divided into minor and major nerve blockade. Minor nerve blockade will include blocking ulnar, radial, or intercostal nerves; while major nerve blockade relates to the deeper nerves or trunks such as brachial plexus.[3]

LA can also be used in the treatment of acute and chronic pain. Acute pain can refer to labour pain, postoperative pain, and trauma. Chronic pain is complex and therefore requires treatment by an expert in pain management. Often LAs are given in these cases with a combination of opioids, non-steroidal drugs, and anticonvulsants.

## Toxicity

Coma, circulatory collapse, cardiac arrest, and apnoea may occur in toxicity.[4,5] Signs and symptoms of CNS toxicity include:

- Light-headedness
- Dizziness and circumoral paraesthesia which may precede visual and/or auditory disturbances which can include difficulty focusing and tinnitus.

Other symptoms of toxicity include:

- Disorientation and feelings of drowsiness
- Respiratory depression.

Signs of CNS toxicity are usually excitatory and include:

- Shivering
- Muscular twitching and tremors initially involving muscles of the face and distal parts of the extremities
- Ultimately, convulsions of a tonic–clonic nature occur.

If a dose of LA is given rapidly IV or the administered dose is too great for an individual, then the initial signs of excitation may progress very quickly to generalized CNS depression and coma.[1] The AAGBI has produced guidelines for management of patients with severe LA toxicity.[5]

Respiratory depression may result in respiratory arrest. CNS toxicity is exacerbated by hypercarbia and acidosis. When injecting LA into vascular areas, great care should be taken to avoid intravascular injection; should accidental intravascular injection occur, signs and symptoms would be convulsions and cardiovascular collapse which can occur rapidly.

## References

1. British National Formulary (2020). Local anaesthesia. Available at: ℗ https://bnf.nice.org.uk/treatment-summary/anaesthesia-local.html

2. Simpson PJ, Popart MT (2002). Understanding anaesthesia (4th ed). Oxford: Butterworth-Heinemann.

3. British National Formulary (2020). Severe local anaesthetic-induced cardiovascular toxicity. Available at: ℗ https://bnf.nice.org.uk/treatment-summary/severe-local-anaesthetic-induced-cardiovascular-toxicity.html

## Further reading

Al-Shaikh B, Stacey S (2018). Essentials of equipment in anaesthesia, critical care and perioperative medicine (5th ed). Edinburgh: Elsevier.

Association of Anaesthetists of Great Britain and Ireland (2010). Guidelines for the management of severe local anaesthetic toxicity. London: Association of Anaesthetists of Great Britain and Ireland.

Pollard B, Kitchen G (eds) (2017). Handbook of clinical anaesthesia (4th ed). London: CRC Press.

Royal College of Anaesthetists (2021). Chapter 11: guidelines for the provision of anaesthesia services for inpatient pain management. London: Royal College of Anaesthetists.

Scarth E, Smith S (2016). Drugs in anaesthesia and intensive care (5th ed). Oxford: Oxford University Press.

# Intravenous conscious sedation

- Intravenous conscious sedation (IVCS) refers to mild-to-moderate depression of levels of consciousness allowing the patient to maintain their own airway.
- IVCS allows patients to respond to commands and/or physical stimulation.
- Patients are normally given sedatives to reduce anxiety and tolerate medical and nursing procedures.
- Sedation can also be used in intensive care for ventilated and spontaneous breathing patients.
- Sedation can be delivered either by continuous infusion or bolus doses through either a central line (for long-term sedation) or an IV line.
- It is essential that the line is secured properly as any disruption of the infusion or delivery of the sedation will result in emergence.
- It must be ensured that the patient is monitored appropriately throughout.[1] This should include:
  - ECG
  - NIBP
  - Respiratory rate
  - $SpO_2$.
- Some degree of respiratory depression may be observed along with fluctuation in BP, heart rate, and rhythm.

Drugs commonly used are:
- IV anaesthetic agents: propofol infusions are commonly used as propofol is controllable—produces rapid changes in consciousness (e.g. can wake patients up to allow them to breath spontaneously and assess neurologically). Propofol, however, can cause hypotension in some patients especially those who are hypovolaemic or dehydrated.
- Benzodiazepines: potent amnesiacs.
- Opioids: these are often used for pain relief, supported sometimes by sedatives.

## Reference

1. Association of Anaesthetists of Great Britain and Ireland (2016). Recommendations for standards of monitoring during anaesthesia and recovery 2015. Anaesthesia, 71(1):85–93.

## Further reading

Al-Rifai Z, Mulvey D (2016). Principles of total intravenous anaesthesia: practical aspects of using total intravenous anaesthesia. British Journal of Anaesthesia Education, 16(8):276–280.

Al-Shaikh B, Stacey S (2018). Essentials of equipment in anaesthesia, critical care and perioperative medicine (5th ed). Edinburgh: Elsevier.

Freedman R, Herbert L, O'Donnell A, et al. (eds) (2022). Oxford handbook of anaesthesia (5th ed). Oxford: Oxford University Press.

Middleton B, Phillips J, Stacey S (2021). Physics in anaesthesia: for FRCA candidates, ODPs and nurse anaesthetists (2nd ed). Banbury: Scion.

Phillips N, Hornacky A (2020). Berry & Kohn's operating room technique (14th ed). St Louis, MO: Elsevier.

Royal College of Anaesthetists (2019–2021). Guidelines for the provision of anaesthetic services. London: Royal College of Anaesthetists.

Thompson J, Moppett I, Wiles M (eds) (2019). Smith and Aitkenhead's textbook of anaesthesia (7th ed). Edinburgh: Elsevier.

# Epidural anaesthesia

- Epidural anaesthesia is achieved by the administration of a LA drug into the epidural space via an epidural catheter.
- The advantages of an epidural over spinal anaesthesia are that the epidural catheter allows for the epidural to be 'topped-up' with a LA, therefore prolonging the duration of action.
- Epidural has a slower onset than spinal anaesthesia and can take up to 45 minutes for surgical anaesthesia to be achieved.
- LA solutions can be delivered through the epidural catheter with a single shot, intermittent top-up, or continuously via a pump.
- Epidural anaesthesia can be used in obstetric, general, gynaecological, and orthopaedic surgery.
- Epidurals can also be used as an on-demand system such as patient-controlled epidural analgesia for postoperative pain relief as per local policy.
- When epidurals are being sited and dressed, a sterile technique must be adhered to and the epidural site dressed according to local policy and practice.
- It must be ensured that the patient is monitored appropriately throughout.[1] This should include:
  - ECG
  - NIBP
  - Respiratory rate
  - $SpO_2$.

Complications of epidural anaesthesia include:
- Hypotension
- Cerebrospinal fluid (CSF)/dural puncture
- Respiratory depression
- Failed block
- Pruritus
- Total spinal effect may occur from accidental dural puncture.

## Reference

1. Association of Anaesthetists of Great Britain and Ireland (2016). Recommendations for standards of monitoring during anaesthesia and recovery 2015. Anaesthesia, 71(1):85–93.

## Further reading

Al-Shaikh B, Stacey S (2018). Essentials of equipment in anaesthesia, critical care and perioperative medicine (5th ed). Edinburgh: Elsevier.

Anaesthesia UK (2005). Conduct of epidural and subarachnoid blockade. Available at: http://www.frca.co.uk/article.aspx?articleid=100445

Anaesthesia UK (2017). Bromage scale. Available at: http://www.frca.co.uk/article.aspx?articleid=100316

Association of Anaesthetists of Great Britain and Ireland (2020). Infection prevention and control. Available at: http://dx.doi.org/10.21466/g.IPAC2.2020

Association of Anaesthetists of Great Britain and Ireland (2020). Safety guideline: neurological monitoring associated with obstetric neuraxial block. Available at: https://doi.org/10.1111/anae.14993

Freedman R, Herbert L, O'Donnell A, et al. (eds) (2022). Oxford handbook of anaesthesia (5th ed). Oxford: Oxford University Press.

Phillips N, Hornacky A (2020). Berry & Kohn's operating room technique (14th ed). St Louis, MO: Elsevier.

Royal College of Anaesthetists (2019–2021). Guidelines for the provision of anaesthetic services. London: Royal College of Anaesthetists.

Thompson J, Moppett I, Wiles M (eds) (2019). Smith and Aitkenhead's textbook of anaesthesia (7th ed). Edinburgh: Elsevier.

# Caudal anaesthesia

- This is described as a low approach to the epidural space through the sacral hiatus, which is an anatomical gap in the sacrum.
- The caudal anaesthesia produces a block of the sacral and lumbar nerve roots.
- This procedure is prominently used in children as higher volumes of LA are needed to produce an effective block in adults.
- As this can be unpleasant for children, caudal anaesthetics are normally performed once the GA has been induced and before surgery.
- There are now caudal anaesthesia kits available with catheters similar to the epidural catheters which allow for the block to be prolonged during the course of surgery.

Complications of caudal anaesthesia are the same as epidural anaesthesia.

## Further reading

Al-Shaikh B, Stacey S (2018). Essentials of equipment in anaesthesia, critical care and perioperative medicine (5th ed). Edinburgh: Elsevier.

Association of Anaesthetists of Great Britain and Ireland (2016). Recommendations for standards of monitoring during anaesthesia and recovery 2015. Anaesthesia, 71(1):85–93.

Freedman R, Herbert L, O'Donnell A, et al. (eds) (2022). Oxford handbook of anaesthesia (5th ed). Oxford: Oxford University Press.

## Spinal anaesthesia

Spinal anaesthesia is also known as a subarachnoid block or spinal analgesia and is the introduction of LA solutions directly into the CSF which produces spinal anaesthesia.

- Spinals usually involve the lower part of the body, with a complete sensory and motor block of the affected area resulting in a total loss of sensation including pain, temperature, and position.
- Spinal anaesthesia can also have the effect of total or partial loss of power in the numb area for the duration of the block.
- Depending on the agent used, and the dose/volume given, the technique is fast onset with the duration of the block lasting anywhere between 1 and 4 hours.
- The area blocked can extend between the nipple levels (T10) to toes.
- It must be ensured that the patient is monitored appropriately throughout.[1] This should include:
  - ECG
  - NIBP
  - Respiratory rate
  - $SpO_2$.
- Patients can become hypotensive because of sympathetic blockade and vasodilation so the circulation system may need supporting with IV fluids.
- Vasoconstrictors such as ephedrine need to be available when this procedure is taking place and patients should be monitored appropriately throughout.
- The level of the spinal anaesthetic is measured for spread and height of the block. This is normally done with ice and/or light touch. Ethyl chloride is no longer commonly used, due to it being an atmospheric pollutant which tests afferent function.
- Motor function is normally tested with the Bromage scale[2] (Table 7.2).
- Spinal anaesthesia is suitable for surgical anaesthesia and is sometimes supported with a combination of epidural anaesthesia. The epidural allows for prolonged block for surgery and/or pain relief post surgery.
- When a spinal injection is being performed and dressed, a sterile technique must be adhered to and the spinal injection site dressed according to local policy and practice.
- Spinal anaesthesia is predominantly used in obstetric, orthopaedic, general, and gynaecological procedures.

### Complications

See Box 7.2.

### Contraindications

- Surgical procedures above the thorax.
- Hypovolaemia.
- Local/systemic infection.
- Raised intracranial pressure.
- Surgical procedures of long duration (i.e. lasting >2 hours).

**Table 7.2** Bromage scale

| Grade | Definition |
| --- | --- |
| 1 | Free movement of legs and feet |
| 2 | Just able to flex knees with free movement of feet |
| 3 | Unable to move knees but with free movement of feet |
| 4 | Unable to move legs or feet |

From Bromage PR. Epidural Analgesia. Philadelphia: WB Saunders; 1978:144.

## Box 7.2 Complications of spinal anaesthesia

- Failure of spinal anaesthesia.
- Uncommon complication is neurological disorder due to trauma.
- Localized bruising and back pain.
- Respiratory depression with opiates.
- PONV.
- High spinal block.
- Bladder distension.
- Bradycardia.
- Infection.
- Spinal headache.
- Hypotension: LA drugs block the sympathetic nerves to the blood vessels therefore causing vasodilatation.

## References

1. Association of Anaesthetists of Great Britain and Ireland (2016). Recommendations for standards of monitoring during anaesthesia and recovery 2015. Anaesthesia, 71(1):85–93.
2. Anaesthesia UK (2017). Bromage scale. Available at: ℜ http://www.frca.co.uk/article.aspx?articleid=100316

## Further reading

Anaesthesia UK (2005). Conduct of epidural and subarachnoid blockade. Available at: ℜ http://www.frca.co.uk/article.aspx?articleid=100445

Association of Anaesthetists of Great Britain and Ireland (2020). Safety guideline: neurological monitoring associated with obstetric neuraxial block. Available at: ℜ https://doi.org/10.1111/anae.14993

Freedman R, Herbert L, O'Donnell A, et al. (eds) (2022). Oxford handbook of anaesthesia (5th ed). Oxford: Oxford University Press.

Royal College of Anaesthetists (2019). Chapter 3: guidelines for the provision of anaesthesia services for intraoperative care. London: Royal College of Anaesthetists.

Royal College of Anaesthetists (2020). Chapter 9: guidelines for the provision of anaesthesia services for an obstetric population. London: Royal College of Anaesthetists.

# Continuous spinal anaesthesia

- Continuous spinal anaesthesia was first described by Edward Tuohy in 1944.
- Small-bore catheters for continuous spinal anaesthesia are available but 'they do not enjoy wide-spread popularity'[1] mainly due to postdural puncture headache[2].
- Once a microspinal catheter has been inserted, it must be clearly labelled to avoid accidental injection of an epidural-style dose.

## Advantages

- Good-quality block with the ability to titrate the dose and avoiding the risk of inadvertent total spinal block.
- Allows repeated boluses (or infusion) of LA.
- Acceptable for patients in labour and operative delivery.
- Decreases the possibility of cardiovascular instability during anaesthesia.
- Can be left in place for postoperative analgesia.
- Smaller decrease in BP and lower incidence of vasopressor use in elderly patients.
- Rapid onset of action, better quality of analgesia, and better muscle relaxation.

## Disadvantages

- It is uncommon in the UK.
- Associated with the development of cauda equina syndrome.
- Handling of the microspinal catheters is difficult.
- Risk of postdural puncture headache.
- Mistaking the microspinal catheter for an epidural catheter.
- Persistent paraesthesia and lower back pain.
- Risk of infection.
- Expensive.

## References

1. Simpson PJ, Popart MT (2002). Understanding anaesthesia (4th ed). Oxford: Butterworth-Heinemann.
2. Veličković I, Pujic B, Baysinger CW, et al. (2017). Continuous spinal anesthesia for obstetric anesthesia and analgesia. Frontiers in Medicine, 4:133. Available at: ℅ https://www.frontiersin.org/articles/10.3389/fmed.2017.00133/full

## Further reading

Anaesthesia UK (2005). Conduct of epidural and subarachnoid blockade. Available at: ℅ http://www.frca.co.uk/article.aspx?articleid=100445
Freedman R, Herbert L, O'Donnell A, et al. (eds) (2022). Oxford handbook of anaesthesia (5th ed). Oxford: Oxford University Press.
Ye M, Seet E, Kumar CM (2017). Myths and mysteries surrounding continuous spinal anaesthesia. Trends in Anaesthesia and Critical Care, 17:5–10.

# Patient positioning for regional anaesthesia

Spinal and epidural anaesthesia are often performed with the patient awake and in a sitting position.

- The sitting position allows for the patient to position themselves in the optimum position for the spinal/epidural anaesthesia to take place.
  - When possible, the patient rounds his/her back to open the gaps between vertebrae.
  - Place chin to chest.
  - The patient leans over a pillow on his/her lap and relaxes shoulders down.
  - Their feet should rest on a stool.
- The patient can also be placed on their side in a fetal position as is required for caudal anaesthesia if sitting is not possible. Lateral position, however, distorts the midline anatomy.
- It is a matter of individual judgement whether the advantages of the sitting position outweigh the discomfort for the patient in cases such as trauma or obstetrics.
- It is essential that one member of the anaesthetic team is solely dedicated to helping the patient maintain their position through the course of the procedure and continually monitors the patient's comfort and safety at all times.

## Further reading

Al-Shaikh B, Stacey S (2018). Essentials of equipment in anaesthesia, critical care and perioperative medicine (5th ed). Edinburgh: Elsevier.

Anaesthesia UK (2005). Conduct of epidural and subarachnoid blockade. Available at: ℜ http://www.frca.co.uk/article.aspx?articleid=100445

Anaesthesia UK (2017). Bromage scale. Available at: ℜ http://www.frca.co.uk/article.aspx?articleid=100316

Association of Anaesthetists of Great Britain and Ireland (2016). Recommendations for standards of monitoring during anaesthesia and recovery 2015. Anaesthesia, 71(1):85–93.

Freedman R, Herbert L, O'Donnell A, et al. (eds) (2022). Oxford handbook of anaesthesia (5th ed). Oxford: Oxford University Press.

Monteiro S, Salman M, Malhotra S, et al. (2019). Analgesia, anaesthesia and pregnancy: a practical guide (4th ed). Cambridge: Cambridge University Press.

# Contraindications for spinal, epidural, and caudal anaesthesia

- Technical/anatomical difficulties: if the spinal/epidural/caudal proves to be technically difficult, as a general rule, after two or three unsuccessful attempts seek more experienced help or an alternative technique. The anaesthetic assistant must be aware how to contact additional support should this be required.
- Lack of patient cooperation or if patient refuses.
- Lack of full resuscitation equipment available.
- If the patient's coagulation means there is heightened risk of haemorrhagic complications:
  - Patient is receiving anticoagulants such as warfarin prior to the spinal/epidural anaesthesia.
  - Here the international normalized ratio (INR) results need to be within acceptable limits to avoid haemorrhagic complications.
  - Normal INR = 1.
  - Acceptable INR = 0.8–1.2.
- Localized skin infection.
- Raised intracranial pressures.
- Patients with fixed cardiac output states.

## Further reading

Anaesthesia UK (2005). Conduct of epidural and subarachnoid blockade. Available at: ℘ http://www.frca.co.uk/article.aspx?articleid=100445

Anaesthesia UK (2017). Bromage scale. Available at: ℘ http://www.frca.co.uk/article.aspx?articleid=100316

Association of Anaesthetists of Great Britain and Ireland (2016). Recommendations for standards of monitoring during anaesthesia and recovery 2015. Anaesthesia, 71(1):85–93.

Freedman R, Herbert L, O'Donnell A, et al. (eds) (2022). Oxford handbook of anaesthesia (5th ed). Oxford: Oxford University Press.

Monteiro S, Salman M, Malhotra S, et al. (2019). Analgesia, anaesthesia and pregnancy: a practical guide (4th ed). Cambridge: Cambridge University Press.

Smith B, Rawlings P, Wicker P, et al. (2007). Core topics in operating department practice: anaesthesia and critical care. Cambridge: Cambridge University Press.

# Essential anaesthetic equipment

# Preparing the anaesthetic room

The checks and preparation detailed in this topic should be carried out before commencing each and every operating session and should be in accordance with the relevant AAGBI recommendations.[1]

## Checking machines

- The anaesthetic machine should be clean and free from damage and debris.
- Check that the machine is directly connected to a mains electrical supply and has a well-charged battery back-up (where appropriate).
- Connect gas pipelines to corresponding mains outlets and perform a 'tug test', ensuring each gas outlet exclusively supplies its corresponding flowmeter.
- The mains supply pressure for each gas should be 400–500 kPa.

## Check the following according to the AAGBI (2019) guidelines for checking anaesthetic equipment

- An audible $O_2$ fail alarm sounds when $O_2$ supply is shut off.
- Anti-hypoxia guard present: you should not be able to deliver a gas mix of >75% $N_2O$:25% $O_2$, and $N_2O$ flow should shut off if $O_2$ supply fails.
- All gas flowmeters move freely throughout ranges.
- Reserve $O_2$ cylinder fitted, functioning, and sufficiently full.
- Additional cylinders fitted and contents checked, as required.
- Emergency $O_2$ bypass control.
- Vaporizer(s) correctly mounted on back bar and locked in place (when one vaporizer is switched on it should lock off all other vaporizers from use).
- Calibrate $O_2$ and gas flow sensors and assess function.
- Circle breathing circuit, and ventilation limb and bag patent, intact, and in date (these are disposable items and have a defined period of use).
- Adjustable pressure-limiting (APL) valve and one-way flow valves function.
- Perform low-pressure breathing circuit leak test.
- Ventilator function.
- Auxiliary/common gas outlet function.
- Soda lime ($CO_2$ absorber) intact.
- Anaesthetic gas scavenging system operational.

  *Don't forget* to sign and date anaesthetic machine log book.
  *Remember*: if the anaesthetic machine fails any of these tests:
- It must be removed from service
- Complete failure documentation
- Inform anaesthetic service team and anaesthetic department.

## Checking equipment

Check availability and function of:
- Operational head-down (Trendelenburg) facility on bed/trolley.
- Essential minimal patient monitoring (ECG, NIBP, $SpO_2$, end-tidal carbon dioxide ($ETCO_2$)).
- Appropriate airway management equipment—➔ see Chapter 10.

- Mains suction with Yankauer sucker and a selection of suction catheter sizes (suction is incorporated into some anaesthetic machine designs).
- Difficult/emergency airway equipment—McCoy laryngoscope blades, intubating laryngeal mask airway (ILMA), fibreoptic laryngoscope, cricothyroidotomy kit.
- Alternative anaesthetic breathing circuit (e.g. Bains, Waters).
- Self-inflating bag and alternative $O_2$ cylinder.
- Peripheral nerve stimulator—for assessing neuromuscular blockade.
- Infusion pressure cuff/rapid infusion devices.
- Temperature monitoring equipment.
- Patient/fluid warming devices.

## Reference

1. Association of Anaesthetists of Great Britain and Ireland (2019). Checklist for draw-over anaesthetic equipment. Available at: ℜ http://dx.doi.org/10.21466/g.CFDAE2.2019

## Further reading

Al-Shaikh B, Stacey S (2018). Essentials of equipment in anaesthesia, critical care and perioperative medicine (5th ed). Edinburgh: Elsevier.

Association of Anaesthetists of Great Britain and Ireland (2018). The anaesthesia team 2018. Available at: ℜ http://dx.doi.org/10.21466/g.TAT.2018

Freedman R, Herbert L, O'Donnell A, et al. (eds) (2022). Oxford handbook of anaesthesia (5th ed). Oxford: Oxford University Press.

Martin A, Allman K, McIndoe A (eds) (2020). Emergencies in anaesthesia (3rd ed). Oxford: Oxford University Press.

Pollard B, Kitchen G (eds) (2017). Handbook of clinical anaesthesia (4th ed). London: CRC Press.

Royal College of Anaesthetists (2021). Chapter 2: guidelines for the provision of anaesthesia services for preoperative assessment and preparation. London: Royal College of Anaesthetists.

## Stocking of essential items

A sufficient stock level of the following consumable items should be kept in each anaesthetic room to cover not only the planned operating session but also any emergencies that may potentially arise.

- Facemasks.
- Oropharyngeal ('Guedel') and nasopharyngeal airways.
- Laryngeal mask airways (LMAs)—sized by patient weight (Table 8.1).
- Endotracheal tubes (ETTs)—selected by internal diameter (ID) (Table 8.2); always have a tube one size below that selected immediately available.
- Laryngoscope handle and blades—Macintosh size 3 and 4 (always check the bulb of the laryngoscope is secure, bright, and focuses on the tip of the blade. Keep spare batteries and bulbs in the anaesthetic room).
- Bougie/introducer and stylet.
- Water-based lubricant for LMA/ETT.
- Tie/tape for securing LMA/ETT.
- Gauze roll throat pack.
- Eye pads/protection.
- Gum guard and petroleum/paraffin jelly for teeth and lip protection.
- Heat and moisture exchange (HME) bacterial/viral filter.
- $O_2$ masks and other airway $O_2$ enrichment devices (e.g. T-piece, T-bag).
- Anaesthetic drugs, emergency drugs, and fluids.
- Syringes and needles—various sizes.
- IV cannulae (various sizes) and giving sets/taps/extensions.

*All of these items are available as single-patient use products.*

### Preparing the anaesthetic tray

After securing the patient's airway, the anaesthetic tray should hold everything you require for intra- and postoperative airway management. Most commonly:

- Laryngoscope
- Magill's forceps
- Syringe—for inflating cuffs on airway devices
- Facemask
- Oro-/nasopharyngeal airway (for post extubation).

**Table 8.1** Guidelines for selection of LMAs

| Size | Patient weight (kg) |
| --- | --- |
| 1 | <5 |
| 1.5 | 5–10 |
| 2 | 10–20 |
| 2.5 | 20–30 |
| 3 | 30–50 |
| 4 | 50–70 |
| 5 | 70–100 |
| 6 | >100 |

**Table 8.2** Guidelines for selection of endotracheal tubes

| ID (mm) | Patient weight (kg) | Patient group |
| --- | --- | --- |
| 2.5 | <1.5 | Premature |
| 3.0 | 1.5–2.5 | Premature |
| 3.5 | 3.5 | Newborn |
| 4.0 | 10 | Age 1 |
| 4.5 | 15 | Age 2–3 |
| 5.0 | 20 | Age 4–6 |
| 5.5 | 30 | Age 7–9 |
| 6.0 | 40 | Age 10–12 (small adult) |
| 6.5 | 50 | Age 13–15 (small adult) |
| 7.0 | >60 | >16 (adult) |
| 7.5 | | Female adult |
| 8.0–9.0 | | Male adult |

## Further reading

Al-Shaikh B, Stacey S (2018). Essentials of equipment in anaesthesia, critical care and perioperative medicine (5th ed). Edinburgh: Elsevier.

Association of Anaesthetists of Great Britain and Ireland (2018). The anaesthesia team 2018. Available at: ℘ http://dx.doi.org/10.21466/g.TAT.2018

Association of Anaesthetists of Great Britain and Ireland (2019). Checklist for draw-over anaesthetic equipment. Available at: ℘ http://dx.doi.org/10.21466/g.CFDAE2.2019

Davey A, Ince CS (2010). Fundamentals of operating department practice. Cambridge: Cambridge University Press.

Freedman R, Herbert L, O'Donnell A, et al. (eds) (2022). Oxford handbook of anaesthesia (5th ed). Oxford: Oxford University Press.

Martin A, Allman K, McIndoe A (eds) (2020). Emergencies in anaesthesia (3rd ed). Oxford: Oxford University Press.

Pollard B, Kitchen G (eds) (2017). Handbook of clinical anaesthesia (4th ed). London: CRC Press.

Royal College of Anaesthetists (2019). Chapter 4: guidelines for the provision of post-operative care. London: Royal College of Anaesthetists.

# Anaesthetic machines

During GA, medical gases are delivered to the patient via the anaesthetic machine and anaesthesia breathing systems. In addition, the modern-day anaesthetic machine has the facility to provide additional monitoring for physiological parameters and ventilation.

Modern anaesthetic machines incorporate a circle breathing system and possess the following features (adapted from Al-Shaikh and Stacey[1]):
- Pressure gauges—colour coded.
- Pressure regulators.
- Flowmeters—colour coded.
- Vaporizers.
- $O_2$ flow meter controlled by a single-touch coded control knob.
- $O_2$ concentration monitor or analyser.
- High-flow $O_2$ flush.
- $N_2O$ cut-off device when $O_2$ pressure is low.
- $O_2$, $N_2O$ ratio monitor, and controller.
- Pin index safety system.
- $O_2$ failure warning alarm.
- Ventilator disconnection alarm.
- Reserve $O_2$ cylinder in case of pipeline failure.

The anaesthetic machine is checked by the anaesthetic practitioner according to the AAGBI checklist for anaesthetic equipment guidelines.[2] This helps to inform standardization of practice. However, all anaesthetists have the responsibility to carry out checks of the anaesthetic equipment prior to commencement of the operating list.

All modern anaesthetic machines have the ability to be connected to an external power supply which means they need to be switched on. When this occurs, some anaesthetic workstations enter into a self-test programme and calibration exercise. These functions do not have to be retested.

## Safety systems
- Piped gases are colour coded and connectors are specific to the gas being used so that, for example, an $O_2$ pipeline (white) cannot be connected to a $N_2O$ outlet (blue).
- On an anaesthetic machine, the cylinder yoke, into which the cylinder fits, is protected by the '*pin index*' system.[3]
- The pin index system is a series of holes and pins designed to make sure that the wrong cylinder cannot be fitted to the wrong attachment.
- The holes drilled in to the cylinder valve must correspond with the pins that are located on the cylinder yoke of the anaesthetic machine.
- Each medical gas cylinder used on the anaesthetic machine has its own unique pin index code so only the correct gas can be connected to the correct cylinder yoke.[3]

# References

1. Al-Shaikh B, Stacey S (2018). Essentials of equipment in anaesthesia, critical care and perioperative medicine (5th ed). Edinburgh: Elsevier.
2. Association of Anaesthetists of Great Britain and Ireland (2019). Checklist for draw-over anaesthetic equipment. Available at: ℘ http://dx.doi.org/10.21466/g.CFDAE2.2019
3. Davey A, Ince CS (2010). Fundamentals of operating department practice. Cambridge: Cambridge University Press.

# Further reading

Freedman R, Herbert L, O'Donnell A, et al. (eds) (2022). Oxford handbook of anaesthesia (5th ed). Oxford: Oxford University Press.
Pollard B, Kitchen G (eds) (2017). Handbook of clinical anaesthesia (4th ed). London: CRC Press.
Royal College of Anaesthetists (2019). Chapter 2: guidelines for the provision of anaesthesia services for preoperative assessment and preparation. London: Royal College of Anaesthetists.

# Ventilators

Ventilation of the lungs can be performed without any equipment at all. Today, artificial ventilation is used on a daily basis as part of an anaesthetic technique. To aid this, a range of ventilators have been developed and many are multifunctional.

During GA, it may be necessary to paralyse and ventilate the patient. Ventilators are used to provide intermittent positive pressure ventilation (IPPV). During spontaneous respiration, gas moves into the lungs by negative intrathoracic pressure but this process is reversed for IPPV. Anaesthetic/medical ventilators should be simple, robust, and economical to purchase and use.[1]

Modern anaesthetic ventilators incorporate the following features (adapted from Al-Shaikh and Stacey[1]):

• Volume cycling—predetermined tidal volume.
• Time cycling—predetermined inspiratory rate.
• Pressure cycling—predetermined pressure is reached.
• Flow cycling—predetermined flow is reached during inspiration when it switches to exhalation.
• Either gas or electrically powered.
• Pressure generator—produces inspiration by generating a predetermined pressure.
• Flow generator—produces inspiration by a predetermined flow of gas.
• Should be easy to clean and sterilize.

Pressure generator ventilators cannot compensate if there is a change in the patient's chest compliance; however, they are able to compensate if a leak is detected. A flow generator can compensate to compliance changes but not leaks within the system.

The modern anaesthetic machine incorporates a 'bag in a bottle ventilator' which is a time-cycled ventilator consisting of bellows that collapse, delivering the fresh gas flow from within the bellows, and then the driving gas (compressed air) returns the bellows to the ascending position in readiness for the next cycle. The ventilator can generate within the chamber a tidal volume of 0–1500 mL. A paediatric version is also available generating a tidal volume of 0–400 mL.

## Safety systems

During anaesthesia, it is vitally important that both the patient and the equipment used are monitored closely. The complexity of anaesthesia depends on a variety of factors including (adapted from Gwinnutt and Gwinnutt[2]):

• Type of operation and surgical technique
• Anaesthetic technique
• Patient's past medical history and/or pre-existing conditions
• Anaesthetist's preferences
• Equipment available and anaesthetist's familiarization with the equipment.

# References

1. Al-Shaikh B, Stacey S (2018). Essentials of equipment in anaesthesia, critical care and perioperative medicine (5th ed). Edinburgh: Elsevier.
2. Gwinnutt M, Gwinnutt CL (2016). Lecture notes: clinical anaesthesia (5th ed). Oxford: Wiley-Blackwell.

# Further reading

Association of Anaesthetists of Great Britain and Ireland (2018). The anaesthesia team 2018. Available at: http://dx.doi.org/10.21466/g.TAT.2018

Association of Anaesthetists of Great Britain and Ireland (2019). Checklist for draw-over anaesthetic equipment. Available at: http://dx.doi.org/10.21466/g.CFDAE2.2019

Freedman R, Herbert L, O'Donnell A, et al. (eds) (2022). Oxford handbook of anaesthesia (5th ed). Oxford: Oxford University Press.

Martin A, Allman K, McIndoe A (eds) (2020). Emergencies in anaesthesia (3rd ed). Oxford: Oxford University Press.

Pollard B, Kitchen G (eds) (2017). Handbook of clinical anaesthesia (4th ed). London: CRC Press.

Royal College of Anaesthetists (2019). Chapter 3: guidelines for the provision of anaesthesia services for intraoperative care. London: Royal College of Anaesthetists.

Royal College of Anaesthetists (2021). Chapter 2: guidelines for the provision of anaesthesia services for preoperative assessment and preparation. London: Royal College of Anaesthetists.

# Vaporizers

Inhalational anaesthetic agents (volatiles) are used for the induction and maintenance of anaesthesia and form the basis of modern-day anaesthetic practice.[1] Historically, in the early days of anaesthesia, vapours were administered without a vaporizer; ether was administered by the drop method where a cloth was placed over the patient's face and the agent was dripped onto it. The invention of the Schimmelbusch mask helped to improve this system which lifted the cloth off the patient's face, enabling air to circulate.[1] However, the use of ether was inaccurate and dangerous, resulting in deaths from overdose and a risk of combustion. This led to the invention of more stable and user-friendly volatiles and the creation of more predictable means of administration, namely vaporizers.[2]

## Basic principles of vaporizers

- A vaporizer[3] is a device that adds the necessary concentration of volatile anaesthetic vapour to the stream of anaesthetic-carrying gas.
- Vaporizers are flow and temperature compensated so they are unaffected by positive pressure ventilation.
- All volatile anaesthetic agents have different physical properties and therefore each vaporizer is agent specific.
- Volatile agents commonly used in practice include sevoflurane, isoflurane, and desflurane.
- A vaporizer functions by dividing the carrying gas flow into two streams. One stream is directed into the vaporizing chamber, the other into the bypass chamber. This is known as the 'splitting ratio'. Gas that leaves the vaporizing chamber is fully saturated with the volatile agent of choice. The dial on the vaporizer, which can be adjusted by the anaesthetist, alters the proportion of gas entering the bypass chamber which in turn can alter the final concentration leaving the outlet.[4]
- All vaporizers used today have a colour-coded 'key filler' system and supply bottle so that each vaporizer can only be replenished with the fluid intended for that particular vaporizer.[5]
- Vaporizers are usually sited on the backbar of the anaesthetic machine. The Selectatec™ system allows the various vaporizers to be removed easily for any reasons, for example, so they can be refilled, changed, or if faulty. It also ensures that only one vaporizer can be used at a time. A combination of vaporizer designs is hazardous and should be strongly discouraged.

## There are four types of vaporizers currently in use

- Plenum.
- Draw-over.
- Gas blenders.
- Computer controlled.

*Plenum vaporizer*

This is the most frequently used vaporizer in the UK. They are agent specific, efficient, variable, and unidirectional. They are used outside the breathing system. Features of modern plenum vaporizers include (adapted from Eales and Cooper[4]):

• Flow and temperature compensated
• Consistent output
• One-hand, easily operated dial
• Clear indication of fill level
• 'Easy-fil™' filler, reduces leaks, agent specific.

*Draw-over vaporizer*

This is mainly used by the armed forces as part of the tri-service anaesthetic equipment and in remote areas. The draw-over vaporizers are used within the breathing circuit. They have a low resistance to flow and are relatively efficient. Examples include the Oxford Miniature Vaporizer (OMV), simple and robust hence its use as tri-service anaesthetic equipment.

*Gas blender*

Gas blenders are used to administer desflurane only, due to the physical properties of the agent. They require an external power supply which enables the desflurane to be heated to 39°C and pressurizes it to 1500 mmHg (about 2 atmospheres). This means that there is a constant stream of vapour under pressure flowing out of the chamber and blending with the fresh gas flow.

*Computer-controlled vaporizer*

Computer-controlled vaporizers are found on certain anaesthetic machines and they consist of a central processing unit, assigned by a magnetic code to each volatile agent, which measures and adjusts the gas flow. The volatile agent of choice is adjusted by regulating the flow of gas through the processor.

## Safety

According to Ince et al. [6] it is important to observe the following important safety precautions:

• Do not carry the vaporizer by the dial.
• Check that the mounting point 'O' rings on the Selectatec™ manifold are intact and undamaged and that the mating surfaces are clean.
• Make sure that the vaporizer control knob is in the 'off' position and the locking lever is in the 'on' position.
• Lower the vaporizer onto the manifold and move the locking lever to the 'lock' position.
• Make sure the vaporizer is properly seated.
• Leak test the system with the vaporizer off and then turned on. A leak from the vaporizer can result in awareness for the patient.[7]

## References

1. Haslam GM, Forrest FC. 2004. Principles of anaesthetic vaporisers. Anaesthesia and Intensive Care Medicine, 5(3):88–91.
2. Huang L, Sang CN, Desai MS (2017). Beyond ether and chloroform—a major breakthrough with halothane. Journal of Anesthesia History, 3(3):87–102.
3. Young J, Kapoor V (2016). Principles of anaesthetic vaporizers. Anaesthesia and Intensive Care Medicine, 17(3):133–136.
4. Eales M, Cooper R (2007). Principles of anaesthetic vaporisers. Anaesthesia and Intensive Care Medicine, 8(3):111–115.
5. Al-Shaikh B, Stacey S (2018). Essentials of equipment in anaesthesia, critical care and perioperative medicine (5th ed). Edinburgh: Elsevier.
6. Ince CS, Skinner AC, Taft E (2000). Scientific principles in relation to the anaesthetic machine. In: Ince CS, Davey A (eds) Fundamentals of operating department practice. London: Greenwich Medical Media.
7. Association of Anaesthetists of Great Britain and Ireland (2019). Checklist for draw-over anaesthetic equipment. Available at: ℰ http://dx.doi.org/10.21466/g.CFDAE2.2019

## Further reading

Association of Anaesthetists of Great Britain and Ireland (2016). Recommendations for standards of monitoring during anaesthesia and recovery 2015. Anaesthesia, 71(1):85–93.

Sherwood M (2010). Vapourisation and vapourisers. Anaesthesia tutorial of the week 171. Available at: ℰ https://www.aagbi.org/sites/default/files/171-Vapourisation-and-vapourisers.pdf

# Breathing systems

To enable an anaesthetic mixture to be delivered to the patient, anaesthetic breathing systems are employed. They are fundamental in coupling the patient's respiratory system to the anaesthetic machine. Different breathing systems exist, including open, semi-closed, and circle systems, but the ideal circuit features should include[1]:

- Efficient elimination of expired $CO_2$
- Low resistance to gas flow
- Safety and robustness
- Low dead space
- Light and easy to use.

### Non-rebreathing systems

Consist of unidirectional valves to direct exhaled gases away from the patient. These systems are seldom used in anaesthesia because of valve problems but are used in the transportation of critically ill patients and within post-anaesthetic care units (PACUs). A common example of a non-rebreathing system is the 'non-rebreather mask' consisting of a facemask and a reservoir bag which continually refills with fresh gas, often an oxygen source. A non-rebreathing or one-way valve separates the reservoir and mask allowing fresh gas to be delivered to the patient upon inspiration but closes upon expiration, preventing the patient from rebreathing the exhaled gases.[2]

### Rebreathing systems

Rebreathing systems are widely used in anaesthesia and in 1954, WW Mapleson described the theory of anaesthetic breathing circuits into open, semi-open, and semi-closed. The six classifications—A, B, C, D, E, and F (Fig. 8.1)—are the mainstay of all modern-day anaesthetic breathing systems. B and C are not commonly used in anaesthesia, although Mapleson C circuits such as the Water's circuit are seen in resuscitation scenarios. The high fresh gas flows required to reduce rebreathing result in these systems not being commonly used for routine anaesthesia.[3]

### Mapleson A

Commonly known as 'Magill' or 'Lack' consists of corrugated tubing or co-axial system with an APL valve at the patient end and with a 2 L reservoir bag at the anaesthetic machine end. A simple system but can prove cumbersome and not suitable for use when ventilation is required. The modern version of this system, the Lack, is coaxial or parallel and the APL valve is at the anaesthetic machine end.

### Mapleson D

Commonly known today as a 'Bain' coaxial system, it is inefficient for spontaneous breathing because the exhaled gas passes into the reservoir bag resulting in the possibility of rebreathing unless fresh gas flow is high. Good for IPPV and is useful if anaesthesia access to the patient is compromised, for instance, during head and neck surgery.

## Mapleson E and F

Commonly known today as Ayre's T-Piece (E) (Phillip Ayre, 1937) and Jackson Rees Modification (F) (Dr Jackson Rees). These systems are used for paediatric patients up to 25–30 kg body weight[4] because of their lack of resistance, limited 'dead space', and their valve-less state. They are suitable for spontaneous and controlled ventilation. As there is no APL valve with these systems, scavenging of waste anaesthetic gases can be problematic. Certain manufacturers have designed paediatric systems with APL valves so that scavenging can occur. However, the use of this particular system is debatable.

## Circle systems

The advantages of using the circle system are that they use very low fresh gas consumption and volatile anaesthetic agents (saves money), absorb $CO_2$ (saves pollution), and they warm and humidify anaesthetic gases (maintain normothermia) (adapted from Fenlon[5]). Appropriate monitoring must be used before this system is utilized.[6]

A diagrammatic version of a circle system is shown in Fig. 8.2.

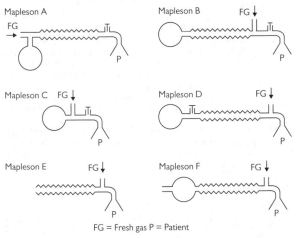

FG = Fresh gas    P = Patient

**Fig. 8.1** Breathing circuits.

Reproduced with permission from Allman KG and Wilson IH (eds) (2016). Oxford Handbook of Anaesthesia (4th ed). Oxford: Oxford University Press.

## $CO_2$ absorption

$CO_2$ absorption[2] is an important requirement for circle systems. Circle systems require an adequate oxygen supply and, provided the patient's exhaled $CO_2$ is removed, the same anaesthetic gasses can be recirculated and reused.

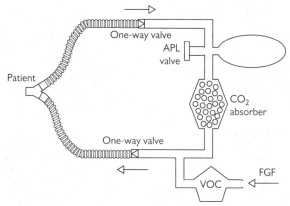

**Fig. 8.2** Circle breathing system with $CO_2$ absorption and vaporizer out of circuit (VOC). FGF, fresh gas flow.

$CO_2$ absorption is commonly achieved using soda lime. Soda lime is a compound of calcium hydroxide (94%), sodium hydroxide (5%), and potassium hydroxide (1%). As the exhaled mixture passes through the soda lime granules, a chemical reaction results in the $CO_2$ binding to the granules, allowing the remaining anaesthetic mixture to be topped up with fresh gases and rebreathed by the patient.

As the chemical reaction and absorption of $CO_2$ takes place, water and heat are produced, which help combat the dehumidifying and cooling effects of the fresh gas flow.

Soda lime needs to be replaced after a period of time, different manufacturers include different colour indicators, whereby the soda lime changes colour as it becomes exhausted. However, a more accurate method of gauging when soda lime needs changing is that 1 kg of soda lime should safely absorb $CO_2$ of an average-build anaesthetized adult for approximately 8 hours.

### References

1. Ince CS, Skinner AC, Taft E (2000). Scientific principles in relation to the anaesthetic machine. In: Ince CS, Davey A (eds) Fundamentals of operating department practice. London: Greenwich Medical Media.
2. Simpson PJ, Popat M (2002). Understanding anaesthesia (4th ed). Oxford: Butterworth Heinemann.
3. Tej KK, Geeta M (2013). Mapleson's breathing systems. Indian Journal of Anaesthesia, 57(5):507–515.
4. Al-Shaikh B, Stacey S (2002). Essentials of anaesthetic equipment. London: Churchill Livingstone.
5. Fenlon S (2005). Equipment for paediatric anaesthesia. In: Davey A, Diba A (eds) Ward's anaesthetic equipment. London: Elsevier Saunders.
6. Association of Anaesthetists of Great Britain and Ireland (2004). Checking anaesthetic equipment. London: Association of Anaesthetists of Great Britain and Ireland.

## Further reading

Association of Anaesthetists of Great Britain and Ireland (2015). Recommendations for standards of monitoring during anaesthesia and recovery. London: Association of Anaesthetists of Great Britain and Ireland.

Lockwood GG (2007). Circle systems. Anaesthesia and Intensive Care Medicine, 10(4):215–221.

Lovell T (2007). Breathing systems. Anaesthesia and Intensive Care Medicine, 8(3):102–106.

# Humidifiers

Dry anaesthetic gases can affect the cells lining the respiratory tract. Humidification devices used in anaesthesia and anaesthetic breathing systems are used as a counter to the heat lost through vaporized water in the airway. The main humidifiers used in anaesthesia are also capable of providing microbiological protection for the patient. They are single-patient use and should be positioned as close to the patient's mouth as possible, normally between the catheter mount, which is connected to the ETT or other airway adjunct, and the anaesthetic breathing system of choice.

The majority of humidifiers used in the clinical area have a provision for connection of a sampling tube for gas and vapour concentration analysers. HME filter humidifiers are compact, passive, inexpensive, and are appropriate for most clinical situations.

HME filters function by allowing condensation of water vapour upon exhalation within the filter. The heat and moisture from the water vapour help to warm and humidify the inspired anaesthetic gases.

The humidifiers contain a hygroscopic or hydrophobic element as well as a bacterial filter.[1]

## Hygroscopic membrane HMEs

Hygroscopic membrane HMEs have the following characteristics (adapted from Poolacherla and Nickells[2]):
- Foam, paper, or wool-like material.
- Coated with moisture-retaining chemicals.
- Impregnated with bactericide.
- Subjected to electrical field to increase its polarity.
- More efficient than hydrophobic HMEs.

## Hydrophobic membrane HMEs

Hydrophobic membrane HMEs have the following characteristics (adapted from Poolacherla and Nickells[2]):
- Folded ceramic fibre.
- Surface area must be high.
- Membrane is pleated.
- Low thermal conductivity.
- Allows passage of water vapour.
- Can use nebulization.
- Performance impaired with high ambient temperatures.

The use of low fresh gas flows in a circle system help to conserve heat and moisture, coupled with the reaction of the soda lime and $CO_2$ producing heat and moisture.[1]

Heated humidifiers are used in the critical care setting when ventilatory assistance may be required for a number of days rather than hours. They utilize the same principles as vaporizers in that they heat (45–60°C), power, and can maintain a constant and stable humidification of fresh gas flows.

## Safety systems

- HMEs must be checked on regular occasions as an accumulation of water in the filter may cause an increase in airway resistance.[2]
- All humidifier systems increase the number of connections within the anaesthetic circuit and potentially increase the risk of disconnection. To minimize this risk, a disconnection alarm should be utilized, and all connections must be checked on regular occasions and pushed home and twisted.[1]
- Disposable HME filters are single-patient use only.

## References

1. McKindoe A (2003). Humidification devices. Anaesthesia and Intensive Care Medicine, 4(11):353–354.
2. Poolacherla R, Nickells J (2006). Humidification devices. Anaesthesia and Intensive Care Medicine, 7(10):351–353.
3. Al-Shaikh B, Stacey S (2002). Essentials of anaesthetic equipment. London: Churchill Livingstone.

## Further reading

Association of Anaesthetists of Great Britain and Ireland (2012). Checking anaesthetic equipment. London: Association of Anaesthetists of Great Britain and Ireland.
Association of Anaesthetists of Great Britain and Ireland (2016). Recommendations for standards of monitoring during anaesthesia and recovery 2015. Anaesthesia, 71(1):85–93.

# Fluid/blood warmers

Fluid/blood warmers are used to infuse warmed fluids to patients. The use of IV fluid warmers is recommended to help reduce the risk of patients developing inadvertent perioperative hypothermia.[1] With reports of a potential fall in patient core temperature of 0.25±C with the administration of 1 L of room temperature fluid.[2] Therefore, it is recommended that blood products and IV fluids of >500 mL should be warmed using a fluid warming device.[1]

Previously, fluid warming was achieved by immersing an infusion coil in a water bath. This is no longer acceptable as they were messy and an excellent medium for bacterial growth.[3] There are a range of fluid warming systems, although there are two systems commonly in clinical use: dry heat warmers and the coaxial fluid heating system.

Due to the range of different devices available, this is a brief overview, it is important to be familiar with the ones in your own clinical practice.

## Dry heat warmers

- These consist of two heated plates in which the plastic insert is sandwiched and primed with a crystalloid.
- Different devices utilize a cassette (Fluido®) which is inserted into the machine and can be transferred with the patient to other areas of care.
- Other dry heat warmers include cylindrical devices which utilize the giving-sets extension.
- These devices increase the resistance to flow and significantly add to the giving-set dead space.[4]
- The added giving-set dead space should be considered when administering medications through the set. Medications should be followed by a flush to ensure the medication has been administered to the patient.

## Coaxial fluid heating system (Hotline®)

- These consist of three lumens within the device with one lumen carrying the infusate to the patient and the other two lumens carrying water heated to 40±C and stored within the heating case.
- The infusate does not come into contact with the circulating water. The coaxial tubing extends to the IV cannula thus ensuring that the tubing is not exposed to room temperature.[4]

Another device involves the use of a preshaped heat exchange coil that is situated within the ducting of a forced air convective warmer.[3]

There are methods for rapidly infusing warm fluids, but this is not discussed in this section; however, further information can be found in the 'Further reading' section and on the Medicines and Healthcare products Regulatory Agency (MHRA) website.[5]

# References

1. National Institute for Health and Care Excellence (2016). Hypothermia: prevention and management in adults having surgery. NICE. Clinical guideline [CG65]. Available at: M https://www.nice.org.uk/guidance/cg65

2. John M, Ford J, Harper M (2014). Peri-operative warming devices: performance and clinical application. Anaesthesia, 69(6):623–638.

3. Diba A (2005). Infusion equipment and intravenous anaesthesia. In: Davey A, Diba A (eds) Ward's anaesthetic equipment. London: Elsevier Saunders.

4. Al-Shaikh B, Stacey S (2002). Essentials of anaesthetic equipment. London: Churchill Livingstone.

5. Medicines and Healthcare products Regulatory Agency. Homepage. Available at: https://www.gov.uk/government/organisations/medicines-and-healthcare-products-regulatory-agency

## Further reading

Association of Anaesthetists of Great Britain and Ireland (2012). Checking anaesthetic equipment. London: Association of Anaesthetists of Great Britain and Ireland.

Association of Anaesthetists of Great Britain and Ireland (2016). Recommendations for standards of monitoring during anaesthesia and recovery 2015. Anaesthesia, 71(1):85–93.

# Patient monitoring

The range of monitoring devices is broad and ever increasing. You should ensure that the monitoring devices used in patient care are fit for purpose whatever the circumstances. In addition to this:

- You should have adequate knowledge of the equipment before its use.
- Calibration of all monitoring equipment should be carried out prior to use when necessary and/or be part of a maintenance programme.
- Monitoring devices are there to keep the team aware of the patient's physiological state, record data, and ensure patient safety.
- Monitors are an adjunct to anaesthesia and are no substitute for patient observation.

> *Remember*: monitor the patient and not the monitor.

The AAGBI[1] has set minimal standards that are acceptable for monitoring patients during anaesthesia and recovery periods and advocate the following:

- Monitoring must be attached before the anaesthetic starts and the patient's physiological state should be continued to be monitored until the patient has recovered.
- All patient physiological data collected must be recorded in the patient's notes. If electronic data is being stored then this should comply with local and national policy including the Data Protection Act.
- If a non-medical member of the perioperative team is recording the patient's vital signs, then it should be ensured they have the competencies to translate the data and act appropriately should the need arise.
- The anaesthetist is responsible for ensuring that the monitoring has been checked, that it is fit for use, and alarm limits have been set and are audible.
- Monitoring that is deemed essential for the safe conduct of anaesthesia are pulse oximeter, NIBP monitor, ECG, airway gases, $O_2$, $CO_2$, vapour and airway pressure, plus having available a nerve stimulator and some means of measuring the patient's temperature.[2]

Patients should also be monitored when receiving a LA/regional anaesthetic or sedative technique when surgical intervention is undertaken. The AAGBI[1] states that the minimum monitoring required in this situation is:

- Pulse oximeter
- NIBP monitor
- ECG.

## References

1. Association of Anaesthetists of Great Britain and Ireland (2016). Recommendations for standards of monitoring during anaesthesia and recovery 2015. Anaesthesia, 71(1):85–93.
2. National Institute for Health and Care Excellence. 2016. Hypothermia: prevention and management in adults having surgery. Clinical guideline [CG65]. Available at: ℘ https://www.nice.org.uk/guidance/cg65

## Further reading

Al-Shaikh B, Stacey S (2018). Essentials of equipment in anaesthesia, critical care and perioperative medicine (5th ed). Edinburgh: Elsevier.

Association of Anaesthetists of Great Britain and Ireland (2012). Checking anaesthetic equipment. London: Association of Anaesthetists of Great Britain and Ireland.

Davey A, Ince CS (2010). Fundamentals of operating department practice. Cambridge: Cambridge University Press.

# Non-invasive monitoring

Non-invasive monitoring that is frequently used within the perioperative environment includes[1]:
- ECG
- NIBP
- Pulse oximetry
- Peripheral nerve stimulators
- Capnography—ETCO$_2$ analyser
- Respiratory rate
- Airway gases
- Vapours
- Nerve stimulator
- Temperature measurement.

## ECG

An ECG monitors the electrical activity of the heart and will determine rate, arrhythmias, conduction defects, and ischaemia.
- ECG monitoring consists of skin electrodes which use silver and silver chloride along with a conducting gel, an amplifier to boost the signal and filter out other frequencies, and an oscilloscope to display the ECG.
- When placing the electrodes on the skin, ensure they are attached properly by first cleaning the skin.
- Attaching the electrodes over bony prominences will reduce the occurrence of artefacts produced by muscular activity such as shivering.
- A three-lead ECG is normally used during the perioperative phase:
  - Although there are many configurations, the three-lead used most widely is left arm, right arm, and left leg and the latter is often placed over the apex; this allows leads I, II, and III to be monitored and the anaesthetist can choose which provides the best amplitude.
- CM5 configuration can be used if cardiac ischaemia is a concern.
- The CM5 configuration consists of one lead over manubrium sterni, the second lead normally placed over the left clavicle on a bony prominence, and the third lead in the V5 position over the left ventricle.
- CM5 configuration will detect left ventricular ischaemia.
- Electrical interference can be caused by other equipment such as diathermy and mobile phones. Most modern monitors are produced with shielding to limit this interference. The MHRA highlights that mobile phones can adversely affect some medical equipment and therefore the Association for Perioperative Practice[2] recommends that all mobile phones should be switched off in the perioperative environment.
- Diathermy burns can occur at the ECG electrode site in the absence of, or misplacement of, a diathermy plate as the passage of the electrical current from the diathermy can pass through the ECG electrodes.

## NIBP

- NIBPs are normally performed with the use of an automatic NIBP measurement device.
- This device gives trend information on systolic, diastolic, mean arterial pressures, and pulse rate.

- It consists of a cuff and tube which connects to an inflation and deflation device.
- A pressure transducer and microprocessor convert the fluctuations in the cuff pressures into a readable BP measurement on the monitor.
- It is essential that the correct size cuff is used, the middle of the cuff bladder should be positioned over the brachial artery, and the cuff should cover at least two-thirds of the patient's upper arm and should be free of kinks and folds. This will ensure the optimum conditions for a correct reading and prevent soft tissue injury to the patient.
- If the cuff is too small it will over-read the BP; equally, if the cuff is large it will under-read the BP, though the error is greater when the cuff is too small.
- Atrial fibrillation and other arrhythmias will affect NIBP readings.
- On the initial BP the cuff will inflate to above the previous systolic pressure.
- As the cuff is inflated and deflated, the transducer senses the oscillations in the cuff from the returning blood flow.
- Mean arterial pressure corresponds to the maximum oscillations at the lowest cuff pressure; systolic pressure corresponds to the rapidly increasing oscillations; and diastolic pressure corresponds to the rapidly decreasing oscillations.

## References

1. Association of Anaesthetists of Great Britain and Ireland (2016). Recommendations for standards of monitoring during anaesthesia and recovery 2015. Anaesthesia, 71(1):85–93.
2. Association for Perioperative Practice (2007). Standards and recommendations for safe perioperative practice. Harrogate: Association for Perioperative Practice.

## Further reading

Abbott H, Booth H (eds) (2014). Foundations for operating department practice: essential theory for practice. Maidenhead: Open University Press.
Al-Shaikh B, Stacey S (2018). Essentials of equipment in anaesthesia, critical care and perioperative medicine (5th ed). Edinburgh: Elsevier.
Davey A, Ince CS (2010). Fundamentals of operating department practice. Cambridge: Cambridge University Press.

# Pulse oximetry

- This measures the arterial blood $O_2$ at the arterioles.
- Pulse oximetry is made up of a probe which consists of two light-emitting diodes on one side, a photodetector on the other, and a microprocessor which displays the $O_2$ saturation, pulse rate, and a waveform.
- Alarm limits can be set for low and high saturation readings and low and high pulse rates.
- Red and infrared light is emitted from the diodes at 660 nm and 940 nm, emitting the light at a high frequency of about 30 times per second.
- The red and infrared light from the diodes passes through the skin, tissue, and bone, and a percentage of this light is absorbed.
- The photodetector detects the returning light transmitted through the tissue which the microprocessor is programmed to mathematically analyse into a readable $O_2$ saturation level.
- Inaccurate readings can be given when the patient is suffering from carbon monoxide poisoning, including smoking, coloured nail varnish, IV injection of certain dyes such as methylene blue, hypoperfusion, and severe vasoconstriction.
- If the oximetry probe becomes disconnected, it can take some time for the peripheral saturation to change; if this occurs, closely observe the patient's colour.
- Inaccurate measurements can be caused by excessive movement, malpositioning of the probe, and external florescent light. Probes have also been known to read a percentage when attached to nothing except a blanket.
- Be aware that probes can also cause pressure damage if left on one site for too long; some manufacturers suggest that the position of the probe should be changed every 2 hours.

## Further reading

Al-Shaikh B, Stacey S (2018). Essentials of equipment in anaesthesia, critical care and perioperative medicine (5th ed). Edinburgh: Elsevier.

Association of Anaesthetists of Great Britain and Ireland (2016). Recommendations for standards of monitoring during anaesthesia and recovery 2015. Anaesthesia, 71(1):85–93.

Aston D, Rivers A, Dharmadasa A (2014). Equipment in anaesthesia and critical care: a complete guide for the FRCA. Banbury: Scion.

Davey A, Ince CS (2010). Fundamentals of operating department practice. Cambridge: Cambridge University Press.

Middleton B, Phillips J, Stacey S (2021). Physics in anaesthesia: for FRCA candidates, ODPs and nurse anaesthetists (2nd ed). Banbury: Scion.

Thompson J, Moppett I, Wiles M (eds) (2019). Smith and Aitkenhead's textbook of anaesthesia (7th ed). Edinburgh: Elsevier.

# Peripheral nerve stimulators

- Peripheral nerve stimulation is used during the anaesthetic phase to monitor the degree of neuromuscular blockade.
- They can also be used to confirm adequate reversal of neuromuscular blockade.
- Two surface electrodes, normally ECG electrodes, are positioned over the nerve and connected via leads to the stimulator which is battery operated. There are also stimulators available with detachable ball electrodes to enable skin contact.
- Supramaximal stimulation is used to stimulate the muscle.
- When supramaximal stimulation is used, contraction of the muscle is observed visually, palpated, or measured by a pressure transducer.
- The most common nerves used are ulna, posterior tibial, facial, and common peroneal.
- There are various methods of monitoring neuromuscular transmission:
  - Twitch—short duration stimulus every 10 seconds.
  - Tetanic stimulation.
  - Train-of-four (ToF)—this is four supra-maximal stimuli of 0.1–0.2 ms duration delivered at 2Hz, that is, 0.5 seconds between.
  - Post tetanic count—is used to assess more profound degrees of block.
  - Double burst.
- It is essential to remember the smaller the muscle group being stimulated, the more sensitive it is to the muscle relaxant; therefore this might not reflect the true picture of the depth of diaphragmatic block.
- Nerve stimulators can also be used to assist in locating the nerve tract when attempting regional anaesthesia.

## Further reading

Al-Shaikh B, Stacey S (2018). Essentials of equipment in anaesthesia, critical care and perioperative medicine (5th ed). Edinburgh: Elsevier.

Association of Anaesthetists of Great Britain and Ireland (2016). Recommendations for standards of monitoring during anaesthesia and recovery 2015. Anaesthesia, 71(1):85–93.

Aston D, Rivers A, Dharmadasa A (2014). Equipment in anaesthesia and critical care: a complete guide for the FRCA. Banbury: Scion.

Davey A, Ince CS (2010). Fundamentals of operating department practice. Cambridge: Cambridge University Press.

Middleton B, Phillips J, Stacey S (2021). Physics in anaesthesia: for FRCA candidates, ODPs and nurse anaesthetists (2nd ed). Banbury: Scion.

Thompson J, Moppett I, Wiles M (eds) (2019). Smith and Aitkenhead's textbook of anaesthesia (7th ed). Edinburgh: Elsevier.

# Respiratory rate

- Respiratory rate is normally monitored by observation of the patient—calculate the rise and fall of the patient's chest on inhalation and exhalation over a period of 1 minute.
- The adequacy of ventilation is judged clinically by the colouring of the patient and the absence of distress associated with breathing difficulties.
- Patients who are recovering from anaesthesia can be particularly prone to airway obstruction due to secretion or blood in the upper airway.
- The following patients are also at risk of reduced respiratory function:
  - Patients following cardiothoracic surgery.
  - Morbidly obese.
  - Heavy smokers.
  - Neuromuscular blockade administration.
  - Patients with pre-existing pulmonary disorders.
- Anaesthetized patients' respiratory rate and volume are normally monitored by:
  - Pneumotachography—measures gas flow.
  - Pressure monitoring during controlled ventilation.
  - Volume monitoring either using pneumotachography or respirometer (measures tidal and minute volume).

## Capnography (ETCO$_2$ analyser)

- Capnography is used to monitor levels of ventilation, confirm tracheal intubation, as a disconnection alarm, and to diagnose lung embolization and malignant hyperpyrexia.
- It can be performed by either mainstream (within the patient's gas stream) or sidestream analysers (at the distal end of the breathing system via a sampling tube).
- Using the principles of infrared absorption for CO$_2$, the rise and fall of CO$_2$ is measure through the respiratory cycle.

## Further reading

Al-Shaikh B, Stacey S (2018). Essentials of equipment in anaesthesia, critical care and perioperative medicine (5th ed). Edinburgh: Elsevier.

Association of Anaesthetists of Great Britain and Ireland (2016). Recommendations for standards of monitoring during anaesthesia and recovery 2015. Anaesthesia, 71(1):85–93.

Aston D, Rivers A, Dharmadasa A (2014). Equipment in anaesthesia and critical care: a complete guide for the FRCA. Banbury: Scion.

Davey A, Ince CS (2010). Fundamentals of operating department practice. Cambridge: Cambridge University Press.

Middleton B, Phillips J, Stacey S (2021). Physics in anaesthesia: for FRCA candidates, ODPs and nurse anaesthetists (2nd ed). Banbury: Scion.

Thompson J, Moppett I, Wiles M (eds) (2019). Smith and Aitkenhead's textbook of anaesthesia (7th ed). Edinburgh: Elsevier.

# Invasive monitoring

## Invasive arterial pressure

- Invasive arterial pressure monitoring allows for beat-by-beat measurement of the BP with continual accuracy.
- Indications for use would be a patient's condition predisposing towards severe changes in BP during the perioperative period and therefore constant measurement of BP is required (e.g. trauma, pre-existing cardiovascular disease).
- Indications for invasive arterial pressure monitoring may include rapid major haemodynamic instability such as blood loss and large fluid shifts. Also, patients undergoing cardiopulmonary bypass as this is the only way to assess if bypass is providing adequate perfusion pressures.
- Arterial blood can also be taken as a sample for ABG analysis.

## Cannula site

- An indwelling arterial cannula is inserted into:
  - Radial artery: first preference if palpable. If radial artery is cannulated then an Allen test should be performed to ensure that there is collateral flow through the ulna artery. In case there is no collateral flow through the ulna artery, radial artery puncture is contraindicated since it can result in a gangrenous finger or loss of the hand from spasm or clotting of the radial artery
  - Brachial artery: if radial not palpable
  - Femoral artery: only if access is limited as this site is a potentially dirty area and a risk of infection
  - Axillary artery: if others unavailable
  - Dorsalis pedis: if access is limited (e.g. neurosurgery).
- The cannula is then attached to a transducer which has previously been zeroed to atmospheric pressure and set at the sternal angle/mid-axillary line of the patient.
- The current generated in the transducer is then measured and converted electronically and displayed on the monitor as systolic, diastolic, and mean arterial pressures.

## Complications

- Infection: as with all invasive procedures strict aseptic technique should be adhered to.
- Arterial injection: arterial lines should be dressed appropriately stating clearly that the line is arterial. Arterial cannulas are specifically designed to eliminate this potential risk as they do not have an injection port.
- Bleeding: it is essential that the cannula is dressed properly and that all connections are tightened to ensure they do not disconnect. Patients can exsanguinate if this goes unnoticed.
- Clotting: though this is reduced with the constant flush device inbuilt to the transducer sets.
- Ischaemia distal to the cannula.
- Haematoma: this is normally related to multiple attempts of insertion.

# Further reading

Al-Shaikh B, Stacey S (2018). Essentials of equipment in anaesthesia, critical care and perioperative medicine (5th ed). Edinburgh: Elsevier.

Association of Anaesthetists of Great Britain and Ireland (2016). Recommendations for standards of monitoring during anaesthesia and recovery 2015. Anaesthesia, 71(1):85–93.

Aston D, Rivers A, Dharmadasa A (2014). Equipment in anaesthesia and critical care: a complete guide for the FRCA. Banbury: Scion.

Davey A, Ince CS (2010). Fundamentals of operating department practice. Cambridge: Cambridge University Press.

Department of Health (2007). High impact intervention no 2: peripheral venous care bundle. Available at: https://www.bsuh.nhs.uk/library/wp-content/uploads/sites/8/2020/09/Peripheral-cannula-care-bundle.pdf

Middleton B, Phillips J, Stacey S (2021). Physics in anaesthesia: for FRCA candidates, ODPs and nurse anaesthetists (2nd ed). Banbury: Scion.

Thompson J, Moppett I, Wiles M (eds) (2019). Smith and Aitkenhead's textbook of anaesthesia (7th ed). Edinburgh: Elsevier.

# Central venous pressure

- CVP measurement is used to closely monitor fluid balance when either significant shifts/losses are anticipated in connection with the planned surgery or if required by the patient's clinical condition.
- It directly measures the filling pressure of the right atrium.
- It can also be used for sampling blood, administering drugs, parental nutrition, and haemofiltration for haemodialysis.
- The Seldinger technique was originally devised for the insertion of venous or arterial catheters for radiological investigations[1] and is now commonly used to insert central venous catheters:
  - A guide wire is inserted into the needle used for venous puncture.
  - The guide wire then allows the needle to be withdrawn and, in succession, dilators and eventually the catheter to be railroaded over the guide wire in to position. The guide wire is then removed.
- Catheters can present as either single lines or up to four ports (quad lines) and can be inserted when the patient is awake under LA; this can be unpleasant and patient support is essential.
- Before the central line is used, confirmation of the placement of the catheter via X-ray should be confirmed.

## Cannula site

- Veins of the arm: these are sometimes described as long lines and are free from complication of direct approaches such as pneumothorax:
  - Median basilica vein.
  - Cephalic vein.
- External jugular vein: can be difficult to place.
- Subclavian vein: high incidence of pneumothorax.
- Internal jugular vein: can produce haematoma if the carotid artery is pierced.
- Femoral vein: high incidence of thrombophlebitis and leg oedema.

## Complications

- Guide wire: when the guide wire is being inserted, the anaesthetic assistant should monitor the patient's ECG. If the guide wire is inserted too far it enters the right atrium of the heart which will cause an increase in cardiac rhythm or ectopic beats; if this occurs, the anaesthetist should be informed immediately.
- Patient positioning: it is essential that the patient is positioned in a head-down tilt as air can be entrained through the cannula causing an air embolus; the head-down position also enlarges the neck veins.
- Pneumothorax with central vein techniques.
- Haematoma.
- Infection: as with all invasive procedures, strict aseptic technique should be adhered to.

## Setting up transducers

- A cannula is attached to a column of bubble-free saline (CVP) or heparinized saline (for arterial line) (manometer line) which flows through a transducer to a bag of saline/heparinized saline that is under approximately 300 mmHg of pressure via a pressure bag.
- The monometer line and the transducer kit are made from a material that reduces compliance. This is important when considering the recordable trace from the transducer as compliant tubing would cause dampening and therefore reduce the trace. Equally, if the materials are too stiff then this would cause resonance.
- Due to the pressure and a constant flushing device, which is built into the transducer set, a constant flush of 3–4 mL/hour of saline/heparinized saline is delivered through the cannula. Therefore, clotting and backflow through the cannula is prevented. There is also the ability to manually flush the cannula.
- Within the transducer is a diaphragm which is an extremely thin membrane that acts as an interface between the transducer and the column of water.
- As the column of fluid moves with the arterial pulsation over the diaphragm it causes changes in resistance which allows current to flow through the wires of the transducer.
- The transducer is attached via cables to an amplifier, oscilloscope.
- Complications with invasive monitoring equipment include:
  - Dampening of the trace which can be related to changes in the patient's position. Raising the transducer above or below the sternal angle/mid-axillary line of the patient will result in error readings
  - Air in the transducer set—this is the most common complication.

## Further reading

Al-Shaikh B, Stacey S (2018). Essentials of equipment in anaesthesia, critical care and perioperative medicine (5th ed). Edinburgh: Elsevier.

Association of Anaesthetists of Great Britain and Ireland (2016). Recommendations for standards of monitoring during anaesthesia and recovery 2015. Anaesthesia, 71 (1):85–93.

Aston D, Rivers A, Dharmadasa A (2014). Equipment in anaesthesia and critical care: a complete guide for the FRCA. Banbury: Scion.

Davey A, Ince CS (2010). Fundamentals of operating department practice. Cambridge: Cambridge University Press.

Department of Health (2011). High impact intervention no 1: central venous catheter care bundle. Available at: 🔗 http://webarchive.nationalarchives.gov.uk/20120118171551/http://hcai. dh.gov.uk/files/2011/03/2011-03-14-HII-Central-Venous-Catheter-Care-Bundle-FINAL.pdf

Middleton B, Phillips J, Stacey S (2021). Physics in anaesthesia: for FRCA candidates, ODPs and nurse anaesthetists (2nd ed). Banbury: Scion.

Pronovost P, Needham D, Berenholtz S, et al. (2006). An intervention to decrease catheter related bloodstream infections in the ICU. New England Journal of Medicine, 355(26):2725–2732.

Thompson J, Moppett I, Wiles M (eds) (2019). Smith and Aitkenhead's textbook of anaesthesia (7th ed). Edinburgh: Elsevier.

# Oesophageal Doppler

- This technique interprets images gained by Doppler in the oesophagus.
- Oesophageal Doppler allows for continuous monitoring of the left and right ventricles as well as the detection of early myocardial ischaemia.
- The probe with manipulation can also view cardiac valves, coronary vessels, and coronary grafts.
- Visualization of the cardiac chambers, the aorta, vena cava, and pulmonary arteries can also be achieved.
- Patients need to be adequately sedated or intubated though a suprasternal probe is available and can be used on awake patients.

## Complications

- The probe can cause damage to the oesophagus and cause burns.
- The readings and their interpretation are dependent on operator expertise.
- Insertion of the probe is not recommended in patients with pharyngo-oesophageal pathology.

## Reference

1. Simpson PJ, Popart MT (2002). Understanding anaesthesia (4th ed). Oxford: Butterworth-Heinemann.

## Further reading

Al-Shaikh B, Stacey S (2018). Essentials of equipment in anaesthesia, critical care and perioperative medicine (5th ed). Edinburgh: Elsevier.

Association of Anaesthetists of Great Britain and Ireland (2016). Recommendations for standards of monitoring during anaesthesia and recovery 2015. Anaesthesia, 71(1):85–93.

Aston D, Rivers A, Dharmadasa A (2014). Equipment in anaesthesia and critical care: a complete guide for the FRCA. Banbury: Scion.

Davey A, Ince CS (2010). Fundamentals of operating department practice. Cambridge: Cambridge University Press.

Middleton B, Phillips J, Stacey S (2021). Physics in anaesthesia: for FRCA candidates, ODPs and nurse anaesthetists (2nd ed). Banbury: Scion.

Thompson J, Moppett I, Wiles M (eds) (2019). Smith and Aitkenhead's textbook of anaesthesia (7th ed). Edinburgh: Elsevier.

# Monitoring obese patients

The AAGBI recommends that monitoring the following is essential at the induction of anaesthesia for *all patients*:

- ECG.
- NIBP.
- $SpO_2$.
- Airway gas.

## ECG

A three-lead ECG, referred to as standard limb leads, is generally used during anaesthesia.

- The electrodes are commonly placed on the right arm (red) and left arm (yellow) with a third, left leg (black/dark green), placed more commonly on the left side of the thorax.
- With obese patients it may be necessary to relocate the electrodes in order to obtain a better trace.
- One alternative to the above is to place the electrodes on the arms of the patient, for example, red to right forearm, with yellow and black either aspect of the left forearm.
- This configuration may also be useful when dealing with agitated patients or children as it is less intrusive than rearranging clothing to apply the electrodes in a more conventional layout.

## NIBP

There are many sizes of cuffs available for today's monitors. They range in length and width to fit babies through to large adults; therefore, a cuff should be chosen that fits the patient comfortably, that is, is long enough to encompass the limb and that the width does not impede joint movement.

- Practitioners should ensure that, whatever the cuff size, it is placed correctly over the artery; failure to do so might cause an incorrect reading, or appear as a fault on the monitor screen.
- Where there is a deep layer of body fat, the NIBP will often be difficult or sometimes impossible to record; in this situation, the practitioner should consider a different size cuff, and/or an alternative placement sites, for example, the patient's forearm in favour of the upper arm, or the calf area where sometimes leaner tissue can be located.
- Failure to obtain readings using this method may result in having to apply invasive monitoring techniques.

When dealing with patients who are agitated, or children, it might be wise not to attach the monitoring (unless medically contraindicated) until immediately after the induction of anaesthesia so as not to further upset the patient.

## $SpO_2$

Obese patients will often have large fingers, which will often lead to inaccurate $SpO_2$ readings of both the pulse and saturation.

- In these situations, alternative probe placement sites should be considered (e.g. the toes).
- The use of a smaller multiuse pulse oximeter probe should also be considered for other areas that may be suitable (e.g. the ear lobe).

## Airway gas

Monitoring the airway gas gives a clear indication that the patient's airway is patent.

- The digitalized waveform of the capnograph signifies that the patent's lung function is good, and that gaseous exchange is taking place.
- The measurement is obtained via the capnograph sensor placed within the patient's anaesthetic circuit and attached to the anaesthetic machine.
- When an obese patient lies in the supine position, their abdominal contents push up their diaphragm, restricting its movement—if this is the case, the patient should be positioned 'sitting up' or tilt the head.

## Further reading

Association of Anaesthetists of Great Britain and Ireland (2010). Preoperative assessment: the role of the anaesthetist. London: Association of Anaesthetists of Great Britain and Ireland.

Association of Anaesthetists of Great Britain and Ireland (2015). Peri-operative management of the obese surgical patient. London: Association of Anaesthetists of Great Britain and Ireland.

Association of Anaesthetists of Great Britain and Ireland (2016). Recommendations for standards of monitoring during anaesthesia and recovery 2015. Anaesthesia, 71(1):85–93.

Association of Anaesthetists of Great Britain and Ireland (2018). The anaesthesia team 2018. Available at: 🔗 http://dx.doi.org/10.21466/g.TAT.2018

Association of Anaesthetists of Great Britain and Ireland (2019). Checklist for draw-over anaesthetic equipment. Available at: 🔗 http://dx.doi.org/10.21466/g.CFDAE2.2019

Bouch C, Cousins J (Eds) (2018). Core topics in anaesthesia and perioperative care of the morbidly obese surgical patient. Cambridge: Cambridge University Press.

National Institute for Health and Care Excellence (2014). Obesity: identification, assessment and management. Clinical guideline [CG189]. Available at: 🔗 https://www.nice.org.uk/guidance/cg189

National Institute for Health and Care Excellence (2015). Obesity prevention. [CG43]. Available at: 🔗 https://www.nice.org.uk/guidance/cg43

National Institute for Health and Care Excellence (2017). Nurse-led ASA grading in pre-operative assessment to guide investigations and risk scoring. Available at: 🔗 https://www.nice.org.uk/sharedlearning/nurse-led-asa-grading-in-preoperative-assessment-to-guide-investigations-and-risk-scoring

Royal College of Anaesthetists (2019–2021). Guidelines for the provision of anaesthetic services for preoperative assessment and preparation. London: Royal College of Anaesthetists.

# Arterial blood gases

An ABG is a set of tests performed on a heparinized sample of arterial blood. Results from this test provide the practitioner with information about:

- Adequacy and extent of gas exchange in the lungs[1]
- Acid–base balance.

Additionally, the test may provide useful information such as fractional oxygen saturation, $SaO_2$, methaemoglobin (MetHb) and carboxyhaemoglobin (COHb), and also serum concentrations of the electrolytes $Na^+$, $K^+$, blood glucose, and serum lactate.

## The sample

A sample of 3–4 mL of arterial blood is drawn into a heparinized syringe (commercially available blood gas syringes are commonly used). The blood sample is obtained in two ways:

- An arterial 'stab' (usually the radial artery).
- From an indwelling arterial catheter.

## Precautions

- If the blood sample is going to a laboratory for analysis, it should be labelled appropriately (see local policy).
- Include fraction of oxygen in inspired air ($FiO_2$) on the request.
- Include patient temperature on the request.
- The sample should be fresh (continued cellular metabolism can affect the result).
- No air bubbles should be present in the sample (air bubbles can dissolve in the plasma which will affect the result).

## Result interpretation

Adoption of a systematic approach makes this readily achievable.

## Normal ranges

$PaO_2$: 12–15 kPa (90–110 mmHg).
$PaCO_2$: 4.5–6 kPa (34–46 mmHg).
$HCO_3^-$: 21–27.5 mmol/L.
$H^+$ ions: 36–44 nmol/L (pH 7.35–7.45).[2]

> *Remember to use your laboratories' values (usually printed on the result slip).*

### A five-step approach to result interpretation

Firstly, ensure that the result is for your patient![3]

- *Step 1*: what is the $PaO_2$, is the patient hypoxic?
- *Step 2*: look at the pH, is the patient acidaemic (pH <7.35) or alkalaemic (pH >7.45)?
- *Step 3*: look at $PaCO_2$, <4 kPa = respiratory alkalosis, >6 kPa = respiratory acidosis.

- *Step 4*: look at $HCO_3^-$, <21= metabolic acidosis, >27.5 = metabolic alkalosis.
- *Step 5*: determine compensation.

The body attempts to maintain pH within the normal range by compensating for acid–base disturbances as follows:
- If the primary cause is metabolic, the respiratory system attempts to compensate by increasing or decreasing excretion of $CO_2$.
- If the primary cause is respiratory, the renal system attempts to compensates by excretion or reabsorption of bicarbonate and acidification of urine.

## References

1. Rempher K, Morton GM (2017). Patient assessment: respiratory system. In: Morton PG, Fonatine DK (eds) Critical care nursing: a holistic approach (11th ed). Philadelphia, PA: Lippincott Williams and Wilkins.
2. Waugh A, Grant A (2018). Ross and Wilson anatomy and physiology in health and illness (13th ed). Edinburgh: Churchill Livingstone.
3. Resuscitation Council UK (2016). Advanced life support (7th ed). London: Resuscitation Council UK.

# Acid–base balance

## Definition

Normal cellular activity within the body requires that the balance between acids and bases in body fluids is tightly controlled.[1] Usefully, the balance between acids and bases is reflected in the pH of the extracellular fluid.[2]

## Measuring pH

- The normal range for the pH of blood is between 7.35 and 7.45.[2]
- Deviation from this range can have major effects on body systems, especially the CNS and the cardiovascular system.[1]

## Common terms

- An acid is a substance that can donate a hydrogen ion when in solution, for example, hydrochloric acid (a strong acid) or carbonic acid (a weak acid).
- A base is a substance that can accept a hydrogen ion from a solution, for example, bicarbonate.
- Acidaemia is said to exist when the pH of the blood is <7.35.
- Alkalaemia is said to exist when the pH of the blood is >7.45.
- The term acidosis refers to the process that is causing the acidaemia.
- The term alkalosis refers to the process that is causing the alkalaemia.[3]
- The relatively constant balance between acids and bases is maintained by three systems:
  - Buffers.
  - The respiratory system.
  - The renal system.

## Determining acid–base balance

Acid–base balance is determined by completing steps 3–5 of the arterial blood gas analysis (→ see Arterial blood gas, p. 248).

## Some common causes of acid–base disturbances

- Acidosis is more common than alkalosis.
- Respiratory acidosis is caused by an increase in $CO_2$—for example, reduced conscious level, head injury, chest trauma, chest infection, inadequate ventilation, atelectasis.
- Respiratory alkalosis is caused by a decrease in $CO_2$—for example, hyperventilation, fear, pain.
- Metabolic acidosis—for example, renal failure, ketoacidosis, severe diarrhoea.
- Metabolic alkalosis—for example, overuse of antacids, GI fistula losses, prolonged nasogastric (NG) free drainage.

## Treatment of acid–base disturbances

The usual treatment is to try and correct the underlying cause, for example, hypoventilation (with a decreased respiratory rate) following early extubation could cause respiratory acidosis. The treatment would be to ensure adequate ventilation to remove excess $CO_2$.

A patient who is hypovolaemic may develop metabolic acidosis because of poor peripheral circulation, resulting in a build-up of metabolic acids (e.g. lactic acid). Administration of fluids to restore an adequate circulation would be the appropriate treatment in this case.

## References

1. Waugh A, Grant A (2018). Ross and Wilson anatomy and physiology in health and illness (13th ed). Edinburgh: Churchill Livingstone.
2. Porth C (2014). Essentials of pathophysiology (4th ed). Philadelphia, PA: Lippincott Williams and Wilkins.
3. Rempher K, Morton GM (2017). Patient assessment: respiratory system. In: Morton PG, Fonatine DK (eds) Critical care nursing: a holistic approach (11th ed). Philadelphia, PA: Lippincott Williams and Wilkins.

# Medical gas cylinders

## Identification of colour-coded cylinders

- All medical gas cylinders make use of a system of a unique colouring which assists in the identification of their contents.
- All medical gas cylinders in the UK are coloured according to the standard BS EN1089-3.
- Colour alone must *never* be used to identify contents of a cylinder.
- Labels on the cylinder/cylinder collar *must* be the primary method of identifying contents.
- *Never* use a cylinder unless the contents can be clearly identified.
- An empty cylinder weight is referred to as 'tare weight'.

## Checking of cylinders and its contents

Every cylinder has a number of other identifying markings on the cylinder shoulder/valve block. These markings contain the following information:
- Name and chemical symbol of the gas/mixture contained.
- Cylinder size/capacity.
- Empty cylinder weight.
- Maximum working pressure and test pressure.

   Cylinders also have plastic collars attached that contain:
- Directions for use
- Storage and handling instructions
- Appropriate hazard warning notice
- Shelf life and expiry date
- Batch number
- Product licence number.

In addition, cylinders are supplied with a red or white plastic safety seal that covers the gas outlet, held in place by clear plastic shrink wrap. This prevents dust or other foreign bodies from entering the gas outlet, and also acts as a visual safety indicator.

## Further reading

Al-Shaikh B, Stacey S (2018). Essentials of equipment in anaesthesia, critical care and perioperative medicine (5th ed). Edinburgh: Elsevier.
Association of Anaesthetists of Great Britain and Ireland (2012). Checking anaesthetic equipment. London: Association of Anaesthetists of Great Britain and Ireland.
Freedman R, Herbert L, O'Donnell A, et al. (eds) (2022). Oxford handbook of anaesthesia (5th ed). Oxford: Oxford University Press.
Royal College of Anaesthetists (2019–2021). Guidelines for the provision of anaesthetic services. London: Royal College of Anaesthetists.

# Attaching cylinders to pin index system on an anaesthetic machine

- The pin index safety system (BS EN 850) is an *almost* foolproof safety system which prevents the connection of cylinders at the wrong location.
- The system comprises a pair of locating holes beneath the gas outlet of the cylinder valve block which correspond to a pair of pins located at the inlet connection of the relevant machine.
- Pin/hole positions are unique for each gas and therefore prevent incorrect connection of cylinders.

To attach a gas cylinder to any piece of equipment—anaesthetic machine, insufflator, or regulator:

- The shrink wrap covered seal is removed.
- The valve is opened momentarily to blow away any foreign bodies or debris.
- The cylinder is then securely attached to the relevant piece of equipment by offering up the pin index holes on cylinder block to the corresponding pins located on the machine yolk taking care not to force the fit.
- The cylinder is then secured to the machine yolk by the appropriate means.
- The valve is slowly opened by two anticlockwise turns of the spindle.

In the event of a leak—usually an audible hiss or an unexplained loss of gas/drop in pressure—then:

- Check that the locking screw is sufficiently tight.
  If the leak remains after tightening:
- The cylinder should be turned off and removed from the piece of equipment.
- The sealing washer between the cylinder and the equipment, that is, the Bodok washer or the rubber 'O' ring, should be checked for damage and replaced as necessary.

If the problem remains, consider replacing the cylinder and/or the particular piece of equipment.

*Never* force an ill-fitting cylinder:

- It may be the incorrect type/size cylinder.
- Attempts to force it may cause the index pins to be bent out of shape or dislodged, preventing the attachment of another cylinder or allowing the connection of an incorrect cylinder with potentially disastrous results.

## Safe storage of cylinders

- Under cover, preferably inside, dry, clean environment avoiding extremes of temperature.
- Not near combustible material or sources of heat.
- Medical gases should be stored separately from other gases.
- Where more than one type of gas is stored in a location, gases should be segregated.

- Under no circumstance should cylinders be repainted, markings on the cylinder/valve block obscured, or labels be removed.
- F-size cylinders should be stored vertically, E-size and smaller should be stored horizontally.

## Pipeline gases

- While cylinders provide a more mobile form of gas supply, the majority of gas supplied within the perioperative setting is by means of pipelines fed by either bulk tanks or large cylinder manifolds.
- The colour coding used on cylinders also extends to pipeline supplies, with pipes and connection points taking on the same colour as the relevant cylinder shoulder.
- Pipeline connections also make use of a unique interface to prevent the incorrect connections.
- Only wall-mounted connection points and associated pipelines that are compliant with Health Technical Memorandum (HTM) 02-01 should be used for delivery of medical gases to patients.

## Further reading

Al-Shaikh B, Stacey S (2018). Essentials of equipment in anaesthesia, critical care and perioperative medicine (5th ed). Edinburgh: Elsevier.

Association of Anaesthetists of Great Britain and Ireland (2012). Checking anaesthetic equipment. London: Association of Anaesthetists of Great Britain and Ireland.

Freedman R, Herbert L, O'Donnell A, et al. (eds) (2022). Oxford handbook of anaesthesia (5th ed). Oxford: Oxford University Press.

Royal College of Anaesthetists (2019–2021). Guidelines for the provision of anaesthetic services. London: Royal College of Anaesthetists.

Simpson J, Popat M (2002). Understanding anaesthesia. Edinburgh: Butterworth-Heinemann.

# Scientific principles

# Heat and humans

### The difference between heat and temperature

Although, in everyday language, heat and temperature are considered to be the same, strictly speaking they are not:

- *Heat* is a measurement of the *total energy* (kinetic and potential) of the molecules or atoms making up a substance. This energy can be transferred from a hotter substance to a colder substance. The heat of a body depends upon both its temperature and mass.
- *Temperature* is a measurement of the *average kinetic energy* of individual molecules or atoms of a substance; temperature can be regarded as the relative degree of 'hotness' or 'coldness' of a body.

### Body temperature

Although normal body temperature is usually regarded as an oral temperature of approximately 37°C, a range of values of temperature can be observed both in, and between, 'normal' individuals (±0.6°C). 'Normal' body temperature also varies with:

- Time of day—up to approximately 1°C between early morning and late afternoon/early evening
- Menstrual cycle—temperature drops immediately prior to ovulation
- Age—temperature declines with age
- External temperature
- Exercise.

Temperature also varies between different regions of the human body, for example:

- Oral body temperature averages between 36.4°C and 37.6°C
- Tympanic temperature is usually between 0.3°C and 0.6°C higher than oral temperature
- Axillary temperature is usually between 0.3°C and 0.6°C lower than oral temperature
- Rectal temperature is usually between 0.3°C and 0.6°C higher than oral temperature.

### The regulation of body temperature

- All heat in the body is produced by processes that occur in the cells— that is, cellular metabolism—in a process known as thermogenesis.
- In thermogenesis, the chemical energy contained in digested food is converted into other forms of energy, substantially heat.
- The amount of heat production in a person at any time is determined by the speed with which energy is released from foods ——the metabolic rate—and is measured in watts.
- All tissues produce heat, but those in which rapid chemical reactions occur (e.g. brain, liver) produce large amounts of heat with the consequence that the temperature of these organs is usually approximately 1°C higher than the rest of the body.
- As the generation of heat within the body is continuous (but not constant), the body must lose heat energy at a rate that ensures no build-up of heat and a corresponding increase in body temperature.

- In normal circumstances the heat lost from the body equals the heat gained from cellular metabolism and other sources—temperature homeostasis.
- Normal regulation of the body's temperature is effected by the thermoregulatory centres in the hypothalamus.
- The temperature of blood pumping through the brain is constantly monitored together with information from temperature receptors in the skin. The body then adjusts its temperature in response to this information and does so in a variety of ways:

*Ways in which body temperature can be increased*
- Vasoconstriction: constriction of fine blood vessels of the skin; this reduces blood flow to the skin and, therefore, reduces the amount of heat lost.
- Shivering: contractions of the skeletal muscles producing heat energy.
- Piloerection: erector pili muscles contract causing body hairs to stand on end, trapping an insulating layer of warm air next to the skin.
- Sympathetic metabolic stimulation: body cells increase the rate of heat production as a result of signals from the nervous system.

*Ways in which body temperature can be decreased*
- Vasodilation: blood vessels in the skin dilate, increasing blood flow to the skin and facilitating heat loss.
- Restriction of heat production mechanisms: for example, shivering, chemical reactions.
- Erector pili muscles relax: lowers skin hairs and allows air to circulate over skin.
- Perspiration: glands in the skin secrete sweat onto the surface of the skin which then evaporates through the action of body heat.

## Thermoregulation abnormalities

Despite the fact that, in normal circumstances, body temperature is regulated to a very high degree, situations can arise where these control mechanisms fail or are inadequate, for example, at extremes of age or as a result of prolonged anaesthesia. These circumstances include:
- Malfunction of the hypothalamus as a result of cerebral trauma (e.g. oedema resulting from head injury, cerebrovascular accidents, brain surgery)
- Effects of toxic substances (e.g. bacterial or viral infections, drugs (including anaesthetic agents))
- Dehydration: with consequent loss of sweating ability
- Prolonged exposure to high/low temperatures.

Such circumstances can give rise to hyperthermia or hypothermia:
- *Hyperthermia*: core body temperature consistently above the normal range.
  - Hyperthermia is usually caused by overexposure to a hot environment or as a result of pathogenic infection.
  - It can also arise, in susceptible patients, as a result of exposure to some anaesthetic agents such as halothane and muscle relaxants (e.g. suxamethonium) and occasionally progresses to the potentially fatal condition of MH.

- *Hypothermia*: core body temperature consistently below the normal range such that normal metabolism is not possible.
  - Hypothermia is a common (particularly at the extremes of age) and potentially serious complication during anaesthesia and surgery.
  - It is associated with numerous perioperative complications including myocardial ischaemia, the impairment of normal coagulation, and a substantially increased risk of wound infection.
  - It arises for a number of reasons, including as a result of GA:
    — Depression of the thermoregulatory centre.
    — Decrease in metabolic rate.
    — Increase in vasodilation.
  - Spinal and epidural anaesthesia can cause hypothermia through vasodilation and loss of muscle tone.
  - Hypothermia also arises as a result of exposure of body surfaces and cavities to the operating theatre environment, which tends to be cool and low in humidity.
  - Hypothermia can also be deliberately induced for some surgery— temperatures 1–3°C below normal provide substantial protection against cerebral ischaemia and hypoxaemia.

### The transmission of heat

There are, essentially, four physical processes by which heat can be transferred (lost or gained):

- *Conduction*: the process by which heat is transmitted through a substance (solid, liquid, gas) or from one substance to another. Conduction is due to molecules colliding with other and transferring their heat energy through the substance or between substances. Conduction varies with the conducting substance; it is greatest in solids and least in gases. For conduction to occur between substances there must be direct contact; in normal circumstances, conduction accounts for approximately 2–3% of the body's heat loss, but it is also possible to gain heat by conduction (e.g. warm bath).
- *Convection*: the process by which heat is transferred in a fluid (liquid or gas) by the movement of molecules from cooler, relatively high-density, regions of the fluid to warmer, relatively low-density regions. Convection does not occur in solids. Normally, convection accounts for approximately 10–15% of the body's heat loss.
- *Radiation*: the process by which heat is lost by the emission of electromagnetic (infrared) radiation from a body. The greater the difference in temperature between the body and the surrounding environment, the greater is the loss of heat from the body by radiation. Radiation does not depend on any substance, that is, it does not depend on the movement of molecules. In normal circumstances, approximately 60% of the body's heat loss is through radiation, but the body may also gain heat by radiation (e.g. sunbathing, proximity to fire).

- *Evaporation*: the process by which heat is transferred by the transformation of a liquid into a vapour and is one of the processes by which the human body loses heat during sweating. Typically, one might expect 20% of the body's total heat loss to be through evaporation although the rate at which evaporation occurs depends upon:
  - Surface area
  - Convection currents
  - Atmospheric humidity
  - The type of liquid
  - Temperature of liquid.

Although heat loss through convection and radiation mainly occurs via the skin, these processes also occur in the lungs. Inhaled air is usually cooler and dryer than the internal surface of the lung; in warming and moisturizing the inhaled air, the body loses heat energy when the air is exhaled.

## Further reading

Chava R, Zviman M, Assis FR, et al (2019). Effect of high flow trans nasal dry air on core body temperature in intubated human subjects. Resuscitation, 134:49–54.

Cheung S, Ainslie PN (2021). Advanced environmental exercise physiology (2nd ed). Champaign IL: Human Kinetics Inc.

Cross ME, Plunkett EVE (2014). Physics, pharmacology and physiology for anaesthetists (2nd ed). Cambridge: Cambridge University Press.

Freedman R, Herbert L, O'Donnell A, et al. (eds) (2022). Oxford handbook of anaesthesia (5th ed). Oxford: Oxford University Press.

Pocock G, Richards CD, Richards DA (2017). Human physiology (5th ed). Oxford: Oxford University Press.

# Electricity

## Static and dynamic electricity

Electricity of all kinds involves electrons—the negatively charged particles found in all atoms—but it is important to distinguish between static electricity and dynamic electricity.

- *Static electricity,* so called because it builds in one place, is caused primarily by friction.
  - As materials are rubbed together, electrons are removed from one material (so that it becomes positively charged) and deposited on the other (which becomes negatively charged).
  - Static electricity builds up on door handles and other metal objects in rooms which have synthetic carpets, on synthetic clothing, and on the bodies of motor vehicles as a result of the friction caused by moving air.
  - The static normally discharges upon touch, causing a spark which can ignite flammable gases, causing explosions and/or fires.
  - To reduce this risk in theatres, cotton clothes are used, and antistatic materials are incorporated into equipment to reduce the build-up of static electricity.
  - Maintaining a high relative humidity also reduces the risks of static electricity accumulating.
  - Static electricity has practical uses, for example, in photocopiers, inkjet printers, in reducing pollution by removing particles of smoke, dirt, and dust from the air, and in paint spraying cars.
- *Dynamic electricity* is caused by the flow of electrons, through a conductor, from a point of higher concentration (higher potential) to a point of lower concentration (lower potential), that is, an electric current—which can be direct current (DC) or alternating current (AC).

## Direct and alternating current

- *DC* is current that travels in a circuit in one direction only.
  - It is produced by sources such as batteries, dynamos, and solar cells and is commonly used to power small electrical devices (e.g. radios, torches, pacemakers).
  - DC can also be produced from an AC supply by using a rectifier.
- *AC* is current that cyclically changes in size and direction, typically at 50 or 60 Hz (cycles per second).
  - It is the form of electricity that is routinely supplied to industry and domestic buildings.
  - AC possesses one main advantage compared with DC: AC allows transformers to be used to increase or decrease voltages depending upon purposes.
  - AC can be converted into DC by using an electrical inverter.

## Some electrical terms

- *Current*: the rate of flow of electrons (electrical charge) between two points in 1 second (measured in amperes).
- *Current density*: current flowing/unit area.

- *Voltage*: also known as potential difference—the difference in electrical charge between two points (measured in volts).
- *Resistance*: the opposition to the flow of electrons (measured in ohms). Resistance of a wire depends upon its diameter, length, and material.
- *Circuit*: the continuous pathway followed by electricity from the source of generation to its destination and back.
- *Electrical power*: the rate of flow of energy, or the work done per second in causing electrical charge to flow (measured in watts).
- *Insulator*: a material that resists the flow of electric current; an object intended to support or separate electrical conductors without current passing through itself.
- *Conductor*: a material that allows the flow of electric charge (current) through it.
- *Semi-conductor*: a substance, usually a solid chemical element or compound, which can conduct electricity under certain conditions only; this property makes it a good medium for the control of electrical current.

## Further reading

Adams S, Allday J (2013). Advanced physics (2nd ed). Oxford: Oxford University Press.
Johnson K, Hewett S, Holt S, et al. (2015). Advanced physics for you (2nd ed). Oxford: Oxford University Press.

# Physiological effects of electricity

- The physiological effects of electricity on the human body depend upon the amount of current flowing and upon the path the current takes through the body (Table 9.1).
- Although the amount of current flowing depends upon the voltage applied and the resistance of the path taken, it is the size of current that is the main factor in classifying the potential hazards.
- The frequency of the current also impacts the physiological effects, with very high frequencies producing heat rather than muscular contractions, a fact that allows their use in electrosurgery.
- Note that the heart is extremely sensitive to frequencies of 50–60 Hz—frequencies at which industrial and domestic supplies are normally delivered.
- The most common type of electric shock received by humans is *macro-shock*, where the electric current travels through body tissues to the heart only after overcoming the relatively high resistance offered by dry, intact skin. In such circumstances, Table 9.1 identifies that currents >10 mA may produce sustained muscular contraction, whereas currents greater than approximately 100 mA have the potential for causing death as a result of inducing ventricular fibrillation.
- *Micro-shock*, on the other hand, occurs when current flows directly to the heart muscle (e.g. via pacemaker wires, catheters). The size of the current necessary to cause ventricular fibrillation in such a situation is many times smaller than in normal circumstances and may be as little as 20 μA.

**Table 9.1** Physiological effects of electricity

| Current (at 60 Hz) | Physiological effect |
| --- | --- |
| 1mA | Threshold of perception |
| 5mA | Considered the maximum harmless current |
| 10–20 mA | Beginning of sustained muscular contraction (cannot let go of electrical contacts) |
| 50mA | Pain, possible fainting, and exhaustion. Cardiac and respiratory functions continue |
| 100–300 mA | Ventricular fibrillation—fatal if sustained. Respiratory function continues |
| 6A | Sustained ventricular contraction followed by normal heart rhythm if current stops (defibrillator). Temporary respiratory paralysis. Potential burns |

## Further reading

Adams S, Allday J (2013). Advanced physics (2nd ed). Oxford: Oxford University Press.
Johnson K, Hewett S, Holt S, et al. (2015). Advanced physics for you (2nd ed). Oxford: Oxford University Press.

# Gases and the gas laws

## Atmospheric pressure

Air is made up of a mixture of gases (Table 9.2).

**Table 9.2** Composition of air

| Component | Percentage by volume | Partial pressure (kPa) |
|---|---|---|
| Nitrogen ($N_2$) | 78.08 | 79.10 |
| Oxygen ($O_2$) | 20.95 | 21.21 |
| Argon (A) | 0.93 | 0.95 |
| Carbon dioxide ($CO_2$) | 0.03 | 0.04 |
| **Total** | 99.99 | 101.30 |

There are other gases present in the atmosphere in very small amounts (e.g. neon, helium, krypton, xenon). Also present is water vapour, which varies in concentration from almost 0% in the cold, dry regions of the Antarctic, for example, to 4% in humid tropical areas.

The term 'partial pressure' refers to the contribution that each gas makes to the total pressure exerted by the atmosphere.

## The gas laws

*Boyle's law* can be expressed as:
The volume of a given mass of gas is inversely proportional to the pressure to which it is subjected provided that the temperature remains constant.

$$\text{Volume}(V) \propto 1/\text{pressure}(P) \text{ (for constant temperature)}$$

$$\text{or} \quad P \times V = \text{constant}$$

Boyle's law is commonly used to predict the result of introducing a change in the volume or pressure of a fixed mass of gas. The original and final volumes ($V_1$ and $V_2$) and pressures ($P_1$ and $P_2$) of the fixed mass of gas are related by the equation:

$$P1 \times V1 = P2 \times V2 = \text{constant}$$

*Charles' law* can be expressed as:
The volume of a given mass of gas is directly proportional to its absolute temperature (in Kelvin), provided that the pressure remains constant.

$$\text{Volume }(V) \propto \text{ temperature }(T) \text{ (at constant pressure)}$$

$$\text{or} \quad V/T = \text{constant}$$

If a change is introduced to the volume or absolute temperature of a fixed amount of gas, then the original and final volumes ($V_1$ and $V_2$) and absolute temperatures ($T_1$ and $T_2$) are related by the equation:

$$V_1/T_1 = V_2/T_2 = \text{constant}$$

*Gay-Lussac's law* can be expressed as:
The pressure of a given mass of gas is directly proportional to its absolute temperature (in Kelvin), provided that the volume is constant.

$$\text{Pressure } (P) \propto \text{temperature } (T) \text{ (at constant volume)}$$

or    $P/T = \text{constant}$

If a change is introduced to the pressure or absolute temperature of a fixed amount of gas, then the original and final pressures ($P_1$ and $P_2$) and absolute temperatures ($T_1$ and $T_2$) are related by the equation:

$$P_1/T_1 = P_2/T_2 = \text{constant}$$

*The general gas law* can be expressed as:
The product of the pressure and volume of a given mass of gas is directly proportional to its absolute temperature (in Kelvin).

$$\text{Pressure } (P) \times \text{volume } (V) \propto \text{temperature } (T)$$

or $P \times V/T = \text{constant}$

If a change is introduced to the pressure, volume, or absolute temperature (in Kelvin) of a fixed amount of gas, then the original and final pressures ($P_1$ and $P_2$), volumes ($V_1$ and $V_2$) and absolute temperatures ($T_1$ and $T_2$) are related by the equation:

$$P_1 \times V_1/T_1 = P_2 \times V_2/T_2 = \text{constant}$$

*Dalton's law* can be expressed as:
The partial pressure of a gas in a gas mixture is the pressure that this gas would exert alone if it occupied the total volume of the mixture in the absence of other components.

$$P_{total} = p_a + p_b + p_c + \ldots$$

where $p_a$, $p_b$, $p_c$ … are the partial pressures of gases in a gas mixture.

*Henry's law* can be expressed as:
The amount of a gas that will dissolve in a given type and volume of a liquid at a given temperature is directly proportional to the partial pressure of the gas in equilibrium with that liquid.

$$\text{Concentration} \propto \text{partial pressure (at constant temperature)}$$

or    $C/p = \text{constant}$

## Further reading

Adams S, Allday J (2013). Advanced physics (2nd ed). Oxford: Oxford University Press.
Franklin K, Muir P, Scott T, et al. (2019). Introduction to biological physics for the health and life sciences (2nd ed). Oxford: Wiley-Blackwell.
Johnson K, Hewett S, Holt S, et al. (2015). Advanced physics for you (2nd ed). Oxford: Oxford University Press.
Johnson T (2016). Introduction to health physics (5th ed). New York: McGraw-Hill.

# The breathing process

During *inspiration*, the sternum moves outwards and upwards, the ribs lift and rotate outwards and the diaphragm contracts, flattens, and descends towards the abdomen.

- The net result of these movements is an increase in the volume of the thoracic cavity, which consequently causes the pressure in the thoracic cavity to decrease (Boyle's law) to below atmospheric pressure.
- The resulting pressure gradient causes air to travel down the trachea and into the lungs until the air within the lungs reaches atmospheric pressure.

During *expiration*, the opposite movements occur:

- This serves to decrease the volume of the thoracic cavity, so that the pressure is increased above atmospheric pressure.
- This increase in pressure creates a pressure gradient and forces the gases in the lungs back into the atmosphere.

*Inhalation* is an active process—involving muscle contraction—and as such involves work being done (the work of breathing). This work can be regarded as consisting of three components: the work necessary to expand the lungs against their elastic forces; the work that is required to overcome the viscosity of the lungs and chest wall; and the work required in moving air into the lungs against the resistance of the airway. Exhalation, however (in normal breathing), is passive—involving muscle relaxation, the recoil of the lungs, ribs, and sternum—and as such does not require work to be done. During exercise, however, exhalation can be an active process.

## Positive and negative pressures

When considering pressures in the lungs and thorax, the terms 'negative pressure' and 'positive pressure' are often used. This is done for convenience and means that all pressures involved are compared with, and expressed relative to, normal atmospheric pressure (101.3 kPa). So:

- Any pressure *above* normal atmospheric pressure is regarded as positive pressure, for example, a pressure of +0.3 kPa is the same as 101.6 kPa
- Any pressure *below* normal atmospheric pressure is regarded as negative pressure, for example, a pressure of –0.3 kPa is the same as 101 kPa.

Although relatively small, these pressure differences are more than enough to form a 'pressure gradient,' and enable the gases involved in inhalation and exhalation to move in the required direction.

## The pressures involved in breathing

*Intra-alveolar pressure* is the same as the pressure everywhere in the lungs, and varies between –0.4 kPa during inspiration to +0.4 kPa during expiration.

*Intrapleural pressure* is the pressure between the lungs and the pleural sac which surrounds them.

- Because of the elastic nature of lung tissue, lungs constantly tend to move towards a state of collapse, and it is the negative pressure in the intrapleural spaces that stops them collapsing.
- Intrapleural pressure normally varies between –1.1 kPa during inspiration and –0.3 kPa during expiration.
- This negative pressure must be maintained at all times (even after expiration, when the lungs are at their smallest, and the alveoli are at

atmospheric pressure) to ensure that atmospheric pressure continues to push the lungs outwards against the pleural sac and chest wall to prevent the lungs from collapsing.

## Gas exchange

See Table 9.3.

- Differences in the partial pressures of inspired, alveolar, and expired air promote free interchange of gases within the lungs—most importantly $O_2$ and $CO_2$.
- The partial pressure of $O_2$ in the atmosphere (i.e. inspired air) is approximately 21.3 kPa, whereas the partial pressure of $O_2$ in the air in the alveoli is approximately 14 kPa. This pressure gradient means that $O_2$ passes from the inspired air to the alveoli.
- The reverse is true for $CO_2$—the partial pressure of $CO_2$ in alveolar air (approximately 5.3 kPa) is much higher than the partial pressure of $CO_2$ in the atmosphere (approximately 0.03 kPa); $CO_2$, therefore, passes from the alveolar air to expired air.
- $O_2$ passes from the alveolar air of the lungs (partial pressure approximately 14 kPa) into the blood in the pulmonary capillaries (partial pressure approximately 5.3 kPa) because of the pressure gradient between alveolar air and that in the capillaries.
- Similarly, there is a pressure gradient between $CO_2$ in the capillaries (partial pressure approximately 6 kPa) and in alveolar air (partial pressure approximately 5.3 kPa) and so $CO_2$ is transferred from blood into air in the alveoli.
- At the tissue capillaries, pressure gradients force $O_2$ from blood (partial pressure approximately 14 kPa) into tissue (partial pressure approximately 5.3 kPa) and $CO_2$ from tissue (partial pressure approximately 6 kPa) back into blood (partial pressure approximately 5.3 kPa).

**Table 9.3** Gas exchange

| Location | Partial pressure $O_2$ (P$O_2$) (kPa) | Partial pressure $CO_2$ (P$CO_2$) (kPa) |
|---|---|---|
| Atmosphere | 21.3 | 0.03 |
| Alveoli | 14.0 | 5.3 |
| Pulmonary artery | 5.3 | 6.0 |
| Pulmonary vein | 14.0 | 5.3 |
| Systemic artery | 14.0 | 5.3 |
| Systemic vein | 5.3 | 6.0 |

## Further reading

Adams S, Allday J (2013). Advanced physics (2nd ed). Oxford: Oxford University Press.

Cheung S, Ainslie PN (2021). Advanced environmental exercise physiology (2nd ed). Champaign IL: Human Kinetics Inc.

Franklin K, Muir P, Scott T, et al. (2019). Introduction to biological physics for the health and life sciences (2nd ed). Oxford: Wiley-Blackwell.

Johnson T (2016). Introduction to health physics (5th ed). New York: McGraw-Hill.

# SI units

All systems of weights and measures are linked through a number of international agreements that support the International System of Units. This system is the SI, derived from the French 'Système international d'unités'.

## Base SI units

Central to the SI are seven base units—for seven base quantities that are assumed to be mutually independent. The base units are able to be defined without reference to any other units (Table 9.4).

**Table 9.4** Base SI units

| Unit | Measure of | Symbol |
| --- | --- | --- |
| Metre | Length | m |
| Kilogram | Mass | kg |
| Second | Time | s |
| Ampere | Electric current | A or amp |
| Kelvin | Temperature | K |
| Mole | Amount of substance | mol |
| Candela | Luminous intensity | cd |

## SI derived units

Other SI units—SI derived units—are able to be defined in terms of the seven base units (Table 9.5).

**Table 9.5** SI derived units

| Unit | Measure of | Symbol |
| --- | --- | --- |
| Square metre | Area | $m^2$ |
| Cubic metre | Volume | $m^3$ |
| Kilogram per cubic metre | Mass density | $kg/m^3$ |
| Cubic metre per kilogram | Specific volume | $m^3/kg$ |
| Mole per cubic metre | Amount of substance concentration | $mol/m^3$ |
| Metre per second | Velocity | m/s |
| Metre per second squared | Acceleration | $m/s^2$ |
| Ampere per square metre | Current density | $A/m^2$ |
| Candela per square metre | Luminance | $cd/m^2$ |

## Special names and symbols

For convenience and to enhance understanding, a number of SI-derived units have been given special names and symbols, see Table 9.6.

**Table 9.6** Special names and symbols

| Unit | Measure of | Symbol | Expressed in terms of other SI units |
|------|-----------|--------|--------------------------------------|
| Newton | Force | N | – |
| Pascal | Pressure | Pa | $N/m^2$ |
| Hertz | Frequency | Hz | $1/s$ |
| Joule | Energy | J | Nm |
| Watt | Power | W | J/s |
| Degree Celsius | Temperature | °C | – |
| Coulomb | Charge | C | – |
| Volt | Potential | V | W/A |
| Farad | Capacitance | F | C/V |
| Ohm | Resistance | Ω | V/A |
| Siemens | Conductance | S | A/V |
| Becquerel | Activity (of a radionuclide) | Bq | $1/s$ |
| Sievert | Dose equivalent | Sv | J/kg |

## Multiplying prefixes

Some of the units used within the SI are either too large or too small to be useful in everyday life (e.g. the metre is too small when measuring very large distances (such as the distance from the Earth to the moon), but too large when measuring very small distances (such as the diameter of a human hair)) so the system employs a standard set of multiplying prefixes to convert units to a more convenient size (Table 9.7).

*Note*: the kilogram is the only SI unit that has a prefix as part of its name and symbol. Because multiple prefixes are not allowed, in the case of the kilogram, prefixes are used with the unit name 'gram' (symbol 'g') so, $10^{-6}$ kg is not written as 1 µkg (1 microkilogram), but as 1 mg (1 milligram). Otherwise, any SI prefix may be used with any SI unit.

**Table 9.7** Multiplying prefixes

| Prefix | Symbol | Multiplying factor |
|---|---|---|
| Tera- | T | 1,000,000,000,000 ($10^{12}$) |
| Giga- | G | 1,000,000,000 ($10^{9}$) |
| Mega- | M | 1,000,000 ($10^{6}$) |
| Kilo- | k | 1000($10^{3}$) |
| Hecto- | h | 100($10^{2}$) |
| Deka- | da | 10($10^{1}$) |
| Deci- | d | 0.1($10^{-1}$) |
| Centi- | c | 0.01($10^{-2}$) |
| Milli- | m | 0.001($10^{-3}$) |
| Micro- | μ | 0.000001($10^{-6}$) |
| Nano- | n | 0.000000001($10^{-9}$) |
| Pico- | p | 0.000000000001($10^{-12}$) |

## Further reading

Adams S, Allday J (2013). Advanced physics (2nd ed). Oxford: Oxford University Press.

Cheung S, Ainslie PN (2021). Advanced environmental exercise physiology (2nd ed). Champaign IL: Human Kinetics Inc.

Franklin K, Muir P, Scott T, Yates P (2019). Introduction to biological physics for the health and life sciences (2nd ed). Oxford: Wiley-Blackwell.

Johnson T (2016). Introduction to health physics (5th ed). New York: McGraw-Hill.

# Airway management

# The importance of airway management

- Maintaining adequate oxygenation is the number one priority for all members of the anaesthetic team.
- Airway management requires that:
  - There is a clear pathway between the $O_2$ supply and the patient's lungs
  - The patient's lungs are protected from the risk of aspiration.

- If there is no respiration or ventilation then subsequently there will be no oxygenation and the patient's circulation and all other vital processes will cease.
- Failure to adequately maintain the airway is responsible for approximately 30% of deaths associated with anaesthesia.
- The chest must rise and fall and allow gaseous exchange to occur in the lungs.

> Remember, it is oxygenation, and not intubation, which keeps patients alive and this can be achieved through simple bag-and-mask hand ventilation.

## Further reading

Association of Anaesthetists of Great Britain and Ireland (2012). Checking anaesthetic equipment. London: Association of Anaesthetists of Great Britain and Ireland.

Association of Anaesthetists of Great Britain and Ireland (2018). The anaesthesia team. Available at: ℘ http://dx.doi.org/10.21466/g.TAT.2018

Association of Anaesthetists of Great Britain and Ireland (2019). Checklist for draw-over anaesthetic equipment. Available at: ℘ http://dx.doi.org/10.21466/g.CFDAE2.2019

Freedman R, Herbert L, O'Donnell A, et al. (eds) (2022). Oxford handbook of anaesthesia (5th ed). Oxford: Oxford University Press.

Pollard B, Kitchen G (eds) (2017) Handbook of clinical anaesthesia (4th ed). London: CRC Press.

Royal College of Anaesthetists (2019–2021). Guidelines for the provision of anaesthetic services. London: Royal College of Anaesthetists.

Royal College of Anaesthetists (2021). Chapter 2: guidelines for the provision of anaesthesia services for preoperative assessment and preparation. London: Royal College of Anaesthetists.

# The role of the anaesthetic practitioner in airway management

It is essential that all equipment is prepared and checked prior to the commencement of all operating lists, even when patients may only require regional anaesthetic or LA techniques.

### Routine checking

This must include the following:
- $O_2$ supply, tug test of pipelines, and cylinder availability with sufficient contents in case of pipeline failure.
- Anaesthetic machine and ventilator checks as per the current AAGBI recommendations.[1]
- The availability and integrity of breathing circuits and HME filters, including a self-inflating resuscitation bag. Self-inflating resuscitation bags can be used to effectively ventilate patients even if the $O_2$ supply fails as most patients can survive if ventilated with air.
- Suction apparatus connected and able to generate a vacuum with all tubing attached and both pharyngeal and bronchial suction catheters available.
- A range of appropriately sized facemasks available. Clear masks are considered advantageous as vomit or secretions can be more quickly detected and managed.
- Airways in a range of types and sizes. Both oral and nasal airways may be used routinely and should remain in their packaging prior to use in order to reduce the risk of cross infection.
- LMAs are essential and all sizes must be available. Disposable LMAs are recommended unless adequate facilities are available for decontamination and sterilization; this is particularly important with the concern of prion disease.
- A prion is an abnormal, transmissible agent that is able to induce abnormal cellular prion proteins in the brain, leading to brain damage and the characteristic signs and symptoms of the disease. Prion diseases usually progress rapidly and are always fatal.
  - Prion diseases, also known as transmissible spongiform encephalopathies (TSEs), are a group of progressive neurodegenerative conditions that exist in both humans and animals.
  - Human prion disease can include Creutzfeldt–Jakob disease (CJD) or variant Creutzfeldt–Jakob disease (vCJD).
  - Animal prion disease can include scrapie, bovine spongiform encephalopathy (BSE) and chronic wasting disease (CWD).
  - While prion disease is not contagious, CNS tissues that include brain, spinal cord, and eye tissue are considered to be extremely infectious and are a cause for concern for those directly handling infected tissue. Although there is no evidence that blood is infectious, special infection precautions should be taken by those handling blood or blood products.
  - A tonsil biopsy is used to diagnose vCJD.
- The move towards single-use devices accelerated following the recognition that prion diseases (causing vCJD) were potentially transmissible despite current disinfection and sterilizing techniques. A

laryngoscope, Macintosh long (size 4) and short (size 3) blades need to be available, their bulbs tested and checked for brightness. The location of a McCoy laryngoscope blade and short laryngoscope handle should be noted.
- Sterile unopened ETTs, of the anticipated size plus one size smaller/larger close to hand. A syringe for cuff inflation is needed and the use of a cuff pressure gauge is recommended to avoid inflation pressures >30 cmH$_2$O causing ischaemia of the tracheal lining with the potential to cause permanent damage.
- A disposable bougie needs to be readily accessible to assist with intubation should the view of the larynx be incomplete or the passage of the ETT be obscured in any way.
- Lubricants should be water based and sterile for the lubrication of airways, LMAs, and ETTs.
- A selection of tapes and ties to secure the position of airway management devices used, noting any patient allergies prior to use.
- Patient monitoring should be switched on and all patient connection devices checked for availability, integrity, and cleanliness. These must include SaO$_2$, NIBP, ECG, and invasive monitoring sets and connectors.
- Gas analysis monitoring devices must be switched on and patient sampling lines connected into the patient breathing circuits, usually via the single-use HME filter or specialist monitoring connection piece.
- Patient beds, trolleys, and operating tables need to be charged if electrically operated; the brakes, rise, and fall mechanism and the head-end tip all in working order.
- Patients must be positioned within easy reach of the anaesthetist at the head end of the bed, trolley, or operating table with the height adjusted to a comfortable working height for the anaesthetist managing the airway.
- All patients will need a pillow positioned just under the head and neck to allow head extension and neck flexion.

Good preoperative preparation, assessment of the operating list, checking of equipment, and planning are all essential for successful outcomes in airway management.

## Reference

1. Association of Anaesthetists of Great Britain and Ireland (2012). Checking anaesthetic equipment. London: Association of Anaesthetists of Great Britain and Ireland.

## Further reading

Association of Anaesthetists of Great Britain and Ireland (2018). The anaesthesia team. Available at: ℛ http://dx.doi.org/10.21466/g.TAT.2018

Association of Anaesthetists of Great Britain and Ireland (2019). Checklist for draw-over anaesthetic equipment. Available at: ℛ http://dx.doi.org/10.21466/g.CFDAE2.2019

Freedman R, Herbert L, O'Donnell A, et al. (eds) (2022). Oxford handbook of anaesthesia (5th ed). Oxford: Oxford University Press.

National Prion Clinic. Homepage. Available at: ℛ https://www.uclh.nhs.uk/our-services/find-service/neurology-and-neurosurgery/national-prion-clinic

Pollard B, Kitchen G (eds) (2017). Handbook of clinical anaesthesia (4th ed). London: CRC Press.

Royal College of Anaesthetists (2019–2021). Guidelines for the provision of anaesthetic services. London: Royal College of Anaesthetists.

Royal College of Anaesthetists (2021). Chapter 2: guidelines for the provision of anaesthesia services for preoperative assessment and preparation. London: Royal College of Anaesthetists.

# Maintaining the airway

One of the top priorities during anaesthetics must be to maintain a patent airway, free from secretions. To this end, the anaesthetic practitioner must be familiar with the following equipment and techniques:

## Patient positioning

- A pillow must be positioned under the patient's head and neck but not too far under the shoulders.
- This position, with the neck flexed and the head extended, commonly referred to as the 'sniffing the morning air' position, will permit a straight line of vision from the patient's mouth to their vocal cords with the aid of a laryngoscope.
- Caution should be applied if potential cervical spine injury exists.

## Head tilt and chin lift

- In the unconscious patient the tongue can obstruct the airway.
- This can usually be avoided by placing one hand on the patient's forehead then tilting the head backwards while lifting the patient's chin firmly with the finger tips of the other hand.

## Jaw thrust

- When obstruction is not alleviated by the simple head tilt and chin lift then the jaw thrust may be needed.
- The practitioner displaces the posterior aspect of the mandible (angle of the jaw) upwards and forwards aiming to get the lower teeth in front of the upper teeth.
- This manoeuvre pulls forward the tongue and lifts it off the back of the pharynx, securing the patient's airway for either spontaneous respiration or bag-and-mask hand ventilation.

## Removal of secretions or vomit

- Suction must be immediately available for use, usually with a Yankauer pharyngeal sucker attached.
- Trauma and bleeding can be avoided by only applying suction to the airway under direct vision.

## Facemasks

- Facemasks are available in a range of paediatric and adult sizes and must be selected to fit over the bridge of the nose onto the cleft of the chin.
- Holding a facemask is a skill, which the anaesthetic practitioner must practise and master.
- The thumb and index finger are used to press the mask against the patient's face and a tight seal is then achieved by the remaining three fingers, placed on the mandible, lifting the patient's face into the mask while maintaining a head tilt and jaw thrust at the same time.
- Holding a facemask may require two hands with a second person, if required to squeeze the bag to provide ventilation.

## Oropharyngeal airway

- The Guedel airway is the most commonly used airway.
- They are colour coded and available in adult and paediatric sizes.
- The appropriate sized airway for an adult patient may be chosen to correspond to the distance from the patient's incisor teeth down to the angle of their jaw.
- Airways should be lubricated prior to use and then, in adults, be inserted into the patient's mouth upside down and then rotated through 180° into the oropharynx.

## Nasopharyngeal airway

- These airways are softer than oropharyngeal airways and typically are better tolerated by the semiconscious patient.
- They are available in a wide range of sizes denoted by their diameter.
- Usual sizing is size 6 for an average-sized female and size 7 for an average-sized male.
- The nasopharyngeal airway needs to be well lubricated prior to the insertion of the bevelled end into the nostril.
- Advancing it requires a gentle twisting action, pushing gently in a posterior direction.
- Do not use excessive force to insert! If there is too much resistance, try the other nostril or go down a size.
- A safety pin inserted through the flanged end of the nasopharyngeal airway prior to insertion can prevent it from slipping too far into the patient's nose.

# Endotracheal tubes: overview

The cuffed ETT is regarded as the most reliable way of maintaining a patient's airway by protecting the trachea from contamination and facilitating IPPV. Cuffed ETTs are all single use and available in sizes 2–10 mm ID and have the following safety features incorporated into their design:

- ETTs have a radiopaque line for X-ray detection.
- At the distal end of the ETT there is an additional hole called Murphy's eye. This will allow ventilation to continue if the end of the tube becomes obstructed. The most common reason for the obstruction is that the tube is inserted too far and impinges on the carina or bronchus wall.
- ETTs now have high-volume, low-pressure cuffs with a pilot balloon, which when inflated seals off the trachea, reducing the risk of tracheal contamination. The low-pressure cuff is designed to reduce the risk of prolonged pressure from the cuff on the tracheal lining, which may cause ischaemia of the tracheal mucosa.

## The role of the anaesthetic practitioner

- An appropriate selection of different sized ETTs must be available for immediate use. One size smaller than anticipated should always be within reach.
- ETTs should be kept sterile within their wrappers until required to minimize the risks of cross infection.
- The lumen of the ETT and the cuff must be checked prior to use.
- The ETT is lubricated with a sterile, water-soluble lubricant immediately prior to insertion.
- When the ETT is situated in the trachea the cuff is inflated with the minimum amount of air to achieve a seal within the trachea with no air leak. The cuff pressure must not exceed 30 cmH$_2$O and can be checked with a pressure gauge designed for the purpose, if available.
- The position of the ETT needs to be secured either with ties or tape according to the anaesthetist's preference.
- Patient documentation must be completed recording the type and size of ETT used, noting the method of insertion, and the type of tape or ties used to secure.

## Further reading

Al-Shaikh B, Stacey S (2018). Essentials of equipment in anaesthesia, critical care and perioperative medicine (5th ed). Edinburgh: Elsevier.

Association of Anaesthetists of Great Britain and Ireland (2012). Checking anaesthetic equipment. London: Association of Anaesthetists of Great Britain and Ireland.

Association of Anaesthetists of Great Britain and Ireland (2018). The anaesthesia team. Available at: ℰ http://dx.doi.org/10.21466/g.TAT.2018

Association of Anaesthetists of Great Britain and Ireland (2019). Checklist for draw-over anaesthetic equipment. Available at: ℰ http://dx.doi.org/10.21466/g.CFDAE2.2019

Cook T, Walton B (2005). The laryngeal mask airway. Anaesthesia, 20:32–42.

Difficult Airway Society (2015). DAS guidelines home. Available at: ℰ https://www.das.uk.com/guidelines

Freedman R, Herbert L, O'Donnell A, et al. (eds) (2022). Oxford handbook of anaesthesia (5th ed). Oxford: Oxford University Press.

Hung OR, Murphy MF (2018). Hung's difficult and failed airway management. London: McGraw Hill.
National Prion Clinic. Homepage. Available at: ℛ http://www.uclh.nhs.uk/OurServices/ServiceA-Z/Neuro/NPC/Pages/Home.aspx
Pollard B, Kitchen G (eds) (2017). Handbook of clinical anaesthesia (4th ed). London: CRC Press.
Royal College of Anaesthetists (2019–2021). Guidelines for the provision of anaesthetic services. London: Royal College of Anaesthetists.
Royal College of Anaesthetists (2021). Chapter 2: guidelines for the provision of anaesthesia services for preoperative assessment and preparation. London: Royal College of Anaesthetists.

# Types of endotracheal tubes

This is only a small selection of the large variety of ETTs available.

## Cuffed ETTs

- Cuffed tubes, when inflated, provide an airtight seal between the seal and the tracheal wall.
- The airtight seal protects the patient's airway from aspiration and allows ventilation during IPPV.
- Following intubation, the cuff is inflated until no gas leak is audible.
- The narrowest point in an adult airway is the glottis so cuffed tubes are used to achieve an airtight seal.[1]

## Uncuffed ETTs

- The paediatric trachea is conical where the narrowest part is at the level of the cricoid ring, and the only part of the airway completely surrounded by cartilage.
- If the tracheal tube is too large, it will compress the tracheal epithelium at this level, leading to ischaemia with consequent scarring and the possibility of subglottic stenosis.[2]
- A correctly sized tube is one where ventilation is adequate but a small audible leak of air is present when positive pressure is applied.
- Avoid the use of catheter mounts for paediatric patients due to the large dead space involved.[2]

## Reinforced ETTs

- These have a nylon or metal spiral embedded within the wall of the ETT.
- These are used to reduce the risk of an obstructed airway caused by the kinking of the ETT (e.g. when turning a patient prone, or during maxilla-facial/neurosurgery).
- They are less rigid than the standard ETTs and may need a stylet to aid insertion.
- Meticulous positioning and fixing of these tubes is essential to ensure the airway is maintained.

## Preformed ETTs

- These can be north or south facing and are used to direct the breathing circuits, when connected to the ETT, away from the surgical site (e.g. ENT or plastic surgery).
- Both are available as cuffed or uncuffed tubes.
- Some paediatric anaesthetists, because of the ease with which they can be made secure, favour the use of uncuffed north-facing ETTs.

## Double-lumen ETTs

- These are exactly what they say they are and are two tubes in one.
- They are available in a large variety of types and sizes, all available as either left- or right-sided tubes.
- They are intended to intubate one or other of the main bronchi as well as the trachea.

- They are designed to facilitate single lung ventilation allowing the collapse of one lung during thoracic surgery or oesophagectomy.
- When inserted their exact position is usually confirmed with the aid of a fibreoptic bronchoscope prior to surgery to ensure that one-lung ventilation is possible when required.
- Additional equipment may be required such as a Y-shaped tube connector, heavy clamps, and a blocker or occluding device. Most of this additional equipment usually comes in the packaging with the tube but check!

## Laser-resistant ETTs

- These are designed for airway management during laser surgery to the larynx.
- These tubes have a metal foil or stainless steel body, which is non-flammable and therefore able to reduce the combustion risk during surgery.
- Sterile saline coloured with methylene blue also needs to be used to inflate the ETT cuff(s) throughout the procedure. This allows any damage to the cuff during surgery to be easily visualized and action taken.
- Most laser tubes have a double cuff for extra protection of the airway in case one cuff becomes damaged during laser surgery.

## References

1. Al-Shaikh B, Stacey S (2018). Essentials of equipment in anaesthesia, critical care and perioperative medicine (5th ed). Edinburgh: Elsevier.
2. Berg S, Campbell S (2022). Paediatric and neonatal anaesthesia. In: Freedman R, Herbert L, O'Donnell A, et al. (eds) Oxford handbook of anaesthesia (5th ed). Oxford: Oxford University Press.

## Further reading

Anaesthesia UK. Homepage. Available at: ꙮ http://www.frca.co.uk/default.aspx
Association of Anaesthetists of Great Britain and Ireland (2012). Checking anaesthetic equipment. London: Association of Anaesthetists of Great Britain and Ireland.
Association of Anaesthetists of Great Britain and Ireland (2019). Checklist for draw-over anaesthetic equipment. Available at: ꙮ http://dx.doi.org/10.21466/g.CFDAE2.2019
Pollard B, Kitchen G (eds) (2017). Handbook of clinical anaesthesia (4th ed). London: CRC Press.

# Laryngeal mask airway

The first LMA was described by Dr Archie Brain, a London anaesthetist, in 1983. The LMA provides a less traumatic alternative to ET intubation but also, when used in place of a facemask, gives better airway control.

It can be used for both spontaneous respiration and positive pressure ventilation, *but it must be remembered that the LMA does not protect the lungs from aspiration.*

- The LMA is available in sizes 1–6 and size selection is based upon the weight of the patient.
- The amount of air needed for cuff inflation increases with tube size. The LMA cuff must be deflated, wrinkle free, and well lubricated on the posterior surface prior to insertion.
- The assistant may be required to open the patient's mouth as widely as possible using a jaw thrust.
- Once in place, the LMA cuff will need inflating gently at which point the LMA will usually lift slightly within the pharynx.
- After this readjustment the LMA can be connected to the breathing filter and circuit.
- Once in position the efficacy of ventilation must be assessed by clinical observation, appropriate tidal volumes, and $ETCO_2$ (Table 10.1).

**Table 10.1** LMA selection and cuff volume guide

| LMA size | Patient weight (kg) | Cuff volume (mL) |
| --- | --- | --- |
| 1 | 0–5 | 2–4 |
| 1.5 | 5–10 | 5–7 |
| 2 | 10–20 | 7–10 |
| 2.5 | 20–30 | 12–14 |
| 3 | 30–50 | 15–20 |
| 4 | 50–70 | 20–30 |
| 5 | 70–100 | 30–40 |
| 6 | >100 | <50 |

## Reinforced laryngeal mask airway

- The reinforced laryngeal mask airway (RLMA) was developed with a coil inside the wall of the LMA to prevent inadvertent kinking of the device when in use.
- It is used when surgery is in close proximity to the airway or when the airway may need to be covered by the surgical drapes.
- The technique for insertion is the same as the standard LMA but meticulous attention must be paid to securing the device once in position.

## Intubating laryngeal mask airway

The ILMA was developed to make a device through which intubation was possible as it was previously impossible through an LMA. It is useful in the management of both anticipated and unexpectedly difficult cases of intubation and such use is now recommended in various difficult airway management algorithms.

• The ILMA is currently a reusable device and is available in adult sizes 3–5.
• The aperture of the ILMA is designed for the insertion of a well-lubricated size 8 mm ETT through it.
• It is also possible to ventilate via the ILMA during the intubation process, if the patient should require it.

## ProSeal™ laryngeal mask airway

• The ProSeal™ laryngeal mask airway (PLMA) is the most recent development of the LMA and has been developed to offer improved performance with IPPV.
• It has a double cuff to allow increased cuff pressures with an improved laryngeal seal.
• The PLMA has an additional drain tube, which is intended to allow the separation of the respiratory and the alimentary tracts, providing a way of escape for any unexpected gastric contents.
• The PLMA is available as a reusable and single-use device in adult sizes 3–5.
• Unlike the other LMAs, the PLMA has an introducer, which when attached gives additional rigidity to aid insertion.
• When the PLMA is correctly inserted, the drain tube should be directly above and in line with the oesophagus allowing a lubricated NG tube to be passed through the drain tube into the stomach through which gastric contents may be aspirated.
• However, it must be noted that there still remains the *risk of gastric aspiration* while the PLMA is *in situ*.

## Further reading

Brain AIJ (1993). The Intravent laryngeal mask: instruction manual (2nd ed). Henley-on-Thames: Intravent.

Calder I, Pearce A (eds) (2004). Core topics in airway management. Cambridge: Cambridge University Press.

Difficult Airway Society (2015). DAS guidelines home. Available at: ℰ https://www.das.uk.com/guidelines

Freedman R, Herbert L, O'Donnell A, et al. (eds) (2022). Oxford handbook of anaesthesia (5th ed). Oxford: Oxford University Press.

Martin A, Allman K, McIndoe A (eds) (2020). Emergencies in anaesthesia (3rd ed). Oxford: Oxford University Press.

Royal College of Anaesthetists (2017). Guidelines for the provision of anaesthetic services. London: Royal College of Anaesthetists.

Van Esch BF, Stegemab I, Smit AL (2017). Comparison of laryngeal mask airway vs tracheal intubation: a systematic review on airway complications. Journal of Clinical Anaesthesia, 36:142–150.

Wharton NM, Gibbison B, Gabbott DA, et al. (2008). I-gel insertion by novices in manikins and patients. Anaesthesia, 63(9):991–995.

# Additional supraglottic devices

## Combitube

This has a dual tube with dual cuffs, designed to straddle the larynx and can allow ventilation from holes between the two cuffs, or act simply as a tracheal tube.[1]

## Laryngeal tube

This is based on the combitube and has a single blind-ending tube, with distal and proximal cuffs; ventilation occurs via holes between the cuffs. It is easy to insert and atraumatic.[1]

## i-gel®

This is a new cuffless polymer airway, similar in design to the PLMA. It is a single-use, supraglottic airway management device designed to create a non-inflatable, anatomical seal of the pharyngeal, laryngeal, and perilaryngeal structures while avoiding compression trauma.

## Streamlined liner of the pharynx airway (SLIPA™)

SLIPA™ is a cuffless airway with the body of the SLIPA™ acting as a reservoir if regurgitation occurs. This airway is sized by matching the external diameter of the patient's larynx to the 'size' of the device.[1]

## Cobra perilaryngeal airway (CobraPLA™)

This is similar to the LT. It has a bullet tip as opposed to a distal balloon and is designed to sit higher in the airway than the LT.[1]

## Reference

1. Jackson K, Cook T (2006). Equipment for airway management. Anaesthesia and Intensive Care Medicine, 7(10):356–359.

## Further reading

Al-Shaikh B, Stacey S (2018). Essentials of equipment in anaesthesia, critical care and perioperative medicine (5th ed). Edinburgh: Elsevier.

Calder I, Pearce A (eds) (2004). Core topics in airway management. Cambridge: Cambridge University Press.

Difficult Airway Society (2015). DAS guidelines home. Available at: ℬ https://www.das.uk.com/guidelines

Freedman R, Herbert L, O'Donnell A, et al. (eds) (2022). Oxford handbook of anaesthesia (5th ed). Oxford: Oxford University Press.

Royal College of Anaesthetists (2019–2021). Guidelines for the provision of anaesthetic services. London: Royal College of Anaesthetists.

Wharton NM, Gibbison B, Gabbott DA, et al. (2008). I-gel insertion by novices in manikins and patients. Anaesthesia, 63(9):991–995.

# Difficult airway assessment

An airway that is difficult to manage is created by both anatomical and clinical factors that complicate, for the skilled practitioner, either ventilation administered via a facemask and/or ET intubation. Predicting which patients will prove difficult to ventilate or intubate, or both, is complex and the subject of much debate. However, airway evaluation is a skill that needs to be learnt for the benefit of patient safety. There are many methods and predictive scoring systems described in the literature. Only one method each for ventilation and intubation will be explored here. It should be noted that these tests while useful are only indicators. They can and often do give false-positive and false-negative results. They should only be regarded as guidance. Experience, clinical judgement, and being well prepared for eventualities will always be a requirement for the anaesthetic practitioner.

It is advisable to know one system well, to remember it, and to use it.

Airway difficulties can be separated into categories:
- Difficult to ventilate.
- Difficult to intubate.
- Both of these.

### Difficult mask ventilation

Difficult mask ventilation (DMV) occurs when the unassisted anaesthetist fails to maintain the oxygen saturation of a patient with bag-and-mask hand ventilation. The incidence of DMV is not uncommon and may occur in approximately 5% of patients. There are five predictors of DMV and the acronym *OBESE* can be used to remember these:
- Obesity.
- Bearded.
- Elderly (>55 years old).
- Snorers.
- Edentulous.

When a patient presents with two or more of these features, then there is a likelihood of DMV.

### Difficult intubation

The incidence of difficult intubation is estimated at 1–3% of patients who require ET intubation. It is important to assess all patients' airways preoperatively to predict possible intubation difficulties prior to anaesthesia. This will ensure that the appropriate skill mix of staff and all necessary equipment will be readily available to implement the planned intubation technique (e.g. awake fibreoptic intubation). One commonly used acronym, *LEMON*, can be a helpful way to remember the predictors for intubation difficulties. The greater the number of unusual anatomical features a patient has, the greater the likelihood of intubation difficulties.
- *Look* externally for any abnormalities to the facial shape. These may include a receding jaw, short or thick neck, protruding teeth, narrow mouth opening, obesity, or other face/neck pathology.
- *Evaluate* the jaw.

- Patients should be able to open their mouths sufficiently to place three of their fingers between their upper and lower teeth.
- Thyromental distance, the distance from the thyroid notch to the tip of the jaw when the patient's head is extended is usually >6.5 cm (Patil test).
- Patients are usually able to place their bottom teeth in front of their top teeth (jaw protrusion).
- *Mallampati* is a scoring system, first described in 1985, based upon the available view of the patient's oropharynx. The patient is sat down with their head held in a neutral position and asked to open their mouth wide and to protrude their tongue maximally. What is then visible is categorized and this is illustrated in Fig. 10.1. The less the anaesthetist is able to view, the greater the likelihood of intubation difficulties.
- *Obstruction* to the airway can be caused by foreign body, tumour abscess, swelling, or haematoma.
- *Neck mobility*, patients should be able to tilt their heads backwards through the movement of the atlanto-occipital (AO) joint. On examination of the patient lying down, one finger of one hand is placed onto the occiput and one finger of the other hand is placed onto the chin; the patient is then asked to tip their head backwards resulting in the finger on the chin usually being lifted higher than the finger placed onto the occiput. Restricted neck movement may be caused by cervical spondylosis, rheumatoid arthritis, or cervical nerve compression.

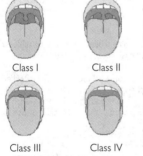

Class I  Class II

**Class I:** visualisation of the soft palate, uvula, fauces, anterior and posterior tonsillar pillars

**Class II:** visualisation of the soft palate, fauces and uvula

**Class III:** visualisation of the soft palate and the base of the uvula

**Class IV:** soft palateis not visible at all

Class III  Class IV

**Fig. 10.1** Mallampati classification.

Reproduced with permission from Allman KG and Wilson IH (eds) (2016). Oxford Handbook of Anaesthesia (4th edn). Oxford University Press: Oxford.

## Further reading

Difficult Airway Society (2015). DAS guidelines home. Available at: ℵ https://www.das.uk.com/guidelines

Freedman R, Herbert L, O'Donnell A, et al. (eds) (2022). Oxford handbook of anaesthesia (5th ed). Oxford: Oxford University Press.

Mallampati SR, Gugino LD, Desai S, et al. (1983). Clinical signs to predict difficult tracheal intubation. Canadian Anaesthetists Society Journal 30(3, Pt 1):316–317.

Martin A, Allman K, McIndoe A (eds) (2020). Emergencies in anaesthesia (3rd ed). Oxford: Oxford University Press.

Royal College of Anaesthetists (2017). Guidelines for the provision of anaesthetic services. London: Royal College of Anaesthetists.

# Rapid sequence induction

- The aim of rapid sequence induction (RSI) is to secure a patient's airway as quickly as possible, avoiding any soiling of the lungs from gastric contents through the application of cricoid pressure or Sellick's manoeuvre as it is sometimes called.
- Pulmonary aspiration of gastric contents, even in quantities as low as 30 mL, is associated with significant morbidity and mortality.
- Cricoid pressure is widely accepted as standard practice in the UK and US but it is controversial and not as widely practised in continental Europe. It is possible that poorly applied cricoid pressure can obscure the anaesthetist's view of the larynx and make intubation in urgent circumstances more difficult.

## Indications

- Inadequate preoperative fasting: <6 hours solid food, <4 hours breast milk, and <2 hours clear fluids.
- Delayed gastric emptying, for example, due to trauma, an acute abdomen, opioids, or poorly controlled diabetes.
- Oesophageal sphincter incompetence, for example, caused by gastric reflux or pregnancy.

## Preparation

Patient monitoring needs to be attached (ECG, NIBP, $SAO_2$) with baseline recording noted. An IV infusion must be sited and connected to a free-flowing infusion.

## Equipment

- Patient needs to be positioned on a tipping trolley or operating table.
- Suction connected, switched on, and easily accessible (e.g. under the pillow by the right hand of the anaesthetist).
- Selection of ETTs, cut if necessary, the cuff of the chosen ETT checked with an air-filled 10 mL syringe attached to the pilot balloon.
- Laryngoscopes (×2) checked with both long and short blades available. The laryngoscope of choice must be placed within easy reach of the left hand of the anaesthetist.
- Bougie must be instantly available to railroad the ETT over it into the trachea in case intubation difficulties occur.
- Stethoscope to identity breath sounds as part of the confirmation of successful intubation.
- Tape or ties to secure the ETT when intubation has been confirmed by the presence of $ETCO_2$, bilateral chest movement, and auscultation.

## Patient preparation

- Explanation of the procedure, any questions answered, and reassurance given.
- Location of the cricoid cartilage by the anaesthetic assistant. If in any doubt, the assistant must confirm with the anaesthetist that the cricoid cartilage has been successfully identified.

- Check that the patient is positioned appropriately at the head end of a tipping trolley or operating table.
- Optimal positioning of the patient's pillow under the head, neck, and just under the shoulders sufficiently to allow the patient to adopt the 'sniffing the morning air' position with their neck flexed and head extended.

## Procedure

- Preoxygenation for a minimum of 3 minutes with 100% $O_2$. In an emergency, four vital capacity breaths may be given, using $O_2$ flush.
- The application of gentle cricoid pressure (approximately 10 N).
- Administration of the anaesthetic induction agent.
- Full application of cricoid pressure: to 30 N (3 kg pressure).
- Administration of suxamethonium.
- Rocuronium *may* be used if suxamethonium is contraindicated. Sugammadex should be immediately available to reverse the blockade in case of an airway emergency. Seek expert advice before commencing this technique.
- No mask ventilation to avoid gastric insufflation, which would increase the risk of gastric reflux and aspiration.
- Wait for the muscle fasciculations to cease.
- Laryngoscopy and intubation with the ETT cuff immediately inflated.
- The positioning of the ETT within the trachea is confirmed by the presence of an $ETCO_2$ trace, bilateral chest movement, and auscultation.
- Cricoid pressure is only released when the anaesthetist confirms that it is safe to do so.
- *Emergence from anaesthesia also presents the same risk of aspiration as induction of anaesthesia.*
  At the end of surgery, the following precautions are necessary:
- Administration of 100% $O_2$.
- Reversal of neuromuscular blockade.
- Patient positioned on their side on a tipping trolley, bed, or operating table.
- Extubation only when the patient is fully awake and able to remove the ETT themselves.

## Cricoid pressure or Sellick's manoeuvre

The cricoid cartilage is the only tracheal ring which is a complete circle. It is located immediately below the thyroid cartilage or 'Adam's apple'. Cricoid pressure is applied: firstly by stabilizing the patient's trachea between the assistant's thumb and middle finger, then secondly by using the index finger to apply posterior pressure to the cricoid cartilage. The amount of pressure required to compress the oesophagus against spines is significant, approximately 30 N or 3 kg of pressure. The circular cricoid cartilage compresses the oesophagus between itself and the vertebral bodies that are located behind it, thus preventing passive regurgitation of gastric contents.

*It must be stressed that cricoid pressure must be released if the patient actively vomits to avoid the risk of oesophageal rupture.*

## Further reading

Association of Anaesthetists of Great Britain and Ireland (2015). Guidance on perioperative fasting for adults and children. Available at: https://www.aagbi.org/news/aagbi-board-has-endorsed-esa-guidance-perioperative-fasting-adults-and-children

Freedman R, Herbert L, O'Donnell A, et al. (eds) (2022). Oxford handbook of anaesthesia (5th ed). Oxford: Oxford University Press.

Martin A, Allman K, McIndoe A (eds) (2020). Emergencies in anaesthesia (3rd ed). Oxford: Oxford University Press.

Royal College of Anaesthetists (2017). Guidelines for the provision of anaesthetic services. London: Royal College of Anaesthetists.

Royal College of Nursing (2005). Perioperative fasting in adults and children: an RCN guideline for the multidisciplinary team. London: Royal College of Nursing.

Sellick BA (1961). Cricoid pressure to control regurgitation of stomach contents during induction of anaesthesia. Lancet, 2(7199):404–406.

# Failed intubation/failed ventilation

The seriousness of the failed intubation cannot be overemphasized but deaths occur when there is a failure to oxygenate a patient as a result of a failure to ventilate. Simple bag-and-mask hand ventilation will keep patients alive when difficulties with intubation are experienced.

Unanticipated airway difficulties can be categorized as follows:
• Difficult or failed intubation.
• Difficult or failed ventilation.
• Both of these.

## Management

The management of airway difficulties can be divided up into four stages.
• *Initial intubation attempt*: when the initial intubation attempt fails then it is important to optimize anaesthesia, the patient position, and the equipment being used. Then to employ external manipulation of the larynx with the help of the assistant and to use a bougie.
• *Secondary intubation attempt*: if the patient can be adequately ventilated by hand, then an LMA or i-gel® could be inserted and these could buy some time; but if intubation is required, then either another attempt is made with more equipment or more experienced staff, or an ILMA could be inserted and an ETT passed through it. The use of video- or fibreoptic-guided devices is recommended to assist intubation.
• *If initial and secondary intubation attempts fail*: ventilation must be maintained with either a bag-and-mask technique or an LMA/PLMA. Consultation with the surgical team must then decide whether to proceed with surgery or to postpone it and wake the patient.
• *The 'can't intubate/can't oxygenate' scenario*: if this scenario occurs then the only option remaining is the use of an invasive tracheal cricothyroidotomy to establish a route through which the patient's lungs may be oxygenated.

## The role of the anaesthetic practitioner

• Keep calm and stay and assist the anaesthetist.
• Request the help of another senior anaesthetist.
• Assist with two-person bag-and-mask hand ventilation.
• Check the patient's position and after discussion reposition the pillow if needed.
• Ensure that all patient monitoring continues to give accurate recordings.
• Request that the difficult intubation equipment be brought into the anaesthetic room immediately.
• This should contain ILMAs, PLMAs in a full range of sizes; a short-handled laryngoscope; McCoy laryngoscope blades (sizes 3 and 4); a range of bougies including extra-long and hollow bougies through which the patient can be ventilated; stylets and guide wires over which an ETT may be passed; ETTs, standard and reinforced in a range of sizes from 5 mm up; emergency cricothyroidotomy kit; and jet ventilation device. A fibreoptic bronchoscope needs to be brought as soon as possible.
• Video laryngoscopes such as C-MAC®, Airtraq®, and Glidescope® may be available in some areas and may be useful in difficult intubation situations or anticipated difficult intubation situations.

## Responsibilities of the anaesthetic practitioner

The anaesthetic practitioner must:
• Be able to locate the operating department's difficult intubation equipment, to fit it together, and understand how it works
• Regularly check, if available, the jet ventilation equipment and be able to connect it to the anaesthetic machine and make sure that there are no missing parts
• Be familiar with the latest guidelines for the management of failed intubation and ventilation. Display them prominently in the clinical areas
• Use date expired equipment for the training of new staff
• Share experiences and reflections with colleagues learning from the available expertise.

## Rescue techniques for the 'can't intubate, can't oxygenate' situation

The Difficult Airway Society (DAS) develops and provides national guidelines for the management of the difficult airway.[1] The DAS 'Management of unanticipated difficult tracheal intubation in adults' guidelines are illustrated in Fig. 10.2.

'Can't intubate, can't oxygenate' is a life-threatening emergency, one which all anaesthetic practitioners must consider and understand. Thankfully, >90% of cases can be resolved with two-person hand ventilation or with the insertion of an LMA, i-gel®, or ILMA. But on the rare occasions when these measures fail, an invasive cricothyroidotomy is a life-saving measure. When the decision is made to undertake a cricothyroidotomy then speed will be essential to prevent brain damage from hypoxia and the anaesthetic practitioner will need to remain calm.

## Reference

1. Difficult Airway Society (2015). Management of unanticipated difficult tracheal intubation in adults. Available at: ℜ https://www.das.uk.com/files/das2015intubation_guidelines.pdf

## Further reading

Freedman R, Herbert L, O'Donnell A, et al. (eds) (2022). Oxford handbook of anaesthesia (5th ed). Oxford: Oxford University Press.

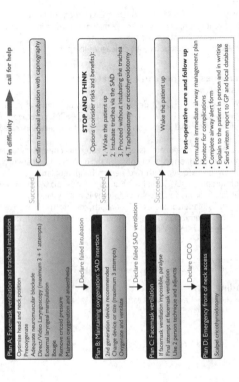

**Fig. 10.2** Management of unanticipated difficult tracheal intubation in adults.

This flowchart forms part of the DAS Guidelines for unanticipated difficult intubation in adults 2015 and should be used in conjuction with the text.

# Complications
# of anaesthesia

# Acid aspiration syndrome

Aspiration is the act of foreign materials inhaled into the lungs which was first described by Mendelson in 1946.[1] Predisposing factors for acid aspiration syndrome include emergency anaesthesia, inadequate anaesthesia, abdominal pathology, and bariatric patients (Table 11.1).[2] Aspiration of solid matter can cause hypoxia, whereas aspiration of acidic gastric fluid can cause a pneumonitis. The risk of mortality and serious morbidity increases with bronchial exposure to greater volumes and acidity of aspirated material.[3,4]

**Table 11.1** Predisposing factors for aspiration under general anaesthesia

| Patient factors | Increased gastric content | Intestinal obstruction |
| --- | --- | --- |
| | | Non-fasted |
| | | Drugs |
| | | Delayed gastric emptying |
| | Lower oesophageal sphincter incompetence | Hiatus hernia |
| | | Gastro-oesophageal reflux |
| | | Pregnancy |
| | | Morbid obesity |
| | | Neuromuscular disease |
| | Decreased laryngeal reflexes | Head injury |
| | | Bulbar palsy |
| | Sex | Male |
| | Age | Older adults |
| Operation factors | Procedure | Emergency |
| | | Laparoscopic |
| | Position | Lithotomy/head-down position |
| Anaesthetic factors | Airway | Gas insufflation |
| | | Difficult intubation |
| | | Topically anaesthetized airway |
| | Maintenance | Inadequate depth |

- When consciousness is lost, the patient with stomach contents may regurgitate gastric material via the oesophagus; this may be aspirated into the lungs causing a severe pneumonitis (inflammation of the lungs) usually called 'aspiration pneumonitis'.
- This is especially severe, and often fatal, if the gastric contents are acidic (pH <2.5).
- As little as 30 mL will cause a severe reaction.

- When solid foods are aspirated, complete obstruction of the airway may occur.
- Normally the specialized junction between the oesophagus and the stomach the oesophagogastric junction acts as a sphincter to prevent material returning to the oesophagus after entering the stomach.
- When the conscious level is depressed, this junction works less efficiently; if the intragastric pressure within the stomach is greater than the closing pressure of the sphincter then regurgitation will occur.
- Regurgitation, which is the flow of stomach content back into the mouth, is the main course of acid aspiration syndrome during anaesthesia.
- Regurgitation is different from vomiting as regurgitation is a passive act and requires no muscle tone and occurs because of reduced or altered levels of consciousness.
- Vomiting is active and requires muscle tone and, therefore, normal or near normal levels of consciousness.
- The aspiration of gastric acid into the lungs followed by bronchospasm, pulmonary oedema, and hypoxia is also referred to as Mendelson's syndrome.
- Aspiration of gastric acid into the lungs then alters the pathology in the lungs, consisting of chemical tracheobronchitis and pneumonia.
- Aspiration of foreign substances into the lungs can also predispose to bacterial pneumonia.
- Acid aspiration is just as likely to happen at induction as extubation and the outcomes can vary from benign consequences to acute respiratory failure leading to death.

Aspiration remains the most significant cause of airway-related mortality. The incidence of aspiration under anaesthesia remains significantly greater with higher ASA status and emergency surgery.[3]

## Prevention

### Fasting
Current guidelines are 2 hours for clear fluids, 4 hours for breast milk, and 6 hours for a light meal, sweets, milk (including formula), and non-clear fluids.[5]

### Reduction of gastric acidity
For obstetric anaesthesia patients, 30 mL of 0.3 molar sodium citrate is normally given prophylactically. Elective patients thought to be at risk of aspiration are routinely prescribed metoclopramide and ranitidine prior to their anaesthetic.

### Rapid sequence induction
For these patient groups, a RSI is part of the routine anaesthesia.

### Cricoid pressure
Compression of the oesophagus between the cricoid ring of cartilage and the sixth cervical vertebral body preventing reflux of gastric contents.

*NG tubes*
Reduces the volume of stomach content. There is no evidence to suggest that NG tubes affect cricoid pressure.[1]

## Early signs and symptoms

Cyanosis.
Tachycardia.
Hypotension.
Massive pulmonary oedema.
Bronchospasm.
Coughing.

## Immediate patient management

- Call for help.
- Head-down tilt:
  - Tilt the patient's head to the side; this enables any foreign material in the mouth to drain away from the patient.
- Oropharyngeal suction.
- 100% $O_2$.
- Apply cricoid pressure and ventilate.
- Deepen anaesthesia/perform RSI.
- Intubate trachea.
- Release cricoid once airway secured.
- Tracheal suction.
- Consider bronchoscopy.
- Bronchodilators if necessary.
- Bronchial aspiration and lavage.

## Later signs and symptoms

- Reduced arterial oxygenation.
- Increased pulmonary artery pressure.
- Reduced compliance of the lungs.
- Chest X-ray can show pulmonary oedema though this will not necessarily diagnose the extent of the pulmonary damage accurately.
- Cardiac failure.

## Therapeutic management

- Corticosteroids.
- Ventilation.
- Fluid management.
- Bronchodilators, diuretics.
- Physiotherapy.
- Treatment for complications as they arise.
- Prophylactic antibiotics are not usually given routinely (unless infected material aspirated) but they may be required for subsequent secondary infections.[2]

## References

1. Mendelson CL (1946). The aspiration of stomach contents into the lungs during obstetric anaesthesia. American Journal of Obstetrics & Gynaecology, 52:191.
2. King W (2010). Pulmonary aspiration of gastric content. Available at: 🔗 http://www.frca.co.uk/Documents/192%20Pulmonary%20aspiration%20of%20gastric%20contents.pdf
3. Robinson M, Davidson A (2014). Aspiration under anaesthesia: risk assessment and decision-making. Continuing Education in Anaesthesia Critical Care & Pain, 14(4):171–175.
4. Kane A, Armstrong R, Nolan JP, et al. (2022). Anaesthetic emergencies. In: Freedman R, Herbert L, O'Donnell A, et al. (eds) Oxford handbook of anaesthesia (5th ed). Oxford: Oxford University Press.
5. Smith I, Kranke P, Murat I, et al. (2011). Perioperative fasting in adults and children: guidelines from the European Society of Anaesthesiology. European Journal of Anaesthesiology, 28(8):556–569.

## Further reading

Crerar-Gilbert AA, MacGregor M (eds) (2018). Core topics in preoperative anaesthetic assessment and management. Cambridge: Cambridge University Press.
NAP4 (2011). Major complications of airway management in the UK. Available at: 🔗 https://www.nationalauditprojects.org.uk/NAP4_home
Pollard B, Kitchen G (eds) (2017). Handbook of clinical anaesthesia (4th ed). London: CRC Press.
Robinson M, Davidson A (2014). Aspiration under anaesthesia: risk assessment and decision-making. Continuing Education in Anaesthesia Critical Care & Pain, 14(4):171–175.
Royal College of Anaesthetists (2020). Chapter 5: guidelines for the provision of emergency anaesthesia. London: Royal College of Anaesthetists.
Vanner R (2004). Preventing regurgitation and aspiration. Journal of Anaesthesia and Intensive Care Medicine, 5(9):293–297.

# High spinal

High/total spinal is defined as a LA depression of the cervical spinal cord and the brainstem.[1] High/total spinal may follow excessive spread of an intrathecal injection of LA, or inadvertent spinal injection of an epidural dose of LA. It may also occur as a complication of some regional anaesthetic blocks (e.g. interscalene blocks on the shoulder or retrobulbar blocks on the eye). It occurs because the needle accidentally enters a sheath surrounding the nerve which allows LA to pass back along the nerve into the CSF. Risk factors are shown in Table 11.2.[2]

**Table 11.2** Factors to consider in order to minimize the risk of high or complete spinal block

| | |
|---|---|
| Drug factors | Block height more dependent on dose than volume (higher dose gives higher risk) |
| | Baricity—cephalad spread easier to control with hyperbaric solution |
| | Prior drug administration—such as epidural LA diffusion (unrecognized/subclinical block gives higher risk) |
| Patient factors | Body morphology—higher BMI or abdominal girth (including pregnancy) may reduce thecal volume and increase the risk of high block |
| | Anatomical or pathological factors—compressed thecal sack (epidural fluid and dilated vessels), spinal canal abnormality can give higher risk |
| Anaesthetic factors | Higher lumbar insertion may increase final block height |
| | Position at and following injection—sitting may minimize cephalad spread |
| | Spinal needle—finer gauge and cephalad direction of needle hole may increase risk of higher block |

## Influencing factors

- High/total spinal occurs when an epidural solution (of LA) is inadvertently given into the CSF while attempting epidural anaesthesia or the spinal anaesthetic does not fix at thoracic vertebra 10 (T10) (nipple level).
- Positioning of the patient is an important factor with all spinal and epidural anaesthetics. If a patient is placed in a head-down position (Trendelenburg position) after the spinal or epidural is performed, especially when using hyperbaric solutions, this could also reproduce the same complication resulting in a high spinal block.
- It is also important to remember that positioning can still affect the block to extend some 20 minutes after the spinal or epidural has been performed.[3]
- The dose, volume, and baricity of the LA can also have an effect on the level of the spinal anaesthesia.

- The technique can be another influencing factor (e.g. type of needle, site of injection, direction of needle, velocity of injection).
- Most spinal and epidural anaesthetics aim to give a maximum upper level block in the region of T10. Anything above this level can produce symptoms that are at least unpleasant and at worst can result in cardiac arrest.

## Early signs and symptoms
- Early warning signs would be numbness and tingling in the little fingers and weakness in the hands and arms. This is an indication that the block has reached the cervicothoracic junction.
- Agitation.
- Difficulty breathing, dyspnoea. The patient will start to complain that they cannot take deep breaths.
- Husky voice. As the phrenic nerves become involved, the patient will start to speak quieter until this eventually becomes a whisper.

## Late signs and symptoms
- If the spinal/epidural solution dissipates as high as the cranial subarachnoid space, 'not only are respiratory muscles paralysed, but also the patient loses use of the cranial nerves',[3] therefore this can progress to:
  - Hypotension
  - Bradycardia
  - Unconsciousness.
- If the solution raises still further, then this might enter the fourth ventricle, paralysing the respiratory and vasomotor centres resulting in cardiorespiratory arrest.[4]

When experiencing the onset of a high spinal, patients very often display increased anxiety. It is absolutely imperative that a member of the perioperative team provides psychological support to the patient at this point. Call for help as extra pairs of hands could be useful.

## Treatment
- Ventilation and protection against aspiration.
- Maintaining the BP, both by physical elevation of the legs and administration of IV fluids.
- Use of vasopressor drugs.
- For obstetric patients, left uterine displacement is also advised to improve circulation due to caval compression and to preserve uteroplacental perfusion.[5]
- It must also be remembered that this condition is self-limiting in the respect that the symptoms will dissipate with the potency of the LA.

## References
1. Dijkema LM, Haisma HJ (2002). Case report—total spinal anaesthesia. Update in Anaesthesia, 14:14. Available at: ℘ www.nda.ox.ac.uk/wfsa/html/u14/u1414_01.htm#tpf
2. Newman B (2010). Complete spinal block following spinal anaesthesia. Available at: ℘ https://www.aagbi.org/sites/default/files/180-Complete-spinal-block-after-spinal-anaesthesia.pdf
3. Ankorn C, Casey WF (2000). Spinal anaesthesia: a practical guide. Update in Anaesthesia, 12:8. Available at: ℘ http://e-safe-anaesthesia.org/e_library/07/Spinal_anaesthesia_a_practical_guide_Update_2000.pdf
4. Simpson PJ, Popat MT (2002). Understanding anaesthesia (4th ed). Oxford: Butterworth-Heinemann.
5. Braveman FR (2006). Obstetric and gynaecological anaesthesia. Philadelphia, PA: Mosby.

## Further reading

Al-Shaikh B, Stacey S (2018). Essentials of equipment in anaesthesia, critical care and perioperative medicine (5th ed). Edinburgh: Elsevier.

Aston D, Rivers A, Dharmadasa A (2014). Equipment in anaesthesia and critical care: a complete guide for the FRCA. Banbury: Scion.

Davey A, Ince CS (2009). Fundamentals of operating department practice. Cambridge: Cambridge University Press.

Freedman R, Herbert L, O'Donnell A, et al. (eds) (2022). Oxford handbook of anaesthesia (5th ed). Oxford: Oxford University Press.

Hocking G, Wildsmith JA. (2004). Intrathecal drug spread. British Journal of Anaesthesia, 93(4):568–578.

Martin A, Allman K, McIndoe A (eds) (2020). Emergencies in anaesthesia (3rd ed). Oxford: Oxford University Press.

Middleton B, Stacey S, Thomas R, et al. (2012). Physics in anaesthesia: for FRCA candidates, ODPs and nurse anaesthetists. Banbury: Scion.

Thompson J, Moppett I, Wiles M (eds) (2019). Smith and Aitkenhead's textbook of anaesthesia (7th ed). Edinburgh: Elsevier.

Yentis S, May A, Malhotra S (2007). Analgesia, anaesthesia and pregnancy: a practical guide. Cambridge: Cambridge University Press.

# Anaphylaxis

- Anaphylaxis is a local or systemic hypersensitivity response to a foreign substance (allergen).[1]
- The localized response causes skin rashes (*urticaria*) and itching (*pruritus*), whereas the more generalized, systemic reaction can also cause wheezing *(bronchospasm)*, swelling of the patient's face and upper airway *(angioedema)*, tachycardia, and severe hypotension. Nausea and diarrhoea may also be present.
- Anaphylactic reactions commonly follow previous sensitization to the allergen and subsequent exposure causes release of histamine from mast cells and basophils *(immunoglobulin E-mediated response)*, leading to bronchospasm, vasodilation, and increased capillary permeability that can redistribute the patient's circulating volume to their tissues (*anaphylactic shock*).
- Anaphylactoid reactions are clinically identical, but do not require previous sensitization.
- These responses may take from between a few minutes to an hour or more to present from the time of contact, and symptoms may recur up to 24 hours after the initial response.

## Common allergens found in the operating department

- Latex.
- Antibiotics.
- Muscle relaxants.
- Anaesthetic induction agents.
- Egg lecithin found in propofol.
- Colloid IV infusions.
- Blood products.

## Management

- Treatment should follow the ABCDE approach as advocated by the Resuscitation Council (UK).[2]
- When possible, contact with the suspected allergen (e.g. blood transfusion) should be terminated immediately.
- Where there is airway involvement, it is imperative that this is managed promptly as complete airway obstruction may develop.
- IM injection is the first-line drug of choice.[2]
- Several doses of adrenaline may be required to relieve the patient's symptoms, and these should be administered at 3–5-minute intervals as necessary.
- Additional salbutamol (nebulized or IV) may be required to combat bronchospasm.
- An antihistamine (e.g. chlorphenamine) should also be given, along with an anti-inflammatory (e.g. hydrocortisone), and IV infusion of crystalloid solution commenced to support the victim's circulation.
- Following severe reactions, observation of the victim should be continued for 24 hours to exclude recurrence.

- Blood is usually taken at specified intervals following anaphylaxis to test for serum tryptase and mast cell histamine.
- Patch tests should be conducted at an allergy clinic to identify the offending allergen and the victim encouraged to wear an appropriate medic-alert bracelet.

## References

1. NICE (2020) Anaphylaxis: assessment and referral after emergency treatment. Available at: https://www.nice.org.uk/guidance/cg134
2. Resuscitation Council UK (2021) Emergency treatment of anaphylactic reactions: Guidelines for healthcare providers. Available at: https://www.resus.org.uk/sites/default/files/2021-04/Anaphylaxis%20Summary%20Document.pdf

## Further reading

National Institute for Health and Care Excellence (2011). Anaphylaxis: assessment and referral after emergency treatment: Clinical guideline [CG134]. Available at: ℘ https://www.nice.org.uk/Guidance/CG134

National Institute for Health and Care Excellence (2020). National Early Warning Score systems that alert to deteriorating adult patients in hospital. Medtech innovation briefing [MIB205]. Available at: ℘ https://www.nice.org.uk/guidance/mib205

Royal College of Anaesthetists (2020). Chapter 5: guidelines for the provision of emergency anaesthesia. London: Royal College of Anaesthetists.

# Laryngospasm

## Definition

Laryngospasm is a temporary spastic paralysis of the vocal cords that causes the complete or partial closure of the laryngeal opening (glottis), thereby preventing the passage of air into or out of the lungs. If not recognized and treated promptly, this condition can lead to hypoxia and, potentially, respiratory and cardiac arrest.

## Causes

- Although laryngospasm can be associated with gastro-oesophageal reflux in some conscious patients, in perioperative practice it is most commonly associated with patients at certain stages of anaesthesia; it is especially common in children.
- Laryngospasm is caused by inadvertent stimuli of the vocal cords (true and false) causing these to go into spasm as a protective reflex against aspiration.
- Stimuli can include the patient's own blood or secretions coming into contact with the cords or can be induced by staff using poor technique when undertaking pharyngeal suction or insertion of airway adjuncts (typically *oropharyngeal or laryngeal mask airways*).
- Patients are particularly at risk of laryngospasm during induction (especially inhalational) and emergence from anaesthesia. At these times, patients are insufficiently 'deep' for them to have lost their other protective airway reflexes (coughing, gagging, swallowing), but too 'light' for them to have conscious control over their airways.
- Patients who have been extubated at deep levels of anaesthesia, for example, following tonsillectomy or maxillo-facial procedures, and those with irritable airways, such as smokers and recent ex-smokers, are at higher risk of laryngospasm.[1]

## Recognition

- Laryngospasm is traditionally accompanied by an inspiratory stridor, described as a 'harsh, crowing noise'.[2]
- The patient will be making obvious respiratory effort, often including the use of accessory muscles (notably the strap muscles of the neck), and paradoxical (see-saw) respirations may be evident.
- Respirations will be ineffective, that is, little or no air will be breathed in or out, and the patient's $SaO_2$ will drop as they become hypoxaemic.

## Treatments

- Call for *help*.
- Use *pharyngeal suction* carefully to remove excess secretions.
- Administer *high-flow oxygen*.
- Apply the '*jaw-thrust*' manoeuvre—place the base of your thumbs on the patient's cheeks and use your middle fingers to lift the angles of the patient's jaw. NB: this technique is very effective in opening the patient's upper airway, but can cause some discomfort which, although it might encourage the patient to fully emerge from their anaesthetic, should not be used once they have regained consciousness.

- Application of *continuous positive airway pressure* (CPAP), using a Waters' circuit (Mapleson C) with the pressure relief valve closed.
- If the laryngospasm is not relieved by these interventions, the anaesthetist may decide to administer small doses of *propofol* or *suxamethonium*. This is a difficult decision to make as laryngospasm might recur as the effect of these drugs wears off.

## References

1. Gavel G, Walker R (2014). Laryngospasm in anaesthesia. Continuing Education in Anaesthesia, Critical Care & Pain, 14(2):47–51.
2. Craig A, Hatfield A (2020). The complete recovery room book (6th ed). Oxford: Oxford University Press.

## Further reading

Freedman R, Herbert L, O'Donnell A, et al. (eds) (2022). Oxford handbook of anaesthesia (5th ed). Oxford: Oxford University Press.

Martin A, Allman K, McIndoe A (eds) (2020). Emergencies in anaesthesia (3rd ed). Oxford: Oxford University Press.

Royal College of Anaesthetists (2019–2021). Guidelines for the provision of anaesthetic services. London: Royal College of Anaesthetists.

# Respiratory arrest

*Respiratory arrest*, the cessation of spontaneous respiratory effort, is a common temporary side effect of GA but may also be seen as a result of critical illness, drug overdose, or trauma. Respiratory arrest leads to a generalized *hypoxia* and *hypercarbia* ($CO_2$ retention) and causes an increase in anaerobic metabolism, contributing to a mixed metabolic and respiratory *acidosis*. Respiratory arrest may be preceded by a period of *respiratory failure* ('Acute impairment in gas exchange between the lungs and the blood causing hypoxia with or without hypercapnia'[1]). If not recognized and managed appropriately, respiratory arrest will almost invariably lead to *cardiac arrest*.

> *Normal respiration* requires stimulation of the diaphragm and intercostal muscles (via the phrenic and intercostal nerves) to inspire air through the upper and lower airways into the alveoli (alveolar ventilation), where gases ($O_2$ and $CO_2$) are exchanged across the alveolar walls to and from the circulation by way of the capillary network of the *pulmonary circulation*. Expiration is normally passive, utilizing the elastic recoil of the thoracic cage, thereby allowing the release of excess $CO_2$ to the atmosphere. The respiratory centre, located in the medulla oblongata, governs the rate and depth of respiration in response to the levels of $CO_2$ detected in blood. Rarely, the body will compensate for chronically high levels of $CO_2$ by responding instead to abnormal levels of $O_2$ (*hypoxic drive*). Effective elimination of $CO_2$ through respiration is integral to the homeostatic mechanism of *acid–base balance*.

## Treatment

Treatment should be both supportive and definitive, and follow the ABCDE principles to *treat first that which kills first*:

### A (airway)

Assess that the patient's airway is patent and free of foreign bodies and excessive secretions; *ensure* that the patient's airway remains open and clear using suction and *airway manoeuvres* (➔ see chapter 10) and adjuncts, including ETTs or surgical airways, as required.

### B (breathing)

Assess the patient's breathing:

- Is it:
  - Normal (regular, symmetrical, suitable depth)?
  - Noisy (wheezy, snoring or crowing)?
  - Absent?
- Noise on inspiration normally indicates partial upper airway obstruction (e.g. presence of foreign body, loss of protective airway reflexes, spasm of vocal cords (laryngospasm) etc.).
- Noise on expiration indicates partial lower airway obstruction (e.g. bronchospasm).
- Silence indicates either complete airway obstruction or respiratory arrest.

- Observe:
  - Rate
  - Rhythm
  - Depth
  - Symmetry (i.e. bilateral air entry).
- Ensure the following:
  - The patient's respiration is sufficient to prevent hypoxia and hypercarbia; *assisted ventilation* with high-flow $O_2$ using either a mechanical ventilator or a self-inflating resuscitator bag, or equivalent, may be required to achieve this. NB: $O_2$ therapy is mandatory in *all* cases of respiratory insufficiency.
  - If *tension pneumothorax* is suspected, needle decompression (➔ see p. 802) must be performed *immediately*.
  - In *bronchospasm*, nebulized bronchodilators (e.g. salbutamol) and IV magnesium and anticholinergics (e.g. ipratropium) may be required,
  - In *laryngospasm*, positive end-expiratory pressure ventilation (PEEP) and small doses of suxamethonium may be required to facilitate adequate ventilation (➔ see p. 308).
  - Continuous pulse oximetry and $ETCO_2$ monitoring (in the anaesthetized patient), along with repeated blood gas analysis (in the critically ill patient) should be employed to monitor the effectiveness of ventilation.

## C (circulation)

- *Assess* the patient's circulation by monitoring:
  - Pulse
  - Capillary refill
  - BP
  - ECG
  - Urine output
  - Invasive techniques may also be employed in high-dependency areas.
- *Ensure* adequacy of the patient's circulation by:
  - Securing IV access (intraosseous access may be required in emergency cases)
  - Administering boluses of crystalloid fluid as required (NB: beware of fluid overload, especially in the young and old, and those with pre-existing heart conditions); in high dependency areas, *inotropes* may be utilized to support the cardiovascular system.

## D (disability)

- *Assess* the patient's level of consciousness; confusion, aggression or coma may all be signs of cerebral hypoxia.

## E (exposure)

- *Assess* and *identify the underlying cause* using the patient's clinical notes and previous history.
- *Initiate* appropriate treatment, such as surgical intervention, drug antagonists (naloxone (opioids), flumazenil (benzodiazepines), neostigmine/glycopyrrolate (muscle relaxants)), and antibiotics.

## Reference

1. Stratton SJ (2018). Acute respiratory failure. Available at: ℘ http://bestpractice.bmj.com/topics/en-gb/853

## Further reading

Davies NJH, Cashman D (2005). Lee's synopsis of anaesthesia (12th ed). Oxford: Butterworth Heinemann.

Freedman R, Herbert L, O'Donnell A, et al. (eds) (2022). Oxford handbook of anaesthesia (5th ed). Oxford: Oxford University Press.

Martin A, Allman K, McIndoe A (eds) (2020). Emergencies in anaesthesia (3rd ed). Oxford: Oxford University Press.

Resuscitation Council (UK). 2016. Advanced life support providers manual. London: Resuscitation Council (UK).

Royal College of Anaesthetists (2019–2021). Guidelines for the provision of anaesthetic services. London: Royal College of Anaesthetists.

# Causes of respiratory arrest

Causes of respiratory failure and arrest may be classified as follows:

## Respiratory drive dysfunction

Caused by, for example:
- Drugs (e.g. anaesthetic agents, alcohol, opioids, sedatives, tranquillizers, etc.)
- Trauma to brain, spinal cord, etc.
- Breath holding (especially in neonates) and obstructive sleep apnoea.

## Impaired function of the chest and lungs

Caused by, for example:
- Obstruction (e.g. by tongue, foreign bodies, tumours, excessive secretions, etc.)
- Trauma—to airway (e.g. burns, blunt trauma), or thoracic cage (flail chest etc.) or soft tissues (pneumothorax, tension pneumothorax, haemothorax, etc.)
- Pulmonary oedema (e.g. due to gastric aspiration, fluid overload, cardiac or liver failure)
- Bronchospasm, laryngospasm
- Infections and other disease processes (e.g. pneumonia, COPD)
- Skeletal abnormality (e.g. scoliosis)
- Muscle weakness—brought on by disease (e.g. myasthenia gravis) or fatigue (especially in acute episodes of asthma and COPD) or drugs (muscle relaxants)
- Gastric/abdominal distension and diaphragmatic splinting
- Pain following trauma, surgery.

## Failure of circulatory gas transport mechanisms

For example:
- Hypovolaemia
- Circulatory failure
- Anaemia
- Poisoning (e.g. carbon monoxide, cyanide).
(NB: this is *not* a definitive list.)

## Further reading

Martin A, Allman K, McIndoe A (eds) (2020). Emergencies in anaesthesia (3rd ed). Oxford: Oxford University Press.

Royal College of Anaesthetists (2020). Chapter 5: guidelines for the provision of emergency anaesthesia. London: Royal College of Anaesthetists.

Stratton SJ (2018). Acute respiratory failure. Available at: ℘ http://bestpractice.bmj.com/topics/en-gb/853

# Malignant hyperpyrexia

## Incidence

- Malignant hyperpyrexia/hyperthermia (MH) is a hereditary condition that results in contracture of the muscle and creates a disruption to metabolic functions during GA.
- It is a rare syndrome that occurs in genetically predisposed patients who are exposed to MH-triggering agents used during GA.
- It results in a series of biochemical changes triggered by volatile anaesthetic inhalation agents and suxamethonium, which alters the calcium ion movement within the sarcoplasmic reticulum of muscle cells during muscle contraction.
- This condition affects 1:100,000 of the population with MH episodes reported to be 1:12,000 paediatric and 1:40,000 adult anaesthetic procedures.[1]

## Recognition

Consider MH if:
- Unexplained, unexpected increase in end tidal $CO_2$ *and*
- Unexplained, unexpected tachycardia *and*
- Unexplained, unexpected increase in $O_2$ consumption
- Rapidly rising body core temperature—rises by 0.6°C (1.0°F) per minute.

## Patient management

*Immediate management*
- *Stop* all trigger agents and maintain anaesthesia.
- *Call for help* and note the time.
- Maintain the airway and administer $O_2$ 100%. Intubate trachea if necessary and ventilate lungs.
- Install clean breathing system and *hyperventilate* with *100% $O_2$ high flow*.
- Maintain anaesthesia with IV agents.
- Abandon surgery if feasible.

*Monitoring and treatment*
- Administer *dantrolene*.
- Initiate active body *cooling* but avoid vasoconstriction.

*Dantrolene*
Give 2.5 mg/kg IV bolus. Repeat 1 mg/kg boluses as required to a maximum of 10 mg/kg.
- *For a 70 kg adult*—initial bolus: nine vials dantrolene 20 mg (each vial mixed with 60 mL sterile water). Further boluses of four vials dantrolene 20 mg repeated up to seven times.

---

**Active body cooling**

Remove warming methods

Apply cooling methods according to need (cold IV fluids, ice to axilla and groins, cold peritoneal lavage)

---

*Continuous monitoring*
Core and peripheral temperature:
- $ETCO_2$.
- $SpO_2$.
- ECG.
- Invasive BP.
- CVP.

*Repeated bloods*
- ABG.
- U&Es (potassium).
- FBC (haematocrit/platelets).
- Coagulation.

*Treat*
- *Acidosis*
*Hyperkalaemia*: calcium chloride, glucose/insulin, $NaHCO_3$.
- *Arrhythmias*: magnesium/amiodarone/metoprolol. *Avoid* calcium channel blockers—interaction with dantrolene.
- *Metabolic acidosis*: hyperventilate, $NaHCO_3$.
- *Myoglobinaemia*: forced alkaline diuresis (may require renal replacement therapy later).
- *DIC*: fresh frozen plasma (FFP), cryoprecipitate, platelets.

## Compartment syndrome

*Later management*
- Continue monitoring on ICU, repeat dantrolene as necessary.
- Monitor for acute kidney injury and compartment syndrome.
- Repeat creatine kinase.
- Consider alternative diagnosis (sepsis, phaeochromocytoma, thyroid storm, myopathy).
- Counsel patient and family members.
- Refer to MH unit.

## Further reading

Association of Anaesthetists of Great Britain and Ireland (2020). Malignant hyperthermia 2020. Available at: https://anaesthetists.org/Home/Resources-publications/Guidelines/Malignant-hyperthermia-2020

Freedman R, Herbert L, O'Donnell A, et al. (eds) (2022). Oxford handbook of anaesthesia (5th ed). Oxford: Oxford University Press.

Martin A, Allman K, McIndoe A (eds) (2020). Emergencies in anaesthesia (3rd ed). Oxford: Oxford University Press.

Royal College of Anaesthetists (2020). Chapter 5: guidelines for the provision of emergency anaesthesia. London: Royal College of Anaesthetists.

# Suxamethonium apnoea

### Incidence

Suxamethonium apnoea is a rare condition that occurs due to an inability to break down the drug suxamethonium. As a result of this, the muscle relaxant effects of the drug last far longer than usual (several hours rather than a few minutes). The enzyme responsible for breaking down suxamethonium is plasma cholinesterase.

This condition can be inherited or appear spontaneously in a person with no family history. In cases where suxamethonium apnoea is inherited, the level of plasma cholinesterase is reduced whereas in the acquired condition the level of plasma cholinesterase is normal but its activity is reduced.

*Suxamethonium*
- Suxamethonium is a depolarizing, fast-acting muscle relaxant and its main use in anaesthesia is to allow the rapid intubation of the trachea.
- Suxamethonium depolarizes skeletal muscle and lasts for approximately 2–6 minutes imitating acetylcholine at the neuromuscular junction where it binds to the postsynaptic membrane.
- As it binds non-competitively at the junction, it cannot be reversed by other drugs.

*Inherited suxamethonium apnoea*
- It is important to identify the possibility of atypical pseudocholinesterase (suxamethonium apnoea) as a genetically inherited condition so a comprehensive family history should be sought.
- Preoperative screening for cholinesterase activity is advised if the patient or a close relative has experienced prolonged paralysis after surgery that required ventilatory support for a significant length of time.
- The action of suxamethonium in inherited incidences can be increased from a few minutes to 2 hours or more.

*Acquired suxamethonium apnoea*
- Plasma cholinesterase is normal in patients with acquired incidence but has reduced activity.
- Acquired incidences in situations such as pregnancy, liver and renal disease, or if the patient may be taking medicines such as methotrexate, the action of suxamethonium can be increased by minutes as opposed to hours.

### Diagnosis

Once suxamethonium has been administered, further muscle relaxants should be avoided until muscle tone returns or if there is a delay in breathing. Look for signs of awareness in an unexpectedly muscle-relaxed patient. Diagnosis can be confirmed by the use of a nerve stimulator to determine the level of neuromuscular transmission.

### Patient management

If diagnosis is confirmed:
- Maintain anaesthesia.
- Maintain ventilation.

- Monitor neuromuscular transmission with nerve stimulator—if nerve stimulator is unavailable, maintain anaesthesia and ventilation and breathing becomes spontaneous.
- Transfer to ICU until metabolism is complete and the patient breathes spontaneously.
- Extubate awake—when the patient is able to obey commands.
- Conduct family studies to determine exposure.

## Further reading

Freedman R, Herbert L, O'Donnell A, et al. (eds) (2022). Oxford handbook of anaesthesia (5th ed). Oxford: Oxford University Press.

Martin A, Allman K, McIndoe A (eds) (2020). Emergencies in anaesthesia (3rd ed). Oxford: Oxford University Press.

Royal College of Anaesthetists (2020). Chapter 5: guidelines for the provision of emergency anaesthesia. London: Royal College of Anaesthetists.

Royal College of Anaesthetists (2018) Suxamethonium Apnoea (SA) Factsheet. Available at: ℘ https://www.rcoa.ac.uk/sites/default/files/documents/2019-11/Factsheet-Suxapnoeaweb.pdf

# Monitoring depth of anaesthesia, including preventing awareness

The prime purpose of GA is twofold:
1. To prevent awareness of unpleasant stimuli.
2. To prevent the body reacting in an unconscious way to noxious stimuli.

These aims, along with muscle relaxation, make up the classic 'triad of anaesthesia'.

The unconscious response of the body's defence systems, in the form of increased sympathetic nervous system activity, can be assessed from such observations as pulse, BP, respiratory rate, sweating, and lachrymation. However, suppression of awareness (and the possibility of subsequent recall) is more difficult to measure.

Until recent times, anaesthetists have relied on their experience and knowledge of drug actions, pharmacodynamics, and pharmacokinetics to deploy an appropriate mix of drugs ('balanced anaesthesia') to address the needs outlined above. However, being able to adjust this balance in response to specific data would be beneficial—in simplistic terms, targeting the use of hypnotic drugs to prevent awareness, and of analgesics and other drugs to limit sympathetic activity.

In recent years, a number of processed electroencephalography (pEEG) monitoring devices have been developed, which measure suppression of cerebral cortex activity (and correlate with cerebral metabolic rate). Examples are BIS, E-Entropy, and Narcotrend-Compact. The aim is to avoid too little anaesthesia (risking awareness) or too much (with consequences discussed below).

## Accidental awareness during general anaesthesia

A 2012 NICE report undertook a cost:benefit analysis of using the monitors listed previously, and recommended their use during certain types of anaesthesia considered to be more likely to risk incidences of awareness.[1]

In 2014, the fifth National Audit Project (NAP5) reviewed accidental awareness under general anaesthesia (AAGA).[2] It reported a lower incidence (1/19,000) than previously thought (1/1000), and identified specific risk factors which made AAGA more likely, and hence pEEG monitoring more desirable, including:
- Obesity
- Previous history of AAGA
- Neuromuscular blockade
- Caesarean section
- During induction and emergence
- Cardiothoracic anaesthesia
- Use of thiopentone
- RSI
- TIVA.

## Excessive anaesthesia

pEEG monitoring has become topical in current studies with regard to reducing postoperative mortality and morbidity, especially in high-risk patients. If these studies confirm previous observations (that a combination of low mean arterial pressure and low BIS in the presence of low MAC is associated with increased postoperative morbidity and mortality, the 'triple low'), then pEEG monitoring, especially in high-risk patients, may become routine.[3,4]

One particular postoperative complication for which the use of pEEG has been promoted is postoperative cognitive dysfunction (POCD).[1,5] POCD has been linked to excessive depth of anaesthesia.[1] Use of pEEG has been shown to reduce POCD in susceptible patients.[6] Risk factors for POCD include[7]:

• Age >75 years
• History of cognitive impairment
• Second procedure
• Long procedure
• Major surgery
• Preoperative confusion or frailty.

Interpretation of pEEG data has been described as an 'intangible art form',[2] but, as with other monitoring, its usefulness is increased by comparison with other concurrent data, and with experience of the user. As an example, when interpreting BIS, it should be remembered that:

• A satisfactory BIS measurement may become unacceptably high following increased surgical stimulation[8]
• A satisfactory BIS measurement may not preclude patient movement, the prevention of which requires twice the depth of anaesthesia needed to prevent awareness[9]
• Awareness is not the same as recall of awareness—BIS was developed to predict recall, and it is possible that a patient could experience awareness with apparently satisfactory BIS readings.[10]

pEEG monitoring is likely to become more prevalent as benefits are revealed by current research programmes.

## References

1. National Institute for Health and Care and Excellence (2012). Depth of anaesthesia monitors – bispectral index (BIS), E-Entropy and Narcotrend-Compact M. London: National Institute for Health and Care and Excellence.
2. Cook TM, Andrade J, Bogod DG, et al. (2014). The 5th National Audit Project (NAP5) on accidental awareness during general anaesthesia: patient experiences, human factors, sedation, consent and medicolegal issues. Anaesthesia, 69(10):1102–1116.
3. Leslie K (2013). Staying alive after surgery: the second POMRC report. Available at: ℘ https://www.hqsc.govt.nz/assets/POMRC/Resources/2013-workshop/04-Kate-Leslie.pdf
4. Sessler DI (2017). Randomized trial of alerts in patients demonstrating a "triple low". Available at: ℘ https://www.clinicaltrials.gov/ct2/show/NCT00998894
5. Avidan MS, Evers AS (2011). Review of clinical evidence for persistent cognitive decline or incident dementia attributed to surgery or general anaesthesia. Journal of Alzheimer's Disease, 24(2):201–216.
6. Ballard C, Jones E, Gauge N, et al. (2012). Optimised anaesthesia to reduce postoperative cognitive decline (POCD) in older patients undergoing elective surgery, a randomised controlled trial. PLoS One, 7(6):e37410.
7. Wilkinson J, Martin IC, Gough MJ, et al. (2010). An age old problem: elective and emergency surgery in the elderly. London: National Confidential Enquiry into Patient Outcome and Death.
8. Schneider G, Wagner K, Reeker W, et al. (2002). Bispectral index (BIS) may not predict awareness reaction to intubation in surgical patients. Journal of Neurosurgical Anesthesiology, 14(1):7–11.

9.  Sebel PS, Lang E, Rampil IJ, et al. (1997). A multicenter study of bispectral electroencephalogram analysis for monitoring anesthetic effect. Anesthesia and Analgesia, 84(4):891–899.
10. Zand F, Hadavi SMR, Chohedri A, et al. (2014). Survey of the adequacy of depth of anaesthesia with bispectral index and isolated forearm technique in elective caesarean section under general anaesthesia with sevoflurane. British Journal of Anaesthesia, 112(5):871–878.

# Chapter 12

# Specialist anaesthesia

# Ear, nose, and throat anaesthesia

The procedures undertaken within this specialty often require a specific ETT and other interventions.

## General considerations

- Position of patient—extended breathing circuits may be required.
- Head ring or other suitable device should be available to aid positioning.
- Potentially difficult intubation. May require additional equipment (e.g. GlideScope®) to improve visualization of the larynx.[1]
- Protection of patient's eyes (e.g. EyeGard®).
- Warming equipment for longer procedures.
- LMAs, RLMAs, and i-gel® devices may be used.

Clear communication is essential during ENT surgery due to the shared airway between the anaesthetist and surgeon.

## Ear surgery

- Bleeding should be kept minimal during surgery of the middle ear, may require hypotensive anaesthesia; 25% below baseline is effective.[2]
- $N_2O$ diffuses into middle ear with the potential to displace surgical grafts; its use should therefore be avoided in middle ear surgery.

## Nasal surgery

- Oral preformed tube (e.g. Ring, Adair, and Elwyn (RAE)) to face away from site of surgery. Sits over bottom lip without kinking.
- May require intranasal vasoconstrictors.
- Throat pack to absorb secretions, precautions include use of throat pack label and leave part of pack protruding. If retained postoperatively, throat pack would cause airway obstruction and potential death, therefore insertion and removal must be recorded as a 'two-person' check.

## Tonsillectomy

- Oral preformed tube to allow surgical access.
- Historically uncuffed ETTs used for paediatrics but now Microcuff tubes are considered advantageous. They have a strong cuff which protects the airway at lower pressures. They also have features which increase the chance of correct placement (i.e. cuff closer to tip of ETT and intubation depth mark).[3]
- Sizes from 3.0 to 7.0 mm ID. Recommended sizes are according to age range.

## Microlaryngoscopy/direct laryngoscopy

- Microlaryngoscopy tube (MLT), available in sizes 4.0, 5.0, and 6.0 mm ID. The smaller diameter will cause high resistance.
- Securing tube to the left allows the surgeon maximum access.
- Cuff size is bigger than a standard tracheal tube of the same ID size to facilitate an adequate seal in an adult trachea.

- It is important not to cut the tube length as it is longer by design to allow nasal intubation if necessary. Also gives greater length outside the mouth to allow circuit to be attached at a safe distance.

## Laser surgery

- Laser-resistant tube required to prevent potential ignition of tube.
- Laser-Flex tube® (Mallinckrodt) consists of a stainless steel body which protects the tube against $CO_2$ laser beams.
- Tube has two cuffs which are inflated with sterile saline. This reduces the risk of an air-filled cuff igniting if penetrated by the laser.
- Some anaesthetists use saline coloured with methylene blue to inflate cuffs so the surgeon is immediately alerted to a ruptured cuff.
- The presence of two cuffs ensures a tracheal seal in the event of damage to one.
- Apply saline-soaked gauze padding to patient's facial area for protection.
- Laser precautions to be followed, including protective spectacles, warning sign on all entrance doors, restrict access, etc.

## Laryngectomy

- Standard or reinforced tracheal tube initially.
- The laryngectomy tube is inserted after the larynx has been removed and when a tracheal stoma has been fashioned.
- When surgeon is ready to insert the laryngectomy/tracheostomy tube, communication must be of paramount importance.
- Surgeon visually locates tracheal tube and withdraws it to just above incision. This allows the tube to be reinserted should airway problems occur.
- Laryngectomy tubes (e.g. Laryngoflex® (sizes 7–9) and Montandon® (sizes 6–10)) have the advantage of allowing the breathing circuit to be attached further from the surgical field, therefore improving access.
- If a laryngectomy tube is used, this will be changed to a tracheostomy tube at the end of surgery, as a shorter tube will reduce both the dead space and the risk of dislodging the tube.

### Thyroidectomy/parathyroidectomy

There is a risk of injury to the recurrent laryngeal nerve. This could cause paralysis of the laryngeal muscles which in turn could lead to loss of speech. Therefore, it is essential to utilize recurrent laryngeal nerve monitoring which is performed via the endotracheal tube.

An electromyogram (EMG) tube is a specialized ETT that has electrodes which, following intubation, are in the vicinity of the vocal cords. If the surgeon stimulates a laryngeal nerve, an audible warning sign is heard. Another method is to use a specific electrode (e.g. Neurosign® Lantern Laryngeal Electrode) which is physically adhered to an ETT prior to intubation.

### References

1. Miller RD, Pardo MC Jr (2011). Basics of anaesthesia (6th ed). Philadelphia, PA: Elsevier.
2. Barash PG, Cullen BF, Stoelting RK, et al. (2013). Clinical anaesthesia (7th ed). Philadelphia, PA: Lippincott Williams & Wilkins.
3. Pollard B, Kitchen G (2018). Handbook of clinical anaesthesia (4th ed). London: CRC Press.

## Further reading

Al-Shaikh B, Stacey S (2018). Essentials of equipment in anaesthesia, critical care and perioperative medicine (5th ed). Edinburgh; Elsevier.

Freedman R, Herbert L, O'Donnell A, et al. (eds) (2022). Oxford handbook of anaesthesia (5th ed). Oxford: Oxford University Press.

Royal College of Anaesthetists (2019). Chapter 3: guidelines for the provision of anaesthesia services for intraoperative care. London: Royal College of Anaesthetists.

Royal College of Anaesthetists (2020). Chapter 12: guidelines for the provision of anaesthesia services for ENT, oral maxillofacial and dental surgery. London: Royal College of Anaesthetists.

# Obstetric anaesthesia

The aim of anaesthesia for caesarean section or any surgery while pregnant is that it should be safe for both the mother and the fetus. The obstetric theatre must always be prepared for immediate use if required and the following points observed:

- Theatre temperature should be between 22°C and 24°C.
- Anaesthetic machine checked and intubation equipment ready.
- Difficult intubation equipment available.
- Spinal/epidural equipment ready.
- IV fluids prepared.
- Many obstetric theatres have pre-drawn-up induction drugs prepared daily and stored in theatre for expediency.
- ECG, BP, pulse oximeter, capnograph, and gas analyser.

## Physiological changes significant to anaesthesia

Circulatory and respiratory changes provide for the metabolic needs of the fetus and the mother.

### Cardiovascular changes

- Increase in cardiac output.
- Increase in blood flow to many organs, biggest being to the uterus.
- Increase in plasma volume causing haemodilution—decrease in Hb leading to anaemia.
- Decrease in BP during first trimester.

### Pre-eclampsia

- Causes problems with circulation which normally show up as high BP, protein in the urine, and swelling.
- Can become serious and affect other systems such as the liver, brain, lungs, or clotting system.
- Haemolysis, elevated liver enzymes, and low platelet count (HELLP) is considered a variant of pre-eclampsia and can be life-threatening.

### Aorto-caval compression

During pregnancy, some women feel faint when lying supine due to the vena cava, and sometimes the aorta, being occluded. A collateral system of veins reaches the heart instead but if this pathway is not effective, the heart is deprived of venous return, output is not maintained, and BP decreases. It must be anticipated in all pregnant women >20 weeks and avoided by uterine displacement. This is done simply by placing a wedge under the patient's right hip causing a tilt to the left and thus preventing the compression.

### Respiratory changes

- Increase in tidal volume due to increased levels of progesterone which has a stimulant effect on the respiratory centre and also an elevated diaphragm from the growing uterus.
- Rapid falls in $O_2$ saturation on induction of GA due to:
  - Increased $O_2$ consumption
  - Decreased cardiac output
  - Decrease in functional residual capacity
  - MAC values decrease in pregnancy increasing susceptibility to anaesthetic agents.

**Box 12.1 Rapid sequence induction for obstetric patients**
- Patient on tilting trolley.
- Intubation equipment ready and to hand—consider smaller ETTs and avoid nasal intubation as the respiratory mucous membrane becomes vascular and oedematous.
- Suction available.
- 100% preoxygenation for 3 minutes.
- Application of cricoid pressure.
- Intubation and inflation of cuff on ETT.
- Check correct placement of tube.
- Release cricoid pressure on instruction of anaesthetist.

## General anaesthesia

The placental barrier is readily crossed by most pharmacological agents used in anaesthesia and may have a potential effect on the fetus. It is fair to assume that all pregnant patients are at risk of inhalation of gastric contents due to regurgitation as a result of:
- 'Big bump': uterus compresses the stomach against the diaphragm
- Heartburn: due to incompetence of lower oesophageal sphincter
- Full stomach: due to delayed gastric emptying.

Post delivery, it can take up to 6 weeks for changes to revert back.

### Prophylaxis and prevention

Raise the pH of gastric contents by administering alkali sodium citrate and block secretion of acid by administering $H_2$ antagonist. Antacids may also be given with regional anaesthesia as it may need to be converted to GA. For RSI, see Box 12.1.

### Risk of difficult intubation
- Full dentition, crowns.
- Laryngeal oedema.
- Large breasts: use polio blade.
- Tilted on their side.

## Regional anaesthesia (spinal/epidural)

Benefit of potentially having partner present in theatre and able to start bonding with the baby straight away.

### Consider
- Epidural may already be in place and just need topping up.
- Preload with IV fluids as risk of hypotension.
- IV ephedrine prepared.
- May be difficult for mother to get or keep in position for insertion.

## Non-obstetric surgery for the pregnant patient
- Only emergency surgery should be performed.
- LA should be considered.
- GA in first trimester should avoid $N_2O$.

- GA in second and third trimester:
  - Avoid aorto-caval compression.
  - RSI.
- Avoid hypotension.
- Equipment available in case of need for emergency caesarean section.

## Further reading

Al-Shaikh B, Stacey S (2018). Essentials of equipment in anaesthesia, critical care and perioperative medicine (5th ed). Edinburgh: Elsevier.

Association of Anaesthetists of Great Britain and Ireland (2019). Checklist for draw-over anaesthetic equipment. Available at: ℘ http://dx.doi.org/10.21466/g.CFDAE2.2019

Association of Anaesthetists of Great Britain and Ireland (2020). Neurological monitoring associated with obstetric neuraxial block. Available at: ℘ https://doi.org/10.1111/anae.14993

Clark V, Van de Velde M, Fernando R (eds) (2016). Oxford textbook of obstetric anaesthesia. Oxford: Oxford University Press.

Freedman R, Herbert L, O'Donnell A, et al. (eds) (2022). Oxford handbook of anaesthesia (5th ed). Oxford: Oxford University Press.

Monteiro R, Salman M, Malhotra S, et al. (2019). Analgesia, anaesthesia and pregnancy: a practical guide (4th ed). Cambridge: Cambridge University Press.

Obstetric Anaesthetists' Association. Clinical guidelines. Available at: ℘ https://www.oaa-anaes. ac.uk/Clinical_Guidelines

Royal College of Anaesthetists (2019). Chapter 3: guidelines for the provision of anaesthesia services for intraoperative care. London: Royal College of Anaesthetists.

Royal College of Anaesthetists (2020). Chapter 9: guidelines for the provision of anaesthesia services for an obstetric population. London: Royal College of Anaesthetists.

# Paediatric and neonatal anaesthesia

Paediatric anaesthesia includes patients from the premature neonate to adolescents (Table 12.1).

**Table 12.1** Definitions of paediatric patients

| | |
|---|---|
| **Neonate** | First 44 weeks of post-conceptual age |
| **Premature infant** | <37 weeks' gestational age |
| **Infant** | Babies from 1 to 12 months old |
| **SGA** | Small for gestational age |
| **Low birth weight** | <2.5 kg (6.5 lbs) |

## Preoperative management

- Preassessment should involve the parents (carers) and children who are given the opportunity to ask questions.
- A designated paediatric intensive care unit (PICU) should be available for children who require intensive care following surgery.
- Day-care surgery should be considered for surgical procedures that are neither complex nor prolonged.
- Preterm or ex-preterm neonates should not be considered for day-case surgery unless they are medically fit and healthy and have reached 60 weeks' post-conceptual age.
- Infants with a history of chronic lung disease or 'apnoea' should be managed in a centre equipped with facilities for postoperative ventilation.
- Parents/carers should be kept informed of their child's progress, especially if there is an unexpected delay in theatre.

Doses of drugs and fluids need to be precisely calculated, and anaesthetic equipment for smaller children differs from that used in older children and adults.[1]

## Anaesthetic management

- Paediatric anaesthesia services must be consultant led.
- Paediatric resuscitation equipment must be available and staff must regularly update their knowledge and competence in paediatric life support.
- Parental presence in the anaesthetic room should be encouraged.
- IV induction:
  - According to anaesthetist's preference, IV cannula should be introduced when the child is sitting on a parent's lap with his/her view obstructed.
  - Induction of anaesthesia with propofol.
  - Thiopental for neonates.
- Gas induction by sevoflurane is recommended while the child is sitting on a parent/carer's lap.

- It may not be possible to attach all monitoring before induction of paediatric patients.
- Monitoring of paediatric patients should include BP, temperature probes, pulse oximetry, and ECG for all patients.
- A defibrillator and resuscitation drugs and equipment must be available wherever children are anaesthetized.
- Anaesthetic machines should incorporate ventilators, which have controls and bellows permitting their use over the entire age range together with the facility to provide pressure-controlled ventilation.[1]
- Volumetric infusion pumps should be used for IV fluids.
- The size of the ETT used for paediatric anaesthesia is important; an ETT that is too large will exert pressure on the internal surface of the cricoid cartilage resulting in oedema which could lead to airway obstruction when the tube is removed (Table 12.2).
- An uncuffed ETT is recommended for use in children <10 years old as it provides a larger ID compared with a cuffed tube.
- ETT should be secured in place.

**Table 12.2** Internal diameter of ETT related to age

| | |
|---|---|
| **Premature** | 2.5–3.0 mm |
| **Neonate–6 months** | 3.0–3.5 mm |
| **6months–1 year** | 3.5–4.0 mm |
| **1–2 years** | 4.0–5.0 mm |
| **>2 years—use the formula** | 4+ (age/4) |

### Thermoregulation
- Paediatric patients, particularly neonates, are prone to heat loss.
- The operating theatre should be warmed up to 26°C prior to surgery.
- A paediatric patient's head should be covered with a cap or gamgee.
- Gamgee can also be used to cover other parts of the patient's body to maintain heat.
- Utilize active warming devices and warm all fluids.

### Equipment
See Box 12.2.

### Postoperative management
- Recovery of a paediatric patient should be on a one-to-one basis.
- Apnoea is a common postoperative complication in neonates who are preterm so provide apnoea monitoring equipment.
- Administer $O_2$ postoperatively if tolerated.
- Allow parents into recovery as soon as airway is maintained.
- Monitor $SpO_2$, pulse, and respiratory rate.
- Analgesia can include NSAIDs and paracetamol; caudal analgesia; nurse-controlled analgesia (NCA) or PCA for severe pain.

**Box 12.2 Equipment that should be available and maintained for use in neonates, infants, and children**

- Airway management and monitoring, including capnography and invasive haemodynamic monitoring.
- Pulse oximetry sensors and BP cuffs.
- Patient warming and fluid warming devices.
- Vascular access equipment, including intraosseous needles.
- Rapid and accurate fluid and drug delivery devices.
- Patient temperature measuring device.
- TIVA pumps with paediatric algorithms.
- Ultrasound devices (for central venous and nerve identification).

*Source:* data from Royal College of Anaesthetists (2020). Chapter 10: Guidelines for the Provision of Paediatric Anaesthesia Services. London: Royal College of Anaesthetists.

## Reference

1. Royal College of Anaesthetists (2020). Chapter 10: guidelines for the provision of paediatric anaesthesia services. London: Royal College of Anaesthetists.

## Further reading

Al-Shaikh B, Stacey S (2018). Essentials of equipment in anaesthesia, critical care and perioperative medicine (5th ed). Edinburgh: Elsevier.

Association of Anaesthetists of Great Britain and Ireland (2016). Recommendations for standards of monitoring during anaesthesia and recovery 2015. Anaesthesia, 71(1):85–93.

Bailey CR, Ahuja M, Bartholomew K, et al. (2019). Guidelines for day-case surgery 2019: guidelines from the Association of Anaesthetists and the British Association of Day Surgery. Anaesthesia, 74(6):778–792.

Freedman R, Herbert L, O'Donnell A, et al. (eds) (2022). Oxford handbook of anaesthesia (5th ed). Oxford: Oxford University Press.

James I, Walker I (eds) (2013). Core topics in paediatric anaesthesia. Cambridge: Cambridge University Press.

National Institute for Health and Care Excellence (2020). Intravenous fluid therapy in children and young people in hospital. NICE guideline [NG29]. Available at: ℘ https://www.nice.org.uk/guidance/ng29

Roberts S (ed) (2019). Paediatric anaesthesia (2nd ed). Oxford: Oxford University Press.

# Neurosurgical anaesthesia

The RCoA states that an anaesthetic clinical service should provide[1]:
- Anaesthesia for neurosurgery including intracranial, complex spinal, and associated surgery
- Anaesthesia for neuroradiology including diagnostic and interventional procedures
- Neurocritical care including pre- and postoperative management of complex elective cases and the management of critically ill patients, for example, severe head injury, intracranial haemorrhage, severe neurological disease, and those who develop systemic complications secondary to their neurological condition.

> Anaesthesia for many neurosurgical factors has common factors, the greatest of which is the prevention of a rise in intracranial pressure (ICP).[2] Neuroanaesthesia for children should include shared responsibility between neuroanaesthetists and paediatric anaesthetists.[1]

## Examples of neurosurgical procedures

These include[3]:
- Cerebral aneurysm repair
- Craniotomy
- Awake craniotomy
- Posterior fossa surgery
- Ventriculoperitoneal shunt
- Laminectomy
- Pituitary surgery
- Evacuation of traumatic intracranial haematoma.

## Preoperative management

- Pre-admission clinics for elective neurosurgery should be available.
- Assessment for signs of raised ICP.
- Assess neurological observations.
- Sedative drugs in patients with raised ICP should be avoided.
- Prophylactic VTE therapy.
- Urinary catheter for surgical procedures of long duration.

## Anaesthetic management

- The incidence of difficult intubation in neurosurgical units carrying out complex cervical spinal surgery is high.
- Difficult airway management equipment must be available.
- Patient monitoring should include:
  - ECG, $SpO_2$, nasopharyngeal temperature
  - CVP and arterial line for invasive BP monitoring for major neurosurgical procedures.
- Preoxygenate for at least 3 minutes.
- Hypertension and tachycardia should be avoided.
- Propofol or thiopental for IV induction administered slowly is recommended with vecuronium as a muscle relaxant.

- Avoid suxamethonium as it raises ICP—only use for RSI in emergency surgery where a full stomach is possible (i.e. head injury).
- An armoured ETT should be use for intubation and secured well.
- Transfer patient from operating theatre table to bed with care to avoid excess movement.
- Patient positions can vary for neurosurgery, so it is essential that all monitoring and ventilatory support are secured.
- Equipment for safe positioning of patients should include:
  - Appropriate sized mattresses
  - Positioning aids to minimize risk of eye injury, nerve injury, and skin damage, for example, pressure sores, during potentially prolonged operations
  - Fixings to prevent accidental movement during the procedure.[1]

## Signs of raised ICP

- Deterioration of levels of consciousness.
- Changes in breathing pattern or respiratory rate.
- Dilated pupil.
- Decreased movement of one side.
- If any of these signs occur, call the anaesthetist and neurosurgeon immediately!

## Postoperative management

- Neurological observations.
- Hypotension decreases cerebral blood flow and may cause hypoxia and fitting.
- Ondine's curse, a complication of neurosurgery, can result from severe brain or spinal trauma; patients can forget to breathe or suffer respiratory arrest so reintubation and ventilation may be necessary.
- Analgesia ± antiemetic therapy.
- Some patients will be transferred immediately to ITU.
- For transfer to ICU—$O_2$, ventilatory support, continuous monitoring, drug infusion pumps, anaesthetic assistance for emergencies, and resuscitation drugs.

## References

1. Royal College of Anaesthetists (2020). Chapter 14: guidelines for the provision of neuro-anaesthetic services. London: Royal College of Anaesthetists.
2. Simpson PJ, Popat M (2002). Understanding anaesthesia (4th ed). Oxford: Butterworth-Heinemann.
3. Leaper DJ, Whitaker I (eds) (2010). Handbook of postoperative complications (2nd ed). Oxford: Oxford University Press.

## Further reading

Association of Anaesthetists of Great Britain and Ireland (2016). Recommendations for standards of monitoring during anaesthesia and recovery 2015. Anaesthesia, 71(1):85–93.
Association of Anaesthetists of Great Britain and Ireland (2019). Safe transfer of the brain-injured patient – trauma and stroke. Available at: ℘ http://dx.doi.org/10.1111/anae.14866
Craig A, Hatfield A (2020). The complete recovery room book (6th ed). Oxford: Oxford University Press.
National Institute for Health and Care Excellence (2018). Brain tumours (primary) and brain metastases in adults. NICE guideline [NG99]. Available at: ℘ https://www.nice.org.uk/guidance/NG99

# Ophthalmic anaesthesia

Ophthalmic surgery encompasses the following areas: intraocular surgery, extraocular surgery, oculoplastic surgery, nasolacrimal surgery, and orbital surgery.[1] Most cataract surgery is performed on an older population, many of whom will also have additional comorbidities and uncommon medical problems; therefore, resuscitation equipment must be readily available.

## Types of anaesthetic

*General*

- Predisposing factors: include age (child), dementia, severe anxiety, surgical duration, LA sensitivity.
- Usually spontaneously breathing using LMA. Follow minimum monitoring guidelines.
- TIVA: used for induction and maintenance in most cases.
- Tape/protect non-surgical eye where appropriate.

*Local*

- Topical: provided by the application of local analgesic eye drops. Short acting, but useful for minor operations on the conjunctiva and cornea. Also required prior to sub-Tenon/peribulbar procedures.
- Surface analgesia: local infiltration of LA is used to good effect for operations on the eyelids.
- Sub-Tenon injection: a technique where the LA is deposited underneath the Tenon's capsule, using a special cannula introduced through a small incision in the conjunctiva.
- Peribulbar infiltration: rarely used now due to risk of nerve damage.

Sharp needle-based LA blocks should be performed or directly supervised by an anaesthetist or surgeon who has been specifically trained.

IV sedation should only be administered under the supervision of an anaesthetist, who must have sole responsibility to that list.

## Anaesthetic equipment required

- Operating table, trolley, or reclining chair.
- Baseline observation recording—heart rate, $O_2$ saturations, BP.
- Monitoring in accordance with local policy for GA.
- Prescribed topical drugs (sterile) tetracaine.
- Sterile gloves.
- Needles, syringes—assorted.
- IV access—anaesthetist preference.

*For anaesthetic*

- Sub-Tenon cannula.
- Lid retractor—speculum.
- Forceps—Moorfields.
- Scissor—Westcott.
- Aqueous povidone iodine, or chlorhexidine—must be aqueous not alcoholic.

*Within theatre*
- Rubens pillow.
- Pillow under knees.
- Heal supports.
- Theatre practitioner or theatre assistant to hold the patient's hand, or patient alert method in place.
- Piped air supply (under drapes) nasal specs can be used for $O_2$ if required/prescribed.

## Other factors for consideration

*Raising intraocular pressure*
- Suxamethonium raises intraocular pressure by the contraction of muscles surrounding orbit.
- Coughing, vomiting, and head-down tilt also raise pressures.

*Oculocardiac reflex*
- Squint surgery inevitably involves some form of traction on the extraocular eye muscles. This may cause cardiac arrhythmias including bradycardia or even asystole.

## Reference

1. Royal College of Anaesthetists (2020). Chapter 13: guidelines for the provision of ophthalmic anaesthesia services. London: Royal College of Anaesthetists.

## Further reading

Al-Shaikh B, Stacey S (2018). Essentials of equipment in anaesthesia, critical care and perioperative medicine (5th ed). Edinburgh: Elsevier.

Association of Anaesthetists of Great Britain and Ireland (2016). Recommendations for standards of monitoring during anaesthesia and recovery 2015. Anaesthesia, 71(1):85–93.

Craig A, Hatfield A (2020). The complete recovery room book (6th ed). Oxford: Oxford University Press.

Denniston AKO, Murray PI (eds) (2018). Oxford handbook of ophthalmology (4th ed). Oxford: Oxford University Press.

Freedman R, Herbert L, O'Donnell A, et al. (eds) (2022). Oxford handbook of anaesthesia (5th ed). Oxford: Oxford University Press.

Royal College of Anaesthetists (2020). Chapter 6: guidelines for the provision of anaesthesia services for day surgery. London: Royal College of Anaesthetists.

Scarth E, Smith S (2016). Drugs in anaesthesia and intensive care (5th ed). Oxford: Oxford University Press.

# Anaesthesia for burns surgery

A burn is an injury to the skin or other organic tissue primarily caused by heat or due to radiation, radioactivity, electricity, friction, or contact with chemicals.[1] See Box 12.3.

A major burn is defined as a burn covering 25% or more of total body surface area. However, any injury over >10% should be treated similarly.

---

**Box 12.3 Key facts about burns**

- An estimated 180,000 deaths every year are caused by burns.
- The majority of burns occur in low- and middle-income countries.
- Non-fatal burn injuries are a leading cause of morbidity.
- Burns occur mainly in the home and workplace.
- Burns are preventable.

---

Rapid assessment is vital as swelling may develop around the airway in the hours after injury and requires intubation. An assessment must be made to identify if the airway is compromised or is at risk of compromise:

- Preoperative assessment of the patient is vital and should include the history and events following the injury.
- It is essential to maintain safety for the individual undergoing treatment; protect vascular access and make appropriate and informed airway care decisions.

The depth of the burn is important for the planning of treatment and can be classified as shown in Box 12.4.

---

**Box 12.4 Classification of burns**

- *Erythema (1°)*: not included in the estimate of the burned area; it will not be blistered but may be painful and usually heals without treatment.
- *Superficial partial thickness (2°), deep partial thickness (2°), and full thickness (3°)* areas are included in the estimate of the burned area. The difference between superficial and deep is that superficial partial thickness burns are more likely to heal without scarring. Under-resuscitation can cause deterioration of burned areas to a more severe grade.
- *Complex burns* are inevitably included in the estimate of the burned area and involve destruction of tissues deep to the skin such as tendon muscle, and bone. Other complex burns include burns to the face, airway, and perineum.

---

## Anaesthetic considerations

Burns or plastics procedures can take many hours and every attempt should be made to ensure the environment is suitable for the needs of patients with burns. Burns patients are susceptible to heat and fluid loss, infection, and airway difficulties, and require specialist pain control. Burn patients are at particular risk of thromboembolic complication.

'Understanding the complexity of surgery for major burns surgery is vital. This includes the need to be prepared for massive blood loss, difficulties with monitoring and venous access, management of heat loss, prevention of thromboembolic events, and sepsis; as well as complex analgesia requirements, and understanding the impact on the patient and their family and of ongoing care for many years ahead.'[2]

### Monitoring

- Patients undergoing extensive burns or microvascular surgical procedures require invasive monitoring during resuscitation, surgery, and intensive care.
- Arterial lines should be inserted in unconscious patients and patients with major burns and/or inhalational injury.
- Vascular access may be compromised by the burn.

### Airway

- Difficult airway equipment must be available where burns patients are treated, including equipment necessary for failed intubation and cricothyroidotomy.
- Patient's airway may be compromised by the oedema of the burn and crystalloid resuscitation—also check mouth and lips.
- Airway difficulties can worsen as the injury matures by scarring and contracture and render conventional laryngoscopy impossible.
- Blind intubation techniques or awake intubation may also be necessary.

### Anaesthesia

- Gas inductions and spontaneous breathing techniques may be considered with the use of an LMA or fibreoptic-aided intubation.
- Caution should be applied with the use of suxamethonium as it can exaggerate hyperkalaemia.
- Consider regional blockade with LA for patients undergoing microvascular surgery.

### Fluid management

- Fluid should be warmed to ensure that the development of hypothermia does not complicate clotting function or cause inappropriate vasoconstriction.
- Signs of inadequate fluid administration include oliguria, haemoconcentration, and hypotension.
- Fluid resuscitation may be performed to:
  - Preserve life
  - Maintain organ function
  - Ameliorate the injury
  - Restrict surgery to necessity and functional restoration
  - Limit psychological damage.

The main objective of fluid administration in thermal trauma is to preserve and restore tissue perfusion and prevent ischaemia.[3]

*Postoperative management*
- If surgery is prolonged, postoperative ventilation may be considered.
- Both acute and chronic pain services will be needed to facilitate optimal pain management.
- Repeated anaesthetic input may be required for debridement and dressings until stable wound coverage and healing is obtained.

## References

1. World Health Organization (2018). Burns. Available at: ℅ https://www.who.int/news-room/fact-sheets/detail/burns
2. Royal College of Anaesthetists (2020). Chapter 17: guidelines for the provision of anaesthesia services for burns and plastic surgery. London: Royal College of Anaesthetists.
3. Guilabert P, Usúa G, Martín N, et al. (2016). Fluid resuscitation management in patients with burns: update. British Journal of Anaesthesia, 117(3):284–296.

## Further reading

Association of Anaesthetists of Great Britain and Ireland (2016). Recommendations for standards of monitoring during anaesthesia and recovery 2015. Anaesthesia, 71(1):85–93.

Freedman R, Herbert L, O'Donnell A, et al. (eds) (2022). Oxford handbook of anaesthesia (5th ed). Oxford: Oxford University Press.

Hettiaratchy S, Papini R (2004). Initial management of a major burn. BMJ, 328(7455):1555–1557.

Grishkevich VM, Grishkevich M (2018). Plastic and reconstructive surgery of burns: an atlas of new techniques and strategies. New York: Springer.

Hung OR, Murphy MF (2018). Hung's difficult and failed airway management. London: McGraw Hill.

Martin A, Allman K, McIndoe A (eds) (2020). Emergencies in anaesthesia (3rd ed). Oxford: Oxford University Press.

National Institute for Health and Care Excellence (2020). Intravenous fluid therapy in children and young people in hospital. NICE guideline [NG29]. Available at: ℅ https://www.nice.org.uk/guidance/ng29

National Institute for Health and Care Excellence (2020). Venous thromboembolic diseases: diagnosis, management and thrombophilia testing. NICE guideline [NG158]. Available at: ℅ https://www.nice.org.uk/guidance/ng158

# Anaesthesia for plastic surgery

Plastic surgery describes a reconstructive procedure designed to restore form and function to the body. It covers all aspects of wound healing and reconstruction after congenital, acquired, or traumatic tissue defects.[1]

> Prolonged plastic surgery procedures are common and require attention to detail regarding positioning, fluid management, blood flow, and prevention of thromboembolic complications.[1]

The range and complexity of anaesthesia during plastic/reconstruction surgery can involve routine and extensive surgical procedures (see Box 12.5 for some examples).

Operative procedures can last many hours, may involve significant blood loss, and can require the presence of more than one anaesthetist.

A burns and plastics service will require provision of anaesthesia for a diverse range of surgical procedures in both emergency and elective situations. Appropriate postoperative care and/or critical care facilities may be required for patients requiring the following procedures:

- Surgery for minor and major hand injuries such as:
  - Replantation following traumatic amputations
  - Minor and routine cosmetic surgery
  - Dressing changes.
- Complex surgical procedures such as surgery for:
  - Head and neck cancers
  - Microvascular techniques
  - Breast reconstructive surgery.
- Other common conditions that can require plastic surgery include reconstruction of large skin defects, pressure sores and other chronic wounds, venous and other leg ulcers, and the results of devastating infections.

> **Box 12.5 Examples of procedures requiring plastic/ reconstructive surgery**
> - Breast augmentation.
> - Breast reduction.
> - Gynaecomastia.
> - Insertion of tissue expander.
> - Liposuction.
> - Correction of prominent ears.
> - Free-flap surgery.
> - Skin grafting.
> - Cranio-facial reconstruction.
> - Abdominoplasty.

## Anaesthetic considerations

- Difficult airway equipment must be available in any area where plastic surgery is performed.
- The patient's airway may be compromised in the case of head and neck surgery and consideration should be given to the shared airway.
- Blind intubation techniques or awake intubation may also be necessary.
- Patients undergoing microvascular surgical procedures may require invasive monitoring.[1]
- Consider regional blockade with LA for patients undergoing microvascular surgery.
- If the operating site is extensive, difficulties may arise with heat conservation, patient monitoring, and vascular access.
- If surgery is prolonged, postoperative ventilation may be considered; additional considerations should be given to:
  - Vascular access
  - Blood loss
  - Fluid balance
  - Thermoregulation
  - Patient positioning
  - VTE prophylaxis
  - Eye care
  - ETT cuff pressure.
- Both acute and chronic pain services will be needed to facilitate optimal pain management.
- A smooth emergence from anaesthesia is recommended to avoid tension on suture lines, which may increase bleeding and the formation of a haematoma.
- Ensure effective postoperative analgesia.

## Reference

1. Royal College of Anaesthetists (2020). Chapter 17: guidelines for the provision of anaesthesia services for burns and plastic surgery. London: Royal College of Anaesthetists.

## Further reading

Association of Anaesthetists of Great Britain and Ireland (2016). Recommendations for standards of monitoring during anaesthesia and recovery 2015. Anaesthesia, 71(1):85–93.

Freedman R, Herbert L, O'Donnell A, et al. (eds) (2022). Oxford handbook of anaesthesia (5th ed). Oxford: Oxford University Press.

Giele H, Cassell O (2016). Plastic and reconstructive surgery. Oxford: Oxford University Press.

Grishkevich VM, Grishkevich M (2018). Plastic and reconstructive surgery of burns: an atlas of new techniques and strategies. New York: Springer.

Leaper DJ, Whitaker I (eds) (2010). Handbook of postoperative complications (2nd ed). Oxford: Oxford University Press.

National Institute for Health and Care Excellence (2020). Venous thromboembolic diseases: diagnosis, management and thrombophilia testing. NICE guideline [NG158]. Available at: ℘ https://www.nice.org.uk/guidance/ng158

Richards A, Dafydd H (2015). Key notes on plastic surgery (2nd ed). Oxford: Wiley-Blackwell.

# Cardiac anaesthesia

Cardiac surgery may involve adult, paediatric, and neonatal patients and can be divided into closed heart procedures and open heart procedures (see Box 12.6 for some examples). Simpson and Popat state that the heart and lungs function normally during closed heart procedures, whereas during open heart procedures, blood to the heart and lungs is diverted or by-passed 'to an extracorporeal circuit comprising a pump and gas exchanger and allowing arrest of lung ventilation and heart beat'.[1]

> **Box 12.6 Examples of cardiac surgical procedures**
> - Coronary artery bypass graft.
> - Aortic valve replacement.
> - Mitral valve replacement.
> - Pulmonary thromboembolectomy.
> - Implantable defibrillators.
> - Thoracic aortic aneurysm surgery.

## Preoperative management
- Comprehensive preassessment should include a 12-lead ECG.
- Assessment of airway.
- Smoking cessation and preoperative physiotherapy is recommended prior to elective cardiac surgery to optimize lung function.
- Dental check for patients with valvar disease and who are at risk of infective endocarditis.
- Diuretic drugs should continue until the day of surgery.

> The aim of induction of anaesthesia for cardiac surgery is to produce unconsciousness while maintaining a stable cardiovascular system in which myocardial $O_2$ demand is minimized and myocardial $O_2$ supply is maximized.

## Anaesthetic management
- Ensure a defibrillator and resuscitation drugs are available in the anaesthetic room.
- Patient monitoring should include:
  - Five-lead ECG
  - $SpO_2$
  - CVP
  - Nasopharyngeal temperature following induction of anaesthesia
  - Arterial line for invasive BP monitoring.
- Preoxygenate for at least 3 minutes.
- Prophylactic antibiotic therapy for some procedures.
- Hypertension and tachycardia should be avoided.

## Cardiopulmonary bypass

- Cardiopulmonary bypass is the joint responsibility of surgeons, anaesthetists, and clinical perfusionists but the safety of the cardiopulmonary bypass remains the primary responsibility of the perfusionist who must be present at all times.
- Only an accredited clinical perfusionist registered with the College of Clinical Perfusion Scientists of Great Britain and Ireland can undertake or supervise the conduct of cardiopulmonary bypass.
- Anticoagulant therapy prior to commencement of bypass.
- Once bypass has commenced, the ventilator should be turned off and IV anaesthesia administered.
- Blood gases and activated clotting time should be checked every 30 minutes.
- It is sometimes necessary to lower the patient's temperature.

> Cardiopulmonary bypass replaces the function of the heart and lungs while the heart is arrested, allowing for a bloodless and stable surgical field.

Although not an exhaustive list, the monitoring equipment identified in Box 12.7 should be used and recorded continuously, according to local protocol.

### Box 12.7 Monitoring equipment for cardiopulmonary bypass

- ECG.
- Systemic arterial pressure.
- CVP.
- Core body temperature.
- Urine output using a freely draining urinary catheter.
- Pulse oximetry.
- Expired $CO_2$ tension/concentration should be continuously displayed when the lungs are being ventilated.
- BIS monitoring should be considered particularly in the presence and use of volatile anaesthetic agents during cardiopulmonary bypass.
- Near infrared spectroscopy for cerebral oximetry monitoring should also be considered for certain procedures requiring cardiopulmonary bypass, for example, paediatric procedures, aortic root/arch surgery, in patients with carotid artery disease, procedures involving the use of retrograde arterial flow.

Source: data from the Society of Clinical Perfusion Scientists of Great Britain & Ireland (2016).

## Postoperative management

- Patients are usually transferred immediately to ITU.
- Adequate postoperative analgesia and physiotherapy is recommended to reduce the incidence of respiratory dysfunction and aid mobilization.
- $O_2$ that is warmed and humidified should be administered postoperatively.

- Close observation of the patient is essential to monitor signs of complications.
- For transfer to ITU:
  - $O_2$.
  - Ventilatory support.
  - Continuous monitoring (ECG, $SpO_2$, BP).
  - Drug infusion pumps.
  - Anaesthetic assistance for emergencies.
  - Sedative, analgesic, and resuscitation drugs.

## Reference

1. Simpson PJ, Popat M (2002). Understanding anaesthesia (4th ed). Oxford: Butterworth-Heinemann.

## Further reading

Association of Anaesthetists of Great Britain and Ireland (2016). Recommendations for standards of monitoring during anaesthesia and recovery 2015. Anaesthesia, 71(1):85–93.

Freedman R, Herbert L, O'Donnell A, et al. (eds) (2022). Oxford handbook of anaesthesia (5th ed). Oxford: Oxford University Press.

Leaper DJ, Whitaker I (eds) (2010). Handbook of Postoperative Complications (2nd ed). Oxford: Oxford University Press.

Martin A, Allman K, McIndoe A (eds) (2020). Emergencies in anaesthesia (3rd ed). Oxford: Oxford University Press.

National Institute for Health and Care Excellence (2020). Intravenous fluid therapy in children and young people in hospital. NICE guideline [NG29]. Available at: ℜ https://www.nice.org.uk/guidance/ng29

National Institute for Health and Care Excellence (2020). Venous thromboembolic diseases: diagnosis, management and thrombophilia testing. NICE guideline [NG158]. Available at: ℜ https://www.nice.org.uk/guidance/ng158

Royal College of Anaesthetists (2020). Chapter 18: guidelines for the provision of anaesthesia services for cardiac and thoracic procedures. London: Royal College of Anaesthetists.

Society of Clinical Perfusion Scientists of Great Britain & Ireland, Association of Cardiothoracic Anaesthetists, Society for Cardiothoracic Surgery in Great Britain & Ireland (2016). Recommendations for Standards of Monitoring during Cardiopulmonary Bypass. Available at: ℜ https://www.scps.org.uk/resources/useful-downloads

Wahba A, Milojevic M, Boer C, et al. (2020). 2019 EACTS/EACTA/EBCP guidelines on cardiopulmonary bypass in adult cardiac surgery. European Journal of Cardio-thoracic Surgery, 57(2):210–251.

# Bariatric anaesthesia

Obesity is an increasingly significant health issue in the UK, with 25% of the population classed as obese, and >3% as class 3 obesity (previously termed morbid obesity).[1]

- An operating table, hoists, beds, positioning aids, and transfer equipment appropriate for the care of bariatric patients should be available and staff should be trained in its use.
- Specialist positioning equipment for the induction of anaesthesia and intubation in the morbidly obese patient should be available.
- Experienced surgeons and anaesthetists are essential for bariatric patients requiring emergency surgery.
- One of the most important criteria for ensuring successful direct laryngoscopy and tracheal intubation is proper patient positioning.

There should be no restriction to treating a patient as a day case based on weight alone. Even morbidly obese patients can safely be managed in expert hands with appropriate resources.[2]

Patients with obstructive sleep apnoea have a higher incidence of postoperative complications including hypoxia, renal failure, unplanned ICU stay, and delayed discharge. Consideration should be given to monitoring these patients in a HDU (level 3) or critical care (level 3) environment postoperatively.[1,3]

- Level 2: patients requiring more detailed observation or intervention including support for a single failing organ system or postoperative care or those 'stepping down' from level 3 care.
- Level 3: patients requiring advanced respiratory support alone, or basic respiratory support together with support of at least two organ systems. This level includes all complex patients requiring support for multiorgan failure.

There must be enough trained and experienced staff in theatre to assist with moving the patient quickly.

The Society for Obesity and Bariatric Anaesthesia[4] has developed an obesity pack to be stored in recovery and available at all times. The pack includes essential equipment to ensure the safe management of bariatric patient (Box 12.8).

Obese patients present a different set of challenges and require specific perioperative care compared with non-obese patients.[5]

In the postoperative period, the safety of obese patients may be improved by:

- Supplemental $O_2$
- Non-invasive ventilation (CPAP)
- Monitoring of sedation
- Continuous pulse oximetry.

The PACU should also have the necessary equipment and staff to provide this.[3]

## Box 12.8 Obesity items for anaesthesia

- Large/XL/XXL BP cuff.
- Difficult airway equipment.
- Airtrach and bougie.
- Awake fibreoptic intubation equipment.
- Sevoflurane/desflurane.
- Neuromuscular block monitor.
- Long epidural and spinal needles.
- Fluid warming equipment.
- Infusion pumps.
- Slide sheet.
- Gel padding.
- Shoulder wedge.

*Source:* data from Society for Obesity and Bariatric Anaesthesia (2015). Guidelines for anaesthesia.

## References

1. Royal College of Anaesthetists (2020). Chapter 5: guidelines for the provision of emergency anaesthesia. London: Royal College of Anaesthetists.
2. Bailey CR, Ahuja M, Bartholomew K, et al. (2019). Guidelines for day-case surgery 2019: guidelines from the Association of Anaesthetists and the British Association of Day Surgery. Anaesthesia, 74(6):778–792.
3. Royal College of Anaesthetists (2019). Chapter 4: guidelines for the provision of postoperative care. London: Royal College of Anaesthetists.
4. Society for Obesity and Bariatric Anaesthesia (2015). Guidelines for anaesthesia. Available at: ℘ https://www.sobauk.co.uk/guidelines-1
5. Association of Anaesthetists of Great Britain and Ireland (2016). Recommendations for standards of monitoring during anaesthesia and recovery 2015. Anaesthesia, 71(1):85–93.

## Further reading

Association of Anaesthetists of Great Britain and Ireland (2015). Peri-operative management of the obese surgical patient. London: Association of Anaesthetists of Great Britain and Ireland.

Bouch C, Cousins J (eds) (2018). Core topics in anaesthesia and perioperative care of the morbidly obese surgical patient. Cambridge: Cambridge University Press.

Leaper DJ, Whitaker I (eds) (2010). Handbook of postoperative complications (2nd ed). Oxford: Oxford University Press.

National Institute for Health and Care Excellence (2014). Obesity: identification, assessment and management. Clinical guideline [CG189]. Available at: ℘ https://www.nice.org.uk/guidance/cg189/

National Institute for Health and Care Excellence (2015). Obesity prevention. Clinical guidance [CG43]. Available at: ℘ https://www.nice.org.uk/guidance/cg43

National Institute for Health and Care Excellence (2016). Surgery for obese adults. Available at: ℘ https://pathways.nice.org.uk/pathways/obesity

Sinha A (ed) (2016). Morbid obesity: anaesthesia and perioperative management. Delhi: Byword Books.

# Thoracic anaesthesia

Patients presenting for thoracic surgery can have limited respiratory reserve and pulmonary function. Successful thoracic anaesthesia requires the ability to control ventilation of both lungs independently, skilled management of the shared lung and airway, and a clear understanding of planned surgery. See Box 12.9 for examples of procedures.

---

**Box 12.9 Examples of thoracic surgical procedures**

- Oesophagectomy.
- Thoracotomy.
- Thymectomy.
- Pneumonectomy.
- Pleurectomy.
- Mediastinoscopy.
- Mediastinotomy.
- Lobectomy.
- Rigid bronchoscopy and stent insertion.
- Lung volume reduction and bulletectomy.
- Repair of broncho-pleural fistula.
- Wedge resection of lung.
- Lung biopsy.

---

## Anaesthetic management

- Comprehensive preassessment should include:
  - Past medical history including cardiac events
  - Assessment of cardiorespiratory reserve
  - Observe colour, signs of cyanosis, breathlessness
  - Monitor vital signs including NIBP
  - 12-lead ECG.
- Assessment of airway.
- Smoking cessation and preoperative physiotherapy is recommended prior to elective thoracic surgery to optimize lung function.

Dedicated equipment for jet ventilation should be available for interventional airway procedures.[1]

## One-lung ventilation

- Double-lumen endobronchial tubes (DLTs) are recommended for intubation.
- A left DLT is advocated for surgery on the right lung.
- A right DLT is advocated for surgery on the left lung.
- Confirmation should be sought to assess the position of a DLT.
- Two-lung ventilation should be recommenced slowly following surgery except where a pneumonectomy has been performed.[1]

Fibreoptic bronchoscopy should be immediately available for all cases where lung isolation is used.[1]

## Postoperative management

- Non-invasive ventilation facilities should be available in the immediate postoperative period, for example, bilevel positive airway pressure (BiPAP), CPAP, and high-flow nasal oxygen therapy (HFNO).
- Postoperative ventilation should be avoided due to excess stress on pulmonary suture lines.
- Adequate postoperative analgesia and physiotherapy is recommended to reduce the incidence of respiratory dysfunction and aid mobilization.
- $O_2$ that is warmed and humidified should be administered postoperatively.
- *Close observation of the patient is essential to monitor signs of complications.* These can include:
  - Bleeding
  - Cardiac arrhythmias
  - Pulmonary oedema
  - Retention of secretions
  - Basal atelectasis/consolidation
- A thoracic epidural should be considered for postoperative analgesia.
- For transfer to ITU:
  - $O_2$.
  - Ventilatory support.
  - Continuous monitoring (ECG, $SpO_2$, BP).
  - Drug infusion pumps.
  - Assistance for emergencies.
  - Sedative, analgesic, and resuscitation drugs.

## Intrapleural drainage

*Indications for use*

- To allow the lung to reinflate.
- To facilitate drainage of air, blood, and fluid from the pleural space.

*Care of chest drains*

- Patients should be monitored closely for any change in respiratory and cardiovascular status. This includes $SpO_2$, respiratory rate and pattern, colour, unequal chest movement, blood gases, BP, and heart rate.
- Ensure patient comfort with upright positioning.
- The drain and drain tubing must remain secure at all times.
- The drain must be well positioned—observe for kinks.
- Clamps must be available close to the patient in case of accidental disconnection.
- The drain must remain below the chest—volume and output must be recorded on a fluid balance chart.

*If a drain becomes disconnected*

- Call for medical assistance.
- Reconnect the drain immediately.
- Encourage coughing to dispel air.
- Arrange for chest X-ray to assess changes in condition.

## Robotic assisted surgery

Robot-assisted thoracic surgery (RATS) is currently undertaken in a small number of UK centres and may provide better surgical outcomes due to improved surgical dexterity and stereoscopic high-definition operating conditions.[1] Surgery using the da Vinci robotic system has been deemed safe, is associated with lower morbidity and mortality rates than thoracotomy, leads to shorter postoperative hospital stays, and ensures improved postoperative quality of life.[2]

## References

1. Royal College of Anaesthetists (2020). Chapter 18: guidelines for the provision of anaesthesia services for cardiac and thoracic procedures. London: Royal College of Anaesthetists.
2. Suda K (2017). Transition from video-assisted thoracic surgery to robotic pulmonary surgery. Journal of Visualised Surgery, 3:55.

## Further reading

Association of Anaesthetists of Great Britain and Ireland (2016). Recommendations for standards of monitoring during anaesthesia and recovery 2015. Anaesthesia, 71(1):85–93.

Freedman R, Herbert L, O'Donnell A, et al. (eds) (2022). Oxford handbook of anaesthesia (5th ed). Oxford: Oxford University Press.

Leaper DJ, Whitaker I (eds) (2010). Handbook of postoperative complications (2nd ed). Oxford: Oxford University Press.

Martin A, Allman K, McIndoe A (eds) (2020). Emergencies in anaesthesia (3rd ed). Oxford: Oxford University Press.

National Institute for Health and Care Excellence (2020). Intravenous fluid therapy in children and young people in hospital. NICE guideline [NG29]. Available at: ℘ https://www.nice.org.uk/guidance/ng29

National Institute for Health and Care Excellence (2020). Venous thromboembolic diseases: diagnosis, management and thrombophilia testing. NICE guideline [NG158]. Available at: ℘ https://www.nice.org.uk/guidance/ng158

Society of Clinical Perfusion Scientists of Great Britain & Ireland, Association of Cardiothoracic Anaesthetists, Society for Cardiothoracic Surgery in Great Britain & Ireland (2016). Recommendations for Standards of Monitoring during Cardiopulmonary Bypass. Available at: ℘ https://www.scps.org.uk/resources/useful-downloads

# Anaesthesia for day surgery

Day surgery is the planned admission of a surgical patient for an elective or semi-elective procedure where the patient is admitted, undergoes surgery, and is discharged on the same calendar day. If the patient remains in a hospital bed overnight on the day of their surgery they are classed as having undergone inpatient surgery.[1]

The AAGBI emphasizes that a condition of day surgery is that pain, nausea, and vomiting must be controlled and that day-case anaesthesia and surgery must be based on proven patient safety and quality of care. Surgical procedures must meet certain criteria for day surgery:

- Minimal blood loss expected.
- Short operating time (<1 hour).
- No expected intraoperative or postoperative complications.
- No requirement for specialist aftercare.

Examples of procedures and pain intensity associated with day-surgery procedures are identified in Table 12.3.[3]

## Anaesthetic management

| No pain | Mild pain | Moderate pain | Severe pain |
|---------|-----------|---------------|-------------|
| Cystoscopy Change of plaster of Paris Examination under anaesthetic of ears IV biological therapy | Adenoidectomy Antral washout Cataract surgery Myringotomy/ insertion of grommets Reduction of nasal fracture Removal of sebaceous cyst/ skin lesion Sigmoidoscopy Termination of pregnancy | Arthroscopy ± meniscectomy Carpel tunnel decompression Cervical and vulval surgery Excision of breast lump Gastric bypass Hysteroscopy/ D&C Laparoscopy Middle ear surgery Vaginal sling Varicose veins stripping/ligation | Anterior cruciate ligament reconstruction Circumcision/ orchidopexy Endometrial ablation Dental extraction (wisdom teeth) Haemorrhoidectomy Inguinal hernia repair Laparoscopic cholecystectomy Shoulder surgery Tonsillectomy |

*Source:* data from Bailey CR et al. (2019). Guidelines for day-case surgery. London: Association of Anaesthetists and the British Association of Day Surgery. Available at: https://anaesthetists. org/Home/Resources-publications/Guidelines/Day-case-surgery

- The anaesthetic technique should induce minimum stress and maximum comfort for the patient.
- Premedication is not recommended except in exceptional circumstances.
- Many anaesthetists advocate propofol-based techniques, due to their beneficial reduction of PONV.

- Prophylactic antiemetic therapy should only be considered in patients with a history of perioperative PONV and some surgical procedures; this might include laparoscopic sterilization, laparoscopic cholecystectomy, and tonsillectomy.
- GA and regional anaesthesia are suitable for day surgery.
- If regional anaesthesia is employed, the patient should be placed at the beginning of the operating theatre list to allow time for the anaesthetic to 'wear off'.
- Caution should be employed if considering femoral nerve blocks in adults; this is due to potential mobility difficulties if sensation is not regained prior to discharge.

## Anaesthetic technique

- Consider TIVA with propofol and incremental doses of fentanyl (without $N_2O$).
- LMA is recommended where possible in place of intubation.
- Consideration must to be given to prevention and treatment of PONV and pain management.
- Consider low-dose spinal anaesthesia for patients who would normally be excluded for GA.
- Fine-bore pencil-point needles reduce the incidence of a post-dural puncture headache.
- If a patient experiences 'no demonstrable block', the British Association of Day Surgery advises that the spinal anaesthetic can be repeated or converted to a GA.[3]
- The advantages of spinal anaesthesia include:
  - Fewer problems with respiratory function and airway management
  - Patients may observe surgery and discuss options with the surgeon
  - Reduction in perioperative venous thromboembolic disease
  - Reduced incidence of PONV
  - Immediate return to normal oral intake—particularly for patients with diabetes
  - NSAIDs as an adjunct to anaesthesia should be considered
  - Morphine can be administered postoperatively if required
  - Reasons why a patient's hospital stay might be extended are identified in Box 12.10.

---

**Box 12.10  Potential reasons for an extended hospital stay**

- Postoperative complications—unexpected.
- Unexpected extensive surgery.
- Inadequate social circumstances.
- Patient does not meet discharge criteria prior to unit closing.
- Uncontrolled pain.
- Uncontrolled nausea and vomiting.

## Older patients

- Older patients are increasingly being listed for day-case surgery as they can safely be operated on in the day surgery environment.
- Admission to hospital for older patients can trigger confusion resulting from disorientation and disruption of their usual routine so day case surgery is usually the optimal pathway for these patients as it is associated with less adverse outcomes.[3]
- *Always check* older patients for signs of dehydration and hypoglycaemia during the perioperative phase.

## Children

A preadmission programme for children should be considered, to decrease the impact and stress of admission to the DSU on the day of surgery.[1]

- Perioperative staff caring for children should be skilled in paediatric and day surgical care and trained in child protection.
- Infants, children, and young people should be managed in a dedicated paediatric unit, or have specific time allocated in a mixed adult/paediatric unit, where they are separated from adult patients.

## References

1. Royal College of Anaesthetists (2020). Chapter 6: guidelines for the provision of anaesthesia services for day surgery. London: Royal College of Anaesthetists.
2. Association of Anaesthetists of Great Britain and Ireland (2016). Recommendations for standards of monitoring during anaesthesia and recovery 2015. Anaesthesia, 71(1):85–93.
3. Bailey CR, Ahuja M, Bartholomew K, et al. (2019). Guidelines for day-case surgery 2019: guidelines from the Association of Anaesthetists and the British Association of Day Surgery. Anaesthesia, 74(6):778–792.

## Further reading

Al-Shaikh B, Stacey S (2018). Essentials of equipment in anaesthesia, critical care and perioperative medicine (5th ed). Edinburgh: Elsevier.
Freedman R, Herbert L, O'Donnell A, et al. (eds) (2022). Oxford handbook of anaesthesia (5th ed). Oxford: Oxford University Press.
Leaper DJ, Whitaker I (eds) (2010). Handbook of postoperative complications (2nd ed). Oxford: Oxford University Press.

# Outreach/out-of-hours anaesthesia

Outreach environments can be challenging for the safe provision of anaesthesia when compared with the main theatre environment.

- There are increasing numbers of surgical diagnostic and therapeutic procedures performed outside of the main operating theatre environment.
- Such procedures may require anaesthetic interventions through monitored care, sedation, regional anaesthesia, or GA.[1]
- Outreach and emergency out-of-hours anaesthesia has always been a fundamental part of perioperative care. As such, patient safety risks are heightened so, where possible, services should be planned in order to deliver high-quality patient care.
- Only immediate or urgent procedures should be conducted after 21.00 hours.

> - Special consideration should be given to the very young, the very old, and the clinically unstable patient who should be operated on during the day where possible.[1]

- The anaesthetist must be accompanied by a suitably skilled anaesthetic assistant when an anaesthetic intervention is planned in all outreach environments. Personnel should be certified resuscitation providers.
- Environments in which patients receive anaesthesia or sedation should have full facilities for resuscitation available, including a defibrillator, suction, $O_2$, airway devices, and a means of providing ventilation.[2]
- Wherever anaesthesia or sedation is undertaken, a full range of emergency drugs including specific reversal agents such as naloxone, sugammadex, and flumazenil should be made available.

> Equipment for monitoring should be available at all sites where patients receive anaesthesia or sedation. This must include pulse oximetry for patients receiving conscious sedation.

## Anaesthesia in ITU

Intensive care is appropriate for patients with severe or life-threatening illnesses, requiring or likely to require:

- Advanced respiratory support
- Support of two or more organ systems
- Patients with chronic impairment of one or more organ systems who also require support for an acute reversible failure of another organ.

The classification of critical care patients is identified in Table 12.4.

In the intensive care setting, it is common to perform a variety of invasive procedures for aiding in both diagnosis and treatment. These procedures (Box 12.11) may require anaesthetic interventions through monitored care, sedation, regional anaesthesia, or GA.[1]

**Table 12.4** Classification of critical care patients

| Level 0 | Patients whose needs can be met through normal ward care in an acute hospital |
| --- | --- |
| Level 1 | Patients at risk of their condition deteriorating, or those recently relocated from higher levels of care, whose needs can be met on an acute ward with additional advice and support from the critical care team |
| Level 2 | Patients requiring more detailed observation or intervention including support for a single failing organ system or postoperative care or those 'stepping down' from level 3 care |
| Level 3 | Patients requiring advanced respiratory support alone, or basic respiratory support together with support of at least two organ systems. This level includes all complex patients requiring support for multiorgan failure |

- Unfortunately, such procedures are not without risk of complications. Patients requiring anaesthesia in an ICU are often critically ill or injured.
- Anaesthetic assistance is not usually required in the ITU environment as a skilled/trained nurse/ODP will be competent to assist the anaesthetist.
- Children should always be managed in accordance with RCoA and Association of Paediatric Anaesthetists of Great Britain and Ireland recommendations.
- Staff should remain as distant from the imaging source as possible.
- Screens or lead gowns should be used to reduce exposure to ionizing radiation.
- Interventional vascular radiology may involve treating unstable patients with severe haemorrhage, for example, GI bleeding, post-partum haemorrhage.
- The following equipment should be available to manage these patients: a variety of intravascular catheters, rapid infusion devices, blood and fluid warming devices, and patient warming devices.

### Box 12.11 Procedures that may require anaesthesia in ITU
- Radiology.
- Percutaneous tracheostomy.
- Intubation.
- Central line insertion.
- Bronchoscopy.
- Pericardiocentesis.
- Paracentesis.
- Lumbar puncture.
- Cardioversion.
- Percutaneous endoscopic gastrostomy tube placement.
- Temporary cardiac pacing.

## Magnetic resonance imaging

- MRI is a widely used diagnostic tool used to investigate many conditions.
- Patients must be accompanied to the scanner by appropriately trained staff members.
- As magnetic field strengths have increased, many patients are now scanned with active implanted medical devices such as neurostimulators, pacemakers, and drug pumps, which augment the challenges for the anaesthetic team.
- If an anaesthetic machine is to be used in the MRI unit, or has the potential to be used, a trained anaesthetic assistant must be present to support the anaesthetist for the duration of the scan.
- The anaesthetic machine and equipment should be checked before transfer or induction.
- The MRI safety checklists for GA, intraoperative MRI, and for transfer of ICU patients should be used in combination with the WHO patient safety checklist:

> - The combination of a continuous strong magnetic field, reduced patient access, and a site frequently remote from the operating theatre suite means that these cases are complex.

- Children and young people may require sedation or GA to enable acceptable images to be produced.
- A child-friendly environment and atmosphere may help minimize the need for sedation.
- Parental presence and/or distraction therapy can be used to improve the compliance of children.
- Performing MRI scans in critically ill patients can be challenging due to the increased risks of the patient's critical condition and the distant location of the scanner.
- Intraoperative MRI can be used to enhance the accuracy and safety of invasive and therapeutic procedures, particularly in neurosurgery, where it has improved the safety and outcomes for tumour resection and epilepsy surgery.

## Emergency department

Patients requiring anaesthesia in the emergency department (ED) are frequently critically ill or injured.

- Emergency airway management in the ED should follow the joint guidance from the RCoA and Royal College of Emergency Medicine.
- Transfer of patients within the hospital to the ICU, radiology, or the operating theatre is not without risk and will require the use of a tipping transfer trolley, $O_2$ cylinders, suction, a transport ventilator, infusion pumps, monitor with adequate battery life, and a portable defibrillator if appropriate.
- The role of the skilled assistant can be undertaken by a number of professionals in the emergency care setting, for example, emergency nurse, anaesthetic nurse practitioner, or an operating department practitioner. They must be formally trained in the role that they will be required to undertake, be that assistance with sedation or assistance with RSI.

- Fasting is not needed for minimal sedation or moderate sedation where verbal contact is maintained.

> - The use of continuous capnography is mandatory wherever deep sedation, dissociative sedation, or GA occurs, and is also recommended at lighter levels of sedation.

- $O_2$ should be given to sedated patients, who may experience a fall in $O_2$ saturation from the baseline level measured on room air. $O_2$ should be given from the start of sedative administration until the patient is ready for discharge from the recovery area.
- Where there is a risk of aspiration, the procedure should be delayed if clinically appropriate.
- Regional anaesthetic techniques may allow the required procedure to be performed with minimal sedation.

## Electroconvulsive therapy

Electroconvulsive therapy (ECT) remains a mainstay treatment option in psychiatry and is used primarily in depression when there is an urgent need for treatment or secondarily after failure or intolerance to pharmacotherapy.
- The aim is to induce a generalized seizure with characteristic EEG changes.
- Contraindications might include raised ICP, recent cerebrovascular accident, untreated cerebral aneurysm, myocardial ischaemia or uncontrolled cardiac failure, unstable major fracture, and severe osteoporosis.

> - The commonest side effects of ECT are confusion, agitation, violent behaviour, amnesia, headache, myalgia, and nausea and vomiting.

- Several modifications have occurred in the last 30 years to increase the safety and patient acceptability of ECT, including GA and muscle relaxation.
- Anaesthesia for ECT is frequently performed in remote locations.
- Anaesthetic techniques including medications are considered to provide adequate therapeutic seizure, simultaneously controlling seizure-induced haemodynamic changes and side effects.
- The level of anaesthesia should not be so deep as to overly suppress the seizure activity which is the goal of the treatment.
- Equipment for managing the airway, including the difficult airway, emergency drugs, resuscitation equipment, and defibrillator should all be available.
- Standards for monitoring and recovery are stipulated by the Association of Anaesthetists and should be adhered to for all ECT cases.
- Succinylcholine is the muscle relaxation of choice due to its rapid onset and short duration. Sevoflurane is the inhalational induction agent used in ECT, as it produces skeletal muscle relaxation and enhances the effects of neuromuscular blocking agents.

## Coronary care unit

Patients with tachyarrhythmias and recent-onset, symptomatic atrial fibrillation (AF) commonly undergo immediate restoration of sinus rhythm by means of pharmacological or electrical (DC) cardioversion.

- AF can sometimes terminate spontaneously.
- Patients may present as an emergency or elective case.
- DC cardioversion requires sedation to facilitate the procedure, as it is painful and distressing for the patient.
- Anaesthesia is usually performed in a specialized cardiac care unit.
- If an anaesthetic machine is to be used, or has the potential to be used, a trained anaesthetic assistant must be present to support the anaesthetist for the duration of the procedure.
- The anaesthetic machine and equipment should be checked before induction.
- Propofol is the preferred anaesthetic induction agent as it is short acting, and produces conscious sedation, to enable rapid recovery after the procedure.

- In older patients with heart disease, etomidate with fentanyl may improve haemodynamic stability.

- Conscious sedation with midazolam for DC cardioversion of AF can be safe and effective as it does not adversely affect respiratory function.
- Anaesthetic or sedative agents that do not have cardiovascular side effects are preferable for cardioversion, as many patients have underlying cardiovascular disease.
- Opiate analgesia may be used in conjunction with anaesthetic agents.
- Atropine is sometimes used before the procedure to reduce the risk of vagus nerve-induced bradyarrhythmia.

## References

1. Royal College of Anaesthetists (2020). Chapter 7: guidelines for the provision of anaesthesia services in the non-theatre environment. London: Royal College of Anaesthetists.
2. Soar J, Nolan JP, Böttiger BW, et al. (2015). European Resuscitation Council guidelines for resuscitation. Section 3: adult advanced life support. Resuscitation, 95:100–147.

## Further reading

Association of Anaesthetists of Great Britain and Ireland (2018). The anaesthesia team. Available at: ℛ http://dx.doi.org/10.21466/g.TAT.2018

Association of Anaesthetists of Great Britain and Ireland (2019). Checklist for draw-over anaesthetic equipment. Available at: ℛ http://dx.doi.org/10.21466/g.CFDAE2.2019

de Oliveira Wafae BG, da Silva RMF, Veloso HH (2019). Propofol for sedation for direct current cardioversion. Annals of Cardiac Anaesthesia, 22(2):113–121.

Faculty of Intensive Care Medicine, Intensive Care Society (2019) Guidelines for the provision of intensive care services. Available at: ℛ https://www.ficm.ac.uk/sites/default/files/gpics-v2.pdf

Freedman R, Herbert L, O'Donnell A, et al. (eds) (2022). Oxford handbook of anaesthesia (5th ed). Oxford: Oxford University Press.

Kadiyala PK, Kadiyala LD (2017). Anaesthesia for electroconvulsive therapy: an overview with an update on its role in potentiating electroconvulsive therapy. Indian Journal of Anaesthesia, 61(5):373–380.

Lewis SR, Nicholson A, Reed SS, et al. (2015). Anaesthetic and sedative agents used for electrical cardioversion. Cochrane Database of Systematic Reviews, 2015(3):CD010824.

Vishal U, Dourish J, Macfarlane A (2010). Anaesthesia for electroconvulsive therapy. British Journal of Anaesthesia, 10(6):192–196.

Wilson SR, Shinde S, Appleby I, et al. (2019). Guidelines for the safe provision of anaesthesia in magnetic resonance units: guidelines from the Association of Anaesthetists and the Neuro Anaesthesia and Critical Care Society of Great Britain and Ireland. Anaesthesia, 74(5):638–650.

# Patient skin preparation

# Surgical site infection

Surgical site infections (SSIs) are one of the commonest healthcare-associated infections. As well as causing distress to patients they are estimated to cost the NHS in excess of 1 billion pounds each year.[1] The incidence of SSI is around 2–5% of patients[2] though this may be underestimated due to a lack of good postoperative surveillance data.

SSIs are classified by their location and can be superficial incisional, deep incisional, or organ/space. The Centres for Disease Control provides detailed definitions for each classification of SSI.[3] A general definition is that an SSI occurs within 30 days of surgery (1 year if there is an implant), exudes pus, swabs positive for organisms, and shows one of the following: pain, localized swelling, redness, or heat. Patients who are immunocompromised may not produce pus, swelling, or redness due to diminished white blood cells but may exhibit fever or pain at the infection site.

## Bacterial sources for SSIs

Most SSIs arise from bacteria, predominantly *Staphylococcus aureus*, entering the wound during the operative phase. The sources of these bacteria are the operating room environment, operating room staff and the surgical team, the surgical procedure, and the patient.

## Risk factors for acquiring an SSI

Several factors affect the risk of patients acquiring an SSI. These relate to bacterial exposure during surgery and the body's ability to fight and overcome the infection. For example, during long surgical procedures there is more opportunity for bacteria from the operating team and the theatre environment to enter the incision site. Hypothermic patients will have reduced blood supply to the incision site and therefore the cellular response will be reduced.

*The following factors affect the risk of patients developing an SSI*
- Patient's overall state of health or increased dependence.
- Increased BMI.
- Increased age.
- More severe surgical wound classification score (see below).
- Pre-existing local or systemic infection.
- *S. aureus* colonization.
- Female sex.
- Poor tissue perfusion—diabetes, vascular disease, hypotensive anaesthesia, hypothermia.
- Increased length of hospital stay and/or use of medical device.[4]

Each patient's risk of developing an SSI can be calculated by using a risk score. Despite recognized limitations from published studies in some surgery types, the most widely used risk tool is the National Nosocomial Infections Surveillance (NNIS) score. This is calculated from the patient's ASA classification, wound class, and duration of operation.[5]

## Surgical wound classification

Surgical wounds are classified as clean, clean contaminated, contaminated, and dirty. Each category is associated with an increasing risk for developing an SSI.

- *Clean*: an uninfected surgical wound where the respiratory, GI, and genitourinary tracts are not incised.
- *Clean contaminated*: surgery where the respiratory, GI, and genitourinary tracts are incised under controlled conditions with minimal spillage.
- *Contaminated*: infected wounds (without pus) or recently traumatized wounds, or with a major spillage from the GI or genitourinary tracts.
- *Dirty/infected*: surgery in infected wounds with pus or involving trauma wounds >4 hours old.

## Practices to reduce SSI

Practices are undertaken to reduce the opportunity for bacteria to be transferred to the surgical site, multiply, and cause infections. Common practices include the following;

- Environmental:
  - Theatre layout design.
  - Minimal traffic through theatres.
  - Specialized ventilation.
- Theatre personnel and the surgical team:
  - Surgical attire.
  - Surgical hand antisepsis.
  - Aseptic techniques.
- Patient preparation:
  - Antiseptic skin preparation.
  - Preoperative hair removal.
  - Total body washing.
- Surgical techniques:
  - Intraoperative antibiotics.
  - Minimally invasive surgery.
  - Shorter procedures.
  - Surgical drapes.
  - Single-use items.

## References

1. Health Protection Agency (2019). English National Point Prevalence Survey on healthcare associated infections and antimicrobial use: preliminary data. London: Health Protection Agency.
2. National Audit Office (2004). Improving patient care by reducing the risk of hospital acquired infection. Report by the Comptroller and Auditor General HC 876 Session 2003–2004. London: The Stationery Office.
3. Mangram A, Horan T, Pearson M, et al. (1999). Guideline for prevention of surgical site infection. Infection Control and Hospital Epidemiology, 20(4):247–278.
4. Korol E, Johnston K, Waser N, et al. (2013). A systematic review of risk factors associated with surgical site infections among surgical patients. PLoS One, 8(12):e83743.
5. National Nosocomial Infections Surveillance (2004). National Nosocomial Infections Surveillance (NNIS) System Report, data summary from January 1992 through June 2004, issued October 2004. American Journal of Infection Control, 32(8):470–485.

## Further reading

National Institute for Health and Care Excellence (2014). Infection prevention and control. Quality standard [QS61]. Available at: ℘ https://www.nice.org.uk/guidance/qs61
National Institute for Health and Care Excellence (2019). Surgical site infections: prevention and treatment. NICE guideline [NG125]. Available at: ℘ https://www.nice.org.uk/guidance/ng125

# Antiseptic skin preparation

Skin is covered by two types of organisms: transient and resident. Resident organisms are the organisms which are normally found on an individual's skin and can include *Staphylococcus epidermidis* and coryneforms. Resident organisms can vary between individuals. For example, around 30% of people are colonized by *S. aureus*. Transient organisms are transferred to the surface of the skin through contact with a source. These organisms are not normally resident on the patient's skin and may include *S. aureus*, enterococci, Clostridia, and *Pseudomonas*. These organisms temporarily contaminate the skin but can be removed through simple hand washing. Resident organisms are harder to remove.

During surgery, transient and resident organisms can enter the incision site where they multiply and cause SSIs. Preoperative patient skin preparation involves using antiseptics and mechanical friction to remove transient organisms, reduce the number of resident organisms, and inhibit organism regrowth.

## Antiseptic solutions

An ideal antiseptic agent should have the following properties:
• A broad range of activity against Gram-negative and Gram-positive bacteria, viruses, and fungi.
• Fast acting.
• Have a residual effect.
• Not be inactivated by organic material.
• Non-irritant.
• Safe to use.

In the UK, the commonest antiseptic agents are povidone-iodine and chlorhexidine gluconate (CHG) in either alcohol or aqueous preparations. It should be noted that alcohol itself is an antiseptic. Choosing which solution to use depends on the area to be incised, the condition of the patient's skin, costs, and potential side effects.

## Alcohol

Alcohol is effective against a wide range of Gram-positive and Gram-negative bacteria, *Mycobacterium tuberculosis*, and many fungi and viruses. Compared with other common antiseptic products alcohol is associated with the most rapid and greatest reduction in microbial count, but it does not remove dirt and is not sporicidal. Alcohols have little or no residual effect but are very fast acting.

## Povidone-iodine

Povidone-iodine is effective against a wide range of Gram-positive and Gram-negative bacteria, *M. tuberculosis*, fungi, and viruses. It is a combination of polyvinylpyrrolidone (povidone) and iodine. Povidone prolongs the activity of iodine by releasing it slowly. Iodophors rapidly reduce transient and resident bacteria but have little residual effect. Iodine is inactivated by organic materials such as blood. Note that povidone-iodine concentrates in breast milk and should be used with caution in nursing mothers.

## Chlorhexidine gluconate

CHG is effective against a wide range of Gram-positive and Gram-negative bacteria, lipophilic viruses, and yeasts. It binds to the outermost layer of skin which results in a persistent activity. Repeated exposure can lead to a cumulative effect where both transient and resident organisms are reduced. CHG is effective in the presence of blood.

## Further reading

Dumville JC, McFarlane E, Edwards P, et al. (2015). Preoperative skin antiseptics for preventing surgical wound infections after clean surgery. Cochrane Database of Systematic Reviews, 4:CD003949.

Joint Formulary Committee (2022). British national formulary. London: BMJ Group and Pharmaceutical Press. Available at: ℘ http://www.medicinescomplete.com

National Institute for Health and Care Excellence (2014). Infection prevention and control. Quality standard [QS61]. Available at: ℘ https://www.nice.org.uk/guidance/qs61

National Institute for Health and Care Excellence (2019). Surgical site infections: prevention and treatment. NICE guideline [NG125]. Available at: ℘ https://www.nice.org.uk/guidance/ng125

# Applying antiseptic solutions

Applying antiseptic solution to the patient's skin immediately before surgery is commonly referred to as 'prepping' the patient. ➲ See p. 373 for infor-mation regarding the application of specific solutions.

### Prepping the patient's skin

- Before applying an antiseptic solution, the patient's skin should be assessed to identify any abrasions or rashes which should be documented. Check allergy status.
- The patient's skin should be clean before applying antiseptic solution as alcohol does not remove dirt and iodine is inactivated by organic material such as blood.
- Most antiseptic solutions are available in multiuse bottles and single-use sachets. Bottles are used more commonly though studies have shown bacteria growing on the inside of bottles.
- Once opened, a bottle of antiseptic solution should be labelled with the date. The length of time an open bottle can be kept varies between solutions; therefore, refer to manufacturers' instructions for this specific information. Bottles should not be refilled to allow tracking in the event of an infection outbreak.
- Try to keep the patient as warm as possible during skin preparation to enhance recovery and reduce SSIs. Most manufacturers advise storing antiseptic solutions at 25°C.
- Skin preparation is usually carried out by a member of the scrub team using an aseptic technique.
- The antiseptic solution can be applied with sterile swabs or sponges specifically manufactured for this process. The swabs and sponges are held with sterile forceps. If swabs are used for prepping, then they should be included in the swab count. ('One-step' prepping systems are also available where a sterile swab is attached to a sterile applicator containing a measured dose of antiseptic solution.)
- The skin should be rubbed gently with the swab to generate the mechanical friction required for cleaning without traumatizing the skin. Special care is needed when prepping skin near malignant cells to prevent dislodging cells.
- The area of skin to be prepped should extend beyond the intended incision site. It must allow for the incision to be extended during surgery, any drains to be sited, and accommodate drapes slipping during the procedure.
- Swabbing should begin at the incision site and move outwards. The principle is to move from 'clean to dirty'. Do not move a swab from an outer area back to the incision site as this may reintroduce bacteria.
- When a contaminated area is to be prepped, the surrounding clean skin should be prepped first. Heavily contaminated areas such as the perineum should be prepped last. This prevents spreading bacteria from dirty areas to clean areas.
- Isolate stoma sites. For example, these can be covered with sterile waterproof dressings.

- Do not dip a used swab back into the pot of antiseptic solution—use a fresh swab for each application.
- Do not allow solutions to pool as this can cause skin irritation and may facilitate a burn injury. Solutions should not come into contact with diathermy plates.
- Solutions should be in contact with the skin as long as possible to allow maximum antiseptic effect. Povidone-iodine should be in contact with the skin for at least 2 minutes as iodine is released slowly from its povidone carrier.
- Alcohol-based solutions should be allowed to air dry completely before draping commences.
- Povidone-iodine does not need to be rinsed off. This removes the active component of the antiseptic. Early preparations of iodine, before povidone iodine, were highly irritant if left in contact with the skin and had to be rinsed.
- The following information should be documented: condition of the skin, antiseptic solution used, reactions to the solution, and postoperative skin assessment.

### Indications, cautions, and contraindications

Solutions containing alcohol can cause drying and should not be applied to mucous membranes or sensitive skin, such as dry 'papery' skin in older patients. Iodine can cross mucous membranes. CHG 0.5% in cetrimide 0.015% is a possible alternative for prepping mucous membranes.

Iodine may be absorbed and it should be used with caution in patients who are pregnant, breastfeeding, or have renal impairment. Iodine is contraindicated in neonates and should not be used regularly for patients with thyroid disorders. If iodine is used on large wounds, it may cause metabolic acidosis, hypernatraemia, and impaired renal function. Iodine and chlorhexidine may cause corneal damage if in contact with eyes. Chlorhexidine should not be applied to the middle ear as it can cause functional impairment.

When preparing graft sites, colourless solutions should be used to allow the vascularity of the skin to be observed.

### Further reading

Association of periOperative Registered Nurses (2016). Guidelines for perioperative practice. Denver, CO: AORN Inc.

Association for Perioperative Practice (2016). Standards and recommendations for safe perioperative practice. Harrogate: Association for Perioperative Practice.

National Institute for Health and Care Excellence (2014). Infection prevention and control. Quality standard [QS61]. Available at: ⅍ https://www.nice.org.uk/guidance/qs61/

National Institute for Health and Care Excellence (2019). Surgical site infections: prevention and treatment. NICE guideline [NG125]. Available at: ⅍ https://www.nice.org.uk/guidance/ng125

# Preoperative hair removal

Hair is removed from the area surrounding the intended surgical site as its presence can interfere with the exposure of the incision, suturing, and the application of adhesive drapes and dressings. In addition, hair is perceived to be unclean and its removal is thought to reduce the risk of SSIs. However, hair removal can cause microscopic cuts and abrasions to skin which can become colonized and result in infections.

There are three methods of hair removal: shaving, clipping, and depilatory creams. Patients should be made aware if hair is to be removed as this may cause some distress. If hair is not removed, skin prep dry-time may need to be increased.

### Shaving

This method uses a sharp blade within the head of a razor, which is drawn over the patient's skin to cut hair close to the surface of the skin. Of the three hair removal methods, razors cause most damage to skin and patients shaved with a razor have the highest risk of developing SSIs.

### Clippers

Clippers use fine teeth to cut the hair close to the patient's skin leaving short stubble of around 1 mm in length. The heads of clippers should be disposed of or sterilized between patients to minimize the risk of cross infection.

### Depilatory creams

Depilatory creams use chemicals to dissolve the hair itself. This is a slower process than shaving or clipping as the cream has to remain in contact with hair for between 5 and 20 minutes. In addition, there is a risk of irritant or allergic reactions to the cream and patch tests should be carried out 24 hours in advance.

### Recommended method of hair removal

- Only remove hair when absolutely necessary.
- If removing hair, use clippers or cream as these cause fewer SSIs than razors.
- When using clippers or razors, hair should be removed as close to the start of the surgical procedure as possible to minimize the amount of time organisms have to colonize any cuts.
- When using cream, it is acceptable to remove hair the day before surgery. Patch tests should be carried out 24 hours before hair is removed.
- If hair is being removed at home using cream, this is likely to be carried out by the patient or carer.
- If hair is being removed in the hospital by razor or clippers, there is no evidence to show who is the best person to do this.
- Hair should not be removed in the operating theatre as loose hair may contaminate the sterile field.

## Further reading

National Institute for Health and Care Excellence (2019). Surgical site infections: prevention and treatment. NICE guideline [NG125]. Available at: ℘ https://www.nice.org.uk/guidance/ng125

Tanner J, Norrie P, Melen K (2011). Preoperative hair removal to reduce surgical site infection. Cochrane Database of Systematic Reviews, 11:CD004122.

# Total body washing

One factor which influences the risk of acquiring a SSI is the patient's bacterial burden, or the amount of bacteria on the patient's skin. Transient and resident bacteria from patients' skin can enter the surgical site where the bacteria then multiply and cause infections. The purpose of a preoperative body washing regimen is to make the skin as clean as possible by reducing transient and resident bacteria, therefore reducing the risk of SSI.

Though there is clear evidence that antiseptic solutions reduce bacteria on skin, evidence of the impact of total body washing in reducing SSIs is inconclusive. Several studies have shown mixed results and a Cochrane systematic review of total body washing to reduce SSI found no clear evidence.[1] However, there are good-quality studies[2] which show the effectiveness of total body washing in eliminating MRSA in patients prior to admission as part of a screening programme. Total body washing is also known as preoperative bathing or showering, or topical eradication.

## MRSA screening

MRSA screening is mandatory for elective and acute admissions to high-risk units and for all patients previously identified as infected or colonized.[3] Some hospitals screen all acute and elective surgical patients for MRSA prior to admission. Ideally, screening is carried out at least 2 weeks before the admission date to allow for results to be processed and treatment to be completed. Swabs are usually taken from the nose, groin/perineum, wound sites if present, urine if the patient is catheterized, and sputum if there is a productive cough. Patients who are MRSA positive will be prescribed a total body washing regimen, such as the one described next. Following completion of the body washing regimen, patients should be tested again for MRSA at least 48 hours after the end of antiseptic and (if applicable) antibiotic therapy.

In hospitals with screening programmes, non-elective patients may commence total body washing prophylactically on admission to hospital until rapid screening swab results can be obtained.

## Total body washing method of application

There is limited evidence to show the most effective method of body washing to reduce SSIs. Current practices range from a single bath or shower with antiseptic solution on the day of surgery to repeated applications in the week before surgery. Body washing protocols to eradicate MRSA, such as the one described here, are more intensive.

- Patients commence body washing 1 week before surgery or immediately after receiving positive identification from an MRSA screening programme.
- The body washing programme lasts 5 consecutive days.
- Patients wash once daily with an antiseptic solution, for example, triclosan or CHG.
- Hair should be washed with antiseptic solution a minimum of two times during the 5-day period.
- Mupirocin should be applied to the anterior nares three times daily for 5 days as the nose is a common site for harbouring MRSA.

## Special instructions

- Patients who show signs of a urinary tract infection and whose urine has tested positive for MRSA can be prescribed systemic antibiotics.
- Total body washing regimens to eradicate MRSA are generally limited to two courses as patients may become resistant to mupirocin.
- Patients with MRSA-positive sputum do not routinely require treatment unless the chest infection is causing an acute illness.

## References

1. Webster J, Osborne S (2015). Preoperative bathing or showering with skin antiseptics to prevent surgical site infection. Cochrane Database of Systematic Reviews, 2:CD004985.
2. Nixon M, Jackson B, Varghese P, et al. (2006). Methicillin-resistant Staphylococcus aureus on orthopaedic wards. Journal of Bone and Joint Surgery, 88(6):812–817.
3. Department of Health (2014). Implementation of modified admission MRSA screening guidance for NHS (2014). Department of Health expert advisory committee on Antimicrobial Resistance and Healthcare Associated Infection (ARHAI). Available at: ℞ https://www.gov.uk/government/uploads/system/uploads/attachment_data/file/345144/Implementation_of_modified_admission_MRSA_screening_guidance_for_NHS.pdf

## Further reading

National Institute for Health and Care Excellence (2019). Surgical site infections: prevention and treatment. NICE guideline [NG125]. Available at: ℞ https://www.nice.org.uk/guidance/ng125

# Chapter 14

# Operating theatre practice

# Theatre preparation: heating, lighting, and humidity

## Heating

There is no ideal temperature for an operating theatre that will be correct in all circumstances as it will depend on the type of surgery undertaken. For example, when operating on babies or young children, the temperature will often be higher to assist in maintaining the patient's core temperature, while in theatres carrying out cardiac surgery the temperature may be low to aid in the cooling of the patient. Consideration must also be made for the elderly patient and those undergoing procedures under LA or regional anaesthesia. The use of warming equipment to maintain the body temperature of the patient will usually mean that the ambient air temperature is less of a consideration and so can be set at a more comfortable working temperature for staff.

The ambient temperature will often be a level that is comfortable for the staff in which to work. The scrub team in particular may request that the temperature is low as they are wearing more protective clothing and are often standing under operating lights which emit heat. The wall-mounted control panel is used to select the desired room temperature. A general principle would be to adjust the temperature using small increments so that a general comfort level is achieved. Many modern operating theatres have a 'setback' control for the ventilation unit that can be used when the theatre is not in use so that the number of air changes within the theatre is reduced, thereby cutting back on electricity consumption. The ventilation system should be placed on to the full setting prior to commencing the operating list in accordance with local guidelines and the manufacturer's instructions.

Ventilation systems:
- Change the air at least fifteen times an hour
- Cause a positive air pressure within the theatre
- Force air in from the ceiling and out through exhaust panels
- Provide a unidirectional airflow to reduce the risk of airborne contamination.

## Lighting

Generally, lighting will be set to full for 'open' operations while some cases, particularly those in which telescopes, microscopes, cameras, and monitors are utilized, may require some of the lighting to be reduced to aid the surgeon's view of the surgical field. The positioning of the operating theatre light is crucial, particularly in surgery in deep cavities of the body. Several centres now have operating theatre lamps with handles which can be sterilized, enabling the surgical team to place the light in the best position to view the surgical field. Where circulating staff are required to position operating lamps, it is advisable for novice staff to familiarize themselves with equipment during a time that no patient is in the operating theatre.

## Humidity

Along with temperature controls many theatre departments have a wall-mounted control panel that controls the atmospheric humidity. This should be set to a level not >60% or <30% as this will minimize static electricity and reduce the potential for bacterial growth, while a higher rate could result in condensation of ambient moisture which may result in damp materials.

## Further reading

Association for Perioperative Practice (2016). Standards and recommendations for safe perioperative practice. Harrogate: Association for Perioperative Practice.

Association of periOperative Registered Nurses (2020). Guidelines for perioperative practice. Denver, CO: AORN Inc.

Australian College of Operating Room Nurses (2020). Standards for perioperative nursing. Adelaide: ACORN Ltd.

Phillips N, Hornacky A (2020). Berry & Kohn's operating room technique (14th ed). St Louis, MO: Elsevier.

Royal College of Ophthalmologists (2018). Ophthalmology service guidance: theatre facilities and equipment. London: Royal College of Ophthalmologists.

Sutherland-Fraser S, Davies M, Lockwood B, et al. (eds) (2021). Perioperative nursing: an introduction (3rd ed). Chatswood: Elsevier Australia.

# Cleaning of the operating theatre

At the end of a day or session the operating theatre must be cleaned in readiness for the following session; this is termed terminal cleaning and practice will vary between departments. All operating theatre departments will have policies for the cleaning process, the basic principles of which are:

• Furniture to be cleaned with an approved disinfectant
• Wheel and casters cleaned and any debris removed
• Horizontal surfaces are cleaned
• The floor is wet-scrubbed once the furniture is removed
• The furniture is replaced once the floor is dry.

The theatre may also be cleaned between cases as required, using a mop to clean spillage onto the floor. The used mop head should be dealt with in accordance with the local cleaning policy. Damp dusting of horizontal surfaces using the approved disinfectant prior to the commencement of the day's operating list may also be carried out to reduce the viable bacterial contamination.

## Further reading

Association for Perioperative Practice (2016). Standards and recommendations for safe perioperative practice. Harrogate: Association for Perioperative Practice.

Association of periOperative Registered Nurses (2020). Guidelines for perioperative practice. Denver, CO: AORN Inc.

Australian College of Operating Room Nurses (2020). Standards for perioperative nursing. Adelaide: ACORN Ltd.

Sutherland-Fraser S, Davies M, Lockwood B, et al. (eds) (2021). Perioperative nursing: an introduction (3rd ed). Chatswood: Elsevier Australia.

# Decontamination and sterilization of instruments

## Decontamination

Decontamination refers to the pre-sterilization process of reusable surgical and anaesthetic instruments which may be performed manually or by machine or, more usually, both. Used instruments are inspected for visible soil and may be manually brushed or washed. Delicate instruments and those with lumens may be decontaminated in an ultrasonic washer. Most instruments are washed in the washer/decontaminator machine which works much like a dishwasher and which would take approximately 1 hour. The purpose of decontamination is to make the instruments safe for the packing staff to handle during the packing process.

## Sterilization

There are nine types of sterilization available, most of which are generally not offered in the hospital setting—steam, ethylene oxide, dry heat, microwaves, formaldehyde gas, hydrogen peroxide plasma, ozone gas, chemical solutions, and ionizing radiation. Only the ones that are either used or commonly encountered will be considered here. To be considered sterile, all microorganisms and bacterial spores should be destroyed. Bacterial spores are the most resistant of all living organisms as they are able to withstand external destructive agents. Packaging is required to indicate that the item within the package is sterile by use of a marker that will have changed colour (e.g. autoclave tape), what method of sterilization has been used, the date of sterilization, and the expiry date, which is when the product can no longer be guaranteed as sterile.

### Steam

This is used in an autoclave with pressure greater than atmospheric to increase the temperature to achieve thermal destruction. The heated, pressurized steam must penetrate to reach the items to be sterilized. During the main sterilization cycle, the time that the steam is in contact with the instrument will depend on the temperature the autoclave reaches. At 130°C it is 3 minutes while at 120°C it is 15 minutes. At the end of the cycle, re-evaporation of water condensate must effectively dry contents of the load to maintain sterility. This method of sterilization is suitable for metal (stainless steel) instruments that are reusable and are designed to withstand the extreme temperature and is available in most UK hospitals.

### Ethylene oxide (EO)

This is suitable for heat- or moisture-sensitive items. EO gas must have direct contact with the organisms on, or in, the item. EO gas is highly inflammable and has to be contained within an explosion-proof chamber. It is also toxic and takes longer than steam sterilization, typically 16–18 hours for a cycle. EO is used commercially and in certain hospitals in the UK.

*Ionizing radiation*

This is the most effective form of sterilization but is only available for commercial use. The process uses beta particles and gamma rays and takes between 10 and 20 hours depending on the strength of the radiation source.

## Further reading

Association for Perioperative Practice (2016). Standards and recommendations for safe perioperative practice. Harrogate: Association for Perioperative Practice.

Association of periOperative Registered Nurses (2020). Guidelines for perioperative practice. Denver, CO: AORN Inc.

Australian College of Operating Room Nurses (2020). Standards for perioperative nursing. Adelaide: ACORN Ltd.

Phillips N, Hornacky A (2020). Berry & Kohn's operating room technique (14th ed). St Louis, MO: Elsevier.

Sutherland-Fraser S, Davies M, Lockwood B, et al. (eds) (2021). Perioperative nursing: an introduction (3rd ed). Chatswood: Elsevier Australia.

# Instrument management

## Checking and packing

After decontamination, the instruments pass into a strictly controlled clean packing environment, sometimes referred to as 'the clean room'. The instruments will usually have been through the washing process in their sets to simplify the checking and packing process. They are then placed onto a prepared instrument tray ready for packaging prior to sterilization. At this time the instruments are inspected for any damage or wear and, if present, are removed and replaced.

Before the tray is finally packed up, the instrument set is checked by the packer and another member of staff against the tray list, and any instrument(s) missing are noted on both the packed list and ideally on the outside of the instrument tray. The instrument trays are packed as dictated by the type of instruments and the local requirements to protect them. The tray is wrapped in a protective sheet made of a single-use non-woven textile in such a way that enables it to be opened without contaminating the inner part of the tray. Some specialist instruments may be packed in a rigid metal container which is designed to withstand the heat of the autoclave while others may be individually wrapped in heat-sealed pouch packaging.

## Reusable instruments

The process described for checking and packing will relate to instruments that are designed to be used a number of times. They are made of stainless steel to the highest standard so that they can withstand the autoclave process. While there is not a maximum number of times they can be used, they do require checking each time they are re-processed and maintained as required. There have been products, such as electrosurgical pens with their accompanying electrical lead, that have a finite life and should only be processed a number of times (typically 50). These products should have a record card with them that is marked off after each use until the item reaches the maximum number after which it is discarded.

## Single-use items

These are produced commercially and may range from large anastomosis guns to small items such as skin marking pens. They often contain plastic material and are usually sterilized using irradiation. They should not be re-sterilized unless the manufacturer has instructed that it is safe to do so and they must also state how reprocessing should be conducted including the method to be used and how long the item can be regarded as sterile and safe to use. Any sterile processing unit or individual re-sterilizing an item that is designed for single use will assume the manufacturer's liability for the sterility and safety of the item when in use.

As a general rule, practitioners should observe the maxim that if you want a reusable item then buy one that is designed to be reused.

## Instrument tracking

In the modern era, this has become an important issue for the protection of patients and to source any processing issues in the event of SSIs so that action can be taken should such an outbreak occur. Instrument sets and sundries should have a unique number to identify them which is placed on the outer wrap or the packaging. This is normally provided as a readable bar code that can be read by a laser scanner in much the same way as products in a supermarket. This system will identify the instrument or the set and will typically be scanned at various stages of the cycle so that the item can be located. It will also indicate the decontamination and sterilization cycles that the item has been through as well as the surgical cases that it has been used in.

There are also marking systems that can be used to place a unique code on the instrument, whether part of an instrument set or a sundry, itself so that if it becomes separated from the packaging, or is taken out of service to go for servicing or repair, it can still be traced until it is taken out of commission entirely.

## Further reading

Association for Perioperative Practice (2016). Standards and recommendations for safe perioperative practice. Harrogate: Association for Perioperative Practice.

Association of periOperative Registered Nurses (2020). Guidelines for perioperative practice. Denver, CO: AORN Inc.

Australian College of Operating Room Nurses (2020). Standards for perioperative nursing. Adelaide: ACORN Ltd.

Phillips N, Hornacky A (2020). Berry & Kohn's operating room technique (14th ed). St Louis, MO: Elsevier.

Sutherland-Fraser S, Davies M, Lockwood B, et al. (eds) (2021). Perioperative nursing: an introduction (3rd ed). Chatswood: Elsevier Australia.

# Management of surgical equipment

The amount of surgical equipment that is not used directly on patients has increased greatly as surgery has developed over recent times. The type of equipment that might commonly be found in operating theatre departments may include:

• Stack systems containing audio equipment, light source, monitor, and insufflator
• Microscopes
• Irrigation equipment
• Specialist drilling equipment
• Cell salvage machine.

As new equipment is purchased, storage space will need to be found to accommodate it when it is not in use in order that it is protected from damage. Staff need to be familiar with the set-up and use of specialist equipment and it may prove necessary to restrict the number of staff that may use the equipment to those who are conversant with it, to minimize damage caused by misuse which may prove expense to repair. Consideration should be given to the provision of regular updates for staff which can be provided by company representatives or staff who are familiar with the equipment. This should include how to set up, use, clean, and store the equipment. Maintenance contracts should also be in place for essential equipment with a specialist contractor.

## Further reading

Association for Perioperative Practice (2016). Standards and recommendations for safe perioperative practice. Harrogate: Association for Perioperative Practice.

Association of periOperative Registered Nurses (2020). Guidelines for perioperative practice. Denver, CO: AORN Inc.

Australian College of Operating Room Nurses (2020). Standards for perioperative nursing. Adelaide: ACORN Ltd.

Phillips N, Hornacky A (2020). Berry & Kohn's operating room technique (14th ed). St Louis, MO: Elsevier.

Sutherland-Fraser S, Davies M, Lockwood B, et al. (eds) (2021). Perioperative nursing: an introduction (3rd ed). Chatswood: Elsevier Australia.

# Maintaining a sterile field

## Definition

The sterile field refers to the area around the surgical site that has been prepared by cleansing with an antimicrobial agent and surrounded with sterile drapes, which separate it from the rest of the patient's body. This is called 'prepping and draping'. The sterile field also includes all furniture covered with sterile drapes, such as the instrument table and the scrub team who are covered in sterile garb.

## Purpose

The purpose of creating and maintaining a sterile field is to protect the patient's wound from microbial contamination during surgery, and to isolate the operative site from the surrounding, unsterile environment.

## Principles

- All items used in a sterile field must be sterile. This includes drapes, instrument trays, sponges, swabs, and basins.
- Items of doubtful sterility are considered unsterile. This includes packaged items that may have been dropped on the floor or when the integrity of the packaging material is in doubt.
- All surgical personnel scrubbed for the case (the scrub team) are gowned and gloved. Gowns are considered sterile in front from chest level to the sterile field, sleeves from 5 cm (2 inches) above the elbow to the stockinette cuff. Once sterile personnel are gowned and gloved, they keep their hands in sight at all times, and at or above waist level or the level of the sterile field.
- Sterile drapes are used to create a sterile field. Once placed, sterile drapes are not moved.
- Tables (once draped) are sterile only at the table level. The edges and sides of the drapes extending below table level are considered contaminated. This rule applies to the operating table edge, once the patient has been prepped and draped.
- Any item falling below the edge is considered contaminated.
- Sterile personnel touch only sterile items or areas; unsterile personnel touch only unsterile items or areas. Members of the scrub team maintain contact with the sterile field by means of sterile gowns and gloves.
- Items must be dispensed to the sterile field by methods that preserve sterility. The edges of anything that enclose sterile contents are considered unsterile; thus, the circulating practitioner must ensure when opening sterile packages that a margin of safety is maintained. For example, the flaps on peel packages should be pulled back not torn, and the contents offered to the scrub practitioner for removal, and not flipped onto the instrument table.
- Unsterile personnel avoid reaching over the sterile field. The unsterile circulating practitioner never reaches over a sterile field to transfer an item. For example, the scrub practitioner sets basins or medicine cups to be filled at the edge of the sterile table, and the circulating practitioner stands at least 30 cm (12 inches) away from the edge of the table to fill them. This distance applies to any part of the sterile field.

- The scrub team keeps well within the sterile field or area. They do not walk around or go outside of the operating room, and they keep movement to a minimum to avoid contamination of sterile items.
- Movement of the scrub team is from sterile area to sterile area, keeping a wide margin of safety when passing an unsterile area. They pass each other back-to-back and turn their backs to an unsterile area or person when passing.
- Unsterile personnel avoid the sterile field and maintain awareness of sterile, unsterile, clean, and contaminated areas and their proximity to each.
- When a sterile area is permeated, it is considered contaminated. Strike-through, the soaking of moisture from an unsterile layer or area to a sterile layer, or vice versa, breaches the integrity of the sterile field, contaminating it. If solution soaks through a sterile drape to an unsterile area, the wet area must be covered with impervious, sterile drapes or towels.
- Every sterile field must be continuously monitored. Someone must remain in the operating room at all times during set up of the sterile field and thereafter, until the surgical procedure is completed.
- The sterile field is created as close as possible to the time of use. Sterile instrument tables are set up immediately prior to the surgical procedure. There is no period of time wherein the table is considered sterile or unsterile and the potential degree of contamination is proportionate to the length of time that sterile items are exposed to the environment. Tables containing sterile items should not be covered; it is impossible to uncover them without risk of contamination.
- Microorganisms must be kept to an irreducible minimum. Sterile technique at the surgical site is an ideal to be approached; it is not an absolute. This is because it is not possible to eliminate all microorganisms from the environment. However, strict application of the measures described here and the exercise of one's surgical conscience are crucial; there is no place for compromise of sterility in the operating room.

## Further reading

Association for Perioperative Practice (2016). Standards and recommendations for safe perioperative practice. Harrogate: Association for Perioperative Practice.

Association for periOperative Registered Nurses (2020). Guidelines for perioperative practice. Denver, CO: AORN Inc.

Australian College of Operating Room Nurses (2020). Standards for perioperative nursing. Adelaide: ACORN Ltd.

Phillips N, Hornacky A (2020). Berry & Kohn's operating room technique (14th ed). St Louis, MO: Elsevier.

Sutherland-Fraser S, Davies M, Lockwood B, et al. (eds) (2021). Perioperative nursing: an introduction (3rd ed). Chatswood: Elsevier Australia.

# Scrubbing up

## Introduction

The patient's surgical outcome is influenced by the establishment and maintenance of an aseptic environment. The wearing of appropriate attire in the operating suite is one of a series of aseptic environmental control measures, which includes scrubbing, gowning, and gloving.

## Purpose

All personnel who work in the semi-restricted or restricted areas of the operating suite must wear theatre attire, which consists of a two-piece pantsuit, head covering, and shoe covers, as appropriate. These items provide an effective barrier that prevents the dissemination of microorganisms shed continuously from the skin and hair of everyone from entering the patient's body. Theatre attire also protects staff from patients' blood and body fluids. Additionally, members of the scrub team wear a mask, protective eyewear, and don sterile gowns and gloves. This is necessary because they are part of the sterile field.

## Using masks and protective eyewear

Prior to scrubbing, members of the scrub team must remove all jewellery and cover their mouth and nose with a single, disposable surgical mask, which conforms to their facial contours and fits closely. Effectively worn, masks will filter inhalations and exhalations, and prevent droplets from the wearer's mouth and nasopharynx contaminating the wound. Eyewear such as goggles or eyeglasses which incorporate top and side shields must also be worn. Alternatives include a combination surgical mask with a visor eye shield or chin-length face shield. Eyewear is worn to protect the wearer from hazardous substances such as blood and body fluids.

## Scrubbing, gowning, and gloving

Before donning a sterile gown and gloves, members of the scrub team must complete a surgical hand wash (called the surgical scrub). Its purpose is to remove as many microorganisms as possible from the hands and arms by a combination of mechanical washing and the use of chemical antiseptic solutions. A standardized procedure, such as the WHO guideline for surgical hand preparation should be used.[1] The first scrub of the day is 5 minutes long; all scrubs thereafter should be 3 minutes.

The two most common forms of hand antisepsis are aqueous scrubs and alcohol rubs. Aqueous scrubs are water-based solutions and contain antiseptic ingredients such as CHG or povidone-iodine.[2]

*Scrubbing up*

- Lay a sterile gown pack on a dressing trolley and open it to expose the contents without touching them, or the inner surface of the wrapping. This becomes a sterile field.
- Peel open the glove packaging and keeping the inside package sterile, tip the inner packet containing the gloves onto the sterile field.
- Place occlusive dressings over any skin lesions and remove jewellery.
- Adjust running water to a comfortable temperature; open a disposable sterile brush, and wet hands and arms to above the elbow. Thereafter, keep the hands above elbow level.

- Hand wash with soap and water first.
- Clean the nails using the supplied nail pick then discard.
- Follow WHO surgical hand rubbing technique guidelines.
- Hands are rinsed from the fingertips to the elbows, while keeping the hands higher than the elbows.
- Taps are turned off using the elbows.
- Hands and arms are dried using a corkscrew movement to dry from the hand to the elbow. The towel should not be returned up the arm to the hand.

*Gowning*

- Pick up gown at top, shake gently to open out without touching anything, and then slip arms in, shrugging gown onto shoulders. Keep hands enclosed in ribbed cuffs while the circulating practitioner ties up gown at the back.

*Gloving*

- Pick up left glove and lay on left hand, thumb to thumb, with glove fingers pointing to elbow. Slip thumb of right hand under cuff of the glove and stretch glove up and over fingers of the left hand and pull on. The cuff of the glove should cover the ribbed cuff of the gown.
- With the gloved hand, remove the right glove from wrapper by placing the left hand inside the folded glove cuff. Repeat the procedure as for the left glove.
- Tug on the sleeves of the gown to adjust gloves for good fit, and then don the second, smaller pair of gloves.
- Hand the tag-enclosed end of the gown's back tie to the circulating member of staff then make a turn to the left. Retrieve the back tie carefully by pulling it out of the tag held by the circulating practitioner then tie it to the other back tie, which has been secured to the front of the gown throughout.

## Notes

- A plastic waterproof apron must be worn under the sterile gown unless an impervious gown is used.
- Artificial nails have been linked to the transmission of bacteria or fungi and are best avoided.
- The use of powder-free or latex-free gloves is recommended.
- At all times, scrub personnel must keep their gloved hands above waist level, hands higher than the elbows, close to the upper, gowned body but away from touching the surgical attire, to avoid contamination.

## References

1. World Health Organization (2018). Appendix 2. WHO guideline summary for surgical hand preparation. In: Implementation manual to support the prevention of surgical site infections at the facility level – turning recommendations into practice. Available at: ℅ https://www.who.int/infection-prevention/publications/implementation-manual-prevention-surgical-site-infections.pdf?ua=1
2. Tanner J, Dumville JC, Norman G, et al. (2016). Surgical hand antisepsis to reduce surgical site infection. Cochrane Database of Systematic Reviews, 1:CD004288.

## Further reading

Association for Perioperative Practice (2016). Standards and recommendations for safe perioperative practice. Harrogate: Association for Perioperative Practice.

Association for Perioperative Practice (2017). A guide to surgical hand antisepsis. Harrogate: Association for Perioperative Practice.

Association of periOperative Registered Nurses (2020). Guidelines for perioperative practice. Denver, CO: AORN Inc.

Australian College of Operating Room Nurses (2020). Standards for perioperative nursing. Adelaide: ACORN Ltd.

Phillips N, Hornacky A (2020). Berry & Kohn's operating room technique (14th ed). St Louis, MO: Elsevier.

Royal College of Ophthalmologists (2018). Ophthalmology service guidance: theatre facilities and equipment. London: Royal College of Ophthalmologists.

Sutherland-Fraser S, Davies M, Lockwood B, et al. (eds) (2021). Perioperative nursing: an introduction (3rd ed). Chatswood: Elsevier Australia.

# Draping of the patient

## Introduction

To create a sterile field, sterile sheets and towels—known as surgical drapes—are strategically placed to isolate the operative site from the remainder of the patient's body. Sterile drapes are used to maintain sterility of the immediate environment. Once placed, they provide a sterile surface on which sterile items such as instruments, sponges, swabs, other sterile equipment, and the gloved hands of the scrub team can rest. Surgical drapes are not placed until the patient's skin has been cleansed with an appropriate antimicrobial solution. Disposable, non-woven or sterile, reusable woven drapes and surgical gowns can be used to prevent SSI.[1] Draping materials are chosen to create and maintain an effective barrier that eliminates the passage of microorganisms between sterile and non-sterile areas. To be effective, they must be blood and aqueous fluid resistant, lint free, antistatic, and penetrable by steam or gas for sterilization purposes. They must also be resistant to tearing, sufficiently porous to eliminate heat build-up, flame resistant, and free of toxic ingredients such as non-fast dyes.

Draping materials are folded and packaged so scrub personnel can handle them easily and safely; large drapes are fan-folded, rolled, or otherwise folded in a way which assists with their subsequent placement on the patient. Large drapes may be fenestrated (have an opening) that, when placed, exposes the incision area. Smaller drapes such as chest sheets, towels, and so forth may be used to 'square drape' a small operative site; they are packaged folded in halves or quarters. Many procedures utilize custom packs. These are sterile, pre-packaged, procedure-specific packs which contain all the draping requirements—and often other disposable items, such as sponges and Ray-Tec® swabs—required for a given surgical intervention such as a joint replacement or a caesarean section. The drapes in these packs are often custom designed.

## Types of drapes

Surgical drapes can be reusable, disposable, or reposable; additionally, there are plastic incisional drapes.

- *Reusable drapes*: these are made of 100%, tightly woven cotton. They are permeable to fluid so a moisture-repellent plastic drape is placed on the patient first. They require sterilized towel clips (ball and socket type) to hold them in place, once they've been laid on the patient. Their use is decreasing because of costs associated with laundering and processing them.
- Increasingly, surgical supply companies are working with perioperative practitioners to design and manufacture customized sterile packs which contain the drapes and consumable requirements necessary for a given procedure, such as a craniotomy or joint replacement procedure.
- *Disposable drapes*: these are soft, lightweight, moisture resistant, and made of antistatic material. They are produced, pre-packaged, and sterilized commercially, and are discarded after one use. They are designed to adhere to the patient's skin, once positioned, and do not require the use of towel clips.

- *Reposable drapes*: these are drapes which are designed for limited reuse and theoretically combine the advantages of reusable drapes (environmentally friendly) with the advantages of disposables (superior quality).
- *Plastic incisional drapes*: these are transparent, self-adherent drapes designed to cover the operative site itself, providing a complete seal between the incision and wound and the skin in the immediate vicinity. They facilitate the draping of irregular body surfaces such as joints.

## Procedure

- Drapes should be handled as little as possible.
- The scrub practitioner protects their gown and gloves by cuffing the drapes over their hands and holding drapes close to body.
- Scrub personnel should carry the folded drape to the operative site, unfold, and then place it.
- Care must be taken to maintain the appropriate distance from non-sterile areas to avoid contamination of scrub gown (30 cm or 12 inches).
- The operative site must always be dry.
- Once placed, drapes should not be removed.
- If drapes fall before or during placement they are discarded.
- If a drape is contaminated or its sterility in question, it is discarded.
- Drapes are applied from sterile area to unsterile area, and the area nearest the scrub person is draped first. Scrub personnel should not reach across or over an unsterile area to drape—they walk around the operating table. Sterile drapes are not passed from one scrubbed person to another across an unsterile surface.
- Drapes should not be flipped, fanned, or shaken. Rapid drape movements create air currents on which dust can migrate. Shaking drapes causes uncontrollable movement and exposes the drape to potential, unseen contamination.
- The area of the incision site is draped first, followed by the peripheral or other areas.
- A drape should never be pulled from an unsterile area to a sterile one.

## Reference

1. World Health Organization (2018). Implementation manual to support the prevention of surgical site infections at the facility level – turning recommendations into practice. Available at: ℬ https://www.who.int/infection-prevention/publications/implementation-manual-prevention-surgical-site-infections.pdf?ua=1

## Further reading

World Health Organization (2018). Web appendix 17. Summary of a systematic review on drapes and gowns. In: Global guidelines for the prevention of surgical site infection. Available at: ℬ https://www.ncbi.nlm.nih.gov/books/NBK536409/

# Role of the circulating practitioner

## Introduction

The circulating practitioner is an integral member of the perioperative team and is vital to the smooth flow of activities before, during, and after the surgical procedure. The ability to multitask is necessary as the circulating practitioner must coordinate patient care, the activities in an operating room, other members of the surgical team, and documentation. The role also demands initiative and good anticipatory skills. The circulating practitioner, as patient advocate, plays a central role in protecting patients from a range of adverse events that may arise in a high-risk environment such as the operative room. The circulating practitioner assists with the preparation of the operating room ensuring all needed equipment, sterile instrumentation, and consumables are available preoperatively. S/he assists intraoperatively working with the scrub practitioner to set up the instrument table, helping with patient transfer to the operating table, managing surgical specimens and consumables, and completing perioperative documentation.

## Activities associated with the circulating practitioner role

During the course of (most) surgical procedures, the circulating practitioner, in conjunction with other surgical team members, or alone, will undertake the following:

- Adhere to standard precautions and, when indicated, transmission-based precautions, at all times.
- Understand and apply the principles of aseptic technique.
- Be accountable for own actions and delegations.

*Preoperatively*

- Ensure the operating room is clean, has the necessary equipment, sterile instruments, and consumables such as sponges and Ray-Tec® swabs.
- Assist in the preparation of scrubbed surgical team members.
- Help the scrub practitioner prepare for the surgical intervention by opening and dispensing sterile supplies.
- Lifting a limb to assist with the application of antiseptic skin preparation. It is important that this is carried out in accordance with accepted lifting techniques to minimize the risk of injury to staff or patient.
- In conjunction with the scrub practitioner ensure all accountable items are counted immediately before the procedure begins; at the commencement of the closure of the body cavity; and at the commencement of skin closure.
- Assist in ensuring the correct patient is admitted for the correct operation, at or on the correct site or side (which is marked, as appropriate).
- Establish that a valid consent has been obtained and that the patient understands the anticipated operation in broad terms.
- Ascertain the patient's fasting status, known allergies, pertinent medical history, and that any necessary preoperative preparation (e.g. bowel preparation) has been completed.
- Confirm patient details with the scrub practitioner.

*Intraoperatively*
- Assist with the transfer of the patient, which must be properly coordinated by staff trained in techniques for safe patient transfer using appropriate lifting devices.
- Ensure the patient is correctly positioned for the anticipated procedure and that pressure areas are protected by the use of gel mattresses, pads, head rings, heel supports, padded boards, stirrups, and so on, as determined by the requirements of the surgical position and status of individual patient.
- If necessary, make sure the patient is secured to the operating table by a reusable belt or by sticking plaster tape, particularly if they are in a lateral position.
- Check if antiembolism stockings are in use and that they are correctly applied, especially those that are thigh length.
- If required, apply the leggings of the sequential calf compression device (DVT prophylactic system) and activate it.
- Apply the disposable, electrosurgery return electrode (diathermy plate) to a clean, muscular, well-vascularized, hairless site on the patient's body. Connect it to the electrosurgical generator (diathermy machine).
- Connect and/or activate other equipment as necessary, such as suction devices, active diathermy electrode, operating lights, other light sources, and so on.
- Supply sterile consumables, additional instruments, and other items as required throughout the course of the procedure.
- Record any use of single instruments that are contaminated and subsequently cleaned and 'flash' sterilized in both the patient's medical record and the department's 'Flash' log.
- Maintain communication with and between the team members in the sterile field, and with other personnel in the perioperative unit/operating department and beyond.
- Exercise a surgical conscience, recognizing and correcting any breaks in aseptic technique throughout the case.
- Support and teach any health professional learners in the environment.
- Document all aspects of perioperative care in the patient's medical record including each of the three counts; position of patient; pressure-relieving devices and DVT prophylaxis, if used; position of the diathermy plate; skin preparation solution used; the operation performed; specimens taken; any implants or prosthesis used; any drains *in situ*, and wound dressings applied.
- Assist with the transfer of the patient on completion of the operation ensuring the medical records, X-rays, and other imaging records (and if necessary, personal belongings) accompany the patient to the recovery unit.
- Oversee the cleaning of the operating theatre in accordance with unit policies and protocols, first ensuring all rubbish, clinical waste, sharps, and soiled linen are removed.
- Check all the requirements for the next case are available.

# Opening of sterile packs

## Introduction

Sterile packs are necessary in order to create and maintain a sterile field, and their use is one of a number of measures taken to protect the patient's wound from microbial contamination during surgery.

Sterile packs contain sterile items such as instruments, draping materials, consumables (e.g. sponges and Ray-Tec® swabs) and other items such as kidney trays. These items may be packed singly or in a combination. For example, most operating departments have standardized instrument tray sets for major and minor procedures, and for each surgical specialty.

Additionally, they have some surgical instruments packed singly. They also have standardized linen (or drape) bundles, as well as single-drape packs; bowl sets; kidney trays; and so forth. These items may be prepared by the operating department's theatre sterile supply unit or the hospital's central sterile supply department.

There is a trend towards the purchase of commercially prepared sterile surgical packs. This is because of the escalating costs associated with 'in house' reprocessing of sterile supplies, necessitated by the need to meet exacting manufacturing standards for items of this nature. Note, some items, such as sponges and Ray-Tec® swabs, are almost always purchased from surgical supply companies, and are not prepared 'in house'.

## Principles

Sterile packs are prepared and manufactured in such a way that they can be opened without touching and thereby contaminating their contents.

- Sterile packs should be opened as close to their time of use as possible.
- Each sterile pack is inspected to check for package integrity, and that the outer wrapping is clean, dry, and intact.
- Each pack is also examined closely to ensure that it has sterilization process (chemical) indicator tape present, which identifies that it has been through a sterilizing process, and one suited to the particular contents of the sterile pack.
- Sterile packs must not have exceeded their shelf life, which is both event related and determined, in part, by the nature and type of packaging used.
- Any outer dust covers are removed before the pack is subsequently opened and offered to the scrub practitioner, or placed on a table top for opening. All heavy items such as instrument trays are placed on a suitable, dry surface.
- Once opened, the edges of a sterile pack are considered unsterile. The contents must be dispensed onto the sterile field in a manner that preserves their integrity, as well as the integrity of the sterile field.
- As the boundaries between sterile and unsterile are often intangible, 2.5 cm (1 inch) is considered standard for wrapped packs, whereas the boundary on a wrapper used to drape a table is at the table edge.
- When opening a sterile pack, the top flap is opened first, away from the circulating practitioner (or non-scrub personnel) opening it. This is followed by opening each of the side flaps, then finally, opening the inside or proximal flap last. As each flap is opened out, it is grasped, pulled down, and held underneath by the hand holding the pack. This

stops the flaps from dangling and contaminating other sterile items. The outer side of the wrapper also serves to cover the circulating practitioner's hand, further protecting the sterile contents.

- The item is then offered to the scrub person so it can be lifted straight up and away from its wrapper.
- On peel-pack pouches, the inner edge of the heat seal is the edge of the sterile boundary. Peel packs should be pulled back evenly, by grasping each edge of the pouch or package top and peeling away smoothly. These packs should not be torn open.
- Peel-pack contents can be retrieved by the scrub practitioner as already described (lifted straight up) or they can be flipped onto the sterile field by the non-scrubbed person. They should not be allowed to slide over the edge of the pack.
- When opening large sterile packs (e.g. packs of drapes) they should be laid on the instrument table because, when opened, the outer wrapper subsequently forms the first sterile covering for the instrument table. When opening the cover of the pack, the hands of the circulating practitioner are kept under the folded pack cuff, thereby protecting the inner, sterile contents, as the practitioner draws the cover back over the table exposing the contents.
- When opening items, the hand and arm motions of the circulating practitioner are always from unsterile to sterile objects.
- If the sterility of the item is in doubt, it should be discarded.

# Movement within the theatre

## Introduction

A further aspect of perioperative care aimed at keeping the patient free from infection is related to movement within the operating theatre, which is a restricted area. Traffic within and out of the operating theatre must be kept to a minimum and only essential personnel should be allowed inside the theatre. This is because the amount of activity in the room increases as the number of persons present increases. In turn, this heightens the potential for contamination as a result of additional shedding and air turbulence that carries microorganisms with it onto the sterile field and the patient's wound. Like many aspects of surgical aseptic technique, the following principles and actions are predicated on the premise that most infections are caused by microorganisms exogenous to the surgical patient's body.

## Principles

- The doors of the operating theatre should be kept closed at all times except when it is necessary to provide a passage for the patient, perioperative personnel involved in the particular procedure, and required supplies and equipment. This ensures the higher positive air pressure in the theatre remains so, and is not allowed to equalize to the lower (or negative) air pressure beyond the theatre, mixing the clean theatre air with that from outer, less clean areas, as well as increasing turbulence.
- Clean and sterile supplies should be separated from contaminated items by time, space, or traffic patterns.
- Movement of personnel within the theatre should be kept to a minimum.
- All members of the surgical team must understand which areas within the theatre are considered sterile and which are considered unsterile, and maintain a continual awareness of them.
- Sterile individuals touch only sterile items or areas; unsterile personnel touch only unsterile items and areas.
- Movement within and around the sterile field must not contaminate the field.
- Scrubbed personnel must guard the sterile field and prevent unsterile items from contaminating the field, or the individuals themselves.
- The circulating practitioner must monitor movement within the theatre and be vigilant for, and address, breaks in aseptic technique.
- Unsterile personnel must not touch or lean over a sterile field.
- Sterile personnel must stay close to the sterile field. If they change position, they turn face-to-face, or back-to-back, while maintaining a safe distance between themselves and other objects.
- The circulating practitioner and other non-sterile personnel face the sterile field when approaching it.
- Unsterile personnel never walk between two sterile fields.
- The circulating practitioner maintains a minimum distance of 30 cm (12 inches) from the sterile field.
- If a solution must be poured into a sterile receptacle on the sterile table, the scrub practitioner holds the receptacle away from the table, or places it near the edge of the waterproof-draped table.

# Further reading

Association for Perioperative Practice (2016). Standards and recommendations for safe perioperative practice. Harrogate: Association for Perioperative Practice.

Association of periOperative Registered Nurses (2020). Guidelines for perioperative practice. Denver, CO: AORN Inc.

Australian College of Operating Room Nurses (2020). Standards for perioperative nursing. Adelaide: ACORN Ltd.

Phillips N, Hornacky A (2020). Berry & Kohn's operating room technique (14th ed). St Louis, MO: Elsevier.

Sutherland-Fraser S, Davies M, Lockwood B, et al. (eds) (2021). Perioperative nursing: an introduction (3rd ed). Chatswood: Elsevier Australia.

# Communication with the surgical team

## Introduction

Good communication is fundamental to the effective management and functioning of the operating department. It involves the exchange of information between patients and staff, between individuals and teams, and within and beyond the operating department. It is necessary for successful interpersonal relationships and to clarify actions. It is effective when the receiver of a message interprets it in the way the sender intended. Communication can be:

- *Verbal*: the most frequently used form of communication
- *Non-verbal*: such as the use of body language
- *Written*: for example, the patient's medical record, perioperative care plans, and theatre department policy manuals
- *Electronic*: increasingly information such as laboratory results, personal (email) communication, and digital imaging (to name but a few) is conveyed this way.

Effective communication is also critical to the formation of functional teams, such as the surgical team. Within the team there must be a shared understanding of the nature and manner of all communication, a shared language, and a commitment to direct and open verbal (and other) interactions. Communication skills can be learned and staff should be supported to access appropriate education, such is the significance of good communication in the operating department.

## Coordinating the operating list

The coordination of the operating list is a crucial activity in the operating department. It involves virtually all perioperative (and other) personnel, and other departments within the hospital, and it can be a complex and fraught task. It is also a shared one. While the details may vary from hospital to hospital (indeed, it may differ within the same organization, if the latter has more than one operating department), it involves a number of key personnel. For example, the operating department manager (or the floor coordinator), a senior anaesthetist/anaesthetic representative, and a member of the surgical staff would be the minimal number of personnel involved in coordinating an operating list. They will be assisted in this endeavour by administrative staff, such as operating department clerks, admissions or outpatient department staff, or the hospital's bed manager.

Ideally, elective surgical lists are determined 2 weeks (or more) ahead of the scheduled day of surgery, and patients on the relevant waiting list are contacted. At this time, they are given the date of surgery and other information pertinent to their procedure. Alternatively, the decision to add patients' names to any given surgical list may be determined during their visit to a preadmission or preoperative clinic, or following a visit to their surgeon. Once an operating list has been compiled and distributed to all stakeholders, it forms an important part of the operating department's records.

- It needs to be printed and posted in several places within the operating department the night before the intended surgical list is to occur.

- Every operating theatre should have its own copy as should each surgical ward, the anaesthetic and surgical departments, the perioperative unit, pathology, X-ray and imaging departments, and any other pertinent departments.
- Any changes to the list must be determined in a collaborative fashion, by the theatre coordinator in conjunction with relevant anaesthetic and surgical personnel. These changes should then be relayed promptly to all key personnel and departments, as well as to the staff in the affected operating room, and the patient(s) concerned, and/or their carers.
- Changes must be noted in the operating department's permanent records.
- There must be a written policy and clear set of guidelines which spell out the manner in which patients will be sent for and by whom, so they are transferred to the operating department in a timely fashion.
- Patients should not be called to the operating department too soon, resulting in them having an excessive wait prior to surgery.
- If patients have pre-medication drugs ordered by the anaesthetist, which are to be given on a phone order from the department, there must be clear guidelines/clinical protocol for this, particularly if perioperative staff are expected to make the phone call, authorizing the dispensation of the ordered drugs.
- Recovery room personnel should ensure that ward staff are notified of the admission of patients immediately following surgery; additionally, they should alert ward staff before transferring the patient back to the ward.

## Effective handover

The Situation, Background, Assessment, Recommendation, Review/response/read back (SBARR) tool was designed as a structured tool for communicating critical information and is recommended as it reduces the need for repetition and the likelihood of errors through miscommunication.

- *Situation* involves a brief couple of sentences to inform about the current situation requiring discussion.
- *Background* involves providing an overview of the patient, including the relevant medical details.
- *Assessment* involves communicating including the vital signs, clinical examination findings, and overall clinical impression of the patient.
- *Recommendation* includes both recommendations for what you believe the next most appropriate steps in management should be and also asking what the person on the phone would recommend.
- *Response/review/read back* ensures that the respondent has understood everything that has been said, allows any further questions, and allows clarification of the expected response.

## Further reading

Association for Perioperative Practice (2016). Standards and recommendations for safe perioperative practice. Harrogate: Association for Perioperative Practice.
Association of periOperative Registered Nurses (2020). Guidelines for perioperative practice. Denver, CO: AORN Inc.
Australian College of Operating Room Nurses (2020). Standards for perioperative nursing. Adelaide: ACORN Ltd.

Health and Care Professions Council (2016). Standards of conduct, performance and ethics London: Health and Care Professions Council.

NHS England, NHS Improvement (2021). SBAR communication tool. Available at: ℗ https://www.england.nhs.uk/wp-content/uploads/2021/03/qsir-sbar-communication-tool.pdf

Nursing and Midwifery Council (2018). The code: professional standards of practice and behaviour for nurses and midwives. London: Nursing and Midwifery Council.

Phillips N, Hornacky A (2020). Berry & Kohn's operating room technique (14th ed). St Louis, MO: Elsevier.

Royal College of Ophthalmologists (2018). Ophthalmology service guidance: theatre facilities and equipment. London: Royal College of Ophthalmologists.

Sutherland-Fraser S, Davies M, Lockwood B, et al. (eds) (2021). Perioperative nursing: an introduction (3rd ed). Chatswood: Elsevier Australia.

# Specimens

## Introduction

During the course of many surgical interventions, samples of the patient's tissue (specimens) are removed for histopathological and other forms of examination. Occasionally, the removal of tissue samples is the main or sole purpose of the surgical procedure. The removal of tissue samples may be invasive and involve the use of local, regional, or general anaesthesia. Correct handling, labelling, and transportation to the laboratory are crucial. Loss of specimens or damage due to incorrect handling, or delay in transporting them, can result in misdiagnosis or patients requiring further surgery to acquire additional specimens for pathology. Alternatively, patients may receive inappropriate or delayed treatment, as a diagnosis cannot always be confirmed in the absence of pathology testing. When a sample of tissue or fluid is removed for pathology, it is referred to as a *biopsy*. In contrast, when all tissue is removed during a surgical procedure, for example, gastrectomy, these tissues are referred to as *surgical specimens* and they are sent to the pathology laboratory for verification of diagnosis.

## Specimen types and tests

Specimens can be categorized into several types:

*Fluid, such as*
- Exudates
- CSF
- Cell washings
- Urine
- Fluid from cysts or abscesses
- Blood
- Bone marrow
- Amniotic fluid
- Semen.

Tests performed on fluid specimens include bacteriology, virology, cytology, cell counts, grouping (blood), and genetic studies.

*Tissue, such as*
- Solid organ biopsy
- Margin of a malignant lesion
- Suspicious lesion or growth
- Skin
- Breast tissue/mass
- Brushings from respiratory or urinary tracts
- Bone
- Muscle
- Ova
- Calculi, such as gallstones.

Tests performed on tissue specimens include histopathological examination of frozen and permanent sections, hormonal assays, and tissue typing (for donor compatibility).

*Non-biological, such as*
- Foreign bodies—fish bones; glass fragments
- Projectiles from a crime scene—bullet
- Explanted items—orthopaedic screws, plates
- Retained surgical swabs
- Clothing from accident or crime victims—underclothes of rape victim.

There are no 'tests' for non-biological material, normally.

> Communication between surgeons and pathologists is essential when a specimen is transferred from an operation theatre to a laboratory. Any errors during transfer of a specimen can lead to serious consequences such as wrong diagnosis, inappropriate treatment, reoperations, and physical and emotional distress.

## Principles

- It is the responsibility of the circulating practitioner to identify, document, and properly care for specimens collected during the course of a surgical procedure.
- Standard and transmission-based precautions should be used to protect individuals handling specimens. Labels should identify the need for precautions as well as the presence of biohazardous material.
- Each specimen must be labelled with the correct (and full) patient's name and medical record number, as well as the specific origin, type, and nature of the specimen. If indicated, the theatre location and phone number should also be included.
- The surgeon must supply clear, descriptive information about the specimen and the circulating practitioner should 'repeat back' this information.
- The specimen details are documented in the patient's medical record; additionally, all specimen details should be entered into the department's specimens' record.
- Specimens should be prepared and cared for in accordance with the specific protocols established by the receiving laboratory.
- As a general rule, specimens should be handled in ways which preserve their integrity, be kept moist, and be transported to the laboratory as soon as possible.
- Formalin is frequently used to preserve specimens that are not taken to the laboratory immediately. Formaldehyde should be handled cautiously to avoid exposure, as it is a hazardous substance which causes watery eyes and respiratory irritation.
- When tissue identification or determination of malignancy is required immediately—that is, a result is required intraoperatively—specimens are taken for a 'frozen section' examination. Such tissue samples are placed in a specimen container, kept dry, and then transported directly to the laboratory. Here they are fast-frozen, sliced, stained, and examined under a microscope immediately. The examining pathologist then phones the operating theatre and conveys the results of the examination to the circulating practitioner.
- If the circulating practitioner receives the phone report, it is imperative that they 'read back' the test result to the pathologist to verify them, before informing the surgical team of the results.

## Further reading

Association for Perioperative Practice (2016). Standards and recommendations for safe perioperative practice. Harrogate: Association for Perioperative Practice.

Association of periOperative Registered Nurses (2020). Guidelines for perioperative practice. Denver, CO: AORN Inc.

Australian College of Operating Room Nurses (2020). Standards for perioperative nursing. Adelaide: ACORN Ltd.

Phillips N, Hornacky A (2020). Berry & Kohn's operating room technique (14th ed). St Louis, MO: Elsevier.

Sutherland-Fraser S, Davies M, Lockwood B, et al. (eds) (2021). Perioperative nursing: an introduction (3rd ed). Chatswood: Elsevier Australia.

# Infection prevention and control

Healthcare-associated infections (HCAIs) can develop as a result of direct contact with a healthcare setting or as a result of a healthcare intervention such as medical or surgical treatment. These have become a significant threat to patient safety. SSI is the commonest form of HCAI in surgical patients. There is increased public and government awareness of the risks associated with acquiring a HCAI and the personal and financial costs incurred.

> Prevention and control of infection in the perioperative area is of paramount importance.
>
> *Patients have a right to be protected from preventable infection and practitioners have a duty to safeguard the well-being of their patients.*

SSI is the commonest form of hospital-acquired infection in surgical patients. SSIs are an avoidable cause of harm and are a significant burden for healthcare organizations.[1] Across all of the surgical specialist categories, Enterobacterales account for 30% of the causative organisms.[2] Patients have a right to be protected from preventable infection and practitioners have a duty to safeguard the well-being of their patients. Control of infection in the perioperative area is of paramount importance. Recommendations for standard precautions are intended primarily for the care of patients in acute hospitals. However, the principles should be applied in any setting where patient care is undertaken.

Best practice recommends that all patients are treated as potentially infected. *Standard precautions* is the term used to describe the approach to infection prevention and control which offers protection to individuals whether or not they carry a known infection risk. Standard Precautions assess the activity to be performed rather than the individual receiving care. The use of appropriate personal protective equipment (PPE) such as gloves, gowns, masks, face shields, eye protection, and aprons are necessary to minimize the risk of SSI and to protect staff from occupational exposure to biohazards.

The precautions constitute a single set of recommendations to be used for the care of all patients regardless of their infection state when exposed to:
• Blood
• Excretions: such as urine, faeces, vomit, but not sweat
• Secretions: such as mucous, seminal fluid, vaginal fluid, lactations, saliva, and sputum
• Other body fluids: such as serum, lymph fluid, and CSF
• Non-intact skin
• Mucous membranes
• Care must be taken with *all* body fluids to avoid skin, mucous membrane, and environmental contamination.

Nine elements of standard infection control precautions have been compiled originally based on Garner's guidance.[3,4] This is the primary strategy for the control and prevention of nosocomial infection:

- Hand hygiene.
- Use of PPE.
- Prevent occupational exposure to infection.
- Manage blood and body fluid spillage.
- Decontamination of patient care equipment.
- Environmental hygiene.
- Safe use and disposal of waste and sharps.
- Safe disposal of used linen.
- Provide care in the most appropriate place.

Transmission-based precautions is a second tier of guidelines designed only for the care of specified patients with documented or suspected infection or colonization with highly transmissible or epidemiologically significant pathogens for which *additional precautions* are necessary to interrupt transmission.
- Airborne precautions: patients with TB, measles, or varicella (chickenpox).
- Droplet precautions: patients with respiratory illness.
- Contact precautions: patients with GI/enteric infection such as hepatitis A, shigellosis, *Escherichia coli*, or *Clostridium difficile*.

## Recommendations include

*Airborne precautions*
Patients with TB, measles, or varicella (chickenpox):
- Respiratory protection.
- Allowing appropriate ventilation air changes in the operating theatre following surgery.

*Droplet precautions*
Patients with respiratory illness:
- Mask wearing when within 1 metre of patients.
- Use of mask for patients during transfer.

*Contact precautions*
Patients with GI/enteric infection (e.g. hepatitis A, shigellosis, *E. coli*, *C. difficile*):
- Wearing gloves when touching the patient.
- Washing hands after removal of gloves.
- Gowning.
- Dedicated equipment if possible.
- Cleaning and disinfecting common equipment.

## References

1. World Health Organization (2018). Implementation manual to support the prevention of surgical site infections at the facility level – turning recommendations into practice. Available at: ℘ https://www.who.int/infection-prevention/publications/implementation-manual-prevention-surgical-site-infections.pdf?ua=1
2. Public Health England (2019). Surveillance of surgical site infections in NHS hospitals in England, April 2018 to March 2019. Available at: ℘ www.gov.uk/phe
3. Garner J (1996). Guideline for isolation precautions. Infection Control and Hospital Epidemiology, 17(1):54–80.
4. Garner JS, Hierholzer WJ, McCormick RD, et al. (1996). Guideline for isolation precautions in hospitals. Part I. Evolution of isolation practices. American Journal of Infection Control, 24(1):24–31.

## Further reading

Centers for Disease Control and Prevention. Guidelines library. Available at: ℘ https://www.cdc.
gov/infectioncontrol/guidelines/index.html

European Centre for Disease Prevention and Control (2014). Safe use of personal protective equipment in the treatment of infectious diseases of high consequence. Available at: ℘ https://www.
ecdc.europa.eu/sites/default/files/media/en/publications/Publications/safe-use-of-ppe.pdf

European Centre for Disease Prevention and Control (2020). Infection prevention
and control and preparedness for COVID-19 in healthcare settings – third update.
Available at: ℘ https://www.ecdc.europa.eu/en/publications-data/infection-prevention-and-
control-andpreparedness-covid-19-healthcare-settings

National Institute for Health and Care Excellence (2019). Surgical site infections: prevention and
treatment. NICE guideline [NG125]. Available at: ℘ https://www.nice.org.uk/guidance/ng125

National Institute for Occupational Safety and Health (2018). Use of respirators and surgical masks
for protection against healthcare hazards. Available at: ℘ https://www.cdc.gov/niosh/topics/
healthcarehsps/respiratory.html

Royal College of Nursing (2017). Essential practice for infection prevention and control.
London: Royal College of Nursing.

# Common infection control terms

- *Alcohol-based hand rub*: a hand decontamination preparation based on alcohol. Can be solution, gel, or wipes.
- *Antimicrobial*: a substance that kills or inhibits the growth of microorganisms.
- *Antiseptic*: a chemical solution which will reduce and prevent growth of microorganisms on skin.
- *Asepsis*: the absence of pathogenic microorganisms.
- *Aseptic technique*: a controlled procedure that aims to prevent contamination by microorganisms.
- *Aseptic non-touch technique (ANTT)*: a framework for aseptic technique based on the concept of defining key parts and key sites to be protected from contamination.
- *Bacteraemia*: the presence of microorganisms in the bloodstream.
- *Bactericidal*: causing the destruction of bacteria.
- *Bacteristatic*: causing the inhibition of bacterial growth.
- *Bacteriuria*: the presence of microorganisms in the urine.
- *Blood-borne virus*: a viral infection transmitted by exposure to blood and/ or bodily fluids. Blood-borne viruses include hepatitis B, hepatitis C, and HIV.
- *Chemical disinfectant*: a chemical solution which may be used to disinfect or sterilize items of equipment.
- *Chlorhexidine*: an antiseptic commonly used as a solution to disinfect the skin.
- *Cleaning*: procedure to physically remove soil, dust, and dirt from the surfaces of hands or equipment.
- *Clinical waste*: waste material consisting of human tissue, blood or body fluids, excretions, drugs, dressings, syringes, needles, or other sharps.
- *Clostridium difficile (C. diff)*: a bacterium that can cause symptoms ranging from diarrhoea to a life-threatening inflammation of the colon.
- *Colonization*: microorganisms that establish themselves in a particular environment, such as a body surface, without producing a disease.
- *Colony-forming unit*: an estimate of the number of viable bacterial cells made by counting visible colonies derived from the replication of a single microbial cell.
- *Contamination*: this occurs when either equipment or articles have been in contact with blood, body fluids, or pathological specimens.
- *Cross infection*: transmission of a pathogenic organism from one person to another.
- *Decontamination*: a procedure that removes the majority of harmful pathogenic organisms from objects and renders them safe to handle.
- *Disinfection*: the removal or destruction of harmful microorganisms but not bacterial spores.
- *Endogenous infection*: microorganisms originating from the patient's own body which cause harm in another body site.
- *Exogenous infection*: microorganisms originating from other people or inanimate objects which are spread by contact or airborne.
- *Extended spectrum beta-lactamase (ESBL)*: an enzyme produced by beta-lactam-resistant bacteria. Antibiotic options in the treatment of ESBLs are extremely limited.

- *Flora*: microorganisms resident in an environment or body site.
- *Gram-negative/positive bacteria*: the type of bacteria identified by a Gram staining method. Gram-positive bacteria appear blue black or purple under a microscope. Gram-negative bacteria appear red under a microscope.
- *Healthcare-associated infection (HCAI)*: infection acquired as a result of the delivery of healthcare in either an acute hospital setting or a community setting.
- *Incidence*: the number of new cases of a disease (or event) occurring in a specified time.
- *Infection*: the damaging of body tissue by microorganisms or by poisonous substances released by the organism.
- *Immunity*: the activation of the body's response to infection.
- *Methicillin-resistant Staphylococcus aureus (MRSA)*: strains of *S. aureus* that are resistant to many of the antibiotics commonly used to treat infection.
- *Methicillin-sensitive Staphylococcus aureus (MSSA)*: strains of *S. aureus* that respond well to antibiotics.
- *Neutropenia*: abnormal decrease in the number of neutrophils in peripheral blood, which results in increased susceptibility to infection.
- *Norovirus*: commonly known as the winter vomiting bug. This is the most common cause of gastroenteritis.
- *Nosocomial infection*: infection acquired during hospitalization, not present or incubating at time of admission to hospital.
- *Outbreak*: two or more cases of the same disease where there is evidence of an epidemiological link between them.
- *Pathogen*: a microorganism capable of causing disease.
- *Personal protective equipment (PPE)*: specialized clothing and equipment worn to protect against substances or situations that present a risk to health and safety.
- *Postexposure prophylaxis*: drug treatment regimen administered as soon as possible after an occupations exposure to reduce the risk of acquiring a blood-borne virus.
- *Prevalence*: the ratio of the total number of individuals who have a disease at a particular time to the population at risk of having the disease.
- *Sepsis*: inflammation and/or pus formation at an infected site.
- *Septicaemia*: the multiplication of microorganisms in the blood stream causing clinical signs of infection.
- *Severe acute respiratory syndrome (SARS)*: a severe form of pneumonia caused by coronavirus.
- *Sharps*: instruments used in delivering healthcare that can potentially inflict a penetrating injury. Examples are needles and scalpels.
- *Spore*: a resistant structure produced by microorganisms that enable it to survive in adverse conditions.
- *Sterilization*: the complete destruction or removal of all living microorganisms including bacterial spores.
- *Surgical mask*: a mask that covers the mouth and nose to prevent droplets from the wearer being expelled into the environment.

- *Surveillance*: a system of collecting, tabulating, analysing, and reporting data on the occurrence of disease.
- *Systemic infection*: an infection where the pathogen is distributed throughout the body rather than being concentrated in one area.
- *Terminal cleaning*: the decontamination of a patient area after a patient has been transferred or discharged, to remove any contamination by potentially pathogenic microorganisms.
- *Transient flora*: microorganisms acquired on the skin through contact with surfaces. They can be easily transferred to other surfaces touched. They can only survive a short time because of the hostile environment of skin and they can be removed by washing with soap and water.
- *Urinary tract infection (UTI)*: the invasion of bladder tissues by microorganisms causing signs and symptoms of infection.
- *Virulence*: the degree of activity of pathogenic organism.

## Reference

1. Loveday HP, Wilson JA, Pratt RJ, et al. (2014). Epic3: national evidence-based guidelines for preventing healthcare-associated infections in NHS hospitals in England. Journal of Hospital Infection, 8651:(Suppl 1):S1–S70.

# Handwashing

Microorganisms are easily transferred directly via hands or indirectly via an environmental source such as a commode or bedpan. Evidence suggests that this is a major contributing factor in the acquisition and spread of infections in healthcare.[1,2] The current spread of antibiotic-resistant organisms can be attributed, in part, to the failure of healthcare workers to wash their hands either as often or as efficiently as the situation requires. A number of outbreak reports have illustrated an association between direct patient contact and contamination.[1,2] National and international guidelines consistently identify that effective hand decontamination results in significant reductions in the transfer of potential pathogens, thus reducing the incidence of HCAI. The importance of handwashing cannot be overemphasized.

Hospital-acquired infections have both a financial and a human cost. Hand hygiene is universally considered to be the most basic but vital infection control measure.

## Guidance for hand hygiene

There is no set frequency for hand washing, it is determined by actions completed and those to be performed.

Hands must be decontaminated:
• Before and after each episode of direct patient care—this includes when carrying out clean and antiseptic procedures
• After contact with body fluids, mucous membranes, and non-intact skin
• After activities or contact with equipment in the clinical environment that may result in the hands becoming contaminated
• After removal of gloves.[1]

## Types of handwashing

Handwashing is decontamination of the hands by one of two methods: handwashing with either an antimicrobial or plain soap and water, or use of an antiseptic hand rub.[4]

Decontamination refers to the process for the physical removal of dirt, blood, and body fluids and the removal or destruction of microorganisms from the hands:
• Social handwash.
• Antiseptic hand disinfection.
• Surgical scrub/antisepsis.

Routine handwashing removes most transient microorganisms from soiled hands (e.g. MRSA). Transient microorganisms can be bacterial or viral. They are located on the surface of the skin and beneath the superficial cells of the stratum corneum. Any damaged skin, moisture, or ring wearing will increase the possibility of colonization. Unlike resident flora, transient microorganisms can be easily removed with handwashing and the risk from cross infection is immediately reduced.

Resident skin flora lives deep within the skin's crevices, in hair, and in sebaceous glands. These are not easily removed by the mechanical action of handwashing. Their numbers can be reduced by a combination of a detergent and a microbicide.

Frequent handwashing and effective handwashing techniques are important in the prevention of nosocomial infection.

## Purpose of surgical hand antisepsis

Surgical hand antisepsis is an extension of hand washing. It is also defined as the antiseptic surgical scrub or antiseptic hand rub performed before donning sterile attire preoperatively. Surgical hand antisepsis is used to destroy transient microorganisms and to inhibit the growth of resident microorganisms. This is routinely carried out before undertaking invasive procedures. The aim is to reduce the number of resident and transient flora to a minimum but also to inhibit their regrowth for as long as possible, not just on the hands but also on the wrists and forearms.

- Remove debris and transient organisms from nails, hands, and forearms.
- Reduce resident microbial count to a minimum.
- Inhibit growth of microorganisms.
- Reduce numbers of microorganisms on hands and reduce contamination of the operative site.

There are three types of antiseptic solution available for surgical hand antisepsis:

- Aqueous scrubs: water-based solutions containing active ingredients (e.g. CHG, povidone-iodine).
- Alcohol rubs: alcohol-based solutions available in preparations of 60% to 90% (e.g. ethanol, isopropanol).
- Alcohol rubs containing additional active ingredients: alcohol-based solutions which contain an additional active ingredient such as CHG.

Active ingredients can be added to water to make aqueous scrubs or added to alcohol to make alcohol rubs with additional active ingredients:

- Iodophors.
- Biguanides.
- Phenolic compounds.

There is evidence from studies in favour of both scrubs and rubs as forms of antisepsis.

### Variables associated with hand antisepsis

- Selection of antiseptic agent.
- Pre-antisepsis handwash.
- Duration of process.
- Use of brushes/sponges/nail picks.

### Guidelines for hand antisepsis

Numerous organizations provide guidelines for hand antisepsis with variations in their recommendations:

- Centers for Disease Control.[3]
- Association of periOperative Registered Nurses.[4]
- Association for Perioperative Practice.[5]
- Australian College of Operating Room Nurses.[6]
- WHO guideline summary for surgical hand preparation.[1]

## References

1. World Health Organization (2018). Implementation manual to support the prevention of surgical site infections at the facility level – turning recommendations into practice. Available at: https://www.who.int/infection-prevention/publications/implementation-manual-prevention-surgical-site-infections.pdf?ua=1

2. Loveday HP, Wilson JA, Pratt RJ, et al. (2014). Epic3: national evidence-based guidelines for preventing healthcare-associated infections in NHS hospitals in England. Journal of Hospital Infection, 8651(Suppl 1):S1–S70.

3. Centers for Disease Control and Prevention. Guidelines library. Available at: https://www.cdc.gov/infectioncontrol/guidelines/index.html

4. Association of periOperative Registered Nurses (2020). Guidelines for perioperative practice. Denver, CO: AORN Inc.

5. Association for Perioperative Practice (2020). Infection control. Available at: ⚙ file://ois.gov.soj/sojdata/HSS_HomeDirs_I-L/JourneauxM/Downloads/afpp-infection-control-0820.pdf

6. Australian College of Operating Room Nurses (2020). Standards for perioperative nursing. Adelaide: ACORN Ltd.

## Further reading

Tanner J, Dumville JC, Norman G, et al. (2016). Surgical hand antisepsis to reduce surgical site infection. Cochrane Database of Systematic Reviews, 1:CD004288.

# Management of a patient with an infection

It is good practice to maintain universal precautions since a patient may have an undiagnosed infection. This will include the use of facial/eye protection, procedure gloves, and gowns to protect staff from being splashed with potentially infected bodily fluids.

## Environment

All unnecessary equipment should be removed before the start of surgery. At the end of a session, the theatre should be cleaned with a chlorine-based detergent.

> To minimize the risk of cross contamination, theatre personnel should be kept to a minimum.

## MRSA

MRSA has been responsible for outbreaks of infection in primary and secondary care. These organisms are not only resistant to all the beta lactams but also to many other antibiotics. It is often introduced into a setting by a colonized or infected patient or healthcare provider.

The main mode of transmission is via hands, usually the hands of healthcare workers.

*Prevention—definition of MRSA carrier*

Consider definite MRSA positive—isolate and screen:

- MRSA positive culture.
- MRSA clearance incomplete.
- MRSA past positive with an unhealed wound.

Consider probable MRSA positive—ideally isolate and screen:

- Transfers from other hospitals.
- Transfer from positive nursing/residential home.

Consider possible MRSA positive—screen on admission:

- Transfer from nursing/residential home.
- Past cleared positive.

*Management*

- Elective patients are best placed at the end of the operating list.
- Known MRSA carriers should be on MRSA suppression therapy 5 days preoperatively and a minimum of 48 hours before surgery.
- Correct handwashing procedures.
- It is not necessary to strip all furniture from the theatre for MRSA patients. However, as with all cases, unnecessary equipment theatre should be removed.
- Disposable aprons and gloves worn by staff transferring.
- Traffic control. There is no need for 'outside' and 'inside' personnel. However, personnel should be kept to a minimum within the theatre.
- Barrier precautions—non-scrubbed surgical team.
- Contaminated instruments taken directly to 'sluice' area/utility room and disposed of in usual manner for hazardous waste.

- Anaesthetic induction should take place within the theatre.
- Recover in PACU using dedicated equipment or in operating theatre.
- Shower and change of attire following procedure—surgical team.
- Operating theatre terminally cleaned. Detergent and hot water should be used for cleaning followed by disinfection using Actichlor™ solution (1000 ppm).
- Operating theatre may be used immediately after cleaning.
- MRSA screening of staff should be part of a coordinated process.

## MSSA Panton–Valentine leukocidin

- Panton–Valentine leukocidin (PVL) is a cytotoxin that destroys white blood cells and is produced by some strains of *S. aureus* (PVL-*S. aureus*).
- Antibiotic prophylaxis should be given.

## Blood-borne viruses

Blood-borne infections pose an occupational risk to perioperative personnel. Risk of occupational transmission of blood-borne pathogens is very low if standard infection control precautions are adhered to. The risk of transmission from a known source with HIV, hepatitis C, and hepatitis B (hepatitis B e-antigen positive or a high hepatitis B DNA load) following a hollow needle stick injury is about 0.3%, 3%, and 30% respectively.

### Hepatitis B

- Hepatitis B (HBV) is also known as serum hepatitis and is easily transmitted percutaneously or permucosally through direct contact with blood and body fluids, needlestick/sharps injury, break in skin, or splash in eye, nose, or mouth.
- Hepatitis B has an incubation period of 6 weeks.
- Immunization is recommended for all high-risk healthcare professionals.

### Hepatitis C

- Hepatitis C virus (HCV) is also known as the silent killer and is usually transmitted through large or repeated exposure to blood.
- Hepatitis C often has no detectable symptoms.
- There is no vaccine for hepatitis C.

### Management of hepatitis B and C

- Use of gloves, gowns, masks, and eyewear.
- Non-sterile gloves readily available to prevent contact with blood or body fluids.
- Sharps safety to prevent injuries from needles, scalpels, and other sharp equipment.
- Double-gloving practice recommended.

### Clostridium difficile

*C. difficile*-associated diarrhoea can be defined as one episode of diarrhoea not attributable to any other cause with a positive *C. difficile* toxin test and/or endoscopic pseudomembranous colitis. *C. difficile* is a species of Gram-positive, anaerobic spore-forming bacteria. It is the most significant cause of pseudomembranous colitis, a severe infection of the colon, often after normal gut flora has been eradicated by the use of antibiotics. *C. difficile* is acquired from contact with humans or objects harbouring the bacteria and occurs through ingestion.

Patients may or may not present with diarrhoea but still need to be managed in the same way.

*Management*
- Consider type of surgery planned and if surgery is necessary or can be postponed. Where possible, surgery should be postponed until diarrhoea has ceased.
- Patients should be placed last on the operating list.
- Withdrawal of antibiotics. In many situations when antibiotics stopped then normal gut flora regrows.
- Anaesthetic induction should take place within the theatre.
- Unscrubbed personnel require disposable gloves and aprons.
- Waste and sharps can be disposed of in the usual manner.
- A double clean using a chlorine-based solution is recommended.

## Pulmonary tuberculosis

TB is an infectious disease that can affect both pulmonary and non-pulmonary sites. The disease is acquired by inhalation of TB bacilli exhaled from the mouth and nose of an infected individual.

TB is the disease caused by *Mycobacterium tuberculosis*. Disease, often similar to TB, can also be caused by non-tuberculous mycobacteria (NTM) otherwise known as atypical mycobacteria. TB usually affects the lungs, but can affect many other parts of the body, including lymph nodes, pleural cavity, bones, and brain.

Patients with a smear-positive pulmonary TB who require assisted ventilation in theatre should have a ventilator fitted with a bacterial filter. Closed suction systems must be used. All respiratory equipment should be single use.
- Patients should preferably be placed last on the operating list.
- Staff should be fitted with FFP3 or N95 facemasks.

## Transmissible spongiform encephalopathy: Creutzfeldt–Jakob disease

Spongiform encephalopathies or prion diseases are caused by prions which are composed mainly of protein and are highly resistant to inactivation by physicochemical agents or normal sterilization techniques. This means that there is the theoretical possibility of transmission of disease during invasive procedures.

There are three categories of Creutzfeldt–Jakob disease (CJD):
- Sporadic.
- Genetic.
- Acquired.

Variant CJD (vCJD) is an acquired form of human prion disease associated with the consumption of bovine spongiform encephalopathy (BSE)-affected meat. It is rare; however, there are likely to be an unquantifiable number of individuals in the population that will now be incubating the disease and will be undergoing surgery. All types of the disease are fatal and once symptoms develop, lead to death within a few months. In order to manage the risk of spreading the disease it is necessary to establish which tissues will be operated on. These are divided into high, medium, or low risk:

- High risk includes brain, spinal cord, and posterior eye.
- Medium risk includes the anterior eye and olfactory epithelium.
- Low risk includes the remainder of the body tissues.

In vCJD cases, lymphoid tissue is regarded as medium risk. It is advisable to utilize disposable instruments for a known vCJD patient; if it proves necessary to use reusable items, these must either be sacrificed or quarantined.

There is thought to be a negligible risk of transmission of CJD prions during fibreoptic endoscopes, in particular gastroscopy, due to the proximity of the tonsils and lymphatic tissue in the gut. Any risk is thought to be from the contamination of biopsy forceps and the biopsy channel of the endoscope. Therefore, the taking of a biopsy on an infected patient should be only be considered if absolutely necessary.

Management of patients infected should follow up-to-date local and national policy and guidelines. The issue of CJD management is under constant review.

## Further reading

Public Health England (2015). Collaborative tuberculosis strategy for England 2015 to 2020. Available at: ℘ https://www.gov.uk/government/publications/collaborative-tuberculosis-strategy-for-england

# Role of the scrub practitioner

The scrub practitioner, who may be a qualified nurse, ODP, or healthcare support worker, is a member of the perioperative team, which also includes (but which is not exhaustive of) a surgeon, a surgical assistant, a circulating practitioner, an anaesthetist, and an anaesthetic practitioner. Depending on training, education, level of competency, and experience, practitioners will perform in more than one role, for example, the scrub practitioner will also practise in the circulating role, and the surgeon in the role of the surgeon's assistant.

The role of the scrub practitioner encompasses the following:
- Donning sterile surgical attire and any additional PPE necessary for the procedure.
- Setting up the surgical instrument tray, including checking all instruments are present, clean, and in good working condition.
- Ensuring checks of all instruments, swabs, needles, blades, sutures, and any other sharps and accessories are correct and accounted for before, during (as necessary), and after the procedure, and that the surgeon is thus informed, therefore reducing the risk of retaining a foreign body.
- Maintaining a sterile operative field throughout the procedure to reduce the risk of SSI.
- Anticipating the surgeon's needs throughout the surgery therefore assisting in its facilitation.
- Ensuring that handling of instruments, sharps, and any associated equipment and accessories avoids injury to the surgical team and/or the patient.
- Ensuring that all medical device equipment, instruments, accessories, and equipment are used in accordance with the manufacturer's recommendations.
- Maintaining a safe operating room environment throughout the procedure.
- Maintaining an awareness of the risks and complications associated with the surgical practice, inclusive of the instrumentation and other equipment and accessories being used (e.g. patient positioning, diathermy, skin preparation solutions, and dressing products).
- Ensuring effective communications with the perioperative team, including checking the patient's identity, consent, allergies, skin integrity, proposed surgical procedure, and surgical site.
- Making sure that the patient's dignity is maintained by the whole perioperative team from entering the operating room to leaving the operating room.
- Ensuring that all specimens are handled, documented, and forwarded to the appropriate department in accordance with local policy.
- Accurately documenting the patient's care in accordance with local policy, inclusive of all instrument and product/implant traceability information.
- Disposing of all contaminated instrumentation, accessories, and associated equipment, including linen and PPE into the appropriate waste receptacles in accordance with local waste disposal guidelines for decontamination or incineration.

- Training and education.
- Adhering to local and national policies, procedures, guidelines, and recommendations in relation to perioperative practice.
- Practising at all times within professional guidelines and legal boundaries.

## Further reading

Association of periOperative Registered Nurses (2020). Guidelines for perioperative practice. Denver, CO: AORN Inc.

Association for Perioperative Practice (2017). Standards and recommendations for safe perioperative practice. Harrogate: Association for Perioperative Practice.

Australian College of Operating Room Nurses (2020). Standards for perioperative nursing. Adelaide: ACORN Ltd.

# Setting up of the surgical instrument tray

The majority of operating departments are supplied with sterile surgical instrument trays and supplementary instruments from a theatre sterile supply unit. Tray sets are usually standardized and named according to specialty and usage (e.g. laparotomy set). Instruments and tray sets should all have a system for tracking and tracing in compliance with decontamination guidelines.

*Pre-set tray systems* are either perforated or solid. Some trays are modified to house specialty-specific instruments (e.g. some orthopaedic sets).

To maintain the sterility of the instruments, trays are often wrapped with a double lining of either reusable or disposable linen. The *outer layer* is non-sterile, and when opened reveals an inner sterile layer, which only the scrubbed practitioner handles. The outer layer is opened away from the body first then towards the circulating practitioner, and the scrub practitioner opens the *inner sterile layer* in the opposite direction, towards the body first then away. If using a trolley set-up system, the trolley should be prepared with a double layer of drapes large enough to cover the surface and sides of the trolley.

The instrument set should be prepared as close to the time of the surgery as possible to maintain sterility. Each tray should have a checklist detailing all the instruments held on the tray. Each instrument should be checked against this list by the scrub and circulating practitioners before each procedure. Each instrument should be inspected to make sure it is in good working order, intact, and free from any contaminants such as dried blood and body tissues. Any instruments which are damaged or contaminated should be removed. If an instrument on the tray set is contaminated, the entire tray should be discarded.

Instruments are usually set on the tray in the order that they will be used and in groups of the same types of instruments. Instruments with ringed handles should be kept together and aligned according to any curves or angles, for example, curved scissors should all point in the same direction. Instruments are laid out beside each other and not on top of each other, and fine instruments, for example, micro-instruments should be treated with extra care. Any tip protectors should be removed. Any sharps should be protected at all times, and blades mounted onto the blade handle using an appropriate instrument, not fingers. Care should be taken to avoid metal-to-metal, as this can increase the chance of instrument damage.

*To maintain sterility*, neither the scrub nor circulating practitioner should lean over the instrument tray/trolley set. The circulating practitioner should hand over any supplementary instruments and other necessary sundries avoiding any contamination either of the tray or the contents of the pack. The outer wrapping of any sterile packs should be opened away from the body then secured allowing the scrub practitioner to take the contents without contamination. Supplementary packs should be presented from the side of the tray/trolley and not dropped onto the tray which may result in contaminating the tray, dropping the pack contents, or displacement of tray instruments.

*Sharps and heavy instruments* should be passed to avoid piercing the tray linen and injury. The circulating practitioner should avoid splashes when pouring liquid solutions into tray pots presented by the scrub practitioner. Wet linen can affect the tray's sterility.

The scrub practitioner is responsible for the instrument tray, and once prepared should stay with it at all times.

## Further reading

Association for Perioperative Practice (2017). Standards and recommendations for safe perioperative practice. Harrogate: Association for Perioperative Practice.

Phillips N, Hornacky A (2020). Berry & Kohn's operating room technique (14th ed). St Louis, MO: Elsevier.

Woodhead K, Fudge L (eds) (2012). Manual of perioperative care: an essential guide. Oxford: Wiley Blackwell.

# Accountability of swabs, sharps, and instruments

The purpose of undertaking instrument and consumable counts is to re-duce the risk of them being retained within the body. Retaining items within the body is considered preventable; therefore, if this occurs, legal proceed-ings may result. If an item is retained within the body it is treated as a foreign body which can cause problems immediately or after a significant period of time; these can include wound infections, infections within body cav-ities, pain (including referred pain), bleeding, delays in wound healing, loss of anatomical structure function, and formation of abscesses, fistulae, and adhesions. Further surgery may be required to remove the foreign body and this may have its associated risks.

All of the surgical team are accountable for the surgical count; however, it is the scrub practitioner who is responsible for implementing the checks of all items being used before, during, and after the surgical procedure, and generally undertakes these checks with the circulating practitioner. This includes checking (but is not exhaustive of), instruments (and any de-tachable parts including screws), swabs, sharps (needles, blades, sutures), clips, slings/sloops, tapes, cotton wool balls, pledgets, ribbon gauze, packs, patties, sponges, diathermy blades, and tips.

If no scrub practitioner is required for the procedure, counts should be undertaken by the surgeon and the circulating practitioner.

All tray instruments are audibly and visually checked against the corres-ponding tray list and counted. Additional consumable items, such as swabs and sutures are visually checked and audibly counted. Consumable items are added onto the theatre wall-mounted swab board. If the count is inter-rupted for any reason, it should be restarted.

## Counts are undertaken

- At the beginning of surgery
- As items are added during surgery
- Before closing a cavity within a cavity
- Before closing the wound/any deep incision
- Before skin closure
- If either the scrub or circulating practitioner is replaced during the surgical procedure
- At any time the scrub practitioner feels it is appropriate to do so.

All counts must be signed for by two practitioners, one of whom must be registered. This is usually the scrub and circulating practitioners, whose names should be added to the theatre register and into the patient's intraoperative record. It is advocated that the two practitioners who under-take the initial count undertake all counts throughout the surgery. If either practitioner is replaced, their names should also be added into the theatre register and in the patient's intraoperative documentation.

All swabs and consumables such as patties, pledgets, and ribbon gauze should be packed and counted in 'fives', and to ensure easy identification at X-ray should they be retained, have an X-ray detectable band.

## Counts discrepancy

Any bundle that does not contain 'five' should be immediately discarded. Items such as blades, sutures, and needles are counted in multiples of 'one'. Any instruments, blades, sutures, or needles which break during surgery should be accounted for and all parts returned. All items, inclusive of waste disposal bags and laundry, used during the surgical procedure should be kept in theatre until surgery is completed. These will be checked if an item goes missing.

If in the case of life-threatening emergency, it may not be possible to perform the count. In this situation, all packaging should be kept, and a count undertaken as soon as is realistically possible.

At every count performed during the procedure, the scrub practitioner should audibly inform the surgeon of the result, and this should be audibly acknowledged by the surgeon. If there is a discrepancy in the count the surgeon should be made aware straight away, as it is the surgeon's responsibility to decide whether to continue or stop until the missing item is found. If the surgical team are unable to find the lost item, an X-ray must be taken either before the patient leaves the operating room or before leaving the theatre suite. Any missing items which have not been found must be recorded in the patient's documentation and an incident form completed.

## Further reading

Association of periOperative Registered Nurses (2020). Guidelines for perioperative practice. Denver, CO: AORN Inc.

Association for Perioperative Practice (2017). Accountable items: swab, instrument and sharp counts. Harrogate: Association for Perioperative Practice.

Association for Perioperative Practice (2017). Standards and recommendations for safe perioperative practice. Harrogate: Association for Perioperative Practice.

Australian College of Operating Room Nurses (2020). Standards for perioperative nursing. Adelaide: ACORN Ltd.

# Administration of drugs during surgery

UK government legislation aims to reduce the incidence of drug errors and ultimately improve patient safety. This legislation includes The Human Medicines Regulations 2012[1] (relates to manufacturing supply, licensing, and sales), and The Misuse of Drugs Regulations 2001[2] (allows identified practitioners within their field of practice to possess, prescribe, and dispense controlled drugs). There should be compliance with local policies and procedures, including guidance on ordering, receipt, storage, and management of controlled and emergency drugs, should further ensure good management in drug administration.

Drug errors can happen at any stage in the process from prescription to administration and some reasons offered for these errors include:
• Failure to cross-reference patient identity with the prescription
• Illegible handwriting
• Fatigue
• Inaccuracies in the prescription dosage
• Use of abbreviations in the prescription
• Administration of the wrong drug
• Discrepancies in the frequency of administration
• Poor communication
• Distractions
• Missing/inaccurate documentation
• Administration of drugs patient is known to be allergic to
• Incorrect labelling.

Drugs within perioperative practice are not just restricted to traditional pharmaceuticals; they are developed from natural, synthetic, and semi-synthetic sources and they come in a variety of different forms including liquids, gases, solids, powders, and creams/ointments. The types of drugs used include antibiotics, analgesics, opiates, gaseous agents (inhalations and IV agents), muscle relaxants, anticoagulants, hormones, laxatives, thrombolytics, diuretics, and antiemetics, and this list is not exhaustive.

Drugs are used locally (via the skin and/or mucous membranes) and systemically (via the digestive system, parenterally, IV, SC and/or through the peritoneal cavity) throughout all three phases of the patient's perioperative journey, for example:
• Preoperatively in an attempt to improve the patient's physical condition to promote a better clinical outcome during and post-surgery, and/or immediately before surgery, for example, to reduce anxiety and provide pain relief.
• Intraoperatively, which often includes some form of local, regional, or general anaesthetic (sometimes a combination of all three).
• Postoperatively, for example to reduce pain and control nausea.

*Perioperative practitioners involved in the administration* of drugs must ensure the right patient receives the right drug, at the right time, in the correct dosage, via the right route. Drugs should not be administered unless the dispensing practitioner has an underlying knowledge of the drug, the strength, its action, the route of administration, the side effects, and knows what to do if the wrong drug is administered or if the patient suffers an allergic reaction. Additional considerations are required for paediatrics; for example, the amount prescribed will depend on the child's body weight and/or the surface area, and the elderly, whose physical condition may, for example, affect the absorption rate.

*Local departments should develop their own policies* to ensure safe drug practices and to encompass incidences when drugs are prepared by one professional and administered by another, as is common practice during anaesthesia and during surgery, for example, the circulating practitioner prepares the medication, and delivers it to the scrub practitioner who hands it to the surgeon to administer. Drugs administered in this way should always be verbally and visually checked to confirm the drug type, the dose, the strength, and the expiry date.

All drugs administered should be labelled correctly, and all drug packaging should stay in the operating room until surgery is complete.

All pharmaceutical preparations used should be clearly documented in the patient records, and any unused medication disposed of appropriately.

## References

1. legislation.gov.uk (2012). The Human Medicines Regulations 2012. Available at: ⅏ https://www. legislation.gov.uk/uksi/2012/1916/contents/made
2. legislation.gov.uk (2001). The Misuse of Drugs Regulations 2001. Available at: ⅏ https://www. legislation.gov.uk/uksi/2001/3998/contents/made

# Handling of surgical instruments

The instruments used during surgery are classified according to what they will be used for, including:
- Cutting
- Dissecting
- Retracting
- Grasping
- Clamping
- Aspirating
- Probing
- Measuring
- Suturing.

The surgical team should know the instruments for the procedure being undertaken, including knowing the instrument's name and what it is used for.

Whether reusable or single-use instruments, to ensure instruments remain fully functioning and in optimum condition for use during surgery they must be handled correctly and with care. Incorrect usage of instruments usually occurs when the correct instrument is unavailable, which can be avoided if instrument sets are preselected appropriately for each procedure.

Appropriate instrument handling also helps to reduce the incidence of injury to the patient and/or the surgical team, including personal injury, and prolongs the life of the instrument.

All surgical instruments should be handled gently, particularly micro-instruments:
- Dropping should be avoided—any dropped instruments should not be returned to the surgical field or instrument tray.
- Heavier instruments should not be placed on top of more delicate instruments.
- Tips and sharps points should be protected with tip protectors (e.g. needles, scissors, and hooks).
- Instruments should be handled either individually or in groups of similar instruments (e.g. artery forceps, scissors).
- Care and attention should be given during the decontamination process (e.g. instruments should not be dropped into wash sinks).
- Used instruments should be sent to a sterile services decontamination unit for reprocessing inclusive of lubricating and drying. (Single-use instrumentation should be discarded in accordance with local and national decontamination guidelines, policies, and procedures.)

Before use, the scrub practitioner should ensure that all tray instrumentation and supplementary instrumentation is sterile. If the sterility is in question, the instrument should be discarded. This includes whether the instrumentation is still within its shelf life, that is, the length of time that the instrument is considered to be sterile.

## Good practice in instrument handling involves

- Passing decisively to the surgeon's operating hand (awareness should be given to whether the surgeon is right- or left-handed), in a manner that allows the surgeon to use immediately without the need for any adjustment. Instruments with curves should be handed over with the curve in the direction of the surgeon's palms. Instruments are often used in sequence, and appropriate to the site, for example, short instruments will be used for superficial wounds and longer instruments for deeper body cavities
- Passing and returning sharps to the hand should be avoided—it is recommended that a 'no-touch' technique is used, for example, sharps instruments are placed into a container such as a kidney dish
- Not placing or leaving instruments on the patient—this increases the risk of injury to the patient and/or surgical team and increases the potential for contamination. All instruments should be returned to the instrument trolley
- Mounting all needles/sutures onto a needle holder before handing over to the surgeon
- Checking all powered instruments, for example, saws and drills for function, and particular attention paid to accidental activation. When not being used, powered instruments should be kept in 'safe' mode.

Instruments should not be used if damaged. Prior to use and during reprocessing all instruments should be checked for any damage including cracks, chips, blunting, and alignment. When instruments become damaged, they should be returned to the manufacturer for repair and/or replacement.

All surgical instrumentation should be stored in an area, which is clean, dust free, and dry. Storage surfaces should be easy to clean with smooth surfaces.

## Further reading

Association for Perioperative Practice (2017). Standards and recommendations for safe perioperative practice. Harrogate: Association for Perioperative Practice.

Clarke P, Jones J (1998). Brigden's operating department practice. Edinburgh: Churchill Livingstone.

Phillips N, Hornacky A (2020). Berry & Kohn's operating room technique (14th ed). St Louis, MO: Elsevier.

# Management of sharps

Sharps can be defined as suture needles, scalpel blades, or any other sharp equipment/instrument with potential to cause injury. Suture needles and scalpel blades have been found to be the leading cause of percutaneous injury. Suture needles alone account for 50% of these injuries. Scalpel injuries have been found to occur most often while passing, disassembling, or disposing of the blade.

Sharps safety is important to prevent injuries which risk the transmission of viruses such as HBV, HCV, and HIV. Percutaneous injuries are usually associated with the occupational transmission of hepatitis B, hepatitis C, and HIV but they are also implicated in the transmission of more than 20 other pathogens.

- A local policy for handling and disposal of sharps should be in place.
- Sharps should not be passed hand to hand. A 'hands-free' technique should be employed when passing sharps. Consider the use of a 'neutral zone'.
- Disposal of sharps is the responsibility of the individual members of the perioperative team.
- An appropriate instrument/device should be used for removal of surgical blades.
- Needles should not be re-sheathed, bent, or broken before disposal.
- A disposable sharps pad should be used to contain sharps and disposed of safely at the end of a procedure.
- Sharps containers should be placed close to the point of use.
- Sharps containers must not be filled to more than three-quarters and should not contain any protruding sharps.
- Sharps containers should be stored off the floor.

## Needlestick injury

A local policy for needlestick injuries should be in place. In the event of injury:

- Encourage bleeding.
- Wash under running water.
- Dry and apply a waterproof dressing.
- Consent must be obtained from the patient to obtain a sample of blood for storage and testing. Patients have the right to refuse this.
- The patient needs to be fully recovered from the effects of GA before they are informed of the incident.
- An incident form should be completed.
- Infection prevention and control team and/or occupational health should be informed as soon as possible.
- Professional counselling and follow-up should be available.

# Clinical waste

All healthcare waste, whether in a hospital or community setting, is assumed to be infectious until it is assessed by the healthcare professional.

## Clinical waste is categorized as

- Healthcare waste
- Medicinal waste
- Infectious waste
- Offensive/hygiene waste.

Infectious waste has been defined as waste with a potential risk of causing infection during handling. Infectious waste has been categorized as:
- Microbiological cultures
- Pathological waste
- Human blood and blood products
- Used sharps.

There is also a revised colour-coded system for the disposal of waste. The Department of Health 'Safe Management of Healthcare Waste' document obliges organizations to segregate waste into specific colour-coded waste streams.[1] Waste should be segregated accordingly into colour-coded bags and containers.
- Yellow stream: infectious waste which requires disposal by incineration and includes diagnostic specimens, reagent or test vials, and kits containing chemicals; all waste from isolation rooms; and all waste from patients undergoing source isolation. Incinerated at 1000°C (holding time 2 minutes).
- Red/orange: anatomical waste such as body parts and any surgical residue.
- Purple stream: cytotoxic and cytostatic waste which must be incinerated in a permitted or licensed facility. Suitable purple/yellow receptacles should be available for this waste. Incinerated at 1000°C (holding time 2 minutes).
- Black stream/white stream: non-infectious/non-hazardous/domestic waste which does not contain infectious materials, sharps, or medicinal materials. Segregation of the potentially hazardous contents such as glass, aerosols and heavy items is important. Incinerated at 800°C (holding time 2 minutes).

## Sharps bins

- Yellow with yellow lids: all sharps other than cytotoxic or cytostatic medicines.
- Yellow with purple lids: sharps contaminated with cytotoxic or cytostatic medicinal products.
- Yellow with blue lids: pharmaceutical products being returned to pharmacy.

## Disposal of waste

- Waste bags should not be overfilled.
- Waste bags should be securely tied.
- Bags must be clearly labelled to indicate the department they came from.
- Waste should be collected promptly and stored securely while awaiting incineration.
- Waste container for storage of waste bags should be easy to clean.
- Spillages from bags should be dealt with immediately.
- Handwashing facilities should be available.
- Adequate provision of sharps' bins.

## Reference

1. Department of Health (2013). Health technical memorandum 07-01. Safe management of health care waste. London: Department of Health.

# Instrument trays

The patient's surgical outcome is dependent on the competence, knowledge, and skills in the application of aseptic technique of practitioners. The basic principles of aseptic technique promote a sterile field in which surgery may be safely performed. Competent preparation and use of equipment is a major investment.

- The type of instrument tray used for a procedure is influenced by the type of surgery to be performed.
- Surgical instruments must be prepared immediately prior to use.
- A designated area should be identified for the purpose of preparing instrument trays for a procedure.
- Equipment should be collected in advance.
- Instrument trays must be checked for sterility, integrity, packaging, and expiry date.
- Instrument trays should be covered with a minimum of two layers of sterile drapes.
- Items/instruments extending over the edge of the trolley are at risk of contamination.
- Instrument trays should be opened away from the body first then towards.
- Prepared instrument trays must be accompanied at all times.
- Staff should adhere to an agreed method of setting the instrument trolley. This facilitates continuity of care for patients and safety for staff if someone else was required to take over for any reason.
- Instruments must always be returned to the trolley when not in use.

## Further reading

Association for Perioperative Practice (2017). Standards and recommendations for safe perioperative practice. Harrogate: Association for Perioperative Practice.

# Decontamination of equipment

All reusable equipment must be decontaminated between use and between patients. Surgical equipment must be cleaned and decontaminated following use in preparation for storage and packaging or disinfection/sterilization. Decontamination is necessary in order to render a reusable instrument safe for handling by staff and for use on patients.

## Decontamination

Decontamination is the term used to describe the process of removing or reducing contamination from infectious organisms or any other harmful substances. Decontamination is the combination of cleaning, disinfection, and sterilization.

### Methods of decontamination

- *Cleaning* is the term used to describe the removal of visible dirt, soil, or organic matter from equipment. Cleaning does not infer killing of microorganisms. Cleaning is necessary before disinfection or sterilization. Failure to adequately clean instruments will render the disinfection or sterilization process ineffective.
- *Disinfection* is the term used to describe a reduction of the number of vegetative microorganisms and viruses to relatively safe levels.
- *Sterilization* is the term used to describe the complete killing or removal of all microorganisms including spores.

The cleaning and decontamination area must be separate from the sterilizing and packing area.

Cleaning/decontamination process:

- Water.
- Mechanical action.
- Detergent or enzymatic products.

### Selection of detergent

- Detergents should facilitate removal of debris without damaging instrument/equipment.
- Detergents should be low sudsing and rinse off without leaving any residue.
- An acidic detergent is preferable for the removal of a combination of organic/ inorganic debris (e.g. urine).
- An alkaline detergent is preferable for the removal of organic debris (e.g. blood and faeces).
- It is important to follow manufacturers' instructions.

### Automated washer-disinfectors

Cleaning by machine is preferable to manual cleaning as it offers greater protection to the worker. Washer decontaminator/disinfectors combine cleaning and heat disinfection and are used to process items for reuse or to render items clean and safe prior to sterilization.

### Ultrasonic cleaners

Ultrasonic cleaners may be used to clean and decontaminate instruments/equipment that may not tolerate the automated washer process.

*Preparation of cleaned and decontaminated instruments*

Cleaned and decontaminated instruments are safe to handle in preparation for storage and packaging or disinfection/sterilization.

- Instruments must be inspected for cleanliness, functioning, defects, sharpness/blunting of cutting edges.
- Lubrication of moving parts is important; a water-based lubricant is recommended.
- Instruments must be dried before storage.

## Further reading

Association of periOperative Registered Nurses (2020). Guidelines for perioperative practice. Denver, CO: AORN Inc.

Association for Perioperative Practice (2017). Standards and recommendations for safe perioperative practice. Harrogate: Association for Perioperative Practice.

# Personal protective equipment

PPE is used to protect both healthcare workers and patients from the risk of infection. The correct and appropriate use of protective clothing has taken on considerable importance in recent years with greater awareness of the risks posed by infectious patients to healthcare workers and the need to reduce transmission of infection from patient to patient.

Health and safety legislation indicates that protective clothing is worn appropriately and correctly to manage the risk of exposure to microorganisms which may be hazardous to health.[1] The principles are underpinned by the Health and Safety at Work Act 1974 and legislation relating to PPE at work.[2]

Healthcare workers have a professional responsibility to ensure that protective clothing is worn appropriately. The NMC states that practitioners are personally accountable for their practice and this involves putting anyone at risk.[3]

The use of protective clothing in preventing cross-infection is extremely important given:
- The morbidity and mortality associated with hospital-acquired infection[4]
- The cost of treating hospital-acquired infections
- The increasing problem of antibiotic-resistant microorganisms.[7]

The primary use of protective clothing in healthcare settings is:
- To protect the skin and mucous membranes of healthcare workers from exposure to blood/body fluids
- To prevent contamination of clothing and to reduce the opportunity of the spread of organisms from patients/fomites to other patients or environments.

## Types of gloves
- Natural rubber latex.
- Neoprene and nitrile gloves.
- Vinyl gloves.

## Gloves

The incorrect use of gloves can lead to undermining hand hygiene initiatives and risks skin problems such as dermatitis. The aim of gloves is to:
- Protect users' hands from becoming contaminated with organic matter and microorganisms
- Protect users' hands from exposure to certain chemicals that may adversely affect the condition of the skin
- Minimize cross infection by preventing the transfer of organisms from staff to patients and vice versa.

Glove use—undertake a risk assessment to determine whether gloves are required:
- Gloves are required for procedures involving contact with blood, body fluids, excretions and secretions, non-intact skin, or mucous membranes.
- Gloves must be changed between patient contacts and between separate procedures on the same patient.
- Change gloves if torn or punctured.

- Gloves are single use and should never be washed or reused.
- Plastic gloves should never be worn for clinical tasks.
- Hands should be decontaminated following the removal of gloves.

## Gowns

Gowns principally perform two functions:
- Single-use fluid-repellent aprons protect the healthcare worker's clothing from contamination with blood, body fluids, or microorganisms.
- Sterile gowns protect the patients from hospital-acquired infections, usually worn by staff when performing invasive procedures (e.g. surgery or the insertion of a central venous catheter).
- The wearing of sterile gowns is necessary in theatres or when performing aseptic invasive procedures in a clinical area.
- Gowns should be disposed of after use as clinical waste and hands decontaminated immediately.

## Masks

Historically, the principal function of a mask has been to:
- Protect patients from the potential shedding of microorganisms from staff
- Protect the healthcare worker from potential exposure to microorganisms.

*Masks should be*
- Worn for all procedures where there is a risk of blood, body fluids, secretions, or excretions splashing into the mucous membranes
- Used as single-use items and disposed of immediately after removing
- Changed if moist or wet
- Appropriate for their purpose
- Worn correctly
- Close fitting
- Handled as little as possible
- Removed by untying and handled only by the ties as they may be heavily contaminated
- Never worn loosely around the neck.

## Eye protection

Eye protection is principally worn to protect the eyes of the healthcare worker from contamination with blood, body fluids, or chemicals.

Eye protection must be readily available in clinical areas where procedures likely to produce splashing are performed. The types commonly used in the healthcare setting are:
- Goggles
- Visors
- Face-shields—single-use surgical facemask with integral eye-shield.

*Goggles/visor/face shield should be worn*
- When splash or spray of blood/body fluids is likely
- When dealing with chemicals
- During aerosol prone procedures.

*Goggles/visor/face-shield should*
- Be comfortable to wear
- Fit correctly
- Allow for clear uncompromised vision.

*Multi-use goggles/visors should*
- Be cleaned with detergent and hot water and dried thoroughly after use
- Be cleaned as above and disinfected with 70% alcohol if contaminated with blood or body fluids
- Be replaced when lenses become scratched/opaque or the elastic ceases to provide a correct fit.

## Caps

Caps are principally worn:
- To reduce the dispersal of hair and skin
- To protect the wearer from contamination from blood or body fluids.

## Disposable plastic aprons

Disposable plastic aprons:
- Provide a physical barrier between clothing and skin
- Prevent contamination and wetting of uniforms during washing of equipment
- Reduce the risk of contamination of uniforms with blood and body fluids.

## References

1. Legislation.gov.uk (2002). The Control of Substances Hazardous to Health Regulations 2002. Available at: ℘ https://www.legislation.gov.uk/uksi/2002/2677/contents
2. Health and Safety Executive (1992). Health and Safety at Work Act 1974. London: HMSO.
3. Nursing and Midwifery Council (2018). The code: professional standards of practice and be-haviours for nurses, midwives and nursing associates. Available at: ℘ https://www.nmc.org.uk/globalassets/sitedocuments/nmc-publications/nmc-code.pdf

## Further reading

Ayliffe GAJ, Fraise AP, Geddes AM, et al. (2000). Control of hospital infection: a practical handbook (4th ed). London: Arnold.
Damani NN (2019). Manual of infection control procedures (4th ed). Oxford: Oxford University Press.
Department of Health (1995). Hospital infection control. Guidance on the control of infection in hospitals. London: Department of Health.
Health and Safety at Work Act (1974). Health Services Advisory Committee. London: The Stationery Office.
Horton R, Parker L (2002). Informed infection control practice (2nd ed). London: Churchill Livingstone.
Infection Control Nurses Association (1999). Glove usage guidelines. Bathgate: Infection Control Nurses Association.
Infection Control Nurses Association (2002). Protective clothing, principles and guidance. Bathgate: Infection Control Nurses Association.
McCulloch J (2000). Infection control, science, management and practice. London: Whurr.
Wilson J (2001). Infection control in clinical practice (2nd ed). London: Balliere Tindall.

# Thermoregulation

The skin maintains the body's normothermic state, that is, at a temperature of 37°C. As the body temperature increases, the peripheral blood vessels dilate, allowing more blood to circulate near the surface. If the body temperature drops then the body will attempt to self-regulate by decreasing the flow of blood near to the surface to conserve internal heat. The loss of heat or the ability to produce heat may directly affect the patient's physiological response to surgery. During surgery the loss of heat is primarily the result of:

- Exposure to the physical environment
- The surgical incision
- The immobility of the patient
- The effect of any existing coexisting circulatory conditions.

## Other causes of hypothermia

Contributory factors that will add to inadvertent hypothermia include:

- Exposure of the skin or body cavities to cool ambient room air or drafts due to operating theatre ventilation air changes
- Patients undergoing longer surgery will be more susceptible to hypothermia as will those who undergo irrigation of body cavities with unwarmed fluids.

## Adverse effects of hypothermia

It has been shown that inadvertent hypothermia:

- Increases postoperative discomfort
- Increases the chance of bleeding
- Increases the incidence of ischaemia and tachycardia
- Can cause impaired wound healing
- Can increase the risk of wound infection which may result in a longer stay in hospital.

## Vulnerable patient groups

### Older patients

While all patients are potentially susceptible to hypothermia during surgery, older patients are more vulnerable due to the ageing process—their metabolic rate is reduced which means they are prone to be more sensitive to cold.

- They have decreased ability to regulate their temperature and they tend to have a lower core temperature.
- The efficiency of the shivering response also reduces the ability to overcome a loss of temperature.

### Paediatric patients

Like older adults, babies and children are also susceptible to heat loss during anaesthesia and surgery and will become hypothermic more quickly than adults. Babies and children will lose body heat in the same way and for the same reasons as adults, but are more at risk for the following reasons:

- In paediatric patients, the head represents a far larger fraction of the total surface area of their body. As the skull and scalp are thin, this allows further loss of heat.
- Because cutaneous heat loss is roughly proportional to surface area, it is relatively easy for infants and children to lose large amounts of heat from the skin surface.[1]

## Further reading

Association for Perioperative Practice (2016). Standards and recommendations for safe perioperative practice. Harrogate: Association for Perioperative Practice.

Australian College of Operating Room Nurses (2020). Standards for perioperative nursing. Adelaide: ACORN Ltd.

Association of periOperative Registered Nurses (2020). Guidelines for perioperative practice. Denver, CO: AORN Inc.

Phillips N, Hornacky A (2020). Berry & Kohn's operating room technique (14th ed). St Louis, MO: Elsevier.

Sutherland-Fraser S, Davies M, Lockwood B, et al. (eds) (2021). Perioperative nursing: an introduction (3rd ed). Chatswood: Elsevier Australia.

# Warming devices and techniques

It is advisable to maintain the patient's body heat which can be helped by keeping the patient warm preoperatively. It is better to prevent heat loss than treat a hypothermic patient.

## Preoperatively
- Check patient's temperature.
- Where possible, use a forced-air warmer for 30 minutes to pre-warm the patient.

## Intraoperatively
Techniques to reduce the inadvertent hypothermia include the following:
- Use blankets to maintain heat pre- and postoperatively.
- Minimize exposure until access is required.
- Increase the anaesthetic room and operating theatre temperature.
- Warm IV and irrigation fluids.
- Use a forced-air warming device during induction of anaesthesia and intraoperatively in accordance with the manufacturer's instructions.
- Monitor and record the patient's temperature throughout the perioperative process.
- Burns are potential complication if warming devices are used inappropriately, particularly in patients who have vascular impairment.

## Postoperatively
- Apply all the pre- and intraoperative measures where possible.
- Avoid the use of excessive layers of ordinary blankets which may cause restriction of movement and respiration and cause discomfort.
- Avoid disturbing the closest layer to the patient's skin as this will result in further heat loss.
- Do not allow the patient to leave the recovery room until normothermic.

## Further reading
Abbott H, Booth H (eds) (2014). Foundations for operating department practice: essential theory for practice. Maidenhead: Open University Press.

Association for Perioperative Practice (2016). Standards and recommendations for safe perioperative practice. Harrogate: Association for Perioperative Practice.

Australian College of Operating Room Nurses (2020). Standards for perioperative nursing. Adelaide: ACORN Ltd.

Association of periOperative Registered Nurses (2020). Guidelines for perioperative practice. Denver, CO: AORN Inc.

Phillips N, Hornacky A (2020). Berry & Kohn's operating room technique (14th ed). St Louis, MO: Elsevier.

Royal College of Anaesthetists (2020). Chapter 10: guidelines for the provision of paediatric anaesthesia services. London: Royal College of Anaesthetists.

Royal College of Anaesthetists (2019). Chapter 4: guidelines for the provision of postoperative care. London: Royal College of Anaesthetists.

Sutherland-Fraser S, Davies M, Lockwood B, et al. (eds) (2021). Perioperative nursing: an introduction (3rd ed). Chatswood: Elsevier Australia.

# Chapter 15

# Patient positioning for surgery

# Principles for selecting patient position

The selection of the position of the patient on the operating table will depend on the type of surgery that is to be undertaken, so that access to the part of the body is maximized for the surgeon while making it possible for the anaesthetist to deliver a safe anaesthetic and monitor the patient.

Most important is that the patient is safe on the operating table and that no harm is done to them while they are moved on or off the operating table and positioned for the procedure.

It is useful when a patient is being positioned on the operating table in the operating theatre, for a member of staff, often the scrub practitioner, to coordinate the positioning by placing themselves where they can oversee the moving and positioning of the patient. The best place to stand is at the foot of the table. It is also important that the patient is positioned anatomically and that limbs in particular are placed in their natural position. This is very important for patients with contractions or deformities of their limbs which must be allowed to remain in their natural position. The same is true for the patient's body alignment, for example, when the patient is placed in the supine position that they are laying in what looks like a comfortable sleeping position.

> Practitioners should be aware that the positioning of the patient can affect BP, venous return, and ventilation.

While overseeing the transfer of the patient, the scrub practitioner should also see that the patient is transferred safely, that the neck and head are supported, and that IV infusions and other lines are safe.

Particular care must also be taken to protect pressure points such as elbows and heels with suitable padding, or pressure-relieving devices such as gel pads, or cushioning such as pillows. Care must also be taken to protect the eyes and consideration may be made by the use of padding where appropriate.

# Supine and Trendelenburg positions

## Supine position

This is probably one of the most widely used and natural positions for the surgical patient and is suitable for many general surgical procedures such as laparotomy, vascular, or breast surgery. The patient is positioned on the operating table on their back with their arms extended on arm boards or alongside their body (Fig. 15.1).

If arm boards are used, the angle of the arms must not exceed 90° with the palms ideally tuned upwards. Hyperabduction of the arm may result in the stretching of the subclavian and axillary blood vessels and stretching of the brachial plexus, ulnar nerve, and superficial nerves of the arm.

The head can be placed on a pillow and the knees are supported by padding. Padding is used to avoid damage caused by pressure to the heels, sacrum, and elbows, and all peripheral nerves such as the ulnar nerve at the elbow and the lateral nerve at the head of the fibula.

## Trendelenburg position

This is a variation of the supine position as already described which involves the tilting of the table to a head-down angle of up to 40°. It is used for abdominal/pelvic gynaecological procedures and operations for varicose veins.

Care must be taken to ensure that the patient does not slip headfirst down the table. This can be achieved by the use of an anti-slip mattress, or securing straps around the patient, or by the use of shoulder pads. In the Trendelenburg position, BP can increase due to the pooling of blood in the upper torso. Care should be taken to return the patient to the supine position slowly to avoid a drop in BP.

The reverse Trendelenburg position is also utilized for head and neck procedures to promote venous drainage away from the operation site.

The use of a footboard may be required in order to prevent the patient slipping feet first. In the reverse Trendelenburg position, there are considerations regarding BP:
- Diminished cardiac return resulting in diminished cardiac output.
- Decrease in brainstem perfusion due to gravity.
- Pooling of blood in lower extremities.
- Possibility of circulatory overload if returned to the supine position too quickly.

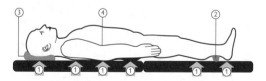

① Pressure points

② Ankle support prevents heel and calf pressure

③ Head support prevents neck hyperextension

④ Access to arm veins restricted: extension to cannula or abduct arm

**Fig. 15.1** Supine position.

Reproduced from Quick C, Thomas P, and Deakin P. Principles of Surgical Management, 2001, ISBN 9780192622303, with permission from Oxford University Press.

# Lloyd-Davies and lithotomy positions

## Lloyd-Davies position

This position is used where access is required to the pelvis and perineum for colorectal, gynaecological, or urological operations and is a modification of the lithotomy position (Fig. 15.2).

The legs are placed in the Lloyd-Davies stirrups at an angle of about 45° with the knee slightly flexed. Care must be taken when placing the legs in position, especially in older patients who may have arthritic problems with hips and knees.

The placing should be coordinated with legs gently lifted at the same time and the anaesthetist informed that the legs are to be lifted. The end of the table is removed and often a tray is attached to the table in the space between the patient's legs for the placement of surgical instruments.

The patient's bottom may also be placed on a pad to further aid access to the pelvic region and the table is usually tipped with the patient's head slightly down.

Great care needs to be taken to ensure that pressure areas and bony prominences are protected. If the patient is kept in this position for >4 hours the risk of compartment syndrome of the calves is increased which can affect the patient's BP and may increase their postoperative pain and may result in significant permanent damage and morbidity.

## Lithotomy position

This is used for operations or examination of the perineum, vagina, or rectum. The patient is placed on the table with their buttocks placed at the lower break in the table with the feet placed in stirrups fixed to either side of the table taking care not to place them in an excessively high position (Fig. 15.3).

The considerations are similar to those for the Lloyd-Davies position but since most procedures that utilize this position are usually shorter, there are generally fewer complications.

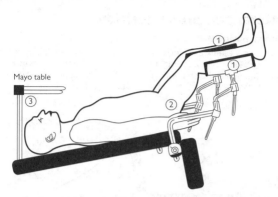

① Pressure on calf may cause venous stasis or compartment syndrome

② Better hip position but hip and femoral vessel injuries still possible

③ Anaesthetic access difficult

**Fig. 15.2** Lloyd-Davis position.

Reproduced from Quick C, Thomas P, and Deakin P. Principles of Surgical Management, 2001, ISBN 9780192622303 with permission from Oxford University Press.

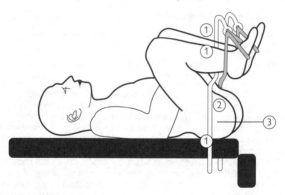

① Danger of touching metal and causing diathermy burn

② Femoral and obturator nerves in danger

③ Hip joint damage and vascular injury possible

**Fig. 15.3** Lithotomy position.

Reproduced from Quick C, Thomas P, and Deakin P. Principles of Surgical Management, 2001, ISBN 9780192622303 with permission from Oxford University Press.

# Lateral and prone positions

## Lateral position

This position can be used for such procedures as hip arthroplasty, kidney surgery, and some chest operations. The patient will be anaesthetized in the supine position and then positioned onto their side using a suitable technique, utilizing slide sheets and other positioning aids (Fig. 15.4).

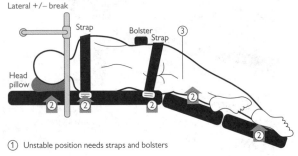

① Unstable position needs straps and bolsters

② Several pressure points

③ Need to separate legs with pillow

④ Needs careful positioning to avoid injury

⑤ Check for contact with metal and all pressure points padded

**Fig. 15.4** Lateral position.

Reproduced from Quick C, Thomas P, and Deakin P. Principles of Surgical Management, 2001, ISBN 9780192622303 with permission from Oxford University Press.

Care must be taken to position the downward shoulder slightly forward to relieve pressure on the brachial plexus while the lower arm can be flexed to rest beside the patient's head on a suitable arm board with a pad under the placed high in the axilla to relieve pressure on the brachial plexus and deltoid muscle. This will also help to prevent axillary artery and vein obstruction.

The upper arm is placed on an adjustable arm rest with the neck not overly extended to avoid stretch damage to the brachial plexus. The patient may need to be secured in position to prevent them from rolling and a pillow or pad is placed between the legs to relieve the pressure of the upper leg and the lower legs which should be slightly flexed to aid stability.

Special care must be taken to provide proper support for the head since necrosis of the ear can be caused by the pressure of the head which can be achieved by use of a soft pillow or a gel headrest.

## Prone position

This is used for procedures on the spine, neck, or the buttocks. Anaesthesia is induced with the patient in the supine position and then the patient is rolled into their front (Fig. 15.5). Techniques to undertake the transfer onto the table should be developed locally and the use of slide sheets and other moving equipment can be useful to ensure staff and patient safety. The arms should be placed along the patient's side and not around the head. The head can be placed on a padded headrest or 'doughnut' and the eyes and nose protected. The lower limbs are supported under the knees and care taken to prevent pressure caused by the feet resting on the table mattress.

A void below the abdomen should be made for the abdominal contents to avoid caval obstruction and hypotension. This can be achieved by use of pillows or a Montreal mattress.

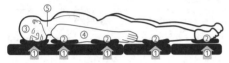

① Pressure points

② Position of padding to keep abdomen clear

③ Turn head to one side to avoid facial and eye congestion

④ Arm position important – see below

⑤ Armoured and secured tube needed

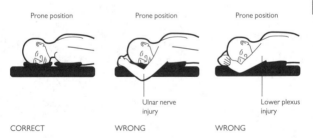

Prone position   Prone position   Prone position

CORRECT   WRONG   WRONG

Ulnar nerve injury

Lower plexus injury

**Fig. 15.5** Prone position.
Reproduced from Quick C, Thomas P, and Deakin P. Principles of Surgical Management, 2001, ISBN 9780192622303 with permission from Oxford University Press.

## Further reading

Adedeji R, Oragui E, Khan W, et al. (2010). The importance of correct patient positioning in theatres and implications of mal-positioning. Journal of Perioperative Practice, 20(4):143–147.

American Society of Anesthesiologists (2018). Practice advisory for the prevention of perioperative peripheral neuropathies 2018: an updated report by the American Society of Anesthesiologists Task Force on Prevention of Peripheral Peripheral Neuropathies. Anesthesiology, 128(1):11–26.

Balen P (2016). Nerve damage due to positioning during surgery. Journal of Patient Safety and Risk Management, 22(3–4):69–75.

Bjøro B, Mykkeltveit I, Rustøen T, et al. (2020). Intraoperative peripheral nerve injury related to lithotomy positioning with steep Trendelenburg in patients undergoing robotic-assisted laparoscopic surgery—a systematic review. Journal of Advanced Nursing, 76(2):490–503.

Kolb B, Large J (2019). An innovative prone positioning system for advanced deformity and frailty in complex spine surgery. Journal of Neurosurgery, 32(2):229–234.

Lall AC, Saadat AA, Battaglia MR, et al. (2019). Perineal pressure during hip arthroscopy is reduced by use of Trendelenburg: a prospective study with randomized order of positioning. Clinical Orthopaedics and Related Research, 477(8):1851–1857.

Mangham M (2016). Positioning of the anaesthetised patient during robotically assisted laparoscopic surgery: perioperative staff experiences. Journal of Perioperative Practice, 26(3):5–52.

Sahay N, Sharma S, Bhadani UK, et al. (2018). Effect of pneumoperitoneum and patient positioning on intracranial pressures during laparoscopy: a prospective comparative study. Journal of Minimally Invasive Gynaecology, 25(1):147–152.

# Chapter 16

# Surgical equipment

# Minimal access surgery

- May also be described as minimally invasive surgery or keyhole surgery.
- Allows access to parts of the body through very small incisions or via natural orifices for:
  - Diagnosis
  - Treatment.

## Advantages over open surgery

- Potentially less postoperative pain as the incisions are small.
- Faster recovery and earlier discharge.
- Patient can return to normal activities more quickly.
- Better cosmetic result as incisions are small.
- Potentially less blood lost during surgery so reduced need for blood transfusion.
- Potential reduction in risk of postoperative wound infection as the incisions are small.
- Opportunities for theatre staff to observe the surgery.
- Useful for teaching.
- Photographs or recordings may easily be made for the patient or for future teaching/presentations (with the patient's consent).

## Disadvantages

- Equipment may be expensive, usually including a large amount and variety of disposable equipment.
- Specific training is required for scrub and circulating staff in safe use of the equipment.
- Instruments are more difficult to clean and decontaminate.
- Difficult technique to learn.
- Can be technically challenging for surgical and scrub staff.
- For these reasons, it can be a longer procedure than open surgery.
- Where appropriate, full consent should be obtained and checked prior to surgery that an open procedure may be required.

## Technique

- Using a traditional approach, at least two incisions are made—one for the telescope and one or more for instruments; however, single incision laparoscopic trocars are now available.
- A telescope attached to a camera is introduced into the area for surgery. The telescope will vary in size and the degree of the angle of the lens will vary the field of vision.
- The operating field is visualized on a monitor, which may include three-dimensional technology.

# Further reading

Association of Perioperative Practice (2009). Surgical smoke: what we know. Harrogate: Association of Perioperative Practice.

Chen JL, Geng W, Xie SX, et al. (2015). Single-incision versus conventional three-port laparoscopic appendectomy: a meta-analysis of randomized controlled trials. Minimally Invasive Therapy, 24(4):195–203.

Foran P (2016). Undergraduate surgical nursing preparation and guided operating room experience: a quantitative analysis. Nurse Education in Practice, 16(1):217–224.

La Chapelle CF, Swank HA, Wessels ME, et al. (2015). Trocar types in laparoscopy. Cochrane Database of Systematic Reviews, 12:CD009814.

Mathews S (2016). Preventing harm from surgical plume. Kai Tiaki Nursing New Zealand, 22(6):26–27.

National Collaborating Centre for Nursing and Supportive Health (2008). Clinical practice guideline. The management of inadvertent perioperative hypothermia in adults. London: National Institute for Health and Care Excellence.

O'Riley M (2010). Electrosurgery in perioperative practice. Journal of Perioperative Practice, 20(9):329–333.

Royal College of Obstetricians and Gynaecologists (2013). Use of adhesion prevention agents in obstetrics and gynaecology. London: Royal College of Obstetricians and Gynaecologists.

Ulmer B (2010). Best practices for minimally invasive procedures. AORN Journal, 91(5):558–575.

# Laparoscopy

- Indicates a procedure involving using a camera to see inside the abdominal cavity.
- May be a diagnostic or an operative procedure.
- Major surgery may be performed this way (e.g. bowel resection).
- May be used alongside other surgical techniques (e.g. laparoscopically assisted vaginal hysterectomy).
- A small incision may be required to remove tissue or an organ surgically incised (e.g. bowel resected laparoscopically).

## Equipment and instruments

A camera stack comprising:
- High-intensity light source
- High-resolution camera system
- Monitor screen
- Recording equipment
- $CO_2$ insufflator
- Fluid and suction to maintain vision.

## Commonly performed laparoscopic procedures

- Cholecystectomy—removal of gall bladder.
- Oophorectomy.
- Appendicectomy.
- Bowel resection.
- Operations on the kidney—pyeloplasty, nephrectomy.

## Technique

- A pneumoperitoneum is achieved using $CO_2$ gas to create space and allow the organs to be visualized.
- Telescope and instruments are used through the ports to perform surgery.

## Risks associated with laparoscopic surgery

*Insufflation*
- A *Verres needle* may be inserted blind through the abdominal wall and gas introduced.
- The first port may be introduced using a *cut down*. A small para-umbilical incision is made into the peritoneal cavity. A blunt trocar is introduced allowing the peritoneal cavity to be visualized during gas insufflation to minimize the risks of perforation.
- Disposable, visual trocars are regularly used; these have a clear tip allowing visualization of each layer during the initial insertion.

*Risks*
- Perforation of blood vessels or organs caused by the needle being wrongly positioned (e.g. into the bowel or into the aorta or vena cava).
- Gas insufflated to the incorrect area potentially causing surgical emphysema if the needle is in the subcutaneous tissue or pneumothorax if in the thoracic cavity.
- Risk of burns from high-intensity light source if placed on skin/drapes.

- Cardiac arrhythmias caused by stimulation of the vagus nerve by the pressure of the gas.
- $CO_2$ embolism caused by insufflation of gas into a blood vessel.
- Respiratory depression caused by upward displacement of the diaphragm by the pressure from the gas leading to reduction in lung capacity, may be associated with patient positioning.
- Inadvertent hypothermia caused by insufflation of cold gas over a period of time.
- Risk of pressure damage to skin due to length of procedure and patient positioning.
- Antiadhesive agents may be introduced to the surgical area post laparoscopy as a measure to reduce the incidence of adhesions.

*Electrosurgery (diathermy) and lasers*
- Breaks in insulation on instruments used for diathermy during surgery may result in damage to tissues or organs out of the visual field (e.g. the bowel). This may not be noticed at the time of surgery and may not become apparent until a postoperative peritonitis occurs.
- Coupling: the live electrode accidentally touches a non-insulated instrument and causes a burn outside of the field of vision.
- Surgical smoke, or 'plume' created by the use of electrosurgery and lasers may obscure the visual field. Surgical plume has also been shown to contain chemicals and biohazardous material which present a potential risk to patients during laparoscopic procedures as well as theatre staff. The use of surgical masks alone is unlikely to provide appropriate protection, therefore, the use of an appropriate filter device to remove smoke, while preventing a loss of pressure in the laparoscopic field, is recommended.

## Further reading

Association of Perioperative Practice (2009). Surgical smoke: what we know. Harrogate: Association of Perioperative Practice.

Chen JL, Geng W, Xie SX, et al. (2015). Single-incision versus conventional three-port laparoscopic appendectomy: a meta-analysis of randomized controlled trials. Minimally Invasive Therapy, 24(4):195–203.

Foran P (2016). Undergraduate surgical nursing preparation and guided operating room experience: a quantitative analysis. Nurse Education in Practice, 16(1):217–224.

La Chapelle CF, Swank HA, Wessels ME, et al. (2015). Trocar types in laparoscopy. Cochrane Database of Systematic Reviews, 12:CD009814.

Mathews S (2016). Preventing harm from surgical plume. Kai Tiaki Nursing New Zealand, 22(6):26–27.

National Collaborating Centre for Nursing and Supportive Health (2008). Clinical practice guideline. The management of inadvertent perioperative hypothermia in adults. London: National Institute for Health and Care Excellence.

O'Riley M (2010). Electrosurgery in perioperative practice. Journal of Perioperative Practice, 20(9):329–333.

Royal College of Obstetricians and Gynaecologists (2013). Use of adhesion prevention agents in obstetrics and gynaecology. London: Royal College of Obstetricians and Gynaecologists.

Ulmer B (2010). Best practices for minimally invasive procedures. AORN Journal, 91(5):558–575.

# Arthroscopy

The term 'arthroscopy' means looking into a joint and is considered to be a diagnostic or an operative procedure.

MRI scanning has largely replaced diagnostic arthroscopy as the quality of the imaging is so good.

## Equipment

See Box 16.1.

> **Box 16.1 Equipment for arthroscopic procedures**
> Equipment consists of a camera stack comprising:
> - High-intensity light source
> - High-resolution camera system
> - Monitor screen
> - Recording equipment.

## Use

- Knee.
- Ankle.
- Hip.

*It may also be used for*
- Elbow
- Wrist
- Big toe.

## Arthroscopy technique

- Two incisions <1 cm long are made in the skin over the joint.
- A port is introduced for the telescope and fluid inflow.
- A telescope attached to a camera is inserted through the port and an instrument through the other incision.
- The instrument may be a probe to assist with visualizing the joint or a punch to remove tissue, such as torn cartilage (meniscectomy).
- Anterior cruciate ligament reconstruction may be performed arthroscopically.

## Further reading

Abbott H, Booth H (eds) (2014). Foundations for operating department practice: essential theory for practice. Maidenhead: Open University Press.

Brignardello-Petersen R, Guyatt GH, Buchbinder R, et al. (2017). Knee arthroscopy versus conservative management in patients with degenerative knee disease: a systematic review. BMJ Open, 7(5):e016114.

Davey A, Ince CS (eds) (2010). Fundamentals of operating department practice. Cambridge: Cambridge University Press.

Garden OJ, Parks RW (eds) (2017). Principles and practice of surgery (7th ed). Edinburgh: Elsevier.

Goodman T, Spry C (2017). Essentials of perioperative nursing (6th ed). Burlington, MA: Jones and Bartlett Learning.

Hamlin L, Davies M, Richardson-Tench M, et al. (2017). Perioperative nursing: an introduction (2nd ed). Chatswood: Elsevier Australia.

Moutrey S (2017). Fundamentals of surgical instruments: a practical guide to their recognition, use and care. Harley: TFM Publishing.

# Endoscopy

- Means looking into the body.
- Uses the body's natural openings without the need for surgical incisions.

## Procedures

See Table 16.1.

**Table 16.1** Commonly performed endoscopic procedures

| | |
|---|---|
| **Gastroduodenoscopy** | To examine the inside of the oesophagus, stomach, and duodenum and take biopsies |
| **Colonoscopy** | To examine inside the colon, take biopsies, and remove polyps |
| **Hysteroscopy** | To examine the cervix and endometrium of the uterus through the vagina, take biopsies, and resect fibroids or the endometrium (TCRE = transcervical resection of endometrium). |
| **Cystoscopy** | To examine the bladder through the urethra, take biopsies, destroy lesions (e.g. cancer) and to resect the prostate gland (TURP = transurethral resection of prostate) |
| **Ureteroscopy** | To examine the ureters via access through the bladder |

## Endoscopy technique

- The picture is viewed on a monitor via a camera.
- Air (gastroscopy and colonoscopy) or fluid (hysteroscopy = warm saline or glycine if operative, and cystoscopy = warm water or glycine if operative) is used to dilate the organ to allow visualization.
- Flexible scopes are widely used for gastroscopy, colonoscopy, and diagnostic cystoscopy and hysteroscopy.
- Rigid scopes are commonly used for resection (TURP, TCRE).

## Further reading

Abbott H, Booth H (eds) (2014). Foundations for operating department practice: essential theory for practice. Maidenhead: Open University Press.

Davey A, Ince CS (eds) (2010). Fundamentals of operating department practice. Cambridge: Cambridge University Press.

Garden OJ, Parks RW (eds) (2017). Principles and practice of surgery (7th ed). Edinburgh: Elsevier.

Goodman T, Spry C (2017). Essentials of perioperative nursing (6th ed). Burlington, MA: Jones and Bartlett Learning.

Hamlin L, Davies M, Richardson-Tench M, et al. (2017). Perioperative nursing: an introduction (2nd ed). Chatswood: Elsevier Australia.

Moutrey S (2017). Fundamentals of surgical instruments: a practical guide to their recognition, use and care. Harley: TFM Publishing.

Paspatis GA, Arvanitakis M, Dumonceau JM, et al (2020). Diagnosis and management of iatrogenic endoscopic perforations: European Society of Gastrointestinal Endoscopy (ESGE) Position Statement. Endoscopy, 52(9):792–810.

# Prostheses

- The definition for a prosthesis is 'the artificial substitute for a missing part of the body for either functional or cosmetic reasons'.
- The most commonly thought of prostheses are those that replace limbs such as legs and arms.
- Other types of prostheses are (but not limited to):
  - Joint replacements
  - Arterial grafts
  - Ophthalmic lenses
  - False teeth
  - Heart valves
  - Reconstructive appliances—breast, chin, penile implants
  - Pacemakers
  - Intervertebral discs
  - Mesh to support muscles walls.

The manufacture and use of prostheses is regulated by the MHRA, who are responsible for ensuring that medical devices, such as prostheses, are fit for use, that is, are safe and perform to the standard expected. The MHRA monitors all medical devices and communicates across healthcare settings any raised concerns regarding devices and suggests action.

The MHRA works closely with NICE to ensure that best practice and clinical effectiveness are used when deciding appropriate selection of a prosthesis.

Prostheses can be made of a variety of materials depending on:

- Anticipated usage after implantation: for example, a young patient receiving a joint replacement would be expected to live longer than the average lifespan of the conventional primary joint prosthesis
- Site of placement: for example, replicate action of natural tissue such as a breast implant. Actions of surrounding tissues or chemical (e.g. dental) implants need to withstand chemical reactions within the mouth
- The majority of prostheses are now made of man-made materials such as metallic alloys, ultra-high molecular weight polyethylene (UHMWPE) and ceramics for joint replacements; expanded polytetrafluoroethylene (ePTFE), Dacron®, and polyurethane (PU) for arterial grafts; although pig valves and human donor grafts have been used for heart valve replacements.

Patients undergoing prosthetic surgery are considered to be at high risk of infection. Therefore, certain precautions have been advocated:

- Prophylactic antibiotics.
- Laminar (ultra clean) theatre with high efficiency particulate air (HEPA) filters.
- Instrumentation and 'scrubbed staff' within the laminar flow.
- Minimal movement of staff during surgery.
- Minimal unnecessary conversation during surgery.

## Further reading

British Orthopaedic Association (2006). Primary total hip replacement: a guide to good practice. London: British Orthopaedic Association.

Hampson FG, Ridgway EJ (2005). Prophylactic antibiotics in surgery. Surgery (Oxford), 23(8):290–293.

Knobben BAS, van Horn JR, van de Mei, HC, et al. (2006). Evaluation of measures to decrease intra-operative bacterial contamination in orthopaedic implant surgery. Journal of Hospital Infection, 62(2):174–180.

Medicines and Healthcare products Regulatory Agency. Homepage. Available at: ℜ https://www.gov.uk/government/organisations/medicines-and-healthcare-products-regulatory-agency

National Institute for Health and Care Excellence. NICE guidelines. Available at: ℜ https://www.nice.org.uk/about/what-we-do/our-programmes/nice-guidance/nice-guidelines

NHS Estates (1994). Health technical memorandum 2025. Ventilation in healthcare premises. Validation and verification. London: Department of Health.

# Electrosurgical equipment

Diathermy is the use of high-frequency electrical current (300 kHz to 3 MHz) to produce heat. This heat is used in the surgical field to cut or destroy tissues. It can also be used to coagulate bleeding vessels. Owing to its high frequency, diathermy does not activate nerves and muscles.

> Diathermy can be defined as either bipolar or monopolar. Because the diathermy is an electrical system, it needs to complete a circuit to be effective.

*Bipolar diathermy* is when the two electrodes within the surgical instrument (e.g. forceps) combine:
- The current passes between the tips of the instrument coagulating the vessels in between and not through the patient; this then completes the circuit.
- Bipolar diathermy is often used when coagulation only is required as cutting can not take place.
- It is also used when very precise or 'micro-coagulation' is required.
- It is suggested to be safer for the patient as the electrical pathway is much shorter.

*Monopolar* uses a 'grounding plate' to complete the circuit:
- This plate or pad is applied to the patient and is known as the return or indifferent electrode.
- Temperature rises at the active electrode (surgical instrument) whenever there is resistance to the flow of currant.
- This rise in temperature is used to produce the cutting and coagulation effects.
- Because the indifferent electrode has a significantly larger surface area with much less resistance, the heat is localized at the instrument tip and not at the plate.
- See Table 16.2.

**Table 16.2** Diathermy plate (grounding plate)

| Ensure plate is placed away from: | Ensure good contact with skin: |
|---|---|
| • Implants | • Remove hair |
| • Scars | • Avoid spirit-based preparation near application site |
| • Bony prominences | • Avoid creases (skin and plate) |

*Diathermy effects*: the effects of the diathermy depend on the current intensity and waveform supplied by the diathermy machine (generator).

## Coagulation

The 'Coag' waveform is produced using short blasts (between 50 and 100 per second) of low-frequency waveforms; this enables slow drying and co-agulation of vessels.

## Cutting

Cutting is achieved through the application of the 'Cut' waveform which generates a continuous current with a sinus waveform at a lower voltage but higher current than 'Coag'. Cell explosion occurs due to the intense heat within the localized area, producing a cutting effect.

### Complications of cutting

- Can interfere with pacemaker function.
- Electrical burns or tissue damage from arcing with surgical instruments and implants.
- Burns under grounding plate if not applied correctly.
- Insulation failure surrounding instrument can cause damage user or surrounding tissues.

## Harmonic scalpel

Used for cutting soft tissue and coagulating blood vessels through ultra-sound vibration, therefore, keeping thermal injury to a minimum. The harmonic scalpel can be used in addition to or as a direct replacement for electrosurgery, standard scalpel, and lasers. Electrical energy produced by the harmonic scalpel generator is converted to a mechanical motion in a dedicated hand piece. The hand piece has a blade tip which moves longitudinally at >55,000 cycles per second. This movement produces enough heat to cause the tissue proteins to change in molecular structure, producing a coagulum. Coagulation occurs when pressure is exerted upon the tissues between the two tips of the handpiece, allowing the coagulum to produce haemostasis. The surgeon can also cut tissues by using different levels of tip pressure, tissue traction, and power level.

### Advantages of harmonic scalpel

- No electrical stimulus to patient.
- Minimal smoke produced, better surgical view.
- Reduces need for ties due to cutting and coagulation effect.
- Lower temperature coagulation: no charring of tissues.

## Further reading

Abbott H, Booth H (eds) (2014). Foundations for operating department practice: essential theory for practice. Maidenhead: Open University Press.

Davey A, Ince CS (eds) (2010). Fundamentals of operating department practice. Cambridge: Cambridge University Press.

Garden OJ, Parks RW (eds) (2017). Principles and practice of surgery (7th ed). Edinburgh: Elsevier.

Goodman T, Spry C (2017). Essentials of perioperative nursing (6th ed). Burlington, MA: Jones and Bartlett Learning.

Hamlin L, Davies M, Richardson-Tench M, et al. (2017). Perioperative nursing: an introduction (2nd ed). Chatswood: Elsevier Australia.

Moutrey S (2017). Fundamentals of surgical instruments: a practical guide to their recognition, use and care. Harley: TFM Publishing.

# Operating microscopes

Operating microscopes may be either fixed to the wall or ceiling of an operating theatre, or freestanding so that they can be moved into the theatre when required. Theatre staff must have an understanding of the use and care of these expensive and complex pieces of theatre equipment and the accessories that accompany them.

---

Microscopes are used in several surgical specialties including:
- Ophthalmology
- ENT
- Neurosurgery
- Microvascular surgery.

---

It is useful if practitioners who work in specialties that use microscopes understand some of the basic principles of the optics:
- Microscopes used in surgery are stereoscopic, which facilitates adjustment of the level of magnification.
- The objective lens is fitted to the bottom of the microscope and the focal length will be determined by the objective length of the lens:
  - Typically, a 400 mm lens is common in neurosurgery while ophthalmology may require a 175 or 200 mm lens.
- The microscope should be wiped over with a mild detergent solution before and after use and then the optics polished with a soft lens cloth prior to storage.
- The lens and eyepieces should be inspected for any damage at this juncture while the light should also be tested prior to use.
- A spare bulb should be kept and practitioners should be aware of how to replace a bulb that has blown.
- The protective cover is then put over the microscope and it is stored away from traffic and free from dust.

Some centres utilize a sterile polythene drape to cover the microscope for specialities such as ENT and neurosurgery while ophthalmology may use sterilized covers which go over the control knobs. It is important that practitioners are conversant with how to prepare the microscope in the manner appropriate for the type of surgery to be undertaken.

## Further reading

Abbott H, Booth H (eds) (2014). Foundations for operating department practice: essential theory for practice. Maidenhead: Open University Press.

Davey A, Ince CS (eds) (2010). Fundamentals of operating department practice. Cambridge: Cambridge University Press.

Moutrey S (2017). Fundamentals of surgical instruments: a practical guide to their recognition, use and care. Harley: TFM Publishing.

Phillips N, Hornacky A (2020). Berry & Kohn's operating room technique (14th ed). St Louis, MO: Elsevier.

# Lasers in surgery

Laser light is an intense narrow beam of light and can be used to vaporize tissue while at the same time sealing small blood vessels and causing minimal damage to surrounding tissues.

---
**'LASER'**
- **L**ight
- **A**mplification by
- **S**timulated
- **E**mission of
- **R**adiation.
---

### Properties of laser light
- Single colour (monochromatic) in a single wavelength. Ordinary, or white light, is a mixture of all colours.
- Laser light is very straight in a parallel beam. Ordinary light spreads out in all directions.
- Laser light is coherent—the waves all run together in phase. Ordinary light is incoherent—the waves are all mixed up.
- Laser light can be concentrated with a lens into a tiny intense spot to cut, coagulate, or vaporize tissue. Ordinary light cannot be concentrated in this way.

### Types of laser
- The colour/wavelength of the light is chosen for absorption of the laser by different tissues in the body.
- The colour of the laser is determined by the medium used to generate the radiation. Common types include:
  - $CO_2$: infrared light.
  - Argon: blue or green light.
  - Nd YAG: infrared.
  - Others—excimer lasers may be argon, krypton, or xenon fluoride and produce ultraviolet pulses used for correcting eye sight.

### Classification of lasers
Ranges from class 1 to class 4. The classification is determined by the potential of damage to the eye caused by the laser, class 1 being the least and class 4 the most hazardous. Class 4 lasers are the ones most usually used in surgery.

### Hazards
*Effects on the eye*
Depend on the wavelength of the light:
- Corneal burns leading to clouding of the cornea.
- Keratitis on the surface of the cornea.
- Retinal damage leading to blind spots.

*Effects on the skin*

A burn is the main hazard:
- Scarring and possible loss of sensation to touch may occur after healing.
- The reflex action of withdrawing from the pain may limit the damage. Anaesthetized patients will not have this reflex.
- Long-term exposure to ultraviolet lasers may result in pigmentation changes and skin cancer.

*Incidental hazards*
- Fire: the beam of a surgical laser is a fire risk if it comes into direct contact with surgical drapes and gowns or flammable skin preparations.
- Reflection of the laser beam from shiny surfaces: such as stainless steel trolleys.
- Laser plume: the smoke generated during vaporization of tissue may contain potentially hazardous substances including toxic chemicals, carbonized tissue, and viral DNA.

## Safety considerations
- Legislation, standards, and guidance govern the safe use of lasers.
- Laser equipment has to have a number of inbuilt safety features including:
  - An audible or visible alarm when the device is being fired
  - Covered foot pedals to prevent accidental firing
  - A removable key to prevent inappropriate use.
- Local rules must be in place wherever lasers are used and include:
  - A safe system of work for operating the laser
  - A list of trained, authorized users
  - The procedure to follow in case of an emergency.
- A laser protection supervisor ensures that the laser is used according to the local rules and usually holds the laser key.
- The laser-controlled area is the room or area where safety precautions specific to that laser apply and may include:
  - Restricted access which may involve the locking of theatre doors
  - Use of appropriate warning signs
  - Window blinds or shields
  - Protective eyewear for staff.

## Further reading
Abbott H, Booth H (eds) (2014). Foundations for operating department practice: essential theory for practice. Maidenhead: Open University Press.

Alberti LR, Vicari EF, De Souza Jardim Vicari R, et al (2017). Early use of CO2 lasers and silicone gel on surgical scars: prospective study. Lasers in Surgery and Medicine, 49(6):570–576.

Davey A, Ince CS (eds) (2010). Fundamentals of operating department practice. Cambridge: Cambridge University Press.

Moutrey S (2017). Fundamentals of surgical instruments: a practical guide to their recognition, use and care. Harley: TFM Publishing.

# Tourniquets

## Indications

Tourniquets are used in the surgical context for three reasons:

- Optimizing the surgeon's view of the site through the provision of a bloodless operating field achieved by the temporary arrest of circulation of blood distal to the point of application.
- Administration and maintenance of regional anaesthesia to a limb, while preventing the release of the LA agent into the general circulation—Bier's block.
- Prevention of systemic toxicity of drugs during IV regional anaesthetic procedures.[1]

## Contraindications

Tourniquets should not be applied to a limb, if the patient suffers the following comorbidities:

- Sickle cell disease.
- Rheumatoid arthritis.
- Regional infection—soft tissue, bone or limb (e.g. cellulitis).
- History of VTE.
- Known or suspected compartment syndrome.
- The patient has a history of vascular disease (absent pulses, poor capillary return). NB: a history of vascular disease or previous surgery on the proposed site for surgery requires *surgical assessment* before application.
- Active malignancy.[1]
- The limb is the site of an arteriovenous fistula for dialysis.

## Equipment

- Pneumatic tourniquets consist of an inflatable cuff, a source of compressed air, and a device to select, control, and maintain the pressure to which the cuff is inflated. There are two types of pneumatic tourniquet:
  - Leak compensating—compensate for any pressure lost automatically.
  - Non-leak compensating—requires continuous observation while in use.
- Non-pneumatic tourniquets take various forms applying the principle of securing a piece of fabric around the limb. The disadvantage of this method is that there is no associated pressure regulator in the device and therefore the pressure to which the soft tissues beneath are subjected is unknown.
- Tourniquets are manufactured in a range of shapes and sizes to meet a range of applications. The details of the product composition and the number of uses for the product are detailed in the manufacturer's instructions.
- Before use, complete the safety checks as identified by the manufacturer and local policy.

## Preparation and application

Before applying the tourniquet, confirm the site of application.

Protection of the patient's soft tissue requires application of both skill and knowledge; practitioners who lack the appropriate level of proficiency should not use tourniquets:

- A risk assessment of the patient's skin integrity, conditions affecting the use of the tourniquet, limb size, wound condition, and placement of the cuff should be undertaken to determine the appropriate device to employ and its subsequent use.
- The skin under the tourniquet should be clean and dry.
- The entire circumference of the limb should be covered with lint-free padding to prevent damage from pinching and shearing forces.
- The ends of the tourniquet cuff should overlap by >7.5 cm and <15 cm.
- If the limb is tapered due to musculature or obesity, a contoured cuff should be used, ensuring adequate skin contact and preventing slippage and shearing forces.
- To prevent maceration and/or chemical burns resulting from the accumulation of fluids between the skin, the padding, and the tourniquet, an occlusive drape should be used.
- Tourniquet inflation pressure can be influenced by limb occlusion pressure (the minimum pressure required to stop the flow of arterial blood distal to the tourniquet cuff), systolic blood pressure, size of limb, or a combination of these factors. The occlusion pressures have been identified as 300–350 mmHg in lower limbs and 200–250 mmHg in upper limbs. Inflation of the cuff should be kept to the minimum effective pressure and be determined by the above-mentioned factors under the direction of the medical team.[1]
- Nerve and tissue damage are a possibility when tourniquets are applied. Consequently, a maximum time limit of 2 hours is suggested.[2,3] The surgeon should be informed after 1 hour of inflation and thereafter at intervals negotiated at the team briefing.[4]
- The inflation time and inflation pressure should be recorded where it is visible to all and a designated member of the team should be responsible for notifying the surgical team of the time elapsed since application.

## Exsanguination

The risk assessment and patient's condition will inform the decision whether to exsanguinate the limb. If exsanguination is required, there are three methods available:

- Elevation of the limb.
- Application of Rhys-Davies exsanguinator—manual compression device.
- Esmarch bandage—use with caution as consistency of pressure applied during use cannot be accurately determined.[5]

## Aftercare

Before deflating the tourniquet, consider the following:

- The anaesthetist and surgeon should be informed that the circulation is about to be restored to the limb.
- Stage of wound closure.

- If the cuff remains inflated at the medical team's request in the recovery area, then the time recorded is a continuation of that in theatre.
- Verbal confirmation and acknowledgement of the release of the tourniquet must be given and received.
- Observation of the patient's vital signs on release/removal of the tourniquet is essential as normal blood flow returns to the limb.
- Regular and frequent observation of the limb's neurovascular status.
- Handover records to the PACU should include the details identified in the following 'Documentation' section and a visual check of the site of application.

## Documentation

The following items should be documented in the patient's record when a tourniquet has been used:
- Equipment used and unique identifying numbers.
- Site of application.
- Duration of inflation including time applied and removed.
- Inflation pressure.
- Condition of the skin before and after application of the tourniquet.
- Tissue protection adjuncts (e.g. orthopaedic wool).
- Method of exsanguination if used.
- Name of person applying and removing the tourniquet.

## Maintenance

- Tourniquets should be clean, dry, and checked regularly for cracks or breaks in the outer fabric and to ensure that the pneumatic bladder, hoses, and joint/connections do not leak.
- Decontaminate tourniquets and manual exsanguinators in line with the manufacturer's instructions.
- Pneumatic regulators should be calibrated according to the manufacturer's instructions.
- Use/reuse of the tourniquet cuff will be dictated by the manufacture's guidance.

## References

1. Association for Perioperative Practice (2016). Standards and recommendations for safe perioperative practice (4th ed). Harrogate: Association for Perioperative Practice.
2. Deloughry JL, Griffith R (2009). Arterial tourniquets. Continuing Education in Anaesthesia, Critical Care and Pain, 9(2):56–59.
3. Malanjum L, Fischer B (2009). Procedures under tourniquet. Anaesthesia and Intensive Care Medicine, 10(1):14–17.
4. World Health Organization (2009). WHO surgical safety checklist. Available at: ℬ https://www.who.int/teams/integrated-health-services/patient-safety/research/safe-surgery/tool-and-resources
5. Desai S, Prashantha PG, Torgal SV, et al. (2013). Fatal pulmonary embolism subsequent to the use of the Esmarch Bandage and Tourniquet: a case report and review of literature. Saudi Journal of Anaesthesia, 7(3):331–335.

## Further reading

Association of periOperative Registered Nurses (2014). Recommended practices for the use of the pneumatic tourniquet in the perioperative practice setting. In: Perioperative standards and recommended practices. Denver, CO: AORN Inc.

Groah LK (1996). Perioperative nursing. London: Appleton & Lange.

McEwan JA (2018). What is limb occlusion pressure (LOP)? Available at: https://tourniquets.org/limb-occlusion-pressure-lop/

Phillips N, Hornacky A (2020). Berry & Kohn's operating room technique (14th ed). St Louis, MO: Elsevier.

Rothrock J (2014). Alexander's care of the patient in surgery. New York: Elsevier.

Royal College of Anaesthetists (2016). Stop before you block. Available at: https://www.rcoa.ac.uk/standards-of-clinical-practice/wrong-site-block

Royal College of Surgeons of Edinburgh (2017). Position statement on the application of tourniquets. Available at: https://fphc.rcsed.ac.uk/media/2276/2017_fphc-position-statement_-tourniquet-application_final.pdf

# Wound management

# Surgical incisions

A surgical incision is when an intentional cut or wound is made on the body usually involving a sharp instrument (scalpel or blade).

A badly placed incision can have a detrimental impact on the healing of the wound, causing haematomas, wound dehiscence (break down), and an increased risk of infections. Also, psychologically, an ugly, inappropriately large or disfiguring scar can influence the patient's perception of the surgery and impact their quality of life afterwards.

## Criteria for placement of incision

A surgeon must take into account when determining the positioning of the incision:

- That it allows adequate access to the operative site
- That the incision can be extended if more extensive surgery is required
- The ease with which the wound can be closed and how secure the wound will be postoperatively
- That it will provide the lowest postoperative complication rate
- That it will reduce postoperative pain
- That it will provide the most aesthetically acceptable appearance when healed
- That an incision along a skin plane is less likely to result in problem scarring.

## Further considerations

The surgeon must also consider the patient's:

- Medical status: for example, diabetes, anaemia, and steroid treatment— as these will have a negative impact on the healing process
- Lifestyle and anticipated length of recovery to 'normal' functions: for example, patient expectation of full recovery will differ depending on their diet and exercise, age, and previous abilities
- Weight: patients who are clinically obese will put more strain on wound closure material and have reduced healing abilities. There may also be impaired healing due to a reduced blood supply caused by the increased amount of adipose tissue
- Reduced nutritional status will impact collagen synthesis, which is part of the basis for wound healing
- Cosmetic expectations: body image and self-esteem post surgery is very important to patients, especially those who have undergone 'enhancement' surgery, and placement of surgical incisions can determine how well a scar heals.

## Classification of surgical wounds

See Fig. 17.1 for common abdominal incisions.

### Clean

Elective, not emergency, non-traumatic, primarily closed, no acute inflammation, no break in technique, respiratory, GI, biliary, and genitourinary tracts not entered.

*Clean-contaminated*

Urgent or emergency that would otherwise be clean, elective opening of respiratory GI, biliary, and genitourinary tracts with minor spillage. Not encountering infected urine or bile. Minor break in technique.

*Contaminated*

Non-purulent inflammation, gross spillage from GI tract, entry into biliary and genitourinary tracts in the presence of infected bile or urine; major break in technique; penetrating trauma <4 hours old.

*Dirty*

Purulent inflammation, preoperative perforation of GI, biliary, and genitourinary tracts; penetrating trauma >4 hours old.

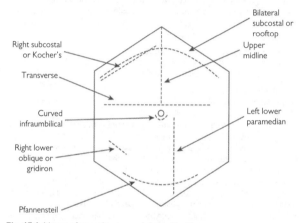

**Fig. 17.1** Names of several common abdominal incisions.

Reproduced with permission from Tulloh B and Lee D (2007). Foundations of Operative Surgery: An Introduction to Surgical Techniques, with permission from Oxford University Press, Oxford.

# Haemostasis

Haemostasis can be described as the arrest of bleeding by either using the physiological process or by surgical means. If haemostasis is not controlled, excessive bleeding can lead to decreasing blood volume and BP, which can eventually result in death.

## Physiological process

*Vasoconstriction*
- Vascular constriction: an immediate response resulting from the contraction of smooth muscle within the vessel wall. Sufficient to close small vessels but only a temporary measure in larger vessels.
- Platelet plug formation: occurs when platelets bind with collagen and then bind with fibrinogen to form a plug. Sufficient to close small tears or cuts.

*Coagulation*
- Required to close large tears or cuts.
- Requires the formation of a blood clot which is a mesh of protein fibres which bind blood cells, platelets, and fluid.

*Surgical methods*
During surgery, providing haemostasis will aid the surgeon maintain visualization of the wound site. It will also assist in the wound healing process as fluid and blood left in the wound site may encourage microbial development leading to infection or prevent direct contact of the wound sides.

Haemostasis during surgery is maintained in a variety of ways:
- *Sutures and ligatures (ties)*: material used to either knot/tie/ligate around medium-to-large bleeding vessels or to bring together sides of a wound. Designed as either absorbable or non-absorbable depending on the requirement. Length of time the material takes to be absorbed is dependent on type of material, patient's health, and speed of wound healing.
- *Metal surgical clips (staples)*: used when a vessel has been identified, clips are placed prior to excision. Though it should not be used as the main haemostatic as they can impede further ligation. Non-absorbable.
- *Bone wax*: a semi-synthetic material used on bone surfaces to halt localized bleeding; absorbable.
- *Electrosurgery (diathermy)*: electrical current which heats the bleeding vessel cauterizing it (➲ see Electrosurgical equipment, p. 470).
- *Ultrasonic*: coagulates blood vessels by vibrating at a frequency of 55,500 cycles/second (55.5 kHz). The human ear may hear sounds from longitudinal waves at frequency range between 20 and 20,000 cycles/second. Heat is generated due to the high-frequency vibration of the tissue.
- *Absorbable haemostats*: various types which are presented in a mesh format to provide a matrix for clot formation used on small blood vessels. Absorbed within 7–10 days.
- *Haemostatic forceps (artery clips)*: presented in various sizes, dependent on potential use, though generally the smaller ones are used to clamp small blood vessels, prior to being ligated or left until blood clot is formed (2–5 minutes).

- *Tissue adhesives*: similar function as glue, used predominantly in head wounds and as a final skin closure material.
- *Chemical*: silver nitrate in an aqueous environment acts as a strong oxidizing agent cauterizing small blood vessels. Predominantly used for epistaxis (nose bleeds).

## Further reading

Erian M, McLaren G (2004). Ultrasonically activated technology in gynaecologic operative laparoscopy. Reviews in Gynaecological Practice, 4(3):194–198.

Goodman T, Spry C (2017). Essentials of perioperative nursing (6th ed). Burlington, MA: Jones and Bartlett Learning.

Lindholm C, Searle R (2016). Wound management for the 21st century: combining effectiveness and efficiency. International Wound Journal, 13(2):5–15.

Lloyd S, Almeyda, J, Di Cuffa R, et al. (2005). The effect of silver nitrate on nasal septal cartilage. Ear, Nose and Throat Journal, 84(1):41–44.

National Institute for Health and Care Excellence (2019). Surgical site infections: prevention and treatment. NICE guideline [NG125]. Available at: https://www.nice.org.uk/guidance/ng125

National Institute for Health and Care Excellence (2020). Sepsis. Quality standard [QS161]. Available at: https://www.nice.org.uk/guidance/qs161

Singh S, Maxwell D (2006). Tools of the trade. Best Practice & Research Clinical Obstetrics & Gynaecology, 20(1):41–59.

# Wound closure

Sutures (stitches) are lengths of material used to either knot/tie/ligate around bleeding vessels or to allow for healing through primary intention, that is, tissues are held in proximity until enough healing occurs to withstand stress without mechanical support. There is no ideal suture—all types have their merits and disadvantages.

## Sutures can be divided into two main categories

- *Absorbable*: loses most of its tensile strength within 60 days of insertion. Ideally loses its strength at the same rate that the tissue regains its strength, being then absorbed into the body leaving no foreign material. Use on stomach, colon, bladder. Absorbable sutures are now used on the skin as a subcuticular closure. They have the advantage of producing better alignment of the wound edges, leave less of a scar, and do not require removal, making them ideal for use in children.
- *Non-absorbable*: retains strength for a long time, sometimes indefinitely. When used as a skin closure they must be removed once healing has taken place to prevent chronic sepsis. Use on skin, fascia, and tendons.

## Sutures can be further divided into

- *Monofilament sutures* have one strand and are considered to be less of an infection risk because the lack of interstices prevents the harbouring of infective organisms. However, frequent handling or tying can create weaker areas causing breakage of the suture.
- *Multifilament sutures* are made up of a number of strands which are twisted or braided which improve the tensile strength, pliability, handling, and knot-tying properties. However, they are associated with higher tissue drag and are therefore coated to ensure relatively smoother passage through the tissues. Avoid in areas of high contamination (e.g. anus).

## Further considerations

- Knot tensile strength: its strength is defined by the force necessary to cause the knot to undo.
- Plasticity, elasticity, and memory are all intertwined, as a suture must be able to allow for wound swelling (plasticity). Though as swelling subsides, the suture should regain its original form and length (elasticity). Memory is related to plasticity and elasticity and enables sutures to return to their original shape after deformation by tying.
- Tissue biocompatibility: suture materials produce varying degrees of tissue reaction, specifically inflammation. Significant inflammation increases the risk of infection and can delay wound healing. Synthetic materials, which are mostly used today, produce a minimal reaction.
- Diameter: sizes of sutures are standardized and relate to a specific diameter range (in mm) of the suture strand that is necessary to produce a certain tensile strength. Sizes are expressed with zeroes, such as 3-0, 4-0, 5-0, and 6-0; more zeroes indicate a smaller size.

## Other types of wound closure

*Steri-Strips™*

These are adhesive skin closures that are sometimes used to close small wounds or in areas where there are cosmetic considerations such as on the face. They might also be used in conjunction with sutures to bring the wound closer together.

*Staples*

These are the fastest method of closing the skin and they have a low level of tissue reactivity. Skin staples come in preloaded different sized dispensers. The edges of the wound should be everted while the stapler is positioned over the line of the incision and a staple placed evenly at each side. Skin staples are removed after 5–7 days using a staple remover and produce an excellent cosmetic result if applied correctly.

## Further reading

Goodman T, Spry C (2017). Essentials of perioperative nursing (6th ed). Burlington, MA: Jones and Bartlett Learning.

Lindholm C, Searle R (2016) Wound management for the 21st century: combining effectiveness and efficiency. International Wound Journal, 13(2):5–15.

Singh S, Maxwell D (2006). Tools of the trade. Best Practice & Research Clinical Obstetrics & Gynaecology, 20(1):41–59.

# Needles

The needles attached to sutures are divided into three main sections:
- Eye: the majority of sutures are now swagged, that is, the suture is attached to the needle. Other eyes are closed and spring.
- Body: part of needle grasped by the needle holder:
  - Straight—generally used by hand.
  - Half curved—allows easy access down trocar ports.
  - Curved needle—most commonly used shape.
  - Compound curve (J-shaped)—used in confined spaces.
- Point: designed to penetrate tissues with minimum damage:
  - Cutting—cutting edge uppermost on the needle.
  - Reverse cutting—cutting edge on the underside of the needle.
  - Taper point.
  - Spatula.
  - Taper cut—round.
  - Blunt.

See Fig. 17.2 for shapes of needles and Fig. 17.3 for examples of types of needles.

## The three main types of cutting needle

- Taper cut: used for tough fibrous tissue.
- Conventional cutting: two opposing cutting edges with a third on the edge on the inside curve of the needle.
- Reverse cutting: two opposing cutting edges with a third edge on the outside curve of the needle. It is a triangular-shaped needle. Only the edges near the tip are sharp.

Taper-cut points are used on delicate tissues that are easily penetrated, such as peritoneum, heart, and intestines. The point is designed so that the shaft gradually tapers to a point which results in a very small hole in the tissue.

Blunt-point needles have a rounded end for use with friable tissue such as the kidney or the liver, when neither piercing nor cutting is suitable.

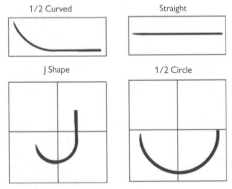

**Fig. 17.2** Shapes of needles.
Courtesy of Ethicon.

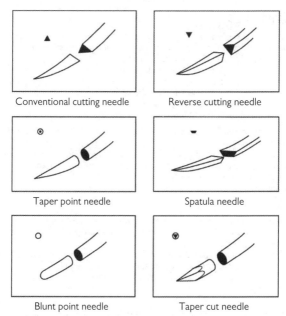

Conventional cutting needle

Reverse cutting needle

Taper point needle

Spatula needle

Blunt point needle

Taper cut needle

**Fig. 17.3** Types of needles.
Courtesy of Ethicon.

# Dressings

The final stage in the operation is the application of the dressing which is a role usually left to the scrub practitioner to perform. A dressing can be said to perform five basic, but important functions:
- To protect the incision from contamination and trauma.
- To absorb exudates.
- To facilitate haemostasis and minimize swelling.
- Provide support, or to splint or immobilize a body part.
- To enhance the patient's physical and psychological comfort.

Dressings should be appropriately selected for the type of wound. For a straightforward skin-wound dressing there are many proprietary makes of occlusive dressing available, the choice of which will often be down to personal preference. Before the surgical procedure is commenced, any allergies that the patient has will have been checked, so care is taken to avoid using an adhesive to which the patient is sensitive.

## Application
- The wound and surrounding area is cleaned by the scrub practitioner with a moistened (if necessary) swab and dried using a swab or sterile dressing towel.
- The dressing is prepared as appropriate for the type of wound using a sterile technique and the dressing applied to the wound.
- The drapes can then be removed from the patient while the dressing is held in place.

'Basic adhesive dressings may be used on closed primary surgical wounds as a pragmatic approach to provide a barrier to the wound and to absorb exudate.'[1]

## Specialist dressings

These include the following:
- Hydrocolloids which contain a matrix and other gel-forming agents such as gelatin and pectin. It promotes autolysis and aids granulation.
- Alginates contain calcium and sodium salts obtained from seaweed. They are useful for heavily exudating wounds.
- Foam dressings can be used for moderately exudating wounds. They deslough by maintaining a moist environment.
- Hydrogels have a high content of water to create a moist wound surface and debride by hydration and autolysis.
- Debriding agents are useful for difficult to heal surgical wounds. They work by removing necrotic tissue and eschar.

## Reference

1. Blazeby J (2016). Do dressings prevent infection of closed primary wounds after surgery? BMJ, 353:i2270.

## Further reading

Grey JE, Harding KG (eds) (2006). ABC of wound healing. Oxford: Blackwell Publishing.

Lindholm C, Searle R (2016). Wound management for the 21st century: combining effectiveness and efficiency. International Wound Journal, 13(2):5–15.

National Institute for Health and Care Excellence (2019). Surgical site infections: prevention and treatment. NICE guideline [NG125]. Available at: ℘ https://www.nice.org.uk/guidance/ng125

Probst S (2020). Wound care nursing: a patient-centred approach (3rd ed). Edinburgh: Elsevier.

# Wound drains

A drain is a means of providing a conduit for internal fluids (or gas) to be removed from the body.

## Main types

- Open: usually corrugated, allows the fluid to drain into a receptacle—either a bag or pads.
- Closed: perforated drainage tube is inserted in area of the drainage site and connected to a bag or bottle.
- Free drainage (passive): relies on differences in pressure between cavities and external environment and the build-up of fluid.
- Low vacuum/suction (active): suction is induced either low or high depending on cavity and drainage site.
- Autologous: patient's own blood is filtered as it drains as can be transfused back into the patient before a nominated time period.

A drain could be a low-vacuum closed drain (e.g. redivac, chest drain); an open passive drain (e.g. Yeates); or a closed passive drain (e.g. urinary catheter).

There is debate surrounding their effectiveness as drains:

*For their use*

- Removes fluid from the wound site which if left could provide a source for bacterial growth.
- Facilitates wound healing by preventing the formation of a haematoma or seroma.
- Provides a means of observing blood loss and early detection of haemorrhage.

*Against their use*

- A conduit for bacteria to enter the cavity, increasing the risk of infection.
- Trauma induced on insertion and removal of the drain.
- Trauma to tissues due to the presence of suction within a cavity.

Some surgeons will use a suture to secure the drain to the skin to prevent accidental displacement of the drain. Through confusion or agitation, patients may inadvertently remove the drain causing further trauma to the wound.

## Urinary catheters

Drains urine from the bladder either transurethrally (via the urethra) or suprapubically (via the abdomen).

*Rationale for use*

- Monitor urine output.
- Allow irrigation of the bladder.
- Bypass an obstruction.
- Obtain a sterile specimen.

Insertion of a catheter is an aseptic technique; despite this, urinary tract infections are the most common infections acquired in hospital. Various sizes, lengths, and materials are used depending on the requirements.

## Nasogastric tubes (also known as Ryles tubes)

- Inserted via the nasal passages and passed into the stomach.
- Remove fluid and gas from GI tract.

*Rationale for use*

- Preparing the patient for emergency surgery such as ectopic pregnancy, ruptured aortic aneurysm; to assist in gastric surgery such as bariatric surgery, keeping the stomach empty to allow the surgeon adequate access to the operative site.
- To drain the gut after surgery during the period of ileus preventing the accumulation of fluid and gas.
- Administer medication and feeding directly into GI tract.
- Obtain specimens of gastric contents.

## Further reading

Chung YS, Lee JY, Nam EJ, et al. (2021). Impact of subcutaneous negative pressure drains on surgical wound healing in ovarian cancer. International Journal of Gynaecological Cancer, 31(2):245–250.

Kumar B (2006). Working in the operating department (2nd ed). Edinburgh: Churchill Livingstone.

National Institute for Health and Care Excellence (2019). Surgical site infections: prevention and treatment. NICE guideline [NG125]. Available at: ℰ https://www.nice.org.uk/guidance/ng125

Parker MJ, Roberts C (2007). Closed suction surgical wound drainage after orthopaedic surgery. Cochrane Database of Systematic Reviews, 4:CD001825.

Wilson J (2003). Infection control in clinical practice. Edinburgh: Bailliere Tindall.

# Specialist surgery

# Cardiothoracic surgery

- Cardiac surgery refers to the heart and great vessels within the mediastinum.
- Thoracic surgery refers to the lungs, pleura, oesophagus, diaphragm, and chest wall.
- Subspecialties include cardiopulmonary transplantation, paediatric cardiac surgery, and mechanical circulatory support (beyond the scope of this chapter).

## Cardiac surgery

*Preoperative preparation*

- The patient is consented for the operation.
- Investigations: FBC, U&Es, cross-match, and coagulation profile.
- Nursing staff prepare the patient for theatre. The operative area is shaved with hair clippers and the patient receives two antiseptic showers using chlorhexidine.
- The patient's identity and consent form are checked before the operation begins.

*Cardiac surgery: general anaesthesia*

- A peripheral cannula and an arterial line are inserted while the patient is awake, so that vasoconstrictors (e.g. metaraminol) can be given to prevent potentially dangerous hypotension on induction of anaesthesia.
- After induction of anaesthesia, an ETT is inserted.
- A triple-lumen central venous catheter and a urinary catheter are inserted.
- ECG monitoring and pulse oximetry are used as standard.
- A transoesophageal echocardiographic probe is inserted for all operations on the cardiac valves.
- A Swan–Ganz catheter is occasionally used, to measure cardiac output, pulmonary artery pressure, and pulmonary capillary wedge pressure.

*Incisions used in cardiac surgery*

Median sternotomy is the standard incision in cardiac surgery, giving excellent access to the heart and great vessels. Minimally invasive incisions have recently gained popularity in aortic and mitral valve surgery.

*Cardiopulmonary bypass*

- Cardiopulmonary bypass is required to maintain the patient's circulation while the heart is arrested for surgery.
- Full body heparinization is necessary, using 300 mg/kg of IV heparin to achieve an activated clotting time of four times the baseline (e.g. 110 seconds baseline to 440 seconds after heparinization).
- Cannulae are inserted into the ascending aorta and right atrium.
- Cardiopulmonary bypass is instituted by the perfusionist, on instruction of the surgeon.
- The temperature is controlled: mild, moderate, or deep hypothermia, depending on the operation.

### Cardioplegia

In order to arrest the heart, it is isolated from the circulation by cross-clamping the aorta proximal to the arterial cannula. Cardioplegia, a potassium- and LA-containing solution, is injected into the aortic root from where it perfuses the coronary arteries. This arrests the heart in diastole and protects it from damage. Topical cooling with iced slush is used. Cold blood cardioplegia is repeated every 20 minutes. The body is typically cooled to 32°C, for brain protection and safety.

### Types of cardiac operations

Once the heart has been arrested, specific operations can be performed, including the following:

### Coronary artery bypass grafting (CABG)

CABG is used to bypass narrowed or blocked coronary arteries, and is highly effective at treating angina and reducing the risk of myocardial infarction.

The conduits used for bypass are the left internal mammary artery and the long saphenous vein, the latter often harvested by a junior surgeon or surgical assistant. The radial artery may also be used. The heart is arrested and the distal anastomosis of the conduits are sutured onto the coronary arteries using a fine polypropylene suture. If the long saphenous vein is used, the proximal anastomosis of the graft is sutured onto the ascending aorta, using a side-biting clamp.

### Aortic valve replacement

Aortic valve replacement is performed for aortic stenosis or aortic regurgitation, the former being very common in the elderly. Aortic valve replacement returns survival to normal and treats the shortness of breath associated with aortic stenosis.

Once the heart is arrested, the diseased aortic valve is excised, and the valve ring (annulus) is decalcified. Sutures are placed in the annulus and the artificial valve, which is then tied in. The artificial valve can be a tissue valve of bovine pericardium (or porcine leaflets), or a mechanical valve made of titanium with pyrolytic carbon leaflets. The aorta is closed, and de-airing manoeuvres are performed to remove all air from the heart, before the cross-clamp is removed and the heart is allowed to beat.

### Mitral valve surgery

Mitral valve surgery is commonly performed for mitral regurgitation, where the valve may be repaired or replaced. Mitral stenosis almost always occurs in rheumatic fever, so is rare is Western countries, but may be present in immigrant populations and the developing world.

Once the heart has been arrested, the mitral valve is exposed directly through the left atrium, or through the right atrium and then atrial septum (*the Guiradon approach*). The mitral valve is then repaired using fine sutures, or replaced, and the heart is de-aired.

In procedures where the heart is opened, the pericardial cavity may be insufflated with $CO_2$, to aid with de-airing. $CO_2$ is more soluble in blood than air, which contains insoluble nitrogen.

*Aortic surgery*
This includes operations on the aortic root, ascending aorta, and aortic arch, often in cases of aortic dissection or aneurysm.

In this type of operation, the site of aortic cannulation may differ, which may be the femoral, subclavian, or axillary artery. In aortic arch surgery, the body circulation may need to be stopped during *deep hypothermic circulatory arrest*, where the body temperature is reduced to 18°C, allowing the circulation to be switched off for 40 minutes, with no neurological sequelae. Further modifications of this technique to perfuse the brain include retrograde (via superior vena cava) or anterograde (through individual aortic arch vessels) perfusion, which can reduce the time of circulatory arrest. Patients who have *deep hypothermic circulatory arrest* have profound coagulopathies at the end of surgery, and require coagulation products, such as platelets, FFP, and fibrinogen.

*Weaning from cardiopulmonary bypass*
After the specific operation is concluded, the heart is allowed to beat, and the patient is weaned from cardiopulmonary bypass. Pacing wires are placed onto the right atrium and right ventricle, in order to achieve an optimum heart rate of 85 bpm. Inotrope medication may be started, which can be either adrenaline or a combination of milrinone and noradrenaline.

*Haemostasis*
- After removal of the venous cannula the heparin is reversed with protamine (1:1 ratio with heparin dose).
- Meticulous haemostasis is essential in cardiac surgery, as a collection of blood outside the heart may compromise diastolic filling, known as cardiac tamponade, which can be lethal. Surgical haemostasis may be aided with coagulation products such as platelets or FFP.
- Once full haemostasis has been complete, chest drains are inserted into the mediastinal, pericardial, and pleural cavities. The sternum is closed with stainless steel wires and absorbable sutures to the subcutaneous layers of the skin. Patients are transferred, ventilated, to the cardiac ICU.

## Thoracic surgery
*Preoperative preparation*
- The patient is consented and routine investigations are performed.
- Preoperative and predicted postoperative lung function is assessed.
- The thoracotomy side is marked with an indelible skin marker.

*General anaesthesia*
- For lung resection, an arterial line and peripheral cannula is needed.
- A rigid and/or flexible bronchoscopy may be performed on induction of anaesthesia.
- A double-lumen ETT is used, enabling one lung to be isolated and the operative lung deflated.
- A central venous catheter may be inserted.
- Analgesia may be performed using an epidural catheter or intrapleural catheter, for intrapleural nerve block.
- The patient is turned laterally, so the operative side is uppermost.

### Incisions

The commonest incision is posterolateral thoracotomy, which divides the latissimus dorsi, but spares the serratus anterior muscle. The scapula is retracted up off the chest wall, and the intercostal space is entered through the fifth or sixth intercostal space. The lung is deflated, before entering the intercostal space with a periosteal elevator. Muscle sparing and mini thoracotomies may be performed. Video-assisted thoracoscopic surgery (VATS) procedures are routinely performed for minor cases such as lung and pleural biopsies. VATS may also be performed for lobectomies with peripheral tumours.

### Operations

#### Lobectomies for lung cancer

The surgeon dissects the fissure, then isolates, ligates, and divides the branches of the pulmonary artery and vein to the lobe, and staples the bronchus. The remaining lung on the operative side is then inflated and the surgeon performs a water test, to check that the bronchial staple line is air tight.

#### Pneumonectomy

Pneumonectomy involves removing the whole lung on either the left or right side. This may be necessary for very central tumours or those affecting all lobes of the lung. Pneumonectomy may need to be performed intrapericardially if the tumour, for example, extends along the pulmonary veins into the left atrium. Pneumonectomy represents a significant physiological challenge for the patient, and the surgeon will make a careful assessment of the patient's ability to tolerate such surgery beforehand.

#### VATS procedures

Lung biopsies, pleural biopsies, and lobectomies can be performed using VATS. Several ports are placed into the chest cavity, with the lung deflated. An operating telescope is inserted through one port and instruments are inserted through the other ports to perform the procedures. This results in less trauma and pain for the patient.

#### Decortication for empyema

Empyema is a collection of pus within the pleural cavity. It can cause the lung to collapse with a thick 'rind' or cortex on the lung surface. Once the pus has been removed from the chest cavity, the cortex must be dissected off the lung to enable full expansion. This can be a time-consuming operation, associated with considerable bleeding.

### Chest drains

After all thoracic operations, chest drains are inserted to drain blood and air. After pneumonectomy, the single chest drain must never be placed on suction, and is removed after 1 day. For all other procedures, chest drains are inserted and placed on suction, with the aim of achieving full expansion of the lung. Once there is no leak of air or significant fluid volume, they are removed.

*Recovery*

Patients are usually extubated on the operating table, and wheeled to the recovery unit. Prolonged ventilation is detrimental to the recovery of thoracic patients.

## Further reading

Association of Anaesthetists of Great Britain and Ireland (2016). Recommendations for standards of monitoring during anaesthesia and recovery 2015. Anaesthesia, 71(1):85–93.

Freedman R, Herbert L, O'Donnell A, et al. (eds) (2022). Oxford handbook of anaesthesia (5th ed). Oxford: Oxford University Press.

Leaper DJ, Whitaker I (eds) (2010). Handbook of postoperative complications (2nd ed). Oxford: Oxford University Press.

National Institute for Health and Care Excellence (2020). Venous thromboembolic diseases: diagnosis, management and thrombophilia testing. NICE guideline [NG158]. Available at: ℘ https://www.nice.org.uk/guidance/ng158

Royal College of Anaesthetists (2020). Chapter 18: guidelines for the provision of anaesthesia services for cardiac and thoracic procedures. London: Royal College of Anaesthetists.

Society of Clinical Perfusion Scientists of Great Britain & Ireland, Association of Cardiothoracic Anaesthetists, Society for Cardiothoracic Surgery in Great Britain & Ireland (2016). Recommendations for standards of monitoring during cardiopulmonary bypass. Available at: ℘ https://www.scps.org.uk/resources/useful-downloads

Suda K (2017). Transition from video-assisted thoracic surgery to robotic pulmonary surgery. Journal of Visualised Surgery, 3:55.

Wahba A, Milojevic M, Boer C, et al. (2020). 2019 EACTS/EACTA/EBCP guidelines on cardiopulmonary bypass in adult cardiac surgery. European Journal of Cardio-thoracic Surgery, 57(2):210–251.

# Urology surgery

Emergency urological surgery can include:
- Trauma to bladder or kidneys
- Testicular torsion
- Removal of foreign bodies
- Fournier's gangrene
- Obstructed urinary tract caused by calculi.

## Testicular torsion

- Testicular torsion can occur at any age but is more frequently seen in adolescents.
- Torsion may be indicated by acute scrotal and lower abdominal pain, redness and swelling of the scrotal area, a lump in the testes, or presence of blood in semen.
- Testicular torsion occurs when blood vessels supplying the testicle become twisted, cutting off the blood supply.
- Prolonged restriction of the blood supply will lead to loss of tissue; therefore, urgent surgical exploration is required and if a torsion is discovered, a fixation (orchidopexy) is required.

## Fournier's gangrene

- Fournier's gangrene is an uncommon but life-threatening condition which generally occurs in men but may also affect women and children and is more common where a patient has an underlying condition, such as diabetes mellitus leading to immunocompromise.
- A form of necrotizing fasciitis, Fournier's gangrene involves tissue of the genitalia and perineum.
- Presenting with redness, pain, and increasing pain in the affected area, patients may also be generally unwell and pyrexial.
- The condition requires administration of broad-spectrum antibiotics and urgent surgical debridement of necrotic areas, which may be extensive, to healthy tissue.

## Further reading

Jeffries MT, Cox AC, Gupta A, et al. (2015). The management of acute testicular pain in children and adolescents. BMJ, 350:h1563.
Shyam DC, Rapsang AG (2013). Fournier's gangrene. Surgeon, 11(4):222–232.
Summers A (2014). Fournier's gangrene. Journal for Nurse Practitioners, 10(8):582–587.

# Bariatric surgery

The purpose of bariatric surgery is to assist with weight loss and reduce the risk of potentially life-threatening weight-related health problems, including:
- Heart disease and stroke
- High blood pressure
- Non-alcoholic fatty liver disease (NAFLD) or non-alcoholic steatohepatitis (NASH)
- Sleep apnoea
- Type 2 diabetes.

There are several surgical procedures that can help a person to lose weight and maintain weight loss. Weight loss surgery minimizes the amount of food a person can eat by reducing the size of the stomach. There are a range of weight loss treatments available which have been designed to aid weight loss, reduce portion sizes, and lead a healthier lifestyle. These can include gastric band, gastric bypass, and sleeve gastrectomy.

## Gastric band surgery

See Fig. 18.1.

Gastric band surgery is a common type of bariatric surgery for people who are very overweight and involves putting an adjustable band around the top part of the stomach, thus reducing the amount of food that can be eaten. It is both a safe and effective weight loss procedure and suitable for those with a BMI between 32 and 45 kg/m$^2$.
- The surgery involves placing an adjustable silicone band around the top of the stomach to create a small pouch just above the band with the larger stomach below.
- This works by restricting the amount of food a person can eat as this new pouch becomes full after only a small portion.
- Tubing that comes off the band connects to an access port stitched to the abdominal wall about an inch below the surface of the skin, close to the belly button.
- The port is not visible but can be accessed by a clinician to adjust the restriction of the band by inflating or deflating it with sterile water.

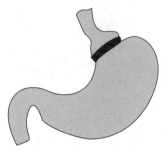

**Fig. 18.1** Gastric band.

## Gastric sleeve surgery

See Fig. 18.2.

This surgical procedure involves removing >80% of the stomach to leave a narrow banana-shaped stomach.

- It offers rapid weight loss and relatively low maintenance.
- It is an effective weight loss procedure and suitable for those with a BMI >40 kg/m$^2$.
- It works by both reducing stomach capacity and by reducing production of ghrelin, a gut hormone which is closely associated with appetite.
- A small tube (called a bougie) is placed through the mouth into the stomach and the surgeon will cut along this using it as a guide to 'size' the new smaller stomach.

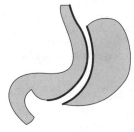

**Fig. 18.2** Gastric sleeve.

## Gastric bypass

See Fig. 18.3.

- The surgeon cuts the small intestine and sews part of it directly onto the pouch.
- The pouch is then connected to the small intestine, bypassing the rest of the stomach.
- It takes less food to make a person feel full and they will absorb fewer calories from the food eaten.

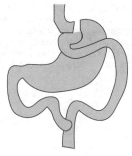

**Fig. 18.3** Gastric bypass.

Although bariatric surgery offers many benefits, all forms of weight loss surgery are major procedures that can pose serious risks and side effects. Patients are also expected to make permanent healthy changes to their diet and take regular exercise to help ensure the long-term success of bariatric surgery.

## Risks associated with bariatric surgery

As with any major procedure, bariatric surgery poses potential health risks, both in the short term and long term. Risks associated with the surgical procedure can include:
- Excessive bleeding
- Infection
- Adverse reactions to anaesthesia
- Blood clots
- Lung or breathing problems
- Leaks in the GI system
- Death (although rare).

Longer-term risks and complications of weight loss surgery vary depending on the type of surgery. They can include:
- Bowel obstruction
- Dumping syndrome
- Gallstones
- Hernias
- Low blood sugar (hypoglycaemia)
- Malnutrition
- Ulcers
- Vomiting
- Acid reflux
- The need for a second, or revision, surgery or procedure
- Death (rare).

> Dumping syndrome can occur as a complication of bariatric surgery. It can cause food (especially food high in sugar) to move from the stomach to the small intestine before the stomach has time to adequately digest it.

Each weight loss surgery has its own advantages and disadvantages, with some being less invasive than others. Table 18.1 outlines the advantages and disadvantages of gastric band, gastric sleeve, and gastric bypass surgery.

The Society for Obesity and Bariatric Anaesthesia (2015) has developed an obesity pack to be available at all times. The pack includes essential equipment to ensure the safe management of bariatric patients (Box 18.1).

**Table 18.1** Advantages and disadvantages of bariatric surgery

| Bariatric procedure | Advantages | Disadvantages |
|---|---|---|
| Gastric band surgery BMI 32–45 kg/m² | Safe and effective procedure<br>Short procedure; approximately 30 minutes' duration<br>Keyhole surgery approach<br>No abdominal incision<br>Day-case surgery<br>Faster recovery<br>Procedure is reversible | Strict changes to diet required GA<br>4 weeks of liquid/soft diet prior to resuming normal food |
| Gastric sleeve surgery BMI >40 kg/m² | Rapid weight loss<br>Low maintenance<br>Keyhole surgery<br>Faster recovery | Longer surgical procedure (1.5 hours) with 80% of stomach removed, leaving a long, tube-like pouch<br>Invasive procedure<br>Hospital stay (1–3 nights)<br>4 weeks of liquid/soft diet prior to resuming normal food<br>Increased risk of complications, e.g. staple line leak |
| Gastric bypass surgery | Positive influence on hypertension and type 2 diabetes<br>Keyhole surgery but may progress to open surgery<br>Rapid weight loss | Long surgical invasive procedure (1–3 hours)<br>Hospital stay (1–3 nights)<br>4 weeks of liquid/soft diet prior to resuming normal food<br>Increased risk of complications<br>Rapid weight loss can result in excess folds of skin<br>Requires major changes to eating habits<br>Susceptibility to anaemia<br>Typically, not reversible |

## Box 18.1 Essential surgical equipment for bariatric patients

- Bariatric operating table.
- Step for patient and theatre personnel.
- Oxford pillow and arm attachments.
- Limb extensions.
- Gel padding.
- Slide sheet.
- Wide hook-and-loop fastener strapping.
- Patient warming equipment.
- Large retractors.
- Plenty of theatre personnel.
- Large calf compressors.
- Hoist.
- Bed for postoperatively.
- Mechanical VTE.

## References and further reading

Association of Anaesthetists of Great Britain and Ireland (2015). Peri-operative management of the obese surgical patient. London: Association of Anaesthetists of Great Britain and Ireland.

Association of Anaesthetists of Great Britain and Ireland (2016). Recommendations for standards of monitoring during anaesthesia and recovery 2015. Anaesthesia, 71(1):85–93.

Bouch C, Cousins J (eds) (2018). Core topics in anaesthesia and perioperative care of the morbidly obese surgical patient. Cambridge: Cambridge University Press.

National Institute for Health and Care Excellence (2014). Recommendations. In: Obesity: identification, assessment and management. Clinical guideline [CG189]. Available at: ℘ https://www.nice.org.uk/guidance/cg189/chapter/1-recommendations

National Institute for Health and Care Excellence (2015). Obesity prevention. Clinical guideline [CG43]. Available at: ℘ https://www.nice.org.uk/guidance/cg43

National Institute for Health and Care Excellence (2016). Surgery for obese adults. Available at: ℘ https://pathways.nice.org.uk/pathways/obesity

National Institute for Health and Care Excellence (2020). Venous thromboembolic diseases: diagnosis, management and thrombophilia testing. NICE guideline [NG158]. Available at: ℘ https://www.nice.org.uk/guidance/ng158

Sinha A (ed) (2016). Morbid obesity: anaesthesia and perioperative management. Delhi: Byword Books.

Society for Obesity and Bariatric Anaesthesia (2015). Guidelines for surgery. Available at: ℘ https://www.sobauk.co.uk/guidelines-1

# Pancreatic cancer surgery

## Aetiology

- Pancreatic cancer is the seventh leading cause of cancer-related deaths worldwide with its toll higher in more developed countries.
- Pancreatic cancer is the fifth most common cause of cancer death in the UK, with an annual incidence of approximately 9600.
- The UK has one of the poorest survival rates in Europe, with average life expectancy on diagnosis just 4–6 months and a relative survival to 1 year of approximately 20%[1]; only 3% of people survive for 5 years or longer.
  - This figure has not improved much in >40 years, and it is not yet clear how the more recent trend of increased surgery and adjuvant chemotherapy will affect survival.
- Pancreatic cancer often doesn't cause any signs or symptoms in the early stages, which can make an early diagnosis difficult.
- Patients seldom exhibit symptoms until an advanced stage of the disease; pancreatic cancer remains one of the most lethal malignant neoplasms that caused 432,242 new deaths in 2018.[2]
- Due to the late diagnosis, only approximately 8% of people with pancreatic cancer are eligible for potentially curative surgery.
- People have up to a 30% chance of surviving 5 years if their tumour can be surgically removed and they have adjuvant chemotherapy.

> Pancreatic cancer develops when cells in the pancreas grow out of control, forming a tumour within the head, body, or tail of the pancreas.

## Treatment

Pancreatic cancer can be difficult to treat so treatment will be dependent on:
- The size and type of pancreatic cancer
- Location of cancer
- If the cancer has metastasized
- It may include surgery, chemotherapy, radiotherapy, and supportive care.

The symptoms of pancreatic cancer (Box 18.2) are often non-specific and patients and their families will require significant psychological support throughout the pancreatic cancer care pathway,[1] particularly in respect of:
- Anxiety and depression
- Pain and fatigue
- GI symptoms
- Nutrition.

## Surgery

There are several surgeries used to treat pancreatic cancer.
- *Potentially curative surgery* is used when the results of examinations and tests suggest that it is possible to resect all the cancer:
  - Surgical resection with adjuvant chemotherapy provides the only chance of long-term survival.

---

### Box 18.2 Symptoms of pancreatic cancer

| | |
|---|---|
| • Nausea and vomiting. | • Jaundice. |
| • Difficulty digesting food. | • Dysphagia. |
| • Altered bowel habit. | • Pyrexia. |
| • Abdominal pain. | • Fever. |
| • Weight loss. | • Fatigue. |

---

- However, only 10–20% of patients with pancreatic cancer are diagnosed with localized, surgically resectable disease.[3]
- The majority of patients present with metastatic disease and are not deemed suitable candidates for surgery.
- *Palliative surgery* usually occurs if the cancer is too widespread to be removed completely:
  - This can relieve symptoms or to prevent certain complications like a blocked bile duct or intestine, but the goal is not to cure the cancer.[1,4]

*Whipple procedure (pancreaticoduodenectomy)*

This is the most common operation to remove a cancer in the head of the pancreas and involves a large abdominal incision.

- Occasionally, this procedure can be undertaken laparoscopically.
- The head of the pancreas and sometimes the body of the pancreas is removed.
- Part of the small intestine, part of the bile duct, the gallbladder, lymph nodes near the pancreas, and sometimes part of the stomach are also removed.
- The remaining bile duct and pancreas are then attached to the small intestine so that bile and digestive enzymes can still go into the small intestine.
- The end pieces of the small intestine are then reattached so that food can pass through the digestive tract.

*Preparation*
- Bowel preparation and carbohydrate loading.
- Clear liquids until 2 hours prior to surgery.
- All patients are considered for the ERAS protocol.
- Prophylactic SC heparin prior to induction.[5]
- Pneumatic mechanical compression boots.
- Arterial line, central venous catheter.

*Surgery*
- Preoperative antibiotics are administered within 1 hour of incision and re-dosed as indicated.
- Oral gastric tube insertion following intubation and removed during surgery.

*Postoperative care*
- Reserve critical care bed.
- Nil orally overnight.
- Sips of water 1 day after surgery.

*Complications*

A Whipple procedure is a very complex operation that carries a high risk of complications that can be life-threatening (Box 18.3).

---

**Box 18.3 Complications of Whipple procedure**

- Leaking from the various connections between organs that the surgeon has to join.
- Fistula.
- Infections.
- Bleeding.
- Trouble with the stomach emptying after eating.
- Trouble digesting some foods (which might require taking some pills to help with digestion).
- Weight loss.
- Changes in bowel habits.
- Diabetes.

---

*Distal pancreatectomy*

- The tail of the pancreas or the tail and a portion of the body of the pancreas is removed.
- The spleen is usually removed also so the patient will be at increased risk of infection.
- Unfortunately, many of these tumours have usually already spread by the time they are found and surgery is not always an option.

*Total pancreatectomy*

- The entire pancreas is removed, in addition to the gallbladder, part of the stomach and small intestine, and the spleen.
- This procedure might be an option if the cancer has spread throughout the pancreas but can still be removed.
- It's possible to live without a pancreas but there are no cells that make insulin and other hormones that help maintain safe blood sugar levels.
- As a result, such patients develop type 1 diabetes, and are dependent on insulin.
- Patients who have had this surgery also need to take pancreatic enzyme pills to help them digest certain foods.[3,4]

# References

1. National Institute for Health and Care Excellence (2018). Pancreatic cancer in adults: diagnosis and management. NICE guideline [NG85]. Available at: ℅ https://www.nice.org.uk/guidance/ng85
2. Rawla P, Sunkara T, Gaduputi V (2019). Epidemiology of pancreatic cancer: global trends, aetiology and risk factors. World Journal of Oncology, 10(1):10–27.
3. Strobel O, Neoptolemos J, Jäger D, et al. (2018). Optimizing the outcomes of pancreatic cancer surgery. Nature Reviews Clinical Oncology, 16(1):11–26.
4. Parks RW (ed) (2019). Hepatobiliary and pancreatic surgery: a companion to specialist surgical practice (6th ed). Edinburgh: Elsevier.
5. Allan BJ, Novak SM, Hogg ME, et al. (2018). Robotic vascular resections during Whipple procedure. Journal of Visualized Surgery, 4:13.

# Further reading

Millis JM, Matthews JB (eds) (2016). Difficult decisions in hepatobiliary and pancreatic surgery: an evidence-based approach. Cham: Springer International Publishing.

National Institute for Health and Care Excellence (2020). Venous thromboembolic diseases: diagnosis, management and thrombophilia testing. NICE guideline [NG158]. Available at: ℜ https://www.nice.org.uk/guidance/ng158

Pancreatic Cancer UK. Homepage. Available at: ℜ https://www.pancreaticcancer.org.uk

Strobel O, Hank T, Hinz U, et al. (2017). Pancreatic cancer surgery. Annals of Surgery, 265(3):565–573.

# Robotic-assisted surgery

- Robotic surgery is considered the future of surgery due to its impact with radical changes obtained in the surgical field in recent years.[1]
- Robotic surgery is usually associated with minimally invasive surgery whereby procedures are performed through small surgical incisions.
- It enables surgeons to perform complex procedures with more precision, flexibility, and control than is usually possible with traditional surgical techniques.[2]

- Robotic-assisted surgery is not intended as a replacement for the surgeon's knowledge, expertise, or judgement.

- The origin of surgical robotics is rooted in the strengths and weaknesses of its predecessors.
- Minimally invasive surgery began in 1987 with the first laparoscopic cholecystectomy.
- Since then, the list of procedures performed laparoscopically continues to grow at a pace consistent with improvements in technology and the technical skill of surgeons.[3]

## Benefits of robotic-assisted surgery

- Small incisions.
- Less surgical trauma.
- Less pain.
- Reduced incidence of postoperative infection.
- Minimal scarring.
- Less blood loss.
- Good patient health outcomes.
- Faster recovery times than with traditional open surgery.
- Cost-effective in the long term.

## Risks/barriers of robotic-assisted surgery

- Similar to open surgery.
- Infection.
- High start-up costs.
- Medical training and additional staff to operate machinery.
- One robotic system cannot meet all surgical needs.
- Loss of force and tactile feedback, natural hand–eye coordination, and dexterity.
- Large footprints with bulky robotic arms, requiring larger operating theatres.

Robotics in surgery is limited only by imagination and cost.

## Procedures

See Table 18.2.

**Table 18.2** Procedures able to use robotic-assisted surgery

| Speciality | Robotic-assisted procedure |
|---|---|
| Orthopaedic surgery | Total hip arthroplasty |
| | Knee arthroplasty |
| Gynaecology | Hysterectomy |
| | Pelvic and lymph node dissection |
| | Myomectomy |
| | Sacrocolpopexy |
| | Tubal anastomosis |
| Urology | Nephrectomy |
| | Partial nephrectomy |
| | Pyeloplasty |
| | Prostatectomy |
| General surgery | Gastric bypass |
| | Bowel resection |
| | Cholecystectomy |
| | Oesophagectomy |
| | Adrenalectomy |
| Cardiothoracic surgery | Coronary artery bypass surgery |
| | Artery harvest |
| | Mitral valve repair |
| | Thymectomy |
| | Lobectomy |
| Neurosurgery | Radiosurgery |
| | Resection of low-grade thalamic tumours |
| Colorectal | Robotic ventral mesh rectopexy |
| | Pelvic organ prolapse |
| Head and neck | Oropharyngeal pathology |
| | Hypopharyngeal and laryngeal disease |
| | Thyroid and parathyroid disease |

## References

1. Zirafa CC, Romano G, Key TH, et al. (2019). The evolution of robotic thoracic surgery. Annals of Cardiothoracic Surgery, 8(2):210–217.
2. Domene CE, Kim KC, Vilallonga P, et al. (eds) (2019). Bariatric robotic surgery: a comprehensive guide. Cham: Springer.
3. Lanfranco AR, Castellanos AE, Desai JP, et al. (2004). Robotic surgery: a current perspective. Annals of Surgery, 239(1):14–21.

## Further reading

Bardakcioglu O (ed) (2019). Advanced techniques in minimally invasive colorectal surgery (2nd ed). Cham: Springer.
Kaye AD, Urman RD (eds) (2017). Perioperative management in robotic surgery. Cambridge: Cambridge University Press.
Tamaki A, Rocco JW, Ozer E (2020). The future of robotic surgery in otolaryngology – head and neck surgery. Oral Oncology, 101:104510.

# Gender reassignment surgery

- Gender dysphoria is a situation where there is incongruence between someone's sex at birth and their personal values, beliefs, and perceptions about their gender. In other words, a patient assigned male at birth may believe that they should be female, or vice versa.[1]
- In order to alleviate this feeling of gender dysphoria and in order to bring gender congruence, some people may choose to undergo gender reassignment surgery (also known as gender-affirming surgery).
- A nurse's role in patients' care should always be in line with the NMC code of professional conduct, which stresses that nurses should employ a non-judgemental approach in patients' care regardless of sex, disability, ethnicity, and socio-economic background, among others.[2]
- It is essential to establish ways of communicating properly with the patient. This means that appropriate terminology needs to be used after having discussed this politely and discreetly with the patient.
- People undergoing gender reassignment surgery might have a number of individual needs and vulnerabilities, so being familiar with various terms during the patient's care is of high importance in order to avoid discrimination.

> Gender reassignment surgery is a life-changing decision where patients need to be treated in a person-centred way with psychological support and education throughout their journey. Communication between the nurse and the patient as well as the nurse with the multidisciplinary team plays a vital role in implementing an individualized care plan for the patient.

## Preoperative management

- Explicit medical and social histories should be taken from the patient before surgery.
- Identify allergies in order to appropriately manage the medications that will be given pre-, peri-, and postoperatively.
- Identify medical conditions that may enhance the morbidity during and/ or after the surgery.
- Liaise with the mental health team including psychiatrist and mental health nurse to plan and implement a person-centred care for the patient.
- Any physical examination that is required before gender reassignment surgery needs to be performed in a sensitive way as patients might feel uncomfortable with their body appearance.[3]
- In accordance with the preoperative care of almost all surgeries, a number of blood tests should be done including FBC, renal and liver function, as well as urine test and urine toxicology.
- Reassure the patient and establish a safe environment for them to disclose any concerns and anxieties.
- Provide the patient with essential information about the actual procedure of gender reassignment surgery and the steps it entails.
- MRSA screening needs to be done after having gained the patient's consent.

- During the preoperative consultation, it is essential to discuss with the patient the surgical interventions and the subsequent changes to their anatomy after surgery and the different aspects of care may include the following:[1]

## Perioperative management

- GA can be administered to patients unless they are allergic to medication.
- Medical history should be taken into consideration, as existing medical conditions can affect the hepatic and renal function of the patient.
- As with every surgery, the patient needs to be closely monitored in order to diagnose and treat potential complications as quickly as possible.

## Postoperative management

- Acute postoperative pain is common among patients after gender reassignment surgery.[3]
- Work collaboratively with the surgical and pain team in order to implement an individualized care plan around pain management.
- Keep monitoring baseline vital signs including temperature, pulse, respiration rate, and BP preferably on an hourly basis until you ensure the patient is stable.
- Liaise with the mental health team to plan a person-centred care for the patient.
- Monitor the patient for potential infection after mammoplasty, genital reconstruction, and mastectomy.[4]
- The vast majority of patients who are immobile are at a high risk of developing DVT. LMWH and antiembolic stockings may prevent DVT during the postoperative period.[5]
- Urinary infections and urinary retention are two common postoperative complications after gender reassignment surgery. Patients should be educated about these and ways to care of their new body.[1]

## References

1. Middleton I, Holden FA (2017). Urological issues following gender reassignment surgery. British Journal of Nursing, 26(18):S28–S33.
2. Nursing and Midwifery Council (2015). The code: professional standards of practice and behaviour for nurses and midwives. Available at: ℘ https://www.nmc.org.uk/globalassets/sitedocuments/nmc-publications/nmc-code.pdf
3. Pisklakov S, Carullo V (2016). Care of the transgender patient: postoperative pain management. Available at: ℘ https://www.nursingcenter.com/cearticle?an=00587875-201606000-00001&Journal_ID=3402523&Issue_ID=3580878
4. Smith F (2016). Perioperative care of the transgender patient. AORN Journal, 103(2):152–163.
5. National Institute for Health and Care Excellence (2010). Venous thromboembolism: reducing the risk of venous thromboembolism (deep vein thrombosis and pulmonary embolism) in patients admitted to hospital. Clinical guideline [CG92]. Available at: ℘ https://www.nice.org.uk/guidance/CG92

## Further reading

McCormack B, McCance, T (2017). Person-centred practice in nursing and health care: theory and practice (2nd ed). Chichester: Wiley Blackwell.
Royal College of Nursing (2016). Fair care for trans patients. Available at: ℘ https://www.rcn.org.uk/professional-development/publications/pub-005575
The Gender Trust. Homepage. Available at: ℘ https://www.gendertrust.org.uk/

# Preparation of the post-anaesthetic care unit

# Preparing the post-anaesthetic care unit (PACU)

Even in major hospitals the majority of recovery's workload will come from routine elective lists during normal operating hours. Good preparation is essential to ensure the unit is safely able to manage patients throughout recovery with varying care requirements. The PACU, therefore, must be fully stocked with the equipment and supplies to manage any unforeseen incidents and critical events. The type of equipment and supplies required will depend on the size of the unit, the type of surgery (elective vs elective and trauma/emergency), and the type of patient cared for and local protocol adopted, for example, if ventilated high dependency patients are recovered or admitted directly to an ICU or HDU.

## Daily

In each PACU there will be emergency equipment which will only be used infrequently during critical incidents and emergency situations. This equipment must be checked on a daily basis to ensure it is fully operational, that all required supplies are present, and that expiry dates have not passed. All checks must be documented and there should be a system of audit to ensure that regular checks are carried out to the required standard[1]:

- Check resuscitation trolley (adults and children) and defibrillator.
- Restock drug cupboard and check for expired drugs.
- Check emergency drugs are correct and in date.
- Check anaesthetic machine.
- Check all monitoring equipment.

The Resuscitation Council (UK)[2,3] guidelines specify the minimum requirements for equipment, drugs required, and recommendations for determining specific requirements based on the dynamics of the unit. Craig and Hatfield[4] additionally outline good practice recommendations for PACU-specific design and equipment requirements. The anaesthetic machine and all monitoring should be checked according to the manufacturers' specifications and in accordance with AAGBI guidelines.[5] Alarms must be audible and parameters set in line with local policy.

## Between patients

Checking and cleaning each individual bay prior to the day's lists and between each patient is essential to maintain safety. Each bay should be readily prepared and fully equipped to receive each patient. Throughout the day bays should be restocked and any supplies used adequately replenished. This may include:

- $O_2$ and tubing
- Suction and tubing
- Oral and nasal airways
- 'T' pieces or 'T' bags
- Ambu bag or water circuit available with facemask and tubing
- Check emergency bell at each bay
- Empty sharps and rubbish containers (as required and in line with local policy).

## Ongoing

Some equipment will be used on a daily basis but not necessarily for every patient. Adequate stock checks should be carried out at the beginning of each day to ensure sufficient levels; these should be re-checked and replenished throughout the day as required. Examples include:

- Consumables such as gloves (latex and latex-free), fluids, giving sets, syringes, needles, dressing supplies, etc.
- Blankets, linen, and gowns
- Equipment such as patient warming system, drip stands, glucometers, etc.

## References

1. Association of Anaesthetists of Great Britain and Ireland (2013). Immediate post anaesthetic recovery. London: Association of Anaesthetists of Great Britain and Ireland.
2. Resuscitation Council (UK) (2018). Quality standards for cardiopulmonary resuscitation and training: acute care. London: Resuscitation Council (UK).
3. Resuscitation Council (UK) (2018). Quality standards for cardiopulmonary resuscitation and training: acute care—equipment and drug lists. London: Resuscitation Council (UK).
4. Craig A, Hatfield A (2020). The complete recovery room book (6th ed). Oxford: Oxford University Press.
5. Association of Anaesthetists of Great Britain and Ireland (2019). Checklist for draw-over anaesthetic equipment. Available at: ℘ http://dx.doi.org/10.21466/g.CFDAE2.2019

## Further reading

Royal College of Anaesthetists (2019). Chapter 4: guidelines for the provision of post-operative care. London: Royal College of Anaesthetists.
Scarth E, Smith S (2016). Drugs in anaesthesia and intensive care (5th ed). Oxford: Oxford University Press.

# PACU personnel

- The provision of care by nurses/ODPs (recovery practitioners) with expertise and experience in the recovery environment is essential.
- Patient care should only be transferred to staff who have been specially trained in recovery procedures and who have been deemed competent in line with locally or nationally agreed prescribed competencies.[1]
- Staffing levels should reflect the number of patients on theatre lists.
- An unconscious patient should receive one-to-one care until consciousness is regained and the patient is able to maintain their own airway.[2]
- There should always be a minimum of two staff on shift when patients are expected to be admitted to the PACU.[2]

## Role of the recovery practitioner

The role of the practitioner in recovery is to:
- Deliver clinically effective care to the patient during the immediate post-anaesthetic period
- Support the patient during anaesthetic emergence, prioritizing patient safety through continuous assessment and clinical evaluation
- Promptly identify adverse postoperative complications of surgery and anaesthesia and manage accordingly
- Implement clinical interventions that facilitate safe and effective recovery, enhancing patient outcomes and experience.

Recovery staff should have a good understanding of anatomy, physiology, and pharmacology related to anaesthesia and surgery. They should also have a rounded knowledge of general medicine as many higher-grade ASA patients present with chronic disease and complex comorbidities.

Specific skills are required in caring for the unconscious and intubated patient with particular emphasis on airway management and, in some cases, extubation. Due to their specialist nature, recovery staff should seek to ensure that proficiency in these skills is maintained, thereby ensuring continuous competence.

All recovery staff should be certified to immediate life support standards as set by the Resuscitation Council (UK).[3] Additionally, the AAGBI[2] recommends that there should always be one certified advanced life support provider on shift and one certified paediatric immediate life support provider on shift if the unit admits children.

*Priorities for the recovery room nurse include*
- Airway management and difficult airway management
- Pain management
- Thermoregulation
- Control of nausea and vomiting
- Haemodynamic management
- Surgical site inspection and postoperative care requirements
- Emotional support.

Box 19.1 identifies additional knowledge and skills required of recovery personnel.

## Box 19.1  Knowledge and skills required of recovery personnel

*Knowledge*
- Principles and practices of anaesthesia.
- Pharmacodynamics.
- Pharmacokinetics.
- Principles and practice of cross-infection.
- Evidence-based practice.

*Skills*
- Excellent interpersonal skills including verbal and non-verbal communication skills.
- Interdisciplinary teamwork.
- Care of catheters, drains, CVP lines, epidural catheters, arterial lines, and peripheral lines.
- Post-anaesthesia care in a range of surgical specialties.
- Care of the ventilated patient.
- Perioperative teaching and information giving.

## References

1. Royal College of Anaesthetists (2019). Chapter 4: guidelines for the provision of post-operative care. London: Royal College of Anaesthetists.
2. Association of Anaesthetists of Great Britain and Ireland (2013). Immediate post anaesthetic recovery. London: Association of Anaesthetists of Great Britain and Ireland.
3. Resuscitation Council (UK) (2018). Quality standards for cardiopulmonary resuscitation and training: acute care. London: Resuscitation Council (UK).

## Further reading

Craig A, Hatfield A (2020). The complete recovery room book (6th ed). Oxford: Oxford University Press.

# Layout of the PACU

The post-anaesthetic recovery period is a critical and potentially vulnerable time for patients.[1]

## Location

The recovery room should be situated in close proximity to the theatre to enable fast contact with medical personnel when needed.

## Observation

- Due to the quick turnover of patients, the PACU should adopt an open plan design, enabling constant observation of all patients.
- Ideally, the layout of the unit should provide 360° visibility,[2] that is, all bays are visible from all points within the room, unhindered by equipment, cupboards, etc.

## Design/size of unit

- There should be two bays for every functioning operating theatre.
- Consideration should be given to the number of theatres and the type of cases/specialties regularly undertaken when deciding on number of bays and need to service lists; for example, the requirements of a PACU that largely admits major and complex cases is significantly different to one that largely admits routine minor and/or quick turnover lists (e.g. day-case surgery). If the unit is major-case focused, it should be positioned relatively close to an ICU, should a transfer be required.
- Consideration should also be given to specialties that require an extended stay in the PACU (e.g. overnight intensive recovery), if these cases are not clinically managed in a separate unit.
- All bays should provide unobstructed access with sufficient space per patient bay for all necessary equipment, supplies, and care delivery activities.
- Adequate space between patient bays is also essential in preventing cross-infection between patients.
- The space between bays should also allow for the use of other equipment as necessary such as ventilators, X-ray machines, resuscitation equipment, etc.
- Clear partitions should be in use to divide bays (e.g. curtains, screens). These maintain patient privacy and dignity and should be portable, cleanable, and lead-lined (if X-ray machines in use).[2]
- The unit should be mechanically ventilated and contain a scavenging system, enabling good airflow and removal of anaesthetic gases. Ideally, it should have access to natural light and 'fresh air'.[3]

## Equipment

- All bays should have facilities to provide immediate access to all necessary equipment (e.g. airways, suction catheters, syringes, dressings, etc.).
- All bays must have piped $O_2$ and suction available.
- Adequate hand-washing facilities must be available and within easy reach of recovery bays.

- An emergency call system must be in place and available from all recovery bays; this should be tested regularly.
- Emergency equipment should be centrally located and easily accessible when required. Equipment drugs, fluid, and equipment required for resuscitation and the management of postoperative complications should be available within 3 minutes.[4]

## Storage

- Adequate, clean storage space should be available for supplies that will be used frequently and need stocking up at individual bays.
- Storage areas for less frequently used equipment/supplies should be close by or readily available when necessary.
- Dirty utility areas should be available within the recovery room for the disposal of soiled and/or contaminated linen and waste.

## Purpose

- Preoperative patients should be separated from and cared for in a different area from postoperative patients at all times.
- If children are admitted to the PACU, there should be an area designated for this purpose; where practicable, preferably away from adult patients.

## References

1. Craig A, Hatfield A (2020). The complete recovery room book (6th ed). Oxford: Oxford University Press.
2. NHS Estates (2004). HBN 26: facilities for surgical procedures, Volume 1. London: Department of Health.
3. Association of Anaesthetists of Great Britain and Ireland (2013). Immediate post-anaesthesia recovery. London: Association of Anaesthetists of Great Britain and Ireland.
4. Royal College of Anaesthetists (2019). Chapter 4: guidelines for the Provision of post-operative care. London: Royal College of Anaesthetists.

# Patient monitoring equipment in the PACU

The AAGBI[1] states that the minimum monitoring requirements for patients in the PACU are:
- Pulse oximeter
- NIBP

It further states that the following should be immediately available[2]:
- Electrocardiograph
- Nerve stimulator
- Thermometer
- Capnograph

In addition to the minimum standards for monitoring, the following equipment should also be freely available as and when required:
- Suction: suction could be seen as the most essential equipment in the PACU. Airway maintenance is the absolute priority for recovery staff and the ability to clear an airway to maintain its patency is vital.
- Resuscitation equipment: the Resuscitation Council (UK) guidelines[3,4] minimum requirements are for airway management equipment, defibrillation equipment, and emergency drugs. Recovery staff should ensure they are familiar with the operation of this equipment and clinically confident with the use of emergency drugs.[5]
- Glucometer: due to the nature of preoperative preparation (e.g. fasting) and the effects of anaesthesia and surgical procedures, hypoglycaemic episodes may be seen frequently in recovery in all patients, not just diabetics. Recovery staff should be vigilant to monitor for the signs and symptoms of low blood sugar and ensure proficiency in using glucose monitoring equipment.
- Infusion devices (volumetric pumps and syringe drivers): many postoperative patients will require IV fluids to replace fluid lost during surgery, or have drug infusions commenced for pre-existing medical conditions, postoperative complications, and/or local analgesia infiltration. Patients must be regularly clinically assessed and monitored in line with local protocols while such devices are in use, ensuring correct infusion rate, physiological integrity, and prevention of adverse effect.
- PCA: PCA may be initiated based on preoperative assessment/surgical procedure, care pathway, or in response to postoperative pain. Pain assessment should always be undertaken before a PCA protocol is initiated. Recovery staff must be competent in the operational function of the device used and have a sound understanding of the physiological effects (relative to the analgesic used). Prompt clinical assessment and device monitoring is required following initiation of PCA to ensure efficacy and prevent adverse effect.
- Epidural infusion and patient-controlled epidural analgesia: epidural infusions are frequently used for postoperative analgesia via continuous infusion. Recovery staff should continually monitor the patient, evaluating analgesic efficacy, physiological integrity and early

identification of adverse effects (e.g. hypotension, bladder distention, ascending block, etc.). The epidural site and device also require frequent monitoring to ensure catheter integrity and site intactness and correct infusion rate and volume reconciliation (i.e. volume infused equals that which is expected).

- Warming blankets: the perioperative experience (surgical preparation/ procedure, anaesthesia, environmental factors) all contribute to hypothermia in postoperative patients. Regular temperature monitoring and prompt intervention to address hypothermia is essential, with warming devices used in line with clinical indications and local protocol. Frequent monitoring, particularly with forced air rewarming blankets, is vital to prevent overwarming.
- X-rays: many surgical and anaesthetic procedures require post-interventional X-rays for clinical verification (e.g. orthopaedic surgery or following central venous catheter insertion). Recovery room staff must be aware of procedures that require this and signs of complications (e.g. pneumothorax). They should also have an awareness of the fundamentals of radiation protection, especially in units where X-rays are commonplace.

## References

1. Association of Anaesthetists of Great Britain and Ireland (2016). Recommendations for standards of monitoring during anaesthesia and recovery. London: Association of Anaesthetists of Great Britain and Ireland.
2. Association of Anaesthetists of Great Britain and Ireland (2013). Immediate post anaesthetic recovery. London: Association of Anaesthetists of Great Britain and Ireland.
3. Resuscitation Council (UK) (2018). Quality standards for cardiopulmonary resuscitation and training: acute care. London: Resuscitation Council (UK).
4. Resuscitation Council (UK) (2018). Quality standards for cardiopulmonary resuscitation and training: acute care—equipment and drug lists. London: Resuscitation Council (UK).
5. Craig A, Hatfield A (2020). The complete recovery room book (6th ed). Oxford: Oxford University Press.

# Managing the post-anaesthesia patient

# Transport to the post-anaesthetic care unit (PACU)

Before transferring the patient to the PACU, it should be confirmed that staff are available to receive the patient and there is a vacant recovery bay.

- Consider that the patient may be starting to regain consciousness and therefore orientation will be required.
- Explain briefly that surgery is complete and that he/she is about to be transferred to the recovery room.
- It is essential that the anaesthetist accompanies a patient who has had a GA to the recovery room, assisted by another member of the theatre team.[1]
- The anaesthetist must remain at the head end of the bed or theatre trolley so that he/she can observe the patient during transfer.
- $O_2$ will be administered to all patients who have had a GA.[2]
- The bed/theatre trolley should therefore be equipped with a portable $O_2$ cylinder, mask, and breathing circuit.
- It must be ensured that the cylinder is secure, switched on, and the flow of $O_2$ is confirmed.

> - Patient safety is of paramount importance during transfer from the operating theatre to the PACU.

- Trolley sides should be in the upright position to prevent falls.
- For paediatrics and restless patients, it is advisable to cover the trolley sides with wipe-clean, protective padding to prevent injury.
- Particular care must also be taken to ensure support equipment (e.g. infusions, drains, catheters, etc.) remain *in situ*.

The anaesthetist should decide upon the need for monitoring during transfer to the PACU.

- Consideration will be given to stability of the patient and proximity of the recovery room to theatre.
- AAGBI guidelines advise that a short interruption of monitoring is only acceptable if the recovery room is adjacent to the theatre.[2]

On arrival in the recovery room, the anaesthetist must provide a comprehensive handover to a qualified theatre practitioner.

## References

1. Phillips N (2016). Berry & Kohn's operating room technique (13th ed). St Louis, MO: Mosby.
2. Association of Anaesthetists of Great Britain and Ireland (2016). Recommendations for standards of monitoring during anaesthesia and 2015. Anaesthesia, 71(1):85–93.

# Patient handover in the PACU

The transfer of the patient from theatre to recovery is a crucial event requiring effective communication, both written and verbally.

It is essential that a formal handover of patient care, both from the anaesthetist and theatre nurse/ODP, is routinely given for every patient. This will aid continuity of care and minimize the risk of omissions.[1]

All relevant details must be verbally communicated and the following points are indicative of the minimum information required. The anaesthetist should always accompany the patient to recovery and provide handover to a trained member of staff.[1]

> An anaesthetist has overall responsibility for the transport of patients from theatre to the PACU.

## Handover from anaesthetist should include

- Name and age of patient
- Procedure performed and name of surgeon
- Type of anaesthetic and drugs given intraoperatively
- Medical and relevant surgical history
- Allergies
- Perioperative vital signs
- Fluid balance—urine output/blood loss/IV fluids administered and prescribed
- Concerns
- Postoperative instructions
- Investigations required (e.g. blood tests, chest X-ray)
- Specific patient information (e.g. communication needs), orders (e.g. 'Do not attempt CPR')
- Does anaesthetist wish to review patient prior to discharge from the PACU?[2]

> In addition to providing this information, all documentation, including the anaesthetic chart and prescription chart, must be handed to the recovery nurse/ODP.

## Handover from theatre nurse/ODP should include

- Patient details should be confirmed
- Procedure performed
- Method of wound closure
- Infiltration of LA
- Dressings
- Drains/packing
- Presence of catheter/stoma
- Blood loss
- Intraoperative events
- Pressure area assessment
- Postoperative instructions.

> The theatre nurse/practitioner should ensure all documentation (e.g. integrated care pathway) has been completed and is handed to the recovery practitioner, along with medical notes and charts.

All documentation are potential legal documents which can be used in dealing with complaints, conduct enquiries, and in court proceedings. They must therefore be an accurate reflection of the care given. Any events should be recorded factually with actions and responses also recorded.[3]

## References

1. Association of Anaesthetists of Great Britain and Ireland (2013). Immediate post-anaesthesia recovery. Anaesthesia, 68(3):288–297.
2. Phillips N (2016). Berry & Kohn's operating room technique (13th ed). St Louis, MO: Mosby.
3. Wicker P, O'Neill J (2010). Caring for the perioperative patient (2nd ed) Blackwell Publishing: Oxford.

## Further reading

Craig A, Hatfield A (2020). The complete recovery room book (6th ed). Oxford: Oxford University Press.
Royal College of Anaesthetists (2019). Chapter 4: guidelines for the provision of postoperative care. London: Royal College of Anaesthetists.

# Patient assessment in the PACU

When there is a patient in recovery who does not meet the discharge criteria, there must be at least two members of staff present, one being a competent and registered practitioner.[1]

The patient must be under close clinical observation at all times[2] and vital signs recorded at 5-minute intervals.

Remember: *follow and correct* ABC before proceeding to DEF.

### Airway

- Is it clear? Obstruction may be partial or total.
- Noisy breathing indicates obstruction but remember total obstruction may be silent—rapid assessment is essential.
- Head tilt, chin lift to clear airway.
- Gentle suction under direct vision may be required to remove secretions.
- Consider use of oral/nasal pharyngeal airway.
- Administer $O_2$ to all patients in recovery.
- Assess patient's level of consciousness.

Occasionally, patients will be handed over to the recovery practitioner with a LMA or other supraglottic airway device in place. The person taking over direct clinical care should be specifically trained in the management of these patients and in the safe removal of the airway device.[1]

### Breathing

- *Look*: is the $O_2$ mask misting? Is the patient's chest rising and falling?
- Observe depth and record rate of respirations—decreased/shallow respirations may not provide sufficient oxygenation.
- Observe skin colour for pallor/cyanosis.
- Monitor and record $O_2$ saturation rate.
- *Listen*: gurgling? Wheezing? Stridor? *Reassess airway.*
- *Feel*: place hand near patient's mouth to feel breath.

### Circulation

- Palpate pulse, noting volume and regularity.
- Record BP. Report hypo/hypertension to anaesthetist.
- ECG monitor to record heart rate and rhythm.
- Maintain circulating volume—administer IV fluids as prescribed.
- Check wound dressing and drains.

It is essential that any problems identified are rectified immediately. Always ask for help if required.

## Drugs

- Note drugs given in theatre and observe for side effects.
- Discuss analgesia prescribed with anaesthetist.
- Assess site and severity of pain—administer analgesia as prescribed and observe patient for effect and side effects (e.g. respiratory depression).
- Consider patient's pre-existing conditions—may need medication or additional monitoring (e.g. blood glucose recording).

## Elimination

- Urine output – record amount and colour if relevant to procedure.
- Record type and amount of vomit—administer antiemetics as prescribed.
- Record type and amount of NG tube drainage/aspirate.
- Record type and amount of wound drainage.

## Further care

- Reassure and orientate patient.
- Observations specific to surgical procedure.
- After regional/spinal anaesthesia, assess sensation and mobility of limbs. Ensure correct alignment.
- Record patient's temperature—consider use of forced air warming. Temperature for discharge should be 36.0°C.[3]
- Record Early Warning Scores[2] to support clinical decisions.
- Ensure patient's skin is clean and dry, document condition of pressure areas.
- Offer patient oral hygiene.
- Replace personal items (e.g. dentures, hearing aid, spectacles), if appropriate to do so.
- Ensure all of the patient's property is returned.

> It is crucial that the written documentation provides a concise, accurate account of the patient's postoperative period

## References

1. Association of Anaesthetists of Great Britain and Ireland (2013). Immediate post-anaesthesia recovery. Anaesthesia, 68(3):288–297.
2. Association of Perioperative Practice (2016). Standards and recommendations for safe perioperative practice (4th ed). Harrogate: Association of Perioperative Practice.
3. National Institute for Health Care and Care Excellence (2017). Inadvertent perioperative hypothermia. Available at: https://pathways.nice.org.uk/pathways/inadvertent-perioperative-hypothermia

## Further reading

Craig A, Hatfield A (2020). The complete recovery room book (6th ed). Oxford: Oxford University Press.
National Institute for Health and Care Excellence (2020). National Early Warning Score systems that alert to deteriorating adult patients in hospital. Available at: https://www.nice.org.uk/guidance/mib205

# Neuromuscular junction blockade

## Definition

A muscle relaxant (or neuromuscular junction blocker) is a drug that acts at the neuromuscular junction and causes paralysis of skeletal muscle through blocking the effects of acetylcholine by binding to its receptor sites.

## Uses

Muscle relaxants are used to[1]:
- Facilitate intubation
- Relax the diaphragm and skeletal muscle in the abdomen to allow the use of lighter anaesthesia
- Facilitate ventilation of patients in intensive care
- Prevent injury to the patient during ECT.

## Classes of muscle relaxant

There are two main classes of muscle relaxants:
- Depolarizing
- Non-depolarizing.

## Depolarizing muscle relaxants

- Suxamethonium (succinylcholine):
  - Is the only depolarizing muscle relaxant.
  - Acts like acetylcholine but is broken down much more slowly.
  - Binds to the acetylcholine receptor sites and causes an action potential (seen as muscle twitches) followed by extended depolarization and flaccid paralysis.
  - Is broken down by plasma cholinesterases.
  - Has a rapid onset of action and a short duration of action (approximately 2–6 minutes).[2]
  - Allows rapid tracheal intubation (useful to prevent aspiration of stomach contents).
  - Cannot be reversed.
  - Normal dose is 1 mg/kg (adult) by IV injection.[2]
  - Individuals with myasthenia gravis are resistant to suxamethonium chloride but can develop dual block resulting in delayed recovery.

Suxamethonium can be responsible for the development of MH. It should be used with caution in patients who are deficient in plasma cholinesterase as this can lead to prolonged apnoea—check family history.[1]

## Non-depolarizing muscle relaxants

Two main classes:
- Benzylisoquoliniums: includes atracurium, cis-atracurium, gallamine, and mivacurium (can promote histamine release, except cis-atracurium).
- Aminosteroids: includes vecuronium, rocuronium, and pancuronium.[2]

Non-depolarizing muscle relaxants:
- Work by competing with acetylcholine at the neuromuscular junction preventing depolarization
- Are administered by IV injection/IV infusion
- Many are excreted unchanged (atracurium and cis-atracurium break down spontaneously—useful in renal failure) in urine
- Are further classified by duration of action:
  - Short acting 15–30 minutes—mivacurium
  - Intermediate acting 30–40 minutes—atracurium, rocuronium, vecuronium, cis-atracurium
  - Long-acting 60–120 minutes—pancuronium
- Can be reversed by anticholinesterases, for example, neostigmine (dose 50–70 mcg/kg with 0.6–1.2 mg atropine sulphate).[2]

## Cautions and care of patients receiving muscle relaxants

- Appropriately trained staff must be available at all times to care for patients who have received a muscle relaxant.
- Advanced airway (e.g. ETT) and mechanical ventilation must be *in situ*.
- Disconnection alarms must be active and set appropriately.
- The patient must be closely monitored (haemodynamically and with pulse oximetry).
- The patient must not be consciously aware therefore adequate sedation and analgesia must be administered.
- Protective reflexes are absent—beware corneal abrasions, no gag reflex, and brachial plexus injuries.

## References

1. Howland RD, Mycek MJ (2006). Lippincott's illustrated reviews: pharmacology (3rd ed) Philadelphia, PA: Lippincott Williams and Wilkins.
2. Joint Formulary Committee (2017). British National Formulary (74 ed). London: BMJ Publishing and RPS Publishing.

## Further reading

Joint Formulary Committee (2022). Neuromuscular disorders. In: British national formulary. Available at: ℜ https://bnf.nice.org.uk/treatment-summary/neuromuscular-disorders.html

# Intubated/ventilated patients in the PACU

The primary goal of the recovery unit is to provide the postoperative patient with the optimum standard of care and to effectively maintain the flow of the surgical list.[1] However, unwanted demands are sometimes placed on a general recovery unit to provide postoperative ventilation. Aps (2004)[2] has often emphasized the increasing concern of recovery practitioners who feel they must care for ventilated patients or to deal with overflows of patients from the ITU into their general recovery wards, without them having the right skills to achieve this. He has also argued that such practice within a recovery unit that is not adequately and properly developed, staffed, and supported does not allow for the safe conduct of postoperative critical care.[2]

The following assessment should be made before accepting a ventilated patient to the recovery room:
- Assess the skill mix.
- Assess the workload.
- Availability of right equipment.
- Assess progress of operating theatre lists, if appropriate.

The recovery room should be equipped with the necessary skills and equipment:
- Appropriate equipment necessary for emergency resuscitation and intubation including difficult airway equipment should easily be accessible within recovery units.
- $O_2$ and suction should be present in every recovery bay.
- Artificial ventilators, CPAP circuits, capnographs,[5] pulse oximetry, cuff pressure manometer, syringe drivers, volumetric pumps, and invasive monitoring.
- A nerve stimulator for assessing neuromuscular blockade, thermometer, patient-warming devices, and glucometer should also be available.[5]
- All drugs, equipment, IV fluids, and emergency algorithms required for resuscitation and management of any complications should be immediately available.[4]
- Recovery practitioners should be appropriately qualified (some with a critical care qualification), experienced, and competent to care for ventilated patients in recovery.
- They should have received appropriate training to nationally recognized standards such as the UK National Core Competencies for Post-anaesthesia Care.[2]
- At least one qualified acute life support provider should be present at all times.[5]
- The standard of nursing and medical care should be equal to that within the ITU.[4]
- If skill mix allows, consideration should be given to a temporary swap in working environments where an ITU nurse will care for the patient and a recovery practitioner will work in ITU so their staff numbers are not depleted.

- A 1:1 patient:practitioner ratio, as for any ventilated patient, is required with the possible attendance of an anaesthetist and/or anaesthetic practitioner at all times.
- When admitting an intubated patient to a recovery room, it is the responsibility of the anaesthetist to formally hand over care of patient to appropriately trained staff.[5] See Fig. 20.1.
- Ventilated patients admitted to the recovery room should remain there for a short period only (normally 2–4 hours).
- Patients who are expected to require complex or prolonged critical care should be admitted directly to the ITU.
- When an ITU patient is admitted to a recovery unit because of bed shortages, the primary responsibility for the patient lies with the critical care team.[5]
- A good working relationship and communication with other clinical areas are essential.

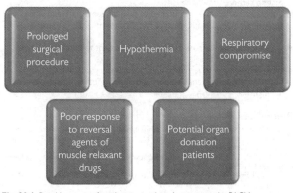

Prolonged surgical procedure

Hypothermia

Respiratory compromise

Poor response to reversal agents of muscle relaxant drugs

Potential organ donation patients

**Fig. 20.1** Possible reasons for admitting intubated patients to the PACU.

On some occasions, it might be necessary to extubate patients in recovery. The patient criteria for extubation in recovery should conform to local policy and may include the following[3]:
- No evidence of confusion or agitation.
- Pain should be controlled to a level that ensures the patient is comfortable and able to cough effectively.
- The patient should be able to breathe spontaneously and adequately and able to protect their own airway against aspiration.
- There should be minimal signs of respiratory depression.
- The patient should have an adequate gas exchange; however, it is vital to establish what is 'normal' for each patient.

## Extubation in recovery

- Extubating patients in the recovery room is the responsibility of the anaesthetist.[4] However, they may delegate this task to an appropriately trained recovery practitioner who is prepared to accept this responsibility.[5]
- Adhere to recommended guidelines and local policy.
- Ensure the patient's pain is adequately managed.
- Ensure relevant equipment including $O_2$ and working suction is ready by the bedside.
- Monitor vital signs and repeat blood gases if necessary.
- Sit the patient in a semi-upright position with a slight tilt to the left side.
- Aspirate the NG/gastric drainage tube (if patient has one) to empty the gastric contents and minimize the risk of pulmonary aspiration.
- Clear oral secretions by applying gentle suction.
- Deflate cuff slowly—in some instances it may be necessary to pass a suction catheter down the ETT.
- The patient should be encouraged to take a deep breath and while applying suction, the anaesthetist can then remove the catheter and ETT together.
- Give $O_2$ therapy via mask and encourage patient to continue to take deep breaths and cough.
- Closely monitor vital signs, especially respiratory rate and $O_2$ saturation levels; patient's colour; and observe for signs of hypoxia or hypercarbia.[3]

## References

1. Association of Anaesthetists of Great Britain and Ireland (2013). UK national core competencies for post-anaesthesia care. Available at: ℘ https://www.aagbi.org/sites/default/files/corecompetencies2013.pdf
2. Aps C (2004). Surgical critical care: the overnight intensive recovery (OIR) concept. *British Journal of Anaesthesia*, 92(2):164–166.
3. Craig A, Hatfield A (2020). The complete recovery room book (6th ed). Oxford: Oxford University Press.
4. Royal College of Anaesthetists (2019). Chapter 4: guidelines for the provision of postoperative care. London: Royal College of Anaesthetists.
5. Witaker DK, Booth H, Clyburn P, et al. (2013). Immediate post-anaesthetic recovery: Association of Anaesthetists of Great Britain and Ireland. *Anaesthesia*, 68(3):288–297.

# Caring for patients following spinal and epidural anaesthesia

Patients in the PACU may have had their surgery under spinal or epidural anaesthesia, or they may have had an epidural inserted for postoperative pain relief alongside a GA or sedation. A combination of LAs and opioids are used.

## Patient assessment and monitoring

Initial assessment of all patients should be the same as for those having GA. Monitoring should include heart rate, respiratory rate, $O_2$ saturation, and BP.

*Specific considerations*
- Ensure the patient remains flat with only one pillow until sensation returns.
- Take care of anaesthetized limbs—ensure they are in alignment and perform passive limb exercises to help prevent DVT.
- Check the injection site for signs of haematoma and leakage.
- Ensure adequate analgesia is given at the first complaint of pain as the effects of the spinal block wear off.
- Make sure the patient is warm and comfortable.
- Observe pressure areas and relieve pressure at vulnerable points (e.g. heels and sacrum).
- Reassure the patient that sensation will return.
- Advise the patient not to try and get out of bed without assistance.

*If an epidural infusion is in place or is to be commenced*
- Ensure a test dose has been given.
- Check the dressing site for leaks and ensure the catheter is not kinked.
- Check the level of the block by asking the patient to move each of their limbs to demonstrate motor function.
- Check effectiveness of epidural analgesia and, if necessary, request top-up bolus doses. If the epidural is not effective, consider other forms of analgesia.
- If patient-controlled epidural analgesia is in place:
  - Explain to patient.
  - Observe and check the pump.
  - Record amounts used.

## Potential problems

*Hypotension*
- Close observation of BP.
- Ensure IV fluids are administered.

*High level of block*
- Assess for any weakness in arms.
- Assess for difficulty in breathing.

*Respiratory depression*
- Observe the respiratory rate carefully.
- Turn off epidural infusion.
- Give $O_2$ therapy.
- Consider administering naloxone.
- Call anaesthetist for advice.

*Local anaesthetic toxicity*

Toxic reactions occur when the concentration of the drug present in the circulation exceeds certain limits either due to incorrect dosage or too rapid uptake into the circulation. In a mild toxic reaction, the patient becomes pale and restless and may feel dizzy and have a tingling sensation of the mouth. In a severe reaction, convulsions followed by cardiorespiratory arrest can occur.

If there is any suspicion of a reaction then:
- Stop any LA infusion
- Call the anaesthetist.

*Urinary retention*

This may be painless due to the effects of the spinal/epidural.
- Monitor urine output.
- Observe abdomen for signs of distension.
- If there is retention, a catheter may be required.

*Post-spinal headache*

This may be caused following post-dural puncture. If this occurs:
- Lie the patient flat.
- Maintain IV fluids.
- Give paracetamol.
- Seek advice from the pain team.

## Discharge from recovery with epidural infusion in progress

Ideally the patient with an epidural should be nursed in a HDU/ITU. If the patient is to return to the ward they should only be discharged from recovery if there are appropriately trained practitioners available to care for them and also when:
- Analgesia is adequate
- There are no serious side effects noted
- Cardiovascular system is stable
- Prescriptions are written for an opioid antagonist (e.g. naloxone), antiemetic, $O_2$, and IV fluids.

## Further reading

Association of Anaesthetists of Great Britain and Ireland (2016). Recommendations for standards of monitoring during anaesthesia and recovery 2015. Anaesthesia, 71(1):85–93.

Association of Anaesthetists of Great Britain and Ireland (2013). Immediate post-anaesthesia recovery. London: Association of Anaesthetists of Great Britain and Ireland.

Craig A, Hatfield A (2020). The complete recovery room book (6th ed). Oxford: Oxford University Press.

National Institute for Health and Care Excellence (2020). National Early Warning Score systems that alert to deteriorating adult patients in hospital. Medtech innovation briefing [MIB205]. Available at: ℘ https://www.nice.org.uk/guidance/mib205

Royal College of Anaesthetists (2019). Chapter 4: guidelines for the provision of postoperative care. London: Royal College of Anaesthetists.

# Caring for children and parents in the recovery room

Children have special needs reflecting fundamental psychological, anatomical, and physiological differences to adults. There should be a designated recovery area that is segregated from the adult areas. It should be child orientated and appropriately decorated. This creates a sense of safety and security. Children should be cared for by appropriately trained and competent staff who have undertaken regular paediatric life support training.

## Parents

> A designated area for parents/guardians should be located in an area close to theatre, where they can be contacted or wait until they are invited by the clinical staff to the recovery area to be reunited with their child as soon as they are awake.[1]

The presence of a parent or guardian in the recovery room should be encouraged. Where possible, the parent should be given a bleep so they can be paged to return to the recovery room at an appropriate time. The parent/guardian should be involved in all aspects of the care of their child. However, it is important to make sure that the parent/guardian is cared for as well by providing them with information about what happens in recovery beforehand and providing them with a chair where they can sit with their child to comfort them.

## Care of the child in recovery

- Provide one-to-one patient care, with another member of staff present.
- Paediatric equipment should be available:
  - Face masks.
  - Breathing systems.
  - Airways.
  - ETTs.
  - Emergency drugs and equipment.
  - Defibrillator.
  - Suction equipment.
  - $O_2$.
- Monitoring equipment—$O_2$ saturation, heart rate, BP.
- $O_2$ administration should be guided by the $O_2$ saturation.
- Be aware of any loose teeth that may become dislodged.
- Ensure any IV cannulas are secured with a dressing and a bandage if necessary, to avoid being pulled out by the child or accidental displacement.
- Observe wound site, dressings, and drains.
- Be aware of any specific observations required depending on surgery, such as:
  - Colour, sensation, and movement of limbs in orthopaedics
  - Bleeding in the airway following dental or ENT surgery.

- Keep the child warm. If they have come to theatre in their own clothes and they had to be taken off, try to put them back on before they wake up so they are not upset at having their clothes removed.
- Ensure that there is padding on the trolley rails to avoid the disorientated child causing themselves injury.

## Potential postoperative problems

### Airway obstruction

Airway obstruction in children rapidly leads to hypoxia due to higher $O_2$ consumption than in adults. Factors that contribute are large floppy tongues, epiglottis, tonsils, and adenoids.

- Recover children in the recovery position.
- If required, gently extend the head by either lifting the mandible by placing fingers under the jaw or through chin lift ensuring that soft tissues are not compressed.
- If necessary, use gentle suction taking care not to stimulate the back of the throat.

### Nausea and vomiting

Frequently affects older children. Increased risk from:

- Inhalational anaesthesia
- Opioid analgesia, especially morphine
- Certain types of surgery (e.g. adenotonsillectomy, appendicectomy, middle ear surgery).

Reassure the child, provide with a vomit bowl, and give antiemetic if indicated. If prolonged, consider IV fluids.

### Pain

It is sometimes difficult to assess if the child is distressed due to anxiety or distressed due to pain.

- Reassure the child through touch and 'cuddles' (if appropriate) involving the parent/guardian if present.
- Ask the child about their comfort using pain assessment scales such as visual analogue scale.
- Observe the child for non-verbal signs of pain such as guarding.
- Avoid IM injections.
- Use PCA for children who are able to understand.

## Discharge from recovery

The child should be discharged from the recovery room when they meet the following criteria:

- Awake with no signs of airway obstruction.
- Clinically stable.
- Little or no pain.
- No nausea or vomiting.
- Warm and comfortable.
- No evidence of bleeding from wound sites.
- Ongoing care prescribed (e.g. pain relief, IV fluids).
- Catheters/drains are patent and drainage is within limits.

The recovery nurse must provide a comprehensive handover to the ward nurse using the SBAR communication tool. These instructions must also be documented in the child's notes and on the postoperative care plan.

## Reference

1. Association of Anaesthetists of Great Britain and Ireland (2013). Immediate post-anaesthesia recovery. London: Association of Anaesthetists of Great Britain and Ireland.

## Further reading

Association of Anaesthetists of Great Britain and Ireland. (2016). Recommendations for standards of monitoring during anaesthesia and recovery 2015. Anaesthesia, 71(1):85–93.

Department of Health (2003). Getting the right start: national service framework for children standard for hospital services. London: Department of Health.

Craig A, Hatfield A (2020). The complete recovery room book (6th ed). Oxford: Oxford University Press.

James I, Walker I (eds) (2013). Core topics in paediatric anaesthesia. New York: Cambridge University Press.

Resuscitation Council UK (2015). Paediatric Basic Life Support. Available at: ℘ https://www.resus.org.uk/library/2021-resuscitation-guidelines/paediatric-basic-life-support-guidelines

Royal College of Anaesthetists (2019). Chapter 4: guidelines for the provision of postoperative care. London: Royal College of Anaesthetists.

Royal College of Anaesthetists (2020). Chapter 10: guidelines for the provision of paediatric anaesthesia services. London: Royal College of Anaesthetists.

Royal College of Nursing (2011). Transferring children to and from theatre: RCN position statement and guideline for good practice. London: Royal College of Nursing.

# Documentation

The documentation of care in the PACU is the final chapter of the patient's operating theatre journey. Many documents are in use and include:
- Observation charts
- Fluid balance charts
- Prescription charts
- Pain relief charts
- Care plans
- Care pathways
- Electronic records.

## What should be documented?

Different units will have their own policies and procedures in place which must be adhered to but consideration should be given to the following:
- Written entries should always be in black ink and signed, name printed, timed, and dated.
- Any errors should be crossed through with a single line and signed with the date and time.
- All care given to the patient in the PACU should be documented:
  - Recording of vital signs, fluid input/output.
  - Assessment of wounds, dressings, and drains.
  - Any medication given, including pain relief.
  - Any nausea/vomiting and whether antiemetics administered.
  - Assessment of pressure areas.
  - Mouth care given.
  - Specific assessments made, such as colour, sensation and movement of limbs, vaginal loss, pedal pulses.
- If regional anaesthesia, record level of sensation return and mobility of limbs.

> Any clinical incident should be recorded in the PACU care plan, nursing notes, and medical records, along with any other departmental reporting mechanisms.

### Integrated care plan/care pathways

Integrated care pathways may also be used in the perioperative area. In this instance, the routine postoperative care of patients is prewritten and only if an action is not met would further documentation be required. This is identified as a variance and the reasons the action had not been met explained. This facilitates a consistent approach to the care given and provides a guideline to evidence-based best practice. Variances can then be audited to establish recurring themes in the perioperative patient's pathway and identify where improvements or changes should be made.

## On discharge to the ward

*Ensure*

- Discharge criteria are met and documented. If there is an exception then this must be reported.
- $O_2$ therapy, pain relief, and IV fluids/blood are prescribed.
- Any invasive lines not required on the ward are documented as removed.
- The patient has an identification band still *in situ*.
- All items returned to patient following surgery (e.g. glasses, dentures) are documented as returned.
- All documentation is returned to the ward with the patient.
- Postoperative instructions are clear and documented.

## Further reading

Association of Anaesthetists of Great Britain and Ireland (2013). Immediate post-anaesthesia recovery. London: Association of Anaesthetists of Great Britain and Ireland.

Craig A, Hatfield A (2020). The complete recovery room book (6th ed). Oxford: Oxford
University Press.

Royal College of Anaesthetists (2019). Chapter 4: guidelines for the provision of postoperative care.
London: Royal College of Anaesthetists.

# Postoperative events and complications

Many surgical episodes are uneventful, although there are a broad range of postoperative risks and complications associated with surgery and anaesthesia.[1,2] These vary in severity, but if incorrectly diagnosed and managed can result in significant harm and even death.[2,3] Most adverse events and complications are likely to occur during the immediate postoperative period following surgery and anaesthesia, even in patients with little/no pre-existing disease, hence this period is associated with the greatest level of risk.[2]

The recovery room or PACU serves as a specialist clinical environment where postoperative patients are cared for and clinically managed. This fit-for-purpose environment provides close clinical observation and monitoring, facilitating safe postsurgical and anaesthetic recovery, and helping to restore the patient back to their preoperative physiological state.[1,2,4,5]

## Incidence

The reported incidence of immediate postoperative adverse events ranges from 1.3% up to 30%, with minor adverse events much more prevalent. Major events and complications arise in between 3% and 17% of inpatient surgical episodes.[2,5,6]

## Common postoperative complications

*Airway and respiratory complications*
- Upper airway obstruction/stridor.
- Laryngospasm.
- Hypoventilation.
- Swelling/oedema.
- Hypoxaemia.
- Loss of/low oropharyngeal muscle tone—mouth and pharynx.
- Bronchospasm.
- Secretions.
- Foreign bodies.
- Atelectasis/pneumothorax.

*Cardiovascular complications*
- Hypotension.
- Hypertension.
- Bradycardia.
- Tachycardia.
- Dysrhythmias.
- Vasodilatation.
- Hypovolaemia.
- MI.
- Cardiac arrest.

*CNS complications*
- Nausea and vomiting.
- Pain.
- Confusion/disorientation/agitation.

*Other complications*
- Hypothermia.
- Hyperthermia.
- Shivering.
- Delayed emergence.
- Prolonged sedation.
- Hypoglycaemia.

## References

1. Royal College of Anaesthetists (2019). Chapter 4: guidelines for the provision of anaesthetic services for postoperative care. London: Royal College of Anaesthetists.
2. Craig A, Hatfield A (2020). The complete recovery room book (6th ed). Oxford: Oxford University Press.
3. Boublik J (2013). Common PACU problems. In: Atchabahian A, Gupta R (eds) The anesthesia guide. New York: McGraw-Hill.
4. Syme P, Craven R (2009). Recovery and post-anaesthetic care. Anaesthesia and Intensive Care Medicine, 10(12):576–579.
5. Preston P, Gregory M (2012). Patient recovery and post-anaesthesia care unit (PACU). Anaesthesia and Intensive Care Medicine, 13(12):591–593.
6. Sewell A, Young P (2003). Recovery and post-anaesthetic care. Anaesthesia and Intensive Care Medicine, 4(10):329–332.

# Respiratory distress

Respiratory or airway complications are common in the PACU. These complications are the most likely to be serious and are of immediate threat to the patient. The nature of surgery influences the likelihood of respiratory complications; it is especially common in patients who have undergone abdominal surgery.[1]

Upper airway obstruction is one of the most common respiratory complications and frequently presents itself in the PACU. Other common respiratory complications are hypoventilation, hypoxaemia, and bronchospasm.[2]

## Causes of upper airway obstruction

Accounts for approximately 30% of adverse events, the most common cause is the tongue falling back causing obstruction of the pharynx in the unconscious patient.
- Laryngospasm.
- Low muscle tone from residual anaesthetic.
- Soft tissue swelling and/or oedema—more common in children.
- Blood, secretions, or vomit—especially after oral and airway surgery.
- Foreign bodies—throat pack, swabs, teeth.

## Causes of hypoventilation

- Defined as respiratory rate of <8 breaths per minute.
- Can be caused by depression of the respiratory centre or impaired respiratory muscles making breathed laboured.

## Depression of the respiratory centre

- Drugs.
- Opioid-induced respiratory depression of both respiratory rate and/or depth.
- Benzodiazepines.
- Volatile or inhalational anaesthetic agents.
- High epidural or total spinal.
- Hypothermia.

## Impaired respiratory muscles

- Airway obstruction.
- Residual or inadequate reversal of muscle relaxant drugs.
- Pre-existing respiratory disease—COPD, asthma.
- Muscle weakness—muscular dystrophies, Guillain–Barré syndrome.
- Splinting of diaphragm due to the nature of surgery, obesity, or pain.

## Causes of hypoxaemia

Low $O_2$ in arterial blood or Hb, demonstrated as $O_2$ saturation of 90% or less.
- Increased $O_2$ consumption—commonly caused by shivering postoperatively.
- Airway obstruction or closure.
- Bronchospasm—more common in patients with an irritable airway (smokers) or pre-existing lung disease—asthma, COPD.

- Laryngospasm.
- Pulmonary oedema—may be due to fluid overload.
- Hypoventilation.
- Diffusion hypoxia—reduction of $O_2$ concentration in the lungs at the end of anaesthesia; the displacement of $O_2$ by $N_2O$ being the major cause of diffusion hypoxia.
- Pneumothorax.
- Atelectasis—collapse of part or all of the lung; anaesthesia increases the risk; secretions can obstruct the airway and may be caused by insufficient analgesia.

## Causes of bronchospasm

Characterized by coughing and wheezing on expiration due to narrowing and obstruction of the airway:
- Most common cause is asthma.
- Anaphylaxis—allergic reaction to drugs or other substances.
- Irritants—irritable airway from smoking or other substances.
- Respiratory infections.

## Treatment of airway obstruction

Manual opening of the airway using head tilt, chin lift procedure:
- Administer high-flow $O_2$—100% $O_2$.
- Using suction or other mechanism clear secretions or remove foreign bodies from the airway.
- Insert an oral/nasal airway.
- If the patient is semiconscious, place in the recovery position.
- If still unresolved, positive airway pressure must be applied via facemask.
- If necessary, intubation must take place—this occurs in only a very small minority of patients.
- Cricothyroidotomy must be performed if all other attempts at relieving the obstruction have failed and the trachea cannot be intubated.

## Treatment of hypoventilation

Appropriate antagonist or reversal must be used[1]:
- Opioids—naloxone.
- Benzodiazepines—flumazenil.
- Residual neuromuscular block—neostigmine and glycopyrronium bromide.

## References

1. Al-Rawi S, Nolan K (2003). Respiratory complications in the postoperative period. Anaesthesia and Intensive Care Medicine, 4(10):332–334.
2. Peskett MJ (1999). Clinical indicators and other complications in the recovery room or postanaesthetic care unit. Anaesthesia, 54(12):1143–1149.

## Further reading

Association of Anaesthetists of Great Britain and Ireland (2013). Immediate post-anaesthesia recovery. London: Association of Anaesthetists of Great Britain and Ireland.
Craig A, Hatfield A (2020). The complete recovery room book (6th ed). Oxford: Oxford University Press.
Royal College of Anaesthetists (2019). Chapter 4: guidelines for the provision of postoperative care. London: Royal College of Anaesthetists.

# Postoperative nausea and vomiting

PONV is one of the most frequently seen side effects following surgery and anaesthesia. It can be very distressing and debilitating for the patient due to its unpleasantness and can cause more concern than pain relief and management of such postoperatively for the patient.

## Incidence

PONV has a reported occurrence of approximately 25–30% although in patients considered high risk, a prevalence as high as 70% has been reported.[1]

## Implications

The detrimental effect on patients can be both physical and psychological and begin immediately postoperatively.

- *Delayed discharge from PACU*: PONV in the recovery room necessitates immediate treatment with antiemetic drugs and discharge will be delayed until the PONV is under control and management is shown to be effective for the patient.
- *Delayed recovery from surgery*: PONV can cause the patient to suffer with dehydration, electrolyte imbalance, wound dehiscence, and can interfere with nutritional needs and other oral treatments which have a vital and essential part in recovering from surgery.
- *Delayed discharge from hospital and impact on hospital costs*: PONV requires an increased amount and level of care and thus carries an economic burden for the patient and the hospital caring for the patient. Further surgery may be required due to complications suffered.

## Risk factors

Predisposing factors for PONV can be identified.

### Patient

- Affects females (post puberty) more than males—ratio 3:1.
- Affects children more than adults—peaks at approximately 11–14 years of age.
- Obesity.
- Previous history of PONV or motion sickness.
- Non-smoker.[2]

### Procedure

The nature of the procedure has more impact on PONV than the type of anaesthetic administered,[3] and all of the following types of surgery increase the incidence of PONV:

- Abdominal.
- Gynaecological.
- ENT.
- Laparoscopic
- Ophthalmic.

The length of surgery also has an influence with the longer the surgery and the longer the anaesthetic, the more likely the patient is to suffer with PONV.

*Anaesthetic*

Some anaesthetic agents influence the likelihood of PONV:

- The use of $N_2O$.
- Use of some inhalational anaesthetic agents—sevoflurane and desflurane less likely to cause PONV than enflurane and halothane.
- Administration of opioids.
- Use of induction agents—propofol less likely to cause PONV than etomidate.
- GA versus regional anaesthesia—GA more likely to cause PONV.

*Postoperative*

- Pain postoperatively is associated with nausea.[2]
- Opioid analgesics—have known emetic properties.
- Hypotension.
- Dehydration.
- Early resumption of oral intake.
- Movement and mobilization.

## Treatment

PONV is multifactorial and management of such is complex, no single treatment is wholly effective at managing PONV. There are four main classes of drugs:

*Anticholinergics*

Atropine/hyoscine—act on the vomiting centre, reduce gastric motility.

*Antihistamines*

Cyclizine/promethazine—useful in middle ear surgery and motion sickness although less effective on agents that stimulate the chemoreceptor trigger zone (CTZ).

*$D_2$ antagonists*

Metoclopramide, droperidol, prochlorperazine—act against agents that stimulate the CTZ, such as opioids, anaesthetic drugs and agents, and chemotherapy.

*$5HT_3$ antagonists*

- Ondansetron, granisetron, dolasetron—effective and successful drug in the prevention of PONV due to blocking of the receptors in the gut; however, it is an expensive treatment.
- Combination therapy is more effective than single therapy and treatment must be prompt.[1]

## References

1. Rahman MH, Beattie J (2004). Post-operative nausea and vomiting. Pharmaceutical Journal, 273:786–788.
2. Taylor R, Pickford A (2003). Postoperative nausea and vomiting. Anaesthesia and Intensive Care Medicine, 4(10):335–336.
3. Hines, R, Barash, PG, Watrous G, et al. (1992). Complications occurring in the postanaesthesia care unit. Anaesthesia and Analgesia, 74(4):503–509.

## Further reading

Craig A, Hatfield A (2020). The complete recovery room book (6th ed). Oxford: Oxford University Press.

# Postoperative sore throat

Postoperative sore throat (POST) is a common adverse event after GA.[1] Although it resolves spontaneously, efforts should be taken to reduce it. POST is often considered a minor complication of anaesthesia, but remains one of the most common patient complaints with an incidence of 20–40%.[2]

- Numerous factors including age, female sex, smoking history, size of the ETT, cuff pressure, time, and manipulations needed to insert the tube, and time of operation and anaesthesia may affect the incidence of POST, with discomfort and dissatisfaction.[3]
- The swelling in the hypopharynx or larynx then affects the vocal cords and the patient experiences POST and hoarseness.[5] GA involves using a variety of techniques and adjuncts to ensure breathing is maintained and compromised.
- The nature of surgery and individual presentation will determine which adjuncts are utilized during anaesthesia and each of these may be part of the cause or contribute to sore throat postoperatively.

## Method of airway management

The incidence of sore throat varies depending on the method used.

- *ETT*: tracheal intubation is associated with the highest incidence of sore throat, which varies from 14% to 50%.[4,5]
- *LMA*: a LMA is less invasive than tracheal intubation and the incidence of sore throat is consistently lower—approximately 4–19%.[4,5]
- *Face mask*: a face mask is usually used to deliver $O_2$ and/or inhalational agents so the incidence of sore throat is minimal.

Consideration of the factors that increase the likelihood of sore throat postoperatively can aid in early detection and treatment which in turn may improve the patient experience. The therapeutic measures that have been used for this condition include topical application of non-steroidal anti-inflammatory agents, topical cortisone, or lidocaine, IV cortisone, inhalation of cortisone agents, or systematic anti-inflammatory medication postoperatively.[5]

## References

1. Scuderi P (2010). Postoperative sore throat: more answers than questions. Anesthesia and Analgesia, 111(4):831–832.
2. Flexman AM, Duggan LV (2019). Postoperative sore throat: inevitable side effect or preventable nuisance? Canadian Journal of Anesthesia, 66(9):1009–1013.
3. Jiang Y, Chen R, Xu S, et al. (2018). The impact of prophylactic dexamethasone on postoperative sore throat: an updated systematic review and meta-analysis. Journal of Pain Research, 11:2463–2475.
4. Tanaka Y, Nakayama T, Nishimori M, et al. (2015). Lidocaine for preventing postoperative sore throat. Cochrane Database of Systematic Reviews, 7:CD004081.
5. Tsintzas D, Vithoulkas G (2017). Treatment of postoperative sore throat with the aid of the homeopathic remedy arnica Montana: a report of two cases. Journal of Evidence-Based Complementary & Alternative Medicine, 22(4):926–928.

# Delayed emergence from anaesthesia

Emergence and extubation are a time of increased risk in all anaesthetics, with more complications occurring then than at induction and intubation.[1]

Patients who undergo surgery and anaesthesia should awaken gradually at the end of the procedure, slowly regaining consciousness. However, some patients will experience delayed emergence from anaesthesia and there are a variety of reasons for this. Patients usually awaken quickly in the postoperative period following the administration of fast-acting anaesthetic agents. The emergence from anaesthesia is affected by the following:

- Patient factors.
- Anaesthetic factors.
- Duration of surgery.
- Painful stimulation.

> Prompt identification and treatment of the underlying cause of delayed emergence is essential to prevent serious morbidity and mortality.[1]

## Causes

The principal factors responsible for delayed awakening following anaesthesia are anaesthetic agents and drugs used during the perioperative period. The residual effect of drugs may be from anaesthetic drugs and agents, and excessive sedative drugs or analgesics.[2]

### Muscle relaxants

Continued muscle relaxation may be due to incomplete reversal or administration of too much drug.

### Benzodiazepines

Midazolam, diazepam, temazepam, and other drugs in this group can be given as pre-medication, all of which enhance the effect of other drugs administered for anaesthesia and may contribute to delayed emergence.

### Analgesics

Opioid drugs, also referred to as narcotic drugs that can be given pre-, peri-, and postoperatively may cause hypoventilation. The consequence of hypoventilation during or after anaesthesia is that there may be a rise in $CO_2$ which if high enough can have a sedative effect or render the patient unconscious.

### Metabolic disorders

- Hypo- or hyperglycaemia.
- Electrolyte imbalance: may be an associated comorbidity in the patient or due to the surgical procedure—TURP syndrome resulting in hyponatraemia.
- Hypothermia: severe hypothermia alters conscious level.

### Neurological complications

Cerebrovascular events or stroke and raised ICP are rare causes of delayed emergence but need to be considered, especially in patients who have undergone carotid or neurosurgery.

## Treatment of residual drugs

Reversal of the effect of the specific drug or likely drug can aid wakening.
- Neuromuscular blockers: reverse using neostigmine and glycopyrronium bromide.
- Benzodiazepines: reverse using flumazenil.
- Opioids: reverse using antagonist naloxone; caution needed as reversal of analgesic effect of opioids may occur.

## Treatment of metabolic disorders

- Hypoglycaemia: once blood sugar level has been ascertained correct using IV dextrose.
- Hyperglycaemia: once blood sugar level has been ascertained, correct using sodium chloride and insulin and supplement with potassium chloride as required.
- Electrolyte imbalance: if TURP syndrome is suspected, surgery must cease immediately with monitoring and correction of electrolytes. Hyponatraemia following TURP: fluid restrict and replace sodium slowly with close monitoring.
- Hypothermia.

## References

1. Foulds L, Dalton A (2018). Extubation and emergence. Anaesthesia and Intensive Care Medicine, 19(9):465–470.
2. Zhang Y, Shan GJ, Zhang YX, et al. (2018). Propofol compared with sevoflurane general anaesthesia is associated with decreased delayed neurocognitive recovery in older adults. British Journal of Anaesthesia, 121(3):595–604.

# Post-anaesthetic shivering

Post-anaesthetic shivering is a common side effect after GA with a reported incidence ranging from 20% to 70%.[1]

Shivering is one of the leading causes of discomfort for postsurgical patients and involves involuntary oscillatory contractions of skeletal muscles; it is a common and challenging side effect of anaesthesia and targeted temperature modulation.[1]

## Causes

- Normal mechanisms for temperature control and regulation are dulled with GA and regional anaesthesia, therefore it is the anaesthetist's responsibility to manage the patient's temperature.
- Perioperative hypothermia is the main cause of post-anaesthetic shivering followed by the impairment of the body's normal mechanism for temperature control.[2]
- Not all post-anaesthetic shivering is due to hypothermia.
- Post-anaesthetic shivering causes distress for the patient but also has potential serious consequences for the patient.

## Risk factors

These include[2]:
- Surgery lasting >1 hour
- Male sex
- Children have an increased risk
- Elderly people have an increased risk
- Patients undergoing combined GA/epidural anaesthesia.

## Key issues to consider

- Shivering causes an increase in $O_2$ demand/consumption.
- Exacerbates postoperative pain.
- Increases heart rate.
- Increases BP.
- Interferes with routine monitoring.

## Treatment

- Active warming methods such as forced-air warming systems.
- Conventional blankets.
- Increasing ambient temperature.
- Warming IV fluids.
- Drug treatment: pethidine, clonidine, or tramadol can be effective in treating post-anaesthetic shivering.
- IV dexamethasone may lower the incidence of postoperative shivering.[3]

## References

1. Lopez MB (2018). Post-anaesthetic shivering – from pathophysiology to prevention. Romanian Journal of Anaesthetic Intensive Care, 25(1):73–81.
2. Buggy DJ, Crossley AWA (2000). Thermoregulation, mild perioperative hypothermia and post-anaesthetic shivering. British Journal of Anaesthesia, 84(5):615–628.
3. Hossain MS, Rashid MM, Islam SA, et al. (2019). Dexamethasone for prevention of postoperative shivering: a prospective clinical study. KYAMC Journal, 10(2):81–84.

# Diaphoresis

Diaphoresis (sweating) can be a symptom of overvigorous warming perioperatively but is also a physical consequence of some postoperative complications or side effects that must be addressed and treated promptly.

Diaphoresis may occur in response to the sympathetic discharge caused by anxiety, pain, hypercarbia, or noxious stimuli in the presence of inadequate anaesthesia. It may also be seen in conjunction with bradycardia, nausea, and hypotension as part of a generalized vagal reaction or as a thermoregulatory response to hyperthermia.

## Causes

- High temperature.
- PONV.
- Hypoglycaemia.
- Opioids.
- Hypoxia.
- High $CO_2$—hypercarbia.
- MH.
- Transfusion reaction.
- Drug reaction.

*Transfusion reaction*

- A transfusion reaction occurs when sensitivity during a blood transfusion is identified.
- The blood transfusion should be stopped if side effects show an elevated temperature and any other associated effects.

## Patient management

- Reassure the patient.
- Inform the anaesthetist.
- Assess pain.
- Monitor vital signs including ECG, $SpO_2$, and BP.
- Monitor blood glucose.
- Administer $O_2$ as prescribed.

## Further reading

Association of Anaesthetists of Great Britain and Ireland (2013). Immediate post-anaesthesia recovery. London: Association of Anaesthetists of Great Britain and Ireland.

Craig A, Hatfield A (2020). The complete recovery room book (6th ed). Oxford: Oxford University Press.

Royal College of Anaesthetists (2019). Chapter 4: guidelines for the provision of postoperative care. London: Royal College of Anaesthetists.

# Hypotension

Postoperative hypotension is a common complication in the PACU which must be addressed and treated. There is no absolute figure that is able to define hypotension as the preoperative reading plus individual patient characteristics and preoperative condition will define the figure.[1]

A baseline BP reading is therefore imperative for all patients[2] as deviation from this reading facilitates a diagnosis of hypotension. Subsequent treatment is indicated if a decrease of 20% or more from the systolic preoperative reading or a mean arterial pressure (MAP) of <60 mmHg lasts for 15 minutes or longer.

Postoperative hypotension is a cardiovascular complication that is frequently seen in PACU and has a wide range of causes.[3,4]

### Key issues to consider

The accuracy of the BP reading *must* be checked as too large or too small a cuff will give a false reading. Monitors are only present to complement visual observation and assessment of the patient.

### Causes

- *Hypovolaemia* is one of the most common causes of hypotension.[5,6]
- *Dehydration*: can occur because of inadequate fluid intake or replacement and prolonged nil by mouth (NBM) status and patients who are generally unwell prior to surgery are more likely to be dehydrated.
  - Certain surgical procedures require patients to undergo bowel preparation prior to surgery which can cause dehydration.
  - Bowel preparation causes huge losses of fluid which if not replaced adequately results in the patient arriving at theatre in a less than optimum state and potentially compromising the patient.
- *Anaesthetic drugs/agents*:
  - Residual effects of drugs and agents can cause hypotension.
  - Regional anaesthesia causes vasodilatation reducing cardiac output.
  - Induction agents—especially propofol cause a decrease in BP proportional to the amount administered.
  - Volatile agents—cause a decrease in BP proportional to the amount administered.
  - Opioids.
  - Non-depolarizing muscle relaxants.

### Cardiovascular disease and medication

Pre-existing cardiovascular disease and associated medication can contribute to hypotension postoperatively. Examples are:

- Ischaemic heart disease, heart failure, dysrhythmias, atrial fibrillation, and complete heart block and patients with valve disease.
- Beta-blockers: reduce cardiac output, ACE inhibitors, and nitrates.

### Other causes

Anaphylaxis causes cardiovascular collapse and therefore hypotension. PE from DVT and air embolus will cause hypotension.

## Treatment

- Cause of the hypotension must be identified and managed[1]:
  - Surgical cause—bleeding.
  - Anaesthetic cause—regional block.
- Oxygenation must be optimized—increase to 100% $O_2$.
- Lay patient down—supine position.
- Fluid challenge with IV fluids—individual patient characteristics and associated comorbidities must be taken into consideration.
- Response to the fluid must be assessed—if hypotension not corrected other causes must be investigated.
- Residual anaesthetic agents and drugs may require vasopressors if fluid bolus is not effective:
  - Ephedrine: 3 mg IV boluses.
  - Metaraminol: 0.5–1.0 mg IV boluses.
  - Phenylephrine: 0.18 mg slow IV injection boluses.
- Inotropes may need to be considered if management necessitates.

## References

1. Beamer JER, Warwick J (2004). Critical incidents: the cardiovascular system. Anaesthesia and Intensive Care Medicine, 5(12):426–429.
2. Osborne A (2006). Hypertension/hypotension in postoperative care. In: Colvin JR (ed) Raising the standard: a compendium of audit recipes for continuous quality improvement in anaesthesia (2nd ed). London: Royal College of Anaesthetists.
3. Kluger MT, Bullock MFM (2002). A review of the anaesthetic monitoring study. Anaesthesia, 57(11):1060–1066.
4. Peskett MJ (1999). Clinical indicators and other complications in the recovery room or post-anaesthetic care unit. Anaesthesia, 54(12):1143–1149.
5. Pescod D (2005). Postanaesthetic care unit complications. Available at: ℗ www.developing an-aesthesia.org/index.php?option=com_content&task=view&id=63&Itemid=45
6. Sewell A, Young P (2003). Recovery and post-anaesthetic care. Anaesthesia and Intensive Care Medicine, 4(10):329–332.

## Further reading

Wesselink EM, Kappen TH, Torn HM, et al. (2018). Intraoperative hypotension and the risk of postoperative adverse outcomes: a systematic review. British Journal of Anaesthesia, 121(4):706–721.

# Postoperative delirium

Delirium is an acute change in cognition and attention, which may include alterations in consciousness and disorganized thinking. While delirium may affect any age group, it is most common in older patients, especially those with pre-existing cognitive impairment.

Proper identification of risk factors is useful for perioperative interventions and can help tailor patient-specific management strategies.

### Risk factors

Some patients are more at risk of developing postoperative delirium. This includes people with:
- Neurological impairment
- Older people of advancing age
- Substance abuse, particularly high alcohol intake
- Functional impairment
- Compromised mobility
- High-risk surgery, particularly trauma and orthopaedic, vascular, and cardiac surgery
- Low mood/depression
- Sensory impairment
- Heart failure.

### Symptoms

See Box 20.1.

---

**Box 20.1 Symptoms of delirium**

Symptoms of delirium can vary considerably; some patients experience agitation and confusion, whereas others could become quiet and withdrawn. Other symptoms might include:
- Disorganized thinking
- Acute disturbance in cognition
- Memory loss
- Speech affectation
- Reversal of sleep patterns
- Emotional changes such as tearfulness, anxiety, anger, or aggression
- Trying to climb out of bed and pulling out drips and tubes
- Paranoia; visual or auditory hallucinations.

---

### Causes of delirium

Causes of delirium are often multifactorial; some specific causes, which may be effectively treated, are:
- Hypoxia—low $O_2$ levels due to the effects of the anaesthesia and opiate analgesia
- Infections, such as wound, urine, and chest infections
- Sepsis
- Poor pain control
- Hypoglycaemia

- Dehydration
- Prolonged constipation
- Sleep disturbance
- Inadequate nutrition
- Sensory impairment can make the symptoms and behaviours of delirium worse.

## Management of delirium

- Reassure the patient.
- Comprehensive neurological examination.
- Provide adequate oxygenation, optimizing the acid–base status, minimizing electrolyte abnormalities.
- Identify and treat its underlying causes.
- Postoperative sedative use should be minimized.
- If a patient is agitated, family members can often serve as a reorienting and reassuring stimulus.

> Benzodiazepines may actually prolong or worsen the course of delirium.

## Further reading

Craig A, Hatfield A (2020). The complete recovery room book (6th ed). Oxford: Oxford University Press.

Royal College of Anaesthetists (2019). Chapter 4: guidelines for the provision of postoperative care. London: Royal College of Anaesthetists.

Royal College of Anaesthetists (2016). Becoming confused after an operation. Available at: ℜ https://www.rcoa.ac.uk/sites/default/files/documents/2020-05/07-Confused2019web.pdf

Rudolph JL, Marcantonio ER (2011). Postoperative delirium: acute change with long-term implications. Anesthesia and Analgesia, 112(5):1202–1211.

Siddiqui N, Harrison JK, Clegg A, et al. (2016). Interventions for preventing delirium in hospitalised non-ICU patients. Cochrane Database System Review, 11(3):CD005563.

# Hypoglycaemia

Diabetes mellitus and other disorders of blood glucose regulation are common in perioperative patients. The optimal management of perioperative dysglycaemia has been shown to improve perioperative outcomes. Patients with diabetes mellitus have increased perioperative morbidity and mortality but it is often found in combination with other significant risk factors, such as a sedentary lifestyle, smoking, and obesity.

Hypoglycaemia occurs when blood glucose levels fall below 4 mmol/L and is quite common among patients who have starved prior to GA. Some patients who have had bariatric surgery will develop hypoglycaemia.

### Risk factors for hypoglycaemia

- Type 1 diabetes.
- Renal failure.
- Cardiac failure.
- Alcohol abuse.
- Sepsis.
- Malnutrition.
- Liver disease.
- Neonates.

Postoperatively, diabetic patients are at increased risk for infection, arrhythmia, acute kidney injury, stroke, myocardial ischaemia, increased length of hospital stay, and death.

### Causes of hypoglycaemia

- Sepsis.
- Trauma.
- Burns.
- Hormonal deficiencies.
- Genetic disorders.

### Symptoms

See Box 20.2.

### Box 20.2 Symptoms of hypoglycaemia in the PACU

- Pale and clammy complexion.
- Sweating.
- Tingling lips.
- Feeling shaky or trembling.
- Dizziness.
- Palpitations and tachycardia.
- Altered state of consciousness.
- Slurring.

## Management

- Inform anaesthetist.
- Immediate treatment should be focused on reversing the hypoglycaemia.
- Measure glucose levels.
- IV dextrose is administered with 25 g boluses of 50% dextrose until the hypoglycaemia has resolved.
- If needed, an infusion of 10% or 20% dextrose can be used to sustain euglycaemia in patients with recurrent episodes of hypoglycaemia.

## Further reading

Bansal N, Weinstock RS (2020). Non-diabetic hypoglycemia. In: Feingold KR, Anawalt B, Boyce A, et al. (eds) Endotext. South Dartmouth, MA: MDText.com, Inc. Available at: 🔎 https://www. ncbi.nlm.nih.gov/books/NBK355894/

Johnston LE, Kirby JL, Downs EA, et al. (2017). Postoperative hypoglycaemia is associated with worse outcomes after cardiac surgery. Annals of Thoracic Surgery, 103(2):526–532.

Rometo D, Korytkowski M (2016). Perioperative glycemic management of patients undergoing bariatric surgery. Current Diabetes Reports, 16(4):23.

Sebranek JJ, Lugli AK, Coursin DB (2013). Glycaemic control in the perioperative period. British Journal of Anaesthesia, 111(Suppl 1):i18–i34.

# Wound dehiscence

## What is it?

Wound dehiscence can be either partial or complete and describes a breakdown of a surgically closed wound. The word dehiscence literally means to split. Be aware that internal wound dehiscence may lead to an incisional hernia forming.

More commonly a late complication of surgery, occurring several days postoperatively; however, complete separation (often known as burst abdomen) can occur at any point postoperatively.

When wound dehiscence is suspected/identified, it should be assumed that the whole wound may be affected until proven otherwise.

## Signs

*Partial*: one part of a surgically closed wound will open up creating a small hole, the remainder of the wound will stay intact. A common precursor to wound dehiscence is a discharge of a 'pinkish' serosanguinous fluid, often seen on the wound dressing. There will be little evidence of systemic disturbance; however, signs of infection may be present.

*Complete*: often called 'burst abdomen' due to the fact that larger wounds (laparotomy) are under greater pressure and therefore have an increased risk of splitting. Obvious signs are a sudden breakdown of the wound, sometimes leading to abdominal contents protruding through. Excessive bleeding can be expected from a complete separation. Patients may experience the feeling of something 'giving way'; however, if they are unable to communicate this, signs of shock/collapse should be looked for.

## Risk factors

Wound dehiscence carries a mortality rate of 15–30% and is classed as a serious complication of surgery.

Predisposing factors include:

- Infection
- Abdominal distension
- Postoperative coughing
- Poor surgical technique
- Inappropriate closure materials
- Malnourishment
- Malignancy—underlying causes
- Smoking.

## Treatment

Depending on the severity of the wound breakdown, treatment will range from observation only in simple partial dehiscence, as these types of wound complications will heal themselves over time, to emergency return to theatre.

If active treatment is needed, consider the following points:

- *Opiate analgesia*: the patient may experience varying degrees of pain dependent upon the severity of the dehiscence.
- *Sterile dressing to wound*:
  - Pressure may also be needed if bleeding occurs.

- For complete separation or where abdominal content is visible, a saline-soaked sterile dressing should be applied.
- *Fluid resuscitation*:
  - Pressure may also be needed if bleeding occurs.
  - For complete separation or where abdominal content is visible, a saline-soaked sterile dressing should be applied.
- *Rapid return to theatre*:
  - Complete dehiscence will need re-closing.
  - This often involves muscle layers so will require the patient to have a GA.
- *Antibiotic administration*: in late dehiscence this may not have an effect but should be considered as prevention of increased chance of infection for ongoing management.

## Further reading

Association of Anaesthetists of Great Britain and Ireland (2013). Immediate post-anaesthesia recovery. London: Association of Anaesthetists of Great Britain and Ireland.

Craig A, Hatfield A (2020). The complete recovery room book (6th ed). Oxford: Oxford University Press.

Royal College of Anaesthetists (2019). Chapter 4: guidelines for the provision of postoperative care. London: Royal College of Anaesthetists.

# Wound dehiscence: images

See Fig. 20.2 and Fig. 20.3.

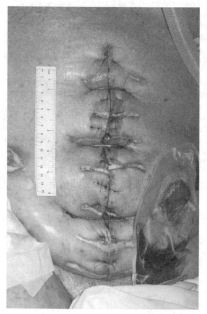

**Fig. 20.2** The warning signs: note pressure around sutures and bruising.
Courtesy of Cardiff & Vale UHB (2006).

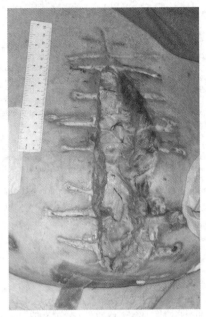

**Fig. 20.3** The burst abdomen.
Courtesy of Cardiff & Vale UHB (2006).

# Pain in the PACU

The majority of patients admitted to the recovery room will experience some level of pain, mainly as a result of their operative procedure. It is important to establish whether the pain is of an acute nature (in response to the surgery) or due to a chronic condition. Acute pain is easier to treat in the recovery room, but often presents more of a problem for patients than chronic pain, due in most part to the sensation of the pain being new.

Appropriate assessment is paramount and the patient's perception of the amount of pain they are in must be believed. Treatment will depend upon the severity of the pain experienced by the patient.

## Signs of pain

Other than verbalizing their level of pain, patients often exhibit non-verbal cues which should alert the practitioner to the fact that the patient may be in pain. They include:

• Hypertension in severe acute pain, but hypotension in chronic pain
• Tachycardia in severe acute pain, but bradycardia in chronic pain
• Increased respiratory rate
• Nausea and vomiting
• Grimacing
• Holding the body rigid
• Sweating
• Pallor
• Reluctance to converse/participate in surroundings.

## Common causes

Aside from the procedure itself, several things can contribute to a patient experiencing pain in the recovery room. Obviously the type of operation the patient undergoes will have an effect as the larger the surgery, the more chance there is of pain as a result.

• Having an anaesthetic can also cause patients to experience pain postoperatively, for example, patients may complain of a sore throat from intubation, or be agitated by a venous cannula.
• It is important to address any aspect of the patient's procedure that may be causing them distress.
• Talking to the patient and keeping them informed will help them to rationalize their pain and hopefully result in a reduction of their perception of the pain.

## Non-surgical-related causes and treatment

Often the pain from the actual wound/procedure is relieved pre-emptively by analgesia given during anaesthesia. However, there are causes of pain which cannot be so easily anticipated, they include angina, positioning, headache, a full bladder, and nerve damage.

• *Angina*: give high-flow $O_2$, reassure the patient, and give glyceryl trinitrate (GTN) sublingually to dilate coronary arteries thus improving $O_2$ supply. Pain relief such as opiates may also be required.
• *Positioning*: assess skin integrity to eliminate open skin sores, ensure the patient is repositioned more comfortably (if appropriate), and offer padding in the form of more pillows. Warm compresses and/or massaging the affected area can also relieve pain.

- *Headache*: if possible, move the patient to a quieter area, dim the lights and provide a cool compress. Paracetamol should be given unless contraindicated.
- *Full bladder*: encourage the patient to pass urine! If this is not possible, catheterization will be required. If the patient experiences bladder spasm, an antispasmodic such as hyoscine hydrobromide 20 mg given IV is an effective remedy.
- *Nerve damage*: the most effective way to treat pain from nerve damage is to inform the patient of the reason for the pain, reassure them, and provide analgesia, the strength of which will depend upon the severity of the pain experienced; however, in most cases this will be a mild-to-moderate level of discomfort alleviated by a weak pain killer.

## Further reading

Association of Anaesthetists of Great Britain and Ireland (2013). Immediate post-anaesthesia recovery. London: Association of Anaesthetists of Great Britain and Ireland.

Craig A, Hatfield A (2020). The complete recovery room book (6th ed). Oxford: Oxford University Press.

Davey A, Ince CS (2010). Fundamentals of operating department practice. Cambridge: Cambridge University Press.

Royal College of Anaesthetists (2019). Chapter 4: guidelines for the provision of postoperative care. London: Royal College of Anaesthetists.

# Hypothermia

Hypothermia occurs when a patient's core body temperature decreases to <36°C, and if left untreated can become a life-threatening complication.

The perioperative aspect of a patient's stay in hospital is one of the most crucial in the possibility of a patient becoming hypothermic, and for this reason it is imperative that measures are taken to prevent its likelihood.

## Causes

- Cold environment.
- Shivering (a way the body warms itself) abolished by GA.
- Vasodilation.
- Scant clothing.
- Evaporative heat loss, particularly of core temperature during intra-abdominal surgery.
- Infusion of cold fluids.
- Cold/dry anaesthetic gases.

Age may be a predisposing factor as older adults and children are more susceptible to hypothermia.

## Effects

*Milder consequences include*
- Patient discomfort
- Impaired wound healing
- Increased risk of infection.

*Serious effects include*
- Reduction in cough reflex, increasing the risk of aspiration
- Tachycardia
- Reduced tissue perfusion
- Atrial fibrillation/ventricular fibrillation
- Delay in metabolism/excretion of drugs
- Increased blood viscosity, impeding flow
- Shivering is significant cause of increased $O_2$ consumption and leads to hypoxia.

If a patient's temperature falls below 33°C they will stop shivering and loss of consciousness is not far away!

## Treatment

- Patients should not be rapidly warmed, and it can take >12 hours to safely rewarm a severely hypothermic patient.
- Monitoring is important to ensure a steady increase in temperature and to identify any cardiovascular changes.

*Monitor*
- Core temperature.
- BP.
- Heart rate/ECG.
- Glucose level.
- Urine output, this will increase as hypothermic kidneys fail to concentrate urine.

Actively warm with the use of a forced air heater. Use fluid warmers for any infusions, the hypothermic patient may also become hypotensive so fluid should be used to maintain circulating volume.

It is important to administer high concentrations of $O_2$ to prevent hypoxia, especially when the patient is shivering, as $O_2$ consumption is increased during the shivering process. Re-warm at a rate no faster than 0.8°C per hour.

Although hypothermia can lead to death, there is a positive chance of successful resuscitation after warming as when a patient is severely hypothermic (temperature below 32°C) some cellular damage is prevented.

## Treatment for hypothermia

*Patient temperature of 35–35.9°C*
- Do not re-expose to cold conditions.
- Keep warm for several hours.
- Watch for a drop in temperature.
- Do not massage cold limbs—this can cause cellular damage.

*Patient temperature of 33–34°C*
- Assess for cardiac arrhythmias.
- Warm only the trunk of the body.
- Give humidified, warmed $O_2$.
- Warm any IV fluids—but do not overload.
- Monitor heart rate, ECG, BP, respiration rate.

*Patient temperature between 30–32°C*
- Any sudden movements of the patient at this stage could induce cardiac arrest.
- NBM.
- Check airway.
- May need to artificially ventilate using bag and mask.
- Intubate if unable to maintain airway.
- Cardiopulmonary resuscitation.
- Defibrillation may be required—but only if core temperature is >30°C.

> Continue to treat—don't give up until the patient is sufficiently warmed.

## Further reading

Association of Anaesthetists of Great Britain and Ireland (2013). Immediate post-anaesthesia recovery. London: Association of Anaesthetists of Great Britain and Ireland.

Craig A, Hatfield A (2020). The complete recovery room book (6th ed). Oxford: Oxford University Press.

Davey A, Ince CS (2010). Fundamentals of operating department practice. Cambridge: Cambridge University Press.

Royal College of Anaesthetists (2019). Chapter 4: guidelines for the provision of postoperative care. London: Royal College of Anaesthetists.

# Post-dural puncture headache

A post-dural headache occurs following spinal or epidural block and is defined as a dural puncture with a 16-gauge needle causing severe headache.[1] Excessive CSF in the epidural space causes traction on the meninges in the brain.[2] The evidence identifying the incidence of this postoperative complication is conflicting but it can occur in up to 2% of patients and sometimes occurs in the recovery room.

## Treatment

- Maintain hydration with fluid therapy.
- Fluid therapy should be continued for 24 hours even if the patient is eating and drinking.
- Simple analgesia.
- If the headache fails to subside, a blood patch is recommended to arrest the CSF leak.

## Postoperative care

- Psychological support should be provided until symptoms subside.
- Maintain fluid therapy.
- Administer analgesia as prescribed.

## Blood patch

- A blood patch should only be undertaken in the absence of sepsis or pyrexia.
- It is effective in the majority of patients.
- Approximately 20 mL of the patient's own blood is injected into the epidural space under sterile precautions.
- This blood should clot and block the CSF leak.
- It is necessary to lay patients flat following this procedure for 2 hours.
- Complications of blood patch can occur if the clot becomes infected within the epidural space.
- Although it is rare, if an abscess develops then paraplegia may occur.

## Further reading

Carpenter M (2003). Postoperative complications related to anaesthesia and intensive care. In: Leaper DJ, Peel ALG (eds) Handbook of postoperative complications. Oxford: Oxford University Press.

Craig A, Hatfield A (2020). The complete recovery room book (6th ed). Oxford: Oxford University Press.

Freedman R, Herbert L, O'Donnell A, et al. (eds) (2022). Oxford handbook of anaesthesia (5th ed). Oxford: Oxford University Press.

# Extravasation

Extravasation occurs when an IV cannula becomes displaced. Occurrence can be reduced by careful siting away from joints.

### Risk factors

Those at increased risk of extravasation include:
- Older people
- Children
- Infants
- Patients with fragile veins
- Confused patients
- Unconscious patients.

### Symptoms

See Box 20.3.

---

**Box 20.3  Symptoms of extravasation**
- Pain.
- Delay in onset of action of the drug administered.
- Swelling.
- Leakage at the site of injection.
- Erythema of the skin around injection site.

---

### Treatment

If extravasation is suspected:
- Stop infusion or administration of IV drug.
- Inspect the site for leakage.
- Inform anaesthetist/medical team.
- Remove cannula and dress accordingly.
- Problems associated with extravasation must be addressed at the earliest opportunity to prevent tissue damage and preserve future venous access.
- Symptoms can be relieved by applying warm or cold compresses.
- Re-site cannula: a different site should be used to administer the remainder of the drug.
- Treatment should be in line with local policy.

### Postoperative care

- Psychological support to the patient should be provided.
- Inform patient that the site may be sore for a few days.
- Observe site regularly.
- Ensure patient's comfort.
- Provide analgesia as prescribed.
- Elevate the limb to reduce swelling.
- Documentation.
- Depending on the severity of the extravasated site and the toxicity of drug injected, plastic surgery may be necessary to remove damaged tissue although this is a very rare occurrence.

# Further reading

Association of Anaesthetists of Great Britain and Ireland (2013). Immediate post-anaesthesia recovery. London: Association of Anaesthetists of Great Britain and Ireland.

Craig A, Hatfield A (2020). The complete recovery room book (6th ed). Oxford: Oxford University Press.

Freedman R, Herbert L, O'Donnell A, et al. (eds) (2022). Oxford handbook of anaesthesia (5th ed). Oxford: Oxford University Press.

Royal College of Anaesthetists (2019). Chapter 4: guidelines for the provision of postoperative care. London: Royal College of Anaesthetists.

# Inadvertent intra-arterial injection

Drugs that are inadvertently administered intra-arterially are irritant and are likely to cause a reaction in the artery and surrounding vessels. It usually occurs when IV injections are attempted in the antecubital fossa region.

## Symptoms

These can include:
- Severe pain.
- Delay in onset of action of the drug administered.
- Blanching of the area affected.

## Treatment

- Treatment should be in line with local policy.
- The drug administered should be diluted.
- Flush the artery with saline.
- If there is marked arterial spasm then a sympathetic block may be helpful as this will produce vasodilation.

## Later care

- The patient should be fully informed and provided with appropriate support.
- Elevation of the arm to reduce oedema.
- Analgesia.
- Detailed documentation listing the chain of events in nursing and medical notes is vital.
- Review by a vascular surgeon may be necessary.

## Further reading

Craig A, Hatfield A (2020). The complete recovery room book (6th ed). Oxford: Oxford University Press.

Royal College of Anaesthetists (2019). Chapter 4: guidelines for the provision of postoperative care. London: Royal College of Anaesthetists.

# Discharge from the recovery room

Clear discharge criteria are essential in the recovery room to enable the safe and timely discharge of patients. A detailed policy outlining such criteria should be in place so that the recovery room nurse can discharge patients who achieve discharge criteria. Policy should also be in place to provide guidance to deal with those patients who do not achieve discharge criteria; this would usually require confirmation from an anaesthetist for discharge.

## Discharge criteria

### Neurological

Anaesthetic agents will impact the patient's neurological functioning and the recovery nurse must be confident that the patient has returned to previous neurological status and is not suffering any after effects of anaesthesia or has experienced any untoward events while in theatre (e.g. CVA). The following criteria should be assessed prior to discharge:

- Eye opening to name.
- Orientated to person and place.
- Obeys commands.
- Muscle strength to sustain head lift for 5 seconds and strong hand grips.
- Neurological assessment consistent with the patient's preoperative status is acceptable if these criteria are not met.

### Respiratory

Anaesthesia, with its sedative drugs and muscle relaxants, impairs breathing. Full recovery of respiratory function is essential prior to discharge, especially as observation on the ward will not be as constant and direct as in recovery. The following criteria should be present prior to discharge:

- Spontaneous breathing at rate between 10 and 24 breaths per minute.
- Able to maintain patent airway without artificial airway, clears oral secretions, and able to cough.
- Room air $O_2$ saturation >93%.
- $O_2$ removed *or* no $O_2$ treatment adjustments for 15 minutes prior to discharge.

### Cardiovascular

Anaesthetic agents can affect cardiovascular function in some way. In addition, most surgical procedures will involve some degree of blood loss and/or potential for blood loss postoperatively. The recovery room nurse must ensure that cardiovascular stability is present prior to discharge:

- Pulse >45 and <120 beats per minute.
- Mean arterial pressure >60 and <120 mmHg.
- Systolic BP >95 and <185 mmHg; diastolic BP <110 mmHg.

### Genitourinary

Particular attention should be given to genitourinary function postoperatively due to the effects of muscle relaxants if undergoing GA, and the loss of sensation and function if given a regional technique. The patient will also have received IV fluids intraoperatively. The bladder should be palpated and not be distended.

*Surgical sites*

Assessment of the patient's surgical site should be carried out prior to discharge to ensure there are no complications. Surgery-specific assessments should be within normal parameters, for example, drain output, wound drainage, perfusion, or swelling. Movement, sensation, and perfusion to extremities should be consistent with surgery, anaesthesia, and the patient's preoperative neurovascular status.

*Pain control*

Pain level should be assessed and be at a level acceptable to the patient. Local policy should determine the minimum stay following analgesia administration, in particular after IM opioid, IV opioid, and bolus epidural medication. Minimum stay following initiation or change in epidural infusion rate should also be identified.

*Thermoregulation*

An adequate temperature is vital for postoperative recovery. Surgical procedures which open the body cavities to the environment, anaesthetic agents which cause vasodilation, cool theatre temperatures, and prep solutions which cool the skin all contribute to a lowered body temperature postoperatively. It can affect pain management as well as impair wound healing and reduce the body's ability to fight infection. Core temperature should be 35.4–38.6°C.

*Discharge procedure*

Once discharge criteria have been met, the patient should be prepared for transfer, for example, positioned safely, drains and catheters emptied and secured, $O_2$ for transfer if required, and any special equipment obtained as required (e.g. monitors, suction).

## Further reading

Association of Anaesthetists of Great Britain and Ireland (2013). Immediate post-anaesthesia recovery. London: Association of Anaesthetists of Great Britain and Ireland.

Association of Anaesthetists of Great Britain and Ireland (2019). Day-case surgery. Available at: ⅏ https://onlinelibrary.wiley.com/doi/10.1111/anae.14639

Craig A, Hatfield A (2020). The complete recovery room book (6th ed). Oxford: Oxford University Press.

Pollard B, Kitchen G (eds) (2017). Handbook of clinical anaesthesia (4th ed). London: CRC Press.

Freedman R, Herbert L, O'Donnell A, et al. (eds) (2022). Oxford handbook of anaesthesia (5th ed). Oxford: Oxford University Press.

Royal College of Anaesthetists (2019). Chapter 4: guidelines for the provision of postoperative care. London: Royal College of Anaesthetists.

# Patient discharge to the intensive care unit

## Why and when?

- Sometimes patients will need to be transferred to the ITU.
- A number of patients will be taken to ITU straight from theatre, sedated and ventilated; while some patients may need to be admitted following deterioration in the recovery room.
- The position of the ITU should be relatively close to the theatre department, ideally on the same floor, to allow for a swift transfer.

## Preparation

- This the key to a successful transfer to ITU.
- The period of transfer is a critical one for a patient; they are often very unwell and therefore need careful management and attention.
- Detailed planning before transfer will ensure as smooth a transition as possible. It is imperative that all healthcare professionals involved in the transfer are informed and ready throughout the process.

## Responsibilities

- The overall responsibility for the transfer lies with the anaesthetist/ intensivist in charge of the patient's care.
- The qualified practitioner caring for the patient has a responsibility to ensure a safe and timely discharge and that all equipment is available and ready for use.
- Communication is vital between perioperative and critical care staff; local policies should be in place regarding transfers and admissions from theatre to ITU and from recovery to ITU.
- The receiving ITU staff have a responsibility to ensure the area is prepared and adequately staffed to safely receive the patient.

## Equipment needed

Equipment must be checked on a daily basis and sufficient stock levels maintained. The basic equipment needed for most patients includes the following:

- Portable ventilator (with adequate $O_2$ for the whole journey).
- Secondary $O_2$ supply.
- Equipment for manual ventilation:
  - Oropharyngeal airways.
  - Ambu bag/waters circuit.
  - Face masks.
- ECG monitor.
- Pulse oximeter.
- Portable suction.
- Emergency drugs and items required for venous access.
- Infusion pumps.

Depending upon the patient's condition and aspects of care, other equipment may be needed during the transfer. It is important that any equipment needed is gathered before moving the patient, preventing any delays/disruption in the care of the patient.

## Handover

Just the same as discharging a patient to a ward, when discharging to the ITU a comprehensive handover of care must be provided to enable continuity of care for the individual patient.

### Medical handover

- Details of cardiovascular status, including relevant history.
- Outline of treatment and reason for the need for ITU care.
- Pharmacological interventions (received and needed).
- Investigations and results.
- Immediate plan of care.

### Nursing handover

- Details of patient, including admitting ward.
- Description of interventions during theatre/PACU/recovery phase.
- Follow local documentation format for a comprehensive but succinct handover, for example, SBAR, NEWS.
- Re-affirm details given during medical handover regarding cardiovascular status, drugs given, fluid balance, and patient history.
- Give details of infusion pumps, drips, drains, and catheters.

Always remember to contact the admitting ward to notify them that the patient has gone to ITU. This will allow the ward staff to inform any relatives or carers of the location of the patient, but may also enable the ward bed to be utilized.

## Further reading

Association of Anaesthetists of Great Britain and Ireland (2013). Immediate post-anaesthesia recovery. Association of Anaesthetists of Great Britain and Ireland.

Association of Anaesthetists of Great Britain and Ireland (2016). Recommendations for standards of monitoring during anaesthesia and recovery 2015. Anaesthesia, 71(1):85–93.

Association of Anaesthetists of Great Britain and Ireland (2019). Checklist for draw-over anaesthetic equipment. Available at: ✍ http://dx.doi.org/10.21466/g.CFDAE2.2019" http://dx.doi.org/10.21466/g.CFDAE2.2019

Association of Anaesthetists of Great Britain and Ireland (2019). Day-case surgery. Available at: ✍ https://onlinelibrary.wiley.com/doi/10.1111/anae.14639

Craig A, Hatfield A (2020). The complete recovery room book (6th ed). Oxford: Oxford University Press.

Davey A, Ince CS (2010). Fundamentals of operating department practice. Cambridge: Cambridge University Press.

Freedman R, Herbert L, O'Donnell A, et al. (eds) (2022). Oxford handbook of anaesthesia (5th ed). Oxford: Oxford University Press.

Pollard B, Kitchen G (eds) (2017). Handbook of clinical anaesthesia (4th ed). London: CRC Press.

Royal College of Anaesthetists (2019). Chapter 4: guidelines for the provision of postoperative care. London: Royal College of Anaesthetists.

# Overnight intensive recovery

## What is it?

- Overnight intensive recovery (OIR) or surgical intensive care (SIC) is, in essence, a recovery space within the PACU that is set up and staffed to provide intensive care for postoperative surgical patients over a short period of time.
- The development of an OIR service can provide a safe period of recovery time for patients who are not well enough to be returned to a ward immediately postoperatively, but may not require an extended period of time in a critical care unit.
- The utilization of such a service can protect critical care beds for elective patients, thus reducing cancellations and preserving ITU beds for acutely ill patients.
- Most recovery units could be adapted to encompass such a service, and the set-up costs would be far less than in the development of a separate stand-alone facility.
- Each OIR bed would need 24-hour staffing and it is imperative that the OIR and ITU collaborate in care provision.
- Recovery nurses should be appropriately qualified (some with a critical care qualification), experienced, and competent to care for those patients requiring OIR, and that the service is not utilized in an inappropriate way.

## Benefits

There are benefits for patients, staff, and the organization in the utilization of an OIR as outlined next:

*Patients*

- A reduced chance of elective surgery cancellations.
- An appropriate level of care postoperatively (one-to-one nurse care opposed to ward-based patient groups).
- A reduction in possible episodes of premature extubation due to lack of critical care beds.
- Appropriately trained staff to care for the patient.

*Staff*

- A clear delineation of role between recovery and intensive recovery staff.
- A reduced likelihood of an over-busy unit which could have resulted in staff needing to stay on past the end of the shift.
- Development opportunities.
- Broader scope of practice.
- Constant nearby availability of an anaesthetist and surgeon.

*Organization*

- Reduced chance of recovery spaces being 'blocked' by ITU patients.
- Extra critical care beds for the acutely sick.
- Reduced chance of cancelled operations, resulting in lowered waiting times.
- A workforce with the appropriate skills to deliver a higher level of postoperative care.

## Considerations

- Although benefits to patients, staff, and the organization have been outlined, it is important to consider the feasibility of creating and running such a service, and the possible drawbacks associated with an OIR unit.
- A major consideration is staffing and skill mix.
- An OIR unit can only be successful if it is properly resourced and the staff working there are competent and confident to care for the type of patient admitted.
- It must be viewed by the organization and its staff as an extra facility and not simply more critical care bed space to fill.
- The criteria of patients only staying overnight (as the name suggests) or 24 hours must be rigidly adhered to.

## Further reading

Aps C (2002). Critical care for the surgical patient. British Journal of Perioperative Nursing, 12(7):258–265.

Aps C (2004). Surgical critical care: the overnight intensive recovery (OIR) concept. British Journal of Anaesthesia, 92(2):164–166.

Association of Anaesthetists of Great Britain and Ireland (2013). Immediate post-anaesthesia recovery. London: Association of Anaesthetists of Great Britain and Ireland.

Association of Anaesthetists of Great Britain and Ireland (2016). Recommendations for standards of monitoring during anaesthesia and 2015. Anaesthesia, 71(1):85–93.

Craig A, Hatfield A (2020). The complete recovery room book (6th ed). Oxford: Oxford University Press.

Freedman R, Herbert L, O'Donnell A, et al. (eds) (2022). Oxford handbook of anaesthesia (5th ed). Oxford: Oxford University Press.

Pollard B, Kitchen G (eds) (2017). Handbook of clinical anaesthesia (4th ed). London: CRC Press.

Royal College of Anaesthetists (2019). Chapter 4: guidelines for the provision of postoperative care. London: Royal College of Anaesthetists.

# Postoperative ward assessment

Postoperative patients should remain in the recovery room until conscious with stable vital signs.

On return to the ward area, a *full comprehensive handover* must be received by the nurse caring for the patient from the recovery staff. This should include:
- Anaesthetic notes
- Operation notes
- Recovery notes
- Full postoperative instructions.

## Monitor immediately: ABC
- Airway.
- Breathing.
- Circulation.

## Assess
- The patient's colour.
- Vital signs.
- $O_2$ saturation levels.
- Level of consciousness.
- CVP/ECG if patient's condition requires.

The frequency of the routine observations will be determined by the nature of the surgery, the predisposing medical condition of the patient, and their recovery.

## Observe and record
- Drains: nature and volume of drainage.
- Wound dressings: for strike through or haemorrhage.
- NG tube: note aspirate, drainage, content, and colour.
- Urinary output: >30 mL/hour.
- Fluid balance: fluid replacement/blood transfusion.
- Pain management.
- $O_2$ therapy via nasal cannula or face mask: encourage deep breathing.

---

NB: observe for complications
- Nausea and vomiting.
- Pulmonary complications.
- Cardiac complications.
- Urinary complications.

---

## The first 24 hours
- Continue to assess, monitor, observe, and record.
- Good communication will help reduce anxiety.
- Regular pain assessment: administration of appropriate prescribed pain relief.

# Further reading

Association of Anaesthetists of Great Britain and Ireland (2013). Immediate post-anaesthesia recovery. London: Association of Anaesthetists of Great Britain and Ireland.

Association of Anaesthetists of Great Britain and Ireland (2019). Day-case surgery. Available at: ℘ https://onlinelibrary.wiley.com/doi/10.1111/anae.14639

Craig A, Hatfield A (2020). The complete recovery room book (6th ed). Oxford: Oxford University Press.

Freedman R, Herbert L, O'Donnell A, et al. (eds) (2022). Oxford handbook of anaesthesia (5th ed). Oxford: Oxford University Press.

Pollard B, Kitchen G (eds) (2017). Handbook of clinical anaesthesia (4th ed). London: CRC Press.

Royal College of Anaesthetists (2019). Chapter 4: guidelines for the provision of postoperative care. London: Royal College of Anaesthetists.

# Chapter 21

# Perioperative pharmacology

# Principles of drug action

Wide ranges of drugs are required throughout the perioperative phase, particularly within the anaesthetic and recovery room, and in some circumstances they are needed urgently. With the growth of interest in the fields of drug interaction, drug surveillance, and clinical pharmacology, knowledge of drug interactions in anaesthesia and post-anaesthesia care should be a mandatory tool ensuring high-quality delivery of care to perioperative patients.[1]

The aim of drug therapy is to prevent, cure, or manage various disease processes. To achieve this goal, adequate drug doses must be delivered to the target tissues so that therapeutic, yet non-toxic levels are obtained. It is essential that clinicians working in anaesthetics and recovery recognize that the speed of onset of drug action, the intensity of the drug's effect, and the duration of drug action are controlled by four fundamental pathways of drug movement and modification in the body.[1]

Pharmacology can be divided into two disciplines:
- *Pharmacokinetics*, which considers medicine disposition and the way the body affects the medicine with time, that is, the factors that determine its absorption, distribution, metabolism, and excretion.
- *Pharmacodynamics*, which deals with the effects of the medicine on the body.

## Pharmacokinetics

The pharmacokinetic phase comprises the medicine absorption, its distribution to the tissues, its biotransformation or metabolism, and its excretion from the body. Individual variations occur because of:
- Difference in body weight
- Age
- Diet and nutrition
- Pathological disease state
- Immunopharmacology
- Psychological and environmental factors
- Genetics.

### Plasma concentration and half-life
- For many medicines, disappearance from the plasma follows an exponential time course characterized by the plasma half-life.
- Plasma half-life, in the simple case, is directly proportional to the volume of distribution, and inversely proportional to the overall rate of clearance.
- With repeated dosages or sustained delivery of a medicine, the plasma concentration approaches a steady value within 3–5 plasma half-lives.

## Reference
1. Whalen K, Feild C, Radhakrishnan R (2019). Lippincott illustrated reviews: pharmacology (7th ed). Philadelphia, PA: Wolters Kluwer.

## Further reading
Rang H, Dale M, Ritter J, et al. (2019). Rang and Dale's pharmacology (9th ed). Edinburgh: Elsevier.

# Absorption and distribution

There are four fundamental pathways of drug movement and modification in the body: absorption, distribution, metabolism, and elimination.[1]

## Medicine absorption

Bioavailability takes into account both absorption and metabolism and describes the proportion of the medicine that passes into the systemic circulation. This will be 100% after IV injection, but following oral administration the following factors affect drug absorption:

- Formulation.
- Stability to acid and enzymes.
- Motility of gut.
- Food in stomach.
- Degree of first-pass metabolism.
- Lipid solubility.

Since medicines must cross membranes in order to enter cells or to transfer between body compartments, medicine absorption will be affected by both chemical and physiological factors, that is, cell membranes, molecular size, and pH.

## Medicine distribution

Following absorption or administration into the systemic blood, a medicine distributes into interstitial and intracellular fluids.

- Cardiac output, regional blood flow, and tissue volume determine the rate of delivery and potential amount of medicine distributed into tissues.
- Initially, liver, kidneys, brain, and other well-perfused organs receive most of the drug, whereas delivery to muscle, most viscera, skin, and fat is slower.
- The second distribution phase may require several hours before the concentration of medicine in the tissues is in distribution equilibrium with that in blood. The second phase accounts for most of the extravascularly distributed medicine.

Tissue distribution is determined by partitioning of medicine between blood and the particular tissue. Lipid solubility and pH are important determinants of such uptake.

## Reference

1. Rang H, Dale M, Ritter J, et al. (2019). Rang and Dale's pharmacology (9th ed). Edinburgh: Elsevier.

# Metabolism and elimination

## Medicine metabolism

Medicines are metabolized in:
- Liver (major site)
- Tissues
- Kidney
- Lung
- GI tract.

The sequential metabolic reactions that occur have been categorized as:
- Phase 1 metabolic reactions including:
  - Oxidation
  - Reduction
  - Hydrolysis
- Phase 2 metabolic reactions:
  - Occur in the liver
  - Involve conjugation of the medicine
  - Conjugates are less active and polar molecules which are readily excreted by kidney.

### Factors affecting metabolism
- *Enzyme induction*: some medicines and pollutants (e.g. polycyclic aromatic hydrocarbons in tobacco smoke) increase activity of drug-metabolizing enzymes (Table 21.1).
- *Enzyme inhibition*: may cause adverse drug interactions. Medicines may inhibit different forms of cytochrome $P_{450}$ and so affect the metabolism only of medicines metabolized by that particular isoenzyme (Table 21.1).
- *Genetic polymorphisms*: the study of determinants that affect medicine action is called pharmacogenetics, for example, 8% of the population have faulty expression of CYP2D6, leading to prolonged responses to medicines such as propranolol and metoprolol.
- *Age*: hepatic microsomal enzymes and renal mechanisms are reduced at birth. In the elderly, hepatic metabolism of medicines may be reduced but declining renal function important for medicine dosages.

## Medicine elimination

Medicines are eliminated from the body either unchanged by the process of excretion (elimination) or converted to metabolites.

Excretory organs eliminate polar compounds more efficiently than substances with lipid solubility. Lipid-soluble medicines thus are not readily eliminated until they are metabolized to more polar compounds.

Excretion of medicines can occur in various ways:
- *Renal excretion*:
  - Glomerular filtration, tubular reabsorption (passive and active), and tubular secretion all determine the extent to which medicine will be excreted by the kidneys.
  - Renal disease will affect excretion of certain medicines.

**Table 21.1** Examples of medicines that induce or inhibit medicine metabolism

| Enzyme inducers | Enzyme inhibitors |
|---|---|
| Antibacterial:<br>• Rifampicin | Antimicrobials/antifungals:<br>• Clarithromycin<br>• Erythromycin<br>• Chloramphenicol<br>• Azoles |
| Antiepileptics:<br>• Phenytoin<br>• Carbamazepine | Cardiovascular:<br>• Amiodarone<br>• Verapamil<br>• Diltiazem |
| Miscellaneous:<br>• Cigarette smoking<br>• St John's wort<br>• Ethanol | GI:<br>• Cimetidine<br>• Proton pump inhibitors |
| | Others:<br>• Ciclosporin<br>• Monoamine oxidase (MAO) inhibitors<br>• Grapefruit juice |

- *GI excretion*:
  - Medicine conjugates excreted into bile.
  - These released into intestines.
  - Hydrolysed back to parent compound and reabsorbed.
  - This 'enterohepatic circulation' prolongs effect of the medicine.
- *Lungs* into exhaled air.
- *Medicines* may also leave body through *breast milk* and *sweat*.

## Further reading

Rang H, Dale M, Ritter J, et al. (2019). Rang and Dale's pharmacology (9th ed). Edinburgh: Elsevier.

# Pharmacodynamics

Pharmacodynamics is the study of the biochemical and physiological effects of medicines and their mechanisms of action.

Two types of effects are delivered by medicines:
- *Primary effect*: reason for which medicine is administered.
- *Secondary effect*: side effect of the medicine that may or may not be desirable.

### Time responses

A period of time after a medicine is administered until the pharmaceutical response is realized is referred to as the medicine's time response. There are three types of time responses:
- Onset: time for the minimum concentration of medicine to cause the initial pharmaceutical response.
- Peak: when the medicine reaches its highest blood or plasma concentration.
- Duration: length of time that the medicine maintains the pharmaceutical response.

All three parameters are used when administering medicines in order to determine the therapeutic range, that is:
- When medicine will become effective.
- When it will be most effective.
- When the medicine is no longer effective.

It also determines when a medicine is expected to reach toxic levels.

### Therapeutic index and therapeutic range

The medicine's therapeutic index identifies the margin of safety of the medicine. Drugs that have a low therapeutic index have a narrow margin of safety, for example, aminoglycosides (gentamicin), anticonvulsants (carbamazepine), immunosuppressants (ciclosporin), digoxin, lithium, and theophylline.

### Peak and trough levels

Plasma concentrations of a medicine must be monitored for medicines that have a narrow/low therapeutic index. Therapeutic index is referred to as the ratio between the toxic dose and the therapeutic dose of a drug, used as a measure of the relative safety of the drug for a particular treatment.
- *Peak level*: highest plasma concentration at a specific time. This indicates the rate the medicine is absorbed in the body and is affected by the route of administration. Blood samples are drawn at the time of estimated peak plasma concentration based on the route of administration. Samples are usually taken 30–60 minutes after medicine administration.
- *Trough level*: lowest plasma concentration of the medicine and measures the rate at which the drug is eliminated. Blood is drawn immediately before the next dose is given.

### Further reading

Rang H, Dale M, Ritter J, et al. (2019). Rang and Dale's pharmacology (9th ed). Edinburgh: Elsevier.

# Medicine response relationships

Drugs are administered by a certain route of administration, at a certain dosage, with the expectation of achieving a desired response. There are many factors that affect the time of onset, the intensity, and the duration of action of a particular drug[1]:

- The concentration of a medicine at the site of action controls the effect of the medicine although this may be non-linear.
- Whether the drug works by binding to a receptor or a chemical interaction, the dose (regardless of route) and the concentration at a cellular level will make the relationship more complex.
- The dose of any medicine should produce a sufficient response but not cause excessive adverse effects.

## Dose response

*Pharmacodynamics*

- There is a hypothetical dose–response curve (Fig. 21.1) where the x-axis plots concentration (dose) and the y-axis plots the response.
- This is related to potency, maximal efficacy (ceiling), and degree of response per unit dose.
- The higher the affinity for the receptor, the lower the concentration at which it produces a given level of occupancy.
- Biological variation (age, weight, general health) will influence response.

*Medicine actions*

- An *agonist* is a medicine that causes a response. If various concentrations of an agonist are administered, the dose–response curve will rise as the concentration increases from low (the left) to high (the right).
- A *full agonist* (A) is a medicine that produces a full response in the tissues. A *partial agonist* provokes a less than maximum response (i.e. less than the *full agonist*).
- An *antagonist* is a medicine that does not cause a response itself but by binding to a receptor will prevent access by the natural *agonist*.

## Drug response definitions

- *Efficacy* refers to the maximum effect that can be produced by a drug.[1]
- *Hyporeactivity* indicates that a person requires excessively large doses of a drug to obtain a therapeutic or desired effect.
- *Potency* refers to the dose required of a particular drug to produce an effect similar to another drug.
- *Tolerance* is a type of hyporeactivity that is acquired during chronic exposure to a drug in which unusually large doses are required to reach a desired effect.
- *Cross-tolerance* occurs when two drugs with similar actions are given to a patient who has developed tolerance to that category of drugs, for example, opioids—the amount of each drug must be increased to achieve the desired effect. One example of this is a diamorphine (heroin) misuser receiving high doses of opioids to maintain minimal analgesia. Another example would be a patient on long-term strong opioid therapy for cancer or persistent pain.

- *Hypersensitivity* refers to a drug-induced antigen–antibody reaction. The particular hypersensitivity reaction can be either a type 1 or anaphylactic reaction or a type 4 delayed reaction.
- *Meta reactivity* is when a drug produces unusual side effects unrelated to the dosage strength. It is also referred to as an idiosyncratic reaction, for example, the occurrence of musculoskeletal pain and increased intraocular pressure following the administration of suxamethonium.

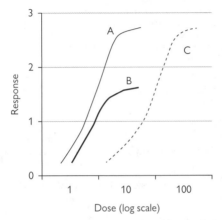

**Fig. 21.1** Dose–response curve: the full agonist (A) is more potent than medicine B. Medicine B is more potent than medicine C, but its maximum efficacy is lower.

## Reference

1. Whalen K, Feild C, Radhakrishnan R (2019). Lippincott illustrated reviews: pharmacology (7th ed). Philadelphia, PA: Wolters Kluwer.

## Further reading

Rang H, Dale M, Ritter J, et al. (2019). Rang and Dale's pharmacology (9th ed). Edinburgh: Elsevier.

# Medicine compatibility

Refers to the possibility of interactions between active medicines and their excipients and includes:
- Chemical and alcohol interactions
- Pharmacokinetic interactions:
  - Affecting absorption
  - Changes in protein binding
  - Affecting metabolism and renal excretion
- Pharmacodynamic interactions:
  - At receptor sites
  - Between medicines affecting the same system
  - Owing to altered physiology.

## IV medicine compatibility

Types of medicines administration includes:
- Continuous IV
- Intermittent IV
- Bolus IV.

Ideally medicines should be infused separately. Most compatibility data is based on physical compatibility. Information on reconstitution and dilution identifies the suitable diluents (e.g. water for injection etc.) and delivery systems (e.g. the need for glass syringes).

Incompatibility of a medicine and its diluent or between two medicines may be identified by:
- Change in colour of the medicine
- Clouding of the medicine
- Development of a haze
- Precipitation.

## pH values

- pH values help predict possible physical incompatibility among medicines where no compatibility data exist.
- It is not advisable to co-administer medicines with divergent pH values as this can lead to precipitation or inactivation of either or both medicines.

## Further reading

Rang H, Dale M, Ritter J, et al. (2019). Rang and Dale's pharmacology (9th ed). Edinburgh: Elsevier.

# Common medicine problems

Medication-related adverse events can be minimized by adhering to the five 'Rs' of safe medicine administration:
* *Right* patient
* *Right* medicine.
* *Right* dose/amount.
* *Right* route—epidural, intrathecal, IV, SC.
* *Right* frequency.

## Adverse reactions

*Sensitivity*

Previous exposure to a medicine or a similar medicine may result in the formation of antibodies. On subsequent administration these antibodies react with the medicine (the allergen) and initiate an allergic reaction by the release of chemicals such as histamine. Sensitivity may manifest as:
* Urticaria
* Pruritus.

*Allergic emergency (anaphylactic shock)*

A severe reaction to an allergen that may manifest itself as a rash, swollen tongue or throat, respiratory distress, shock, pallor, or cyanosis and may lead to a cardiac arrest. Treatment for anaphylaxis includes:
* Airway management
* Adrenaline (epinephrine) IM stat which may need to be repeated.

➔ See Types of shock, p. 743 for practical guidance.

*Idiosyncrasy*

An abnormal reaction owing to a genetic abnormality, for example, the lack of the enzyme cholinesterase prolongs the action of the muscle relaxant suxamethonium.

## Adverse events related to injected medicines

Inappropriate site selection and poor technique may result in:
* Pain
* Distress
* Nerve injury
* Bleeding
* Abscess formation.

## Tolerance, dependence, addiction, and withdrawal

*Tolerance*

Diminished response to the same dose of the same medicine taken on a regular basis. Often seen with opioids (e.g. oxycodone, morphine, and diamorphine) where dose escalation is needed on a regular basis.

*Dependence*

* Psychological: intense mental cravings occur if the medicine is unavailable or withdrawn.
* Physical: a person is dependent on taking the medicine to achieve everyday functions (activities of daily living) or an endpoint. Abrupt cessation of the medicine would lead to withdrawal within 8 hours that may last for 7 days.

*Addiction*

Addiction is defined as compulsive drug-seeking behaviour that results from recurring drug intoxication.

*Withdrawal*

Signs and symptoms include, but are not limited to:

- Restlessness
- Runny nose and sweating
- Aggressive behaviour and restless sleep
- Backache and muscle spasm
- Hypertension and hypotension
- Nausea, vomiting, and diarrhoea.

## Dose adjustment

It may be necessary to adjust the dose in some populations for some medicines. Therefore, it might be necessary to check the following prior to administration:

- Infants and children—age and weight.
- Pregnancy status.
- Breastfeeding status.
- Presence of hepatic or renal disease.

The older person has undergone physical changes, such as an alteration in body fat content, therefore dose adjustment may be necessary. Since the older person usually takes more medicines, this increases the risk of adverse effects and interactions.

## Further reading

Bisson DL, Newell SD, Laxton C (2018). Antenatal and postnatal analgesia. Scientific impact paper no. 59. Royal College of Obstetricians and Gynaecologists. Available at: ℘ https://www.rcog.org.uk/en/guidelines-research-services/guidelines/sip59/

Quinlan J, Cox F. Acute pain management in patients with drug dependence syndrome. Pain Reports, 2017;2(4):e611.

Rang H, Dale M, Ritter J, et al. (2019). Rang and Dale's pharmacology (9th ed). Edinburgh: Elsevier.

# Suspected adverse reactions

This is an unwanted effect of the medicine and is also known as an adverse effect or side effect (Box 21.1). Since medicines are distributed throughout the body, their actions are unlikely to be restricted to a single organ or tissue.

---

### Box 21.1 Yellow card system

Suspected adverse reactions related to one or more drugs/vaccines/complementary remedies should be reported using the yellow card system.

The yellow card system may be used by all health professionals and patients and may be submitted:
- Online accessible via ℘ https://yellowcard.mhra.gov.uk/
- Via post—copy of form in the back of BNF. Completed form to be sent to FREEPOST YELLOW CARD (no other address details required)
- Via the Yellow Card app.

---

## Suspected adverse reactions

*Adverse event*

An adverse event refers to any untoward occurrence in a patient to whom a medicine has been given. This includes occurrences which are not necessarily caused by, or related to, the medicine.

*Adverse reaction*

An adverse reaction refers to any untoward and unintended response in a patient which is related to any dose of a medicine that has been administered.

*Unexpected adverse reaction*

This is known to be an adverse reaction that is 'unexpected' if its nature and severity are not consistent with the information about the medicine found in the summary of product characteristics.

*Serious adverse reaction/event*

An adverse reaction is 'serious' if it:
- Results in death
- Is life-threatening
- Requires prolongation of existing hospitalization
- Results in persistent or significant disability or incapacity.

*Suspected serious adverse reaction (SSAR)*

Any adverse reaction that is classed as serious and which is consistent with the information listed in the summary of product characteristics (SPC).

*Suspected unexpected serious adverse reaction (SUSAR)*

Any adverse reaction that is classed as serious and is suspected to be caused by a medicine that is *not* consistent with the information in the SPC.

## Risk of adverse reactions

This may be reduced by:
- Checking sensitivities and allergies
- Checking use of herbal remedies and supplements
- Do not use the medicine unless there is a good indication
- Use as few medicines as possible
- Dose adjustment may be needed in patients with extremes of age or who have hepatic or renal impairment.

## Types of adverse reactions

These vary in intensity. Clinically relevant side effects of all licensed medicines are listed in the BNF.

Examples of side effects and associated medicines include:
- Nausea and vomiting (e.g. opioids especially tramadol)
- Constipation (e.g. $5HT_3$ antagonists, codeine, strong opioids)
- Ulceration of the oral mucosa (e.g. NSAIDs, chemotherapy)
- Teeth staining (e.g. chlorhexidine)
- Dry mouth (e.g. opioids)
- Extrapyramidal effects (e.g. metoclopramide)
- Rashes
- Drowsiness (e.g. opioids)
- GI side effects including discomfort, bleeding, and ulceration (e.g. NSAIDs)
- Hypersensitivity reactions (e.g. aspirin)
- Renal failure (e.g. NSAIDs).

## Further reading

Rang H, Dale M, Ritter J, et al. (2019). Rang and Dale's pharmacology (9th ed). Edinburgh: Elsevier.

# Routes of medicine administration

'The route of drug administration is determined primarily by the properties of the drug such as water or lipid solubility and ionization, and by the therapeutic objectives which is the desirability of a rapid onset of action or the need for long-term administration or restriction to a local site.'[1]

See Fig. 21.2 for examples of medicine administration routes.

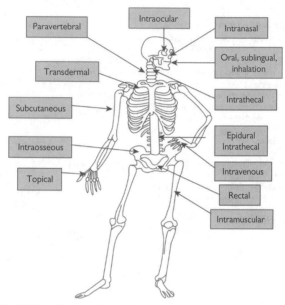

**Fig. 21.2** Examples of medicine administration routes.

### Reference

1. Whalen K, Feild C, Radhakrishnan R (2019). Lippincott illustrated reviews: pharmacology (7th ed). Philadelphia, PA: Wolters Kluwer.

# Medicine administration: enteral

The administration of medicines can be achieved by a variety of routes but there are two major routes of drug administration:
- Enteral drug administration.
- Parenteral drug administration.

> Enteral pertains to the intestinal tract and is commonly used to mean medicines administered by the oral (including via NG or nasojejunal tubes) and rectal routes.

## Enteral drug administration

Enteral drug administration includes drugs given by the following routes:
- Oral (e.g. tablets, capsules, linctus).
- Sublingual (e.g. tablets, sprays).
- Buccal (e.g. mucosal linings of the nasal, rectal, vaginal, ocular, and oral cavity).
- Rectal (e.g. enemas, suppositories, creams).

The enteral (oral) route is preferred wherever possible as it is the simplest, most convenient, and usually cheapest route. The choice of route will be dependent upon the patient's tolerability and the pharmacodynamics (what the drug does to the body) and pharmacokinetics (what the body does to the drug) of the medicine.

## Oral drug administration

Oral preparations are those which are administered via the mouth and sub-sequently swallowed. This is the preferred route in patients able to tolerate oral fluids. Absorption of medicines from this route usually occurs in the small intestine and is dependent upon:
- The formulation of the medicine as this will affect the disintegration and dissolution of tablets or capsules—plain versus coated, drug particle size
- Stomach contents
- Gastric motility
- Splanchnic blood flow—gut perfusion.

The absorption process can also be affected by the alteration of the gastric volume and pH caused by preoperative drugs or anaesthesia and surgery.

Regular oral paracetamol reduces opioid requirements thus reducing the incidence of opioid induced side effects. Other drugs that may be given by the oral route include NSAIDs, immediate-release opioids, and antiemetics (cyclizine, ondansetron, granisetron). The oral route is contraindicated for patients experiencing nausea and vomiting or who have delayed gastric emptying.

The choice of analgesic agent requires careful thought if there is some evidence of impaired renal function. Dose reduction may be necessary in some patients as drug and active metabolite may accumulate. Codeine, dihydrocodeine, and morphine should be avoided in patients with renal dysfunction. Fentanyl and oxycodone should be used in preference.

Modified-release strong opioids are contraindicated in the first postoperative 24 hours because of the risk of dumping secondary to delayed gastric emptying. Oral pethidine should be avoided due to the accumulation of the metabolite *norpethidine* which is toxic.

Oral drugs given in recovery have some distinct disadvantages; nausea and vomiting may occur which reduces the amount of the drug available for absorption by the small intestine.[1] Oral drugs given in recovery include paracetamol, tramadol, codeine, morphine sulfate, and oxycodone solution.

See Box 21.2.

### Box 21.2 First-pass metabolism

Once a drug has been absorbed from the gut it must pass through the liver (where it may be metabolized) before reaching the systemic circulation. Some drugs are almost completely metabolized during this time. These medicines (such as naloxone) are said to undergo complete first-pass metabolism thus making them unsuitable for oral administration. First-pass metabolism varies between individuals.

# Medicine administration: transmucosal (buccal and sublingual)

## Sublingual drug administration

- The medicine is placed under the tongue which avoids first-pass metabolism and allows for rapid absorption.
- One of the most commonly used sublingual analgesics is buprenorphine (which should be used with caution as it is a partial opioid agonist and can displace more effective opioids from their receptor sites).
- The sublingual route allows the drug to diffuse into the capillary network and therefore to enter the systemic circulation directly.
- Administration of a drug by this route means that the drug bypasses the intestine and liver and is not inactivated by first-pass metabolism.[1]
- Drugs such as fentanyl, nifedipine, GTN, and buprenorphine are given sublingually.
- Both the sublingual and the rectal routes of administration have the additional advantage that they prevent the destruction of the drug by intestinal enzymes or by low pH in the stomach.[1]

## Rectal drug administration

- This route of administration relies on passive diffusion like medicines in the upper GI tract.
- Medicines are usually given in the form of a fatty suppository which facilitates transport of the drug to the rectal fluid.
- The rectum has a good blood supply but venous drainage occurs into both the portal (mostly the upper part of the rectum) and systemic (the lower part of the rectum) circulations.
- Owing to individual variations in rectal venous drainage, an unpredictable proportion of an absorbed drug will escape first-pass metabolism.
- Therefore, a suppository (e.g. diclofenac) placed low in the rectum will have a higher proportion of its drug delivered directly to the systemic circulation.
- Patient consent is required for the administration of rectal medicines.
- Rectal medicines (e.g. paracetamol) are often available in a variety of doses for infant, child, and adult use.
- The rectal route is useful if a drug induces vomiting when given orally or if the patient is already vomiting. Drugs given rectally include diclofenac, paracetamol, metronidazole, and occasionally antiemetics.

## Buccal drug administration

The medicine is placed between the upper lip and lining of the upper gum and left in place where it forms a gel. The drug is absorbed transmucosally into the systemic circulation, thus bypassing first-pass metabolism. Rapid absorption can be achieved if medicines are lipophilic (fat soluble), such as fentanyl. Prochlorperazine is available in a buccal preparation for the treatment of nausea and vomiting. This is a useful route for patients who are unable to tolerate oral medicines (NBM) but should be used with caution in patients who have oral ulceration (e.g. post chemotherapy).

## Transmucosal drug administration

The medicine is absorbed through the oral mucosa rather than swallowed. Fentanyl is available as a lozenge which is 'painted' onto all surfaces of the mouth and tongue over a 10–15-minute period. This route is useful for managing procedural and breakthrough cancer pain but should be avoided in patients with a dry mouth or who have mucosal ulceration. Buccal and transnasal fentanyl preparations are available.

## Reference

1. Whalen K, Feild C, Radhakrishnan R (2019). Lippincott illustrated reviews: pharmacology (7th ed). Philadelphia, PA: Wolters Kluwer.

## Further reading

Craig A, Hatfield A (2020). The complete recovery room book (6th ed). Oxford: Oxford University Press.

Lister S, Hofland J, Grafton H, et al. (eds) (2021). The Royal Marsden Hospital manual of clinical nursing procedures (10th ed). Oxford: Wiley Blackwell.

# Parenteral drug administration: 1

Parenteral refers to the administration of medicines other than via the GI tract.

- Parenteral drug administration is used for drugs that are poorly absorbed from the GI tract and for agents such as insulin that are unstable in the GI tract.[1]
- Parenteral administration is used perioperatively in unconscious patients and under circumstances that require a rapid onset of action.
- It provides the most control over the actual dose of the drug delivered to the body.
- The three major parenteral routes most commonly used within the perioperative environment include:
  - IV
  - IM
  - SC.

## IV drug administration

The administration of medicines via the IV route allows rapid therapeutic blood levels as the drug is delivered directly into the systemic circulation, bypassing the first-pass metabolism.

The IV route is commonly used for the bolus administration of analgesia in the recovery room and for continuing postoperative opioid PCA. Repeated bolus administration or a continuous infusion results in steady plasma analgesic concentrations within the 'therapeutic window' (Fig. 21.3).

This route is suitable for most patients (including paediatrics and the elderly) but should be used with expert input in the known or suspected substance misuser.[2] Examples of drugs given IV in the perioperative environment include:
- Anaesthetic induction agents
- Muscle relaxants
- Opioids *and* antagonists
- Antiemetics
- Antibiotics
- Resuscitation drugs
- Reversal agents *and* respiratory stimulants.

*Commonly administered IV analgesics include*
- Morphine
- Fentanyl
- Remifentanil
- Oxycodone
- Paracetamol
- Parecoxib—a selective COX-2 inhibitor.

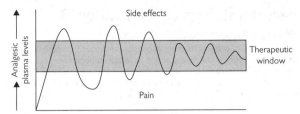

**Fig. 21.3** Achievement of analgesic therapeutic window by repeat bolus administration.

## References

1. Whalen K, Feild C, Radhakrishnan R (2019). Lippincott illustrated reviews: pharmacology (7th ed). Philadelphia, PA: Wolters Kluwer.
2. Quinlan J, Cox F (2017). Acute pain management in patients with drug dependence syndrome. Pain Reports, 2017;2(4):e611.

# Parenteral drug administration: 2

### IM drug administration

The intermittent delivery of drugs into muscular tissues for continuing analgesia after surgery is out of vogue due to local complications—pain, nerve damage, haematoma formation, and scarring (also see Box 21.3). The use of an indwelling cannula for repeated injections can lessen the risk of these, but does not avoid the peaks and troughs of analgesia associated with intermittent IM delivery.

- Drugs administered via the IM route are absorbed relatively slowly into the bloodstream.
- It reaches quite a high peak level and then declines over the next 2–3 hours. This means that pain relief is slow, and lasts a short time.
- The result is a pattern of severe pain, injection, side effects, and short-lived analgesia.
- IM drug administration in the perioperative environment is now uncommon with the exception of anti-D which is given to patients following and evacuation of retained products of conception (ERPC). This is very often administered in theatre when the patient is still un/semiconscious.
- IM drug administration also requires absorption and is slower than the IV or SC route.
- It requires simple diffusion from the site of injection into the systemic circulation.
- It does not provide a reliable rate of systemic absorption.

---

**Box 21.3 Warning!**

'A drug administered by IM or SC injection to a patient who is hypothermic will probably not achieve the desired effect as hypothermia causes vasoconstriction. When a patient is re-warmed, the drug can be rapidly liberated from the injection site, causing large concentrations of the drug into the systemic circulation. This can be dangerous especially when opiates are administered.'[1]

---

### SC drug administration

A hypodermic needle is used to deliver drugs under the horny keratinous layer of the skin. Administration may be intermittent or continuous. Used commonly in palliative care for symptom control the SC route is sometimes used for acute pain when patients are unable to take oral preparations. An indwelling butterfly cannula may be used. If swelling or a local reaction occurs the cannula site will need rotation. PCA can be administered by this route.

*Commonly used SC medicines include*
- Oxycodone
- Diamorphine
- Levomepromazine
- Midazolam
- Cyclizine
- Heparin
- Insulin.

# Reference

1. Whalen K, Feild C, Radhakrishnan R (2019). Lippincott illustrated reviews: pharmacology (7th ed). Philadelphia, PA: Wolters Kluwer.

# Further reading

Craig A, Hatfield A (2020). The complete recovery room book (6th ed). Oxford: Oxford University Press.

Lister S, Hofland J, Grafton H, et al. (eds) (2021). The Royal Marsden Hospital manual of clinical nursing procedures (10th ed). Oxford: Wiley Blackwell.

# Neuraxial analgesia

Neuraxial analgesia refers to the administration of medicines into the epidural (peridural, extradural) or intrathecal (subarachnoid, spinal) spaces to provide relief from pain.

The vertebral column consists of seven cervical, 12 thoracic, and five lumbar vertebrae together with the sacrum and the coccyx. The spinal cord lies in a protective tunnel within the vertebral column and is surrounded by three layers of membrane (also known as meninges): the dura mater (on the outside), the arachnoid mater (middle layer), and the pia mater (inside layer).

## Epidural analgesia

### Indications

- Management of surgical and postoperative pain.
- Management of the pain of labour.
- Amelioration of the stress response to surgery.

### Contraindications to epidural analgesia

- Central or spinal neurological disease.
- Systemic sepsis or local (in the region of the catheter) sepsis.
- Coagulation disorders (e.g. haemophilia, von Willebrand's disease).
- Severe hypovolaemia.

### Precautions with epidural analgesia

- Patients receiving thromboprophylaxis:
  - The smallest dose should be administered.
  - Thromboprophylaxis should be delayed as long as possible for at least 12–24 hours postoperatively.
- Patients receiving treatment doses of heparin.
- Patients receiving antiplatelet therapy: antiplatelet or oral anticoagulant medications should not be given in combination with LMWH due to increased risk of spinal haematoma.
- Patients receiving oral anticoagulation, for example, warfarin, direct oral anticoagulants (dabigatran, rivaroxaban, apixaban).
- Presence of a dural puncture.

### Identifying the epidural space

The epidural space lies outside the protective dural membrane. It is a potential space composed of fat, nerves, lymph tissue, and blood vessels. The most common way to identify the epidural space is the loss of resistance to saline technique. The epidural catheter is advanced through the internal lumen of the Tuohy needle until 3–5 cm of catheter is in the epidural space. The needle is then withdrawn leaving the catheter *in situ*. The catheter is connected to a bacterial and particulate filter and is affixed to the skin using a clear occlusive dressing.

*Medicines used in epidural analgesia*

Most commonly, two types of drugs are used to provide epidural analgesia: LAs and opioids. A combination of both produces a synergistic effect thus reducing the required dose of each. It is recommended that these infusions are commercially prepared and that a limited number of combinations are provided to reduce confusion. The specific drugs and concentrations should be clearly stated in local protocols and on the epidural prescription. An example would be levobupivacaine 0.125% + fentanyl 4 mcg/mL, 0–12 mL/hour.

*Local anaesthetics*

- Reversibly block the sodium channels of nerve cell membranes thus inhibiting nerve conduction.
- Amide LAs with a long duration of action are used in preference.
- Ropivacaine and levobupivacaine are recommended in preference to bupivacaine as they are considered to be less cardiotoxic.

LA effects include:

- Sympathetic blockade (resulting in vasodilatation) which may unmask hypovolaemia
- A high, low, or patchy block
- Urinary retention
- Reduction in the stress response
- LA toxicity.

*Opioids*

- Bind to opioid receptors in the substantia gelatinosa in the dorsal horn of the spinal cord and in the brain.
- Lipophilic (fat-soluble) opioids, for example, fentanyl is most commonly used but has a short duration of action.
- Lipophilicity determines the onset and duration of action but lipophilic drugs need to be delivered close to the incision.

Opioid effects include:

- Pruritus
- Nausea and vomiting
- Drowsiness which may lead to oversedation
- Urinary retention.

Rarely, a patient may experience back pain and a change in sensation in limb sensation and motor function. An epidural haematoma or abscess must be ruled out by the use of MRI.

*Other agents used to potential epidural analgesia*

Clonidine and dexmedetomidine may be added to epidural infusions to enhance analgesia.

## Intrathecal analgesia

- The intrathecal space lies beneath the dura and contains the spinal cord and nerve roots which are bathed in CSF.
- The indications and precautions of spinal analgesia are similar to that for epidurals.

- Opioids are most commonly used as a single dose.
- Opioids IV infusions can be used for postoperative analgesia.
- Doses are small and a single dose of preservative-free morphine 0.5 mg may provide analgesia for 24 hours.

## Further reading

Australian and New Zealand College of Anaesthetists & Faculty of Pain Medicine (2020). Acute pain management: scientific evidence (5th ed). Available at: ℘ https://www.anzca.edu.au/re-sources/college-publications/acute-pain-management/apsme5-draft/4-0-analgesic-medicines-watermarked.pdf

Rang H, Dale M, Ritter J, et al. (2019). Rang and Dale's pharmacology (9th ed). Edinburgh: Elsevier.

Whalen K, Feild C, Radhakrishnan R (2019). Lippincott illustrated reviews: pharmacology (7th ed). Philadelphia, PA: Wolters Kluwer.

# Respiratory medicine administration

Refers to the administration of medicines via the respiratory tract and includes:
• Inhalation
• Intranasal
• Intratracheal.

## Indications

See Box 21.4.

> ### Box 21.4 Indications for respiratory medicines administration
>
> Indications for inhaled opioids are unclear and unlicensed. However, these routes have the advantage of avoiding first-pass metabolism.
>
> The factors that must be considered for these routes include:
> • Medicine absorption and bioavailability
> • Speed of onset of analgesia, efficacy.
>
> Duration of action and side effects—both systemic and related to the route of administration.

## Intranasal

The nasal mucosa is very vascular and permits rapid absorption of drugs into the bloodstream. The maximum volume that can be administered by this route is limited to 150 µL. Medicines that are lipophilic are preferred.

Any swallowed component will be absorbed from the stomach or small intestine and be subject to first-pass metabolism. Some medicines have a bitter taste.

*Medicines include*
• Sufentanil—premedication and PCA for postoperative pain
• Fentanyl—PCA for postoperative pain
• Alfentanil.

## Pulmonary

Medicines are delivered as a nebulized aerosol. Absorption is dependent on the size of the molecule which should be <20 µm to be absorbed. New drug delivery systems increase the bioavailability of opioids up to 100%.

*Medicines include*
• Morphine
• Fentanyl
• Diamorphine.

## Intratracheal route

Suitable for the administration of lipid-soluble drugs only, including lidocaine, adrenaline (epinephrine), atropine, and naloxone (which has the mnemonic 'LEAN'). The drug must be diluted up to 5 mL to aid absorption.

*Indications*

Resuscitation in patients with no IV access. Five adequate tidal breaths must be given after medicine administration.

## Inhalational drug administration

- Inhalation provides the rapid delivery of a drug across the large surface area of the mucous membranes of the respiratory tract and pulmonary epithelium.[1]
- It produces an effect almost as quickly as IV injection.
- This route is used for drugs that are gases or those that can be expelled in an aerosol.
- It is effective for patients with respiratory complaints such as asthma or COPD.
- Inhalation drugs are delivered directly to the site of action and systemic side effects are minimized. Drugs commonly used in the perioperative environment include:
  - Anaesthetic volatile agents
  - Bronchodilators
  - $O_2$
  - $N_2O$
  - Entonox.

## Reference

1. Rang H, Dale M, Ritter J, et al. (2019). Rang and Dale's pharmacology (9th ed). Edinburgh: Elsevier.

## Further reading

Craig A, Hatfield A (2020). The complete recovery room book (6th ed). Oxford: Oxford University Press.

Lister S, Hofland J, Grafton H, et al. (eds) (2021). The Royal Marsden Hospital manual of clinical nursing procedures (10th ed). Oxford: Wiley Blackwell.

# Topical analgesia

Topical refers to the transdermal administration of medicines and in-cludes LAs and opioids (e.g. buprenorphine and fentanyl). Both have a low molecular weight, are lipophilic, and avoid first-pass metabolism as they are taken up directly into the systemic circulation.

## Indications

The management of pain including:
- Pre-emptive, for example, the application of EMLA® at least 60 minutes prior to cannulation or 10 minutes prior to ablation of genital warts
- Treatment, for example, severe opioid responsive pain.

## Contraindications/precautions for transdermal opioids

Management of acute postoperative pain in an opioid-naïve patient. This is because of:
- The lack of opportunity for dosage titration in the short term
- Possibility of significant respiratory depression
- Products may be unlicensed for postoperative pain
- The elderly
- Patients with renal or hepatic dysfunction.

## Medicines

*Local anaesthetics*
- Lidocaine (lignocaine), for example, Versatis® 5% medicated plaster licensed for post-herpetic neuralgia and neuropathic pain but must not be applied to wounds or broken skin.
- EMLA® cream 5% is a mix of lidocaine 2.5% and prilocaine 2.5% and should be applied under an occlusive dressing for most uses. It has been used to provide analgesia for split-skin grafting.

*Opioids*
Buprenorphine is available in two transdermal matrix presentations neither of which is licensed for postoperative pain:

*BuTrans® (5 mcg/hour, 10 mcg/hour, 15 mcg/hour, 20 mcg/hour)*
- Treatment for severe opioid-responsive pain conditions which are not adequately responding to non-opioid analgesics.
- The patch should be changed every 7 days.

*Transtec® (35 mcg/hour, 52.5 mcg/hour, 70 mcg/hour)*
- Licensed for moderate to severe cancer pain and severe pain not responding to non-opioid analgesics.
- Not suitable for acute pain.
- The patch should be changed twice weekly.

Fentanyl is available as a matrix patch. It is indicated for the treatment of chronic intractable pain only and is contraindicated for acute pain because of the lack of opportunity for dosage titration in the short term and the resultant possibility of significant respiratory depression.

# Further reading

Rang H, Dale M, Ritter J, et al. (2019). Rang and Dale's pharmacology (9th ed). Edinburgh: Elsevier.
Whalen K, Feild C, Radhakrishnan R (2019). Lippincott illustrated reviews: pharmacology (7th ed).
Philadelphia, PA: Wolters Kluwer.

# Patient-controlled analgesia

PCA is defined as the administration of analgesia (usually opioids) by a patient to manage pain. Although PCA delivery may occur by a variety of routes (e.g. epidural, transdermal, SC, or intranasal) it usually refers to the IV route, although the SC route may be used.

## Definitions
See Box 21.5.

## IV opioid PCA
*Indications*
The management of acute pain including:
- Acute (e.g. sickle cell crisis)
- Postoperative.
- Procedural (e.g. dressing changes).

*Contraindications/precautions for opioid PCA*
- The possibility of significant respiratory depression if additional opioids are administered by a different route.
- Concomitant administration with sedative or long-acting opioids medicines may lead to opioid-induced hypoventilatory impairment (OIVI).
- Some products are unlicensed for postoperative pain.
- The elderly.
- Patients with renal or hepatic dysfunction.

## Epidural PCA

Epidural PCA combines the benefits of a continuous epidural with the advantage of the patient being in control.

*Indication*
The management of acute postoperative pain.

*Contraindications/precautions to epidural PCA*
- Central or spinal neurological disease.
- Systemic sepsis or local (in the region of the catheter) sepsis.
- Coagulation disorders (e.g. haemophilia, von Willebrand's disease).
- Severe hypovolaemia.

*Advantages*
- Patient controlled.
- Improved patient satisfaction.
- Synergistic effect of low-dose opioid and LA.

For examples see Table 21.2.

## Box 21.5 PCA terminology

- *Loading dose*: a single dose usually administered intraoperatively or in the recovery room before PCA maintenance therapy is commenced.
- *Bolus dose*: the amount of drug a patient receives when they press the demand button. This is measured in milligrams or micrograms.
- *Background infusion*: a continuous infusion of analgesic that may be administered concurrently through the PCA.
- *Lockout time*: a predetermined time when the PCA device will not deliver a dose if requested. Range 4–10 minutes.
- *Four-hour limit*: offers the possibility to pre-set a maximum amount of PCA that a patient may receive in any 4-hour period.

**Table 21.2** PCA examples

| PCA examples | Bolus dose | Lockout time | Comments |
|---|---|---|---|
| Morphine: 100 mg in 100 mL NaCl 0.9% | 1 mg | 5 minutes | Gold standard Metabolites may accumulate |
| Fentanyl: 1000 mcg in 100 mL NaCl 0.9% | 10 mcg | 3–5 minutes | No metabolites |
| Oxycodone: 200 mg in 100 mL NaCl 0.9% | 2–3 mg | 5 minutes | No metabolites |

## Further reading

Electronic Medicines Compendium. Homepage. Available at: ℘ https://www.medicines.org.uk/emc [for further guidance on SPCs for individual drugs]

Levy N, Quinlan J, Boghdadly K, et al. (2021). An international multidisciplinary consensus statement on the prevention of opioid-related harm in adult surgical patients. Anaesthesia, 76(4):520–536.

McGavock H (2017). How drugs work: basic pharmacology for healthcare professionals (4th ed). Boca Taton, FL: CRC Press.

Rang H, Dale M, Ritter J, et al. (2019). Rang and Dale's pharmacology (9th ed). Edinburgh: Elsevier.

Whalen K, Feild C, Radhakrishnan R (2019). Lippincott illustrated reviews: pharmacology (7th ed). Philadelphia, PA: Wolters Kluwer.

# Continuous nerve and wound infusions

Continuous wound infusions use LA medicines to provide relief from pain.

The use of LAs as continuous peripheral nerve blocks and surgical wound infusion as an analgesic technique utilizes a multiholed catheter placed in or alongside the nerves/wounds and a portable infusion device such as an elastomeric balloon.

Placement of the catheter is usually performed by the surgeon and this technique avoids the risks associated with neuraxial blockade.

### Indications

- Management of surgical and postoperative pain (e.g. hepatobiliary and thoracic surgery).

### Contraindications to continuous wound infusion

- Allergy to (amide) LAs.
- Systemic sepsis or local (in the region of the catheter) sepsis.
- Local haematoma.

### Precautions with continuous wound infusion

- Sensitivity to LAs.
- Systemic sepsis or local (in the region of the wound) sepsis.
- Debilitated, elderly, or acutely ill patients may have lower tolerance to elevated blood levels, dose adjustment is recommended.
- Increased risk of developing toxic plasma concentrations in severe hepatic disease.
- Cardiac arrhythmia and cardiac arrest have occurred after unintended intravascular administration.
- Pregnancy and breastfeeding—medication dependent—consult local pharmacy department.

### Indications

- Upper limb peripheral nerve infusions may be used following orthopaedic and plastic surgery on the upper limb, forearm, or hand.
- Lower limb peripheral nerve blocks (e.g. femoral, sciatic) and infusions may be used following major surgery on the lower limbs; hips, knees, ankles or leg including amputation.
- Thoracic paravertebral nerve infusions are indicated for postoperative pain management following thoracic surgery, breast and axillary surgery, or rib fractures (➔ see epidural (p. 203) and paravertebral analgesia protocols (p. 632)).
- Transverse abdominal plane (TAP) catheters are indicated for postoperative pain management following surgery on the abdominal wall including laparotomy, appendectomy, hernia repair, or hysterectomy.
- LA wound catheters allow infiltration of LAs into the wound area and are indicated for hepatobiliary, open nephrectomy, and bowel surgery.

## Local anaesthetics

- Reversibly block the sodium channels of nerve cell membranes thus inhibiting nerve conduction.
- Amide LAs with a long duration of action are used in preference.
- Ropivacaine and levobupivacaine are recommended in preference to bupivacaine as they are considered to be less cardiotoxic.

## Local anaesthetic effects include

- Reduction in the stress response.
- LA toxicity.

## Other agents used to potentiate analgesia

- Clonidine may be added to the LA infusion for single-shot peripheral nerve or plexus blocks prolonged duration of analgesia and motor block. Increased risk of hypotension, fainting and sedation may limit its usefulness.

## Further reading

Rang H, Dale M, Ritter J, et al. (2019). Rang and Dale's pharmacology (9th ed). Edinburgh: Elsevier.
Whalen K, Feild C, Radhakrishnan R (2019). Lippincott illustrated reviews: pharmacology (7th ed).
    Philadelphia, PA: Wolters Kluwer.

# Pain management

# Acute pain

## Principles of acute pain management

Pain is a subjective experience and we are reliant upon patients to report their experience. There is no objective measure. Acute pain can be defined as pain that occurs as a result of an injury and lasts for <3 months. The pain is predominantly nociceptive and self-limiting.

Acute pain management should aim to:
- Improve the patient journey and reduce hospital length of stay
- Provide evidence-based relief from pain
- Minimize or effectively treat analgesia-related side effects
- Minimize the risk of complications from immobility
- Facilitate early discharge
- Reduce the risk of persistent pain after surgery.

*Pain assessment*

Pain assessment is fundamental to managing pain effectively and the patient's report should be believed. It may be performed using a unidimensional (e.g. numerical rating scale or Wong–Baker FACES pain rating scale) or multidimensional pain assessment tool (e.g. Brief Pain Inventory, McGill Pain Questionnaire). See Box 22.1.

> ### Box 22.1 Use a structured approach to basic pain assessment
> - Location—where is it, does it radiate?
> - Pattern—is it continuous, intermittent, or brief?
> - Intensity—how strong is it? See numerical rating scale (Fig. 22.1).
> - Onset—when did it start?
> - Triggers—what makes it worse?
> - Relievers—what makes it better, what has worked in the past?

*Pain should be assessed and recorded as the fifth vital sign*
- On arrival in recovery and at regular intervals—for example, every 15 minutes.
- After every pain-relieving intervention.
- On the ward—minimum 4-hourly.
- Until discharge from hospital.

*Unidimensional pain assessment (pain intensity)*

As a minimum, pain intensity may be assessed and recorded. This may take the form of the use of numbers, text, or a combination of both (Fig. 22.1). If patients are pre-verbal or are cognitively impaired, an alternative would be to use a pain assessment tool with faces that indicate pain intensity.

*Multidimensional pain assessment tools*

The British Pain Society provides open access to assessment tools in a variety of languages and scripts on its website.

| 0 | 1 | 2 | 3 |
|---|---|---|---|
| No pain | Mild pain | Moderate pain | Severe pain |

**Fig. 22.1** A numerical rating scale with intensity descriptors.

## Pain ladder

The WHO devised the original pain ladder >30 years ago for cancer pain but this has been adapted for acute pain and is widely used. If an analgesic or analgesic combination results in inadequate analgesia (pain persists or increases), the prescriber should move up the ladder (Fig. 22.2).

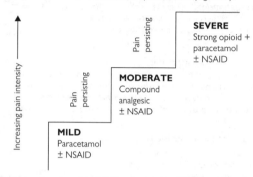

**Fig. 22.2** An adaptation of the WHO analgesic ladder. NSAID, non-steroidal anti-inflammatory drug; compound analgesic, mixture of paracetamol + a mild opioid (e.g. codeine or dihydrocodeine).

## Further reading

Association of Anaesthetists of Great Britain and Ireland (2013). Immediate post-anaesthesia recovery. London: Association of Anaesthetists of Great Britain and Ireland.

British Pain Society. Homepage. Available at: ℞ https://www.britishpainsociety.org/

Cox F (2018). Advances in the pharmacological management of acute and chronic pain. Nursing Standard, 33(3):37–42.

Craig A, Hatfield A (2020). The complete recovery room book (6th ed). Oxford: Oxford University Press.

Royal College of Anaesthetists (2019). Chapter 4: guidelines for the provision of postoperative care. London: Royal College of Anaesthetists.

Royal College of Anaesthetists (2021). Chapter 11: guidelines for the provision of anaesthesia services for inpatient pain management. London: Royal College of Anaesthetists.

# Chronic pain after surgery

## Principles of chronic pain management

These are similar to those for acute pain management. The prevalence of chronic pain after surgery is widely underestimated. Pain that persists for >3 months is described as chronic. Some potential causes of chronicity are listed in Box 22.2 There is scant evidence for the use of pre-emptive analgesia in humans.

> **Box 22.2 Causes of chronic pain after surgery**
> - Unrelieved (poorly managed) acute pain.
> - Certain forms of surgical exposure or surgery such as thoracotomy, inguinal hernia repair, amputation, and mastectomy.
> - Pre-existing chronic painful conditions.

*Multidimensional pain assessment*

Patients with chronic pain or at risk for chronicity require multidimensional pain assessment noting the words used to describe the pain (descriptors) as shown in Table 22.1. This will identify patients experiencing persistent post-acute (nociceptive) pain rather than neuropathic pain which results from nerve injury.

## Diagnosis of neuropathic pain

- Pain history to ascertain underlying cause.
- Examination especially skin changes.
- MRI for central lesions.
- Diagnostic LA blocks.
- Electrophysiological studies (e.g. nerve conduction).
- Sural nerve biopsy where involved.

## Treatment options for neuropathic pain

*Pharmacological*

- Topical agents (e.g. lidocaine plasters, capsaicin cream).
- Opioids (e.g. tramadol, oxycodone—neuropathic pain is only partially responsive to opioids).
- Anticonvulsants (e.g. pregabalin, carbamazepine).
- Tricyclic antidepressants (e.g. amitriptyline, nortriptyline, dosulepin).
- NMDA receptor antagonists (e.g. ketamine).
- Membrane stabilizers (e.g. lidocaine).

*Interventional*

- Cognitive behavioural therapy (CBT).
- Transcutaneous electrical nerve stimulation (TENS).
- Acupuncture.
- Massage.
- Exercise.
- Trigger point injections with LA.
- Regional blockade such as intercostal nerve block with LA or neurolysis with alcohol or phenol.

- Radiofrequency ablation of nerve root.
- Neuraxial blockade.
- Spinal cord (dorsal horn) stimulation.

**Table 22.1** Characteristics of acute nociceptive and neuropathic pain

| Acute nociceptive (<3 months) | Neuropathic (any duration) |
| --- | --- |
| Sharp | Numb |
| Stabbing | Pins and needles |
| Lancinating | Burning |
| Splitting | Pricking |
| | Stinging |
| | Shooting |

## Further reading

Association of Anaesthetists of Great Britain and Ireland (2013). Immediate post-anaesthesia recovery. London: Association of Anaesthetists of Great Britain and Ireland.

British Pain Society. Homepage. Available at: ℗ https://www.britishpainsociety.org/

Cox F (2018). Advances in the pharmacological management of acute and chronic pain. Nursing Standard, 33(3):37–42.

Craig A, Hatfield A (2020). The complete recovery room book (6th ed). Oxford: Oxford University Press.

Royal College of Anaesthetists (2019). Chapter 4: guidelines for the provision of postoperative care. London: Royal College of Anaesthetists.

Royal College of Anaesthetists (2021). Chapter 11: guidelines for the provision of anaesthesia services for inpatient pain management. London: Royal College of Anaesthetists.

# Non-pharmacological pain management

Non-pharmacological approaches to managing pain includes but is not limited to CBT, acupuncture, TENS, aromatherapy, and hypnotism. The combination of pharmacological (medicines) and non-pharmacological strategies is often more successful than a single strategy.

## Cognitive behavioural therapy

CBT is a biopsychosocial approach to pain management based on behavioural and cognitive theories which can help patients manage their pain more effectively. Psychologists commonly use this technique for patients with chronic painful conditions (e.g. back pain, sickle cell anaemia).

### Cognitive theory
The principle of this theory is that early experiences shape our core beliefs from which we develop rules for life (assumptions).

### Behavioural theory
This theory consists of two principles:
- Classical conditioning such as a response initiated by a stimulus—Pavlov's dogs.
- Operant conditioning where a behaviour results in a reward.

## Acupuncture

This technique involves piercing the skin with fine metal needles in order to relieve symptoms, cure disease, and promote health. Two main contemporary approaches to acupuncture exist in UK practice.

### Traditional Chinese
This complex system results from the influence of a number of philosophies and concepts including *yin and yang* and *qi* (life energy or vital force). Needling points along *qi* meridians can exert a therapeutic effect.

### Western medical approach
This approach requires an orthodox clinical diagnosis with points chosen on neurophysiological principles. This includes the needling of trigger points and segmental needling.

## Transcutaneous electrical nerve stimulation

TENS is the safe application of electrical current from a hand-held generator via self-adhesive electrodes through intact skin to activate nerve fibres in tissues underneath the electrodes. This current produces physiological actions that lead to relief from pain. TENS can also be used to reduce postoperative nausea and vomiting and postsurgical symptoms.

## Aromatherapy

This approach uses plant-derived essential oils to enhance physical and psychological well-being.

### Lavender oil
Patients in recovery who received lavender oil therapy expressed greater satisfaction with pain management and had a reduced opioid consumption.

*Peppermint oil*
Patients received peppermint oil had less intense postoperative nausea and vomiting.

## Hypnotism

The power of suggestion is one of the oldest therapeutic tools. Hypnosis can be defined as the induction of a subjective state in which perception or memory can be elicited by suggestion.

*Breast surgery*
The combination of analgesia and preoperative hypnosis has been shown to provide superior analgesia and reduced fatigue, discomfort, and nausea in patients scheduled for breast surgery.

*Oral and maxillofacial surgery*
Adult patients who received intraoperative hypnosis during oral and maxillofacial surgery under LA expressed greater postoperative satisfaction.

*Children*
Children can be easier to hypnotize than adults. Hypnotism has been successfully used for procedural pain associated with bone marrow aspiration and lumbar puncture.

## Further reading

Association of Anaesthetists of Great Britain and Ireland (2013). Immediate post-anaesthesia recovery. London: Association of Anaesthetists of Great Britain and Ireland.

British Pain Society. Homepage. Available at: ℘ https://www.britishpainsociety.org/

Cox F (2018). Advances in the pharmacological management of acute and chronic pain. Nursing Standard, 33(3):37–42.

Craig A, Hatfield A (2020). The complete recovery room book (6th ed). Oxford: Oxford University Press.

Moss D, Willmarth E (2019). Hypnosis, anaesthesia, pain management, and preparation for medical procedures. Annals of Palliative Medicine, 8(4):498–503.

Royal College of Anaesthetists (2019). Chapter 4: guidelines for the provision of postoperative care. London: Royal College of Anaesthetists.

Royal College of Anaesthetists (2021). Chapter 11: guidelines for the provision of anaesthesia services for inpatient pain management. London: Royal College of Anaesthetists.

# Role of the pain management service

The development of the majority of acute pain services in the UK was stimulated by the publication of the report by the RCoA and the Faculty of Anaesthetists in 1990.

## An effective pain management service will

*Be multidisciplinary with input from*
- Nurses
- ODPs
- Recovery staff
- Anaesthetists
- Surgeons
- Physiotherapists
- Pharmacists
- Psychologists
- Patients.

*Educate*
- Patients and carers with information about the choices, risks, and benefits of different perioperative pain management techniques
- Provide targeted education to all members of the multidisciplinary team to meet specific needs including:
  - Sessions on the principles of pain assessment, physiology, pharmacology, and the management of analgesia-related side effects
  - Study days that focus on acute and chronic pain
  - Epidural study days for staff involved in the care of patients receiving epidural analgesia; attendance is mandatory and competency must be assessed and recorded; an update session is essential at least every 3 years.

*Advise*
Provide staff with an expert opinion on the biopsychosocial management of pain in individual patients.

*Modernize*
Ensure prompt access to modern, standardized:
- Equipment—including infusion devices and administration sets
- Infusions—opioid and LA
- Labels
- Guidelines, protocols, and policies.

*Measure quality using audit*
Undertake regular audits of pain standards to demonstrate compliance with local protocols for:
- Staff competency
- Pain assessment documentation
- Pain intensity
- Analgesia consumption
- Patient satisfaction
- Adverse event reporting
- Specific patient groups (e.g. children, the elderly, the pregnant patient).

*Guide*

Ensure that evidence-based policies, procedures, and guidelines are in place to support the care delivered to patients in acute and chronic pain.

## Further reading

Association of Anaesthetists of Great Britain and Ireland (2013). Immediate post-anaesthesia recovery. London: Association of Anaesthetists of Great Britain and Ireland.

British Pain Society. Homepage. Available at: ℘ https://www.britishpainsociety.org/

Cox F (2018). Advances in the pharmacological management of acute and chronic pain. Nursing Standard, 33(3):37–42.

Craig A, Hatfield A (2020). The complete recovery room book (6th ed). Oxford: Oxford University Press.

Moss D, Willmarth E (2019). Hypnosis, anaesthesia, pain management, and preparation for medical procedures. Annals of Palliative Medicine, 8(4):498–503.

Royal College of Anaesthetists (2019). Chapter 4: guidelines for the provision of postoperative care. London: Royal College of Anaesthetists.

Royal College of Anaesthetists (2021). Chapter 11: guidelines for the provision of anaesthesia services for inpatient pain management. London: Royal College of Anaesthetists.

# Perioperative drugs

# Overview of perioperative drugs

A broad range of perioperative drugs are used in the surgical setting. Each has a role in manipulating physiological factors and facilitating anaesthetic and surgical procedures. Due to the fact that the vast majority of these drugs are administered via the IV route, their modes of action occur rapidly, thus requiring knowledgeable and skilled practitioners.

## Premedication

- These are usually given orally and aim to reduce patient anxiety, which facilitates the induction of anaesthesia.
- Benzodiazepines tend to be the premedication of choice as these reduce anxiety and produce amnesic effects preoperatively, some examples include:
  - Temazepam
  - Diazepam
  - Lorazepam.
- Other premedications may be given for other effects, such as *ranitidine* to reduce gastric pH for those with a history of gastric reflux.
- Osmotic (*lactulose*) or stimulant laxatives (*sodium picosulfate*, *bisacodyl*) may be given prior to bowel surgery, although this may be down to individual surgeon preference.

## Local anaesthetics

- These drugs are used to perform minor procedures, avoiding the need to anaesthetize the patient.
- The site of the procedure is infiltrated with a LA thus enabling the tissue to be incised or sutures to be sited. LAs are also used around surgical sites at the end of a procedure as they aid in reducing surgical site pain postoperatively.
- These drugs work by blocking sodium channels in nerve axons, thus preventing the propagation of action potentials. Therefore, the patient does not feel any pain, but they will still feel pressure and touch.
- Examples of LAs include:
  - Lidocaine
  - Bupivacaine
  - Levobupivacaine.

## Sedatives

- Sedatives form the triad of anaesthesia, and can also be used to produce a state of semi-consciousness. This is useful in very anxious patients who are undergoing a surgical procedure with spinal anaesthesia, regional anaesthesia, or LA.
- These drugs are also used in critical care patients and also as premedication, an example is *midazolam*.

## Anaesthetic agents

- These agents produce the loss of consciousness associated with GA, and form one part of the triad of anaesthesia.

*IV anaesthetic agents*

- These drugs produce rapid loss of consciousness when administered in sufficient doses, thus forming the sedative part of the triad of anaesthesia.
- Induction of anaesthesia varies slightly between the drugs, with rapidity and smoothness of induction being factors. These drugs do have vasodilatory effects, which may require the use of fluids or vasopressors to counter.
- Examples of these drugs include:
  - Propofol
  - Etomidate
  - Thiopental sodium
  - Ketamine.

*Inhalational anaesthetic agents*

- These are used for maintenance of anaesthesia, but can also be used to induce anaesthesia; however, this technique is most commonly used in paediatric anaesthesia.
- These volatile agents are added in the air and $O_2$ blend within the anaesthetic circuit; to wake a patient, the volatile agent is turned off and the $O_2$ concentration increased.
- These volatile agents also have a vasodilatory effect and are also the cause of MH.
- Examples of volatile agents include:
  - Sevoflurane
  - Desflurane
  - Isoflurane.

## Analgesics

- Analgesics form part of the triad of anaesthesia and effective pain management is vital in aiding postoperative recovery, as it aids patients in mobilizing early, doing deep breathing exercises, and returning to their activities of daily living.
- There are multiple groups of analgesics used preoperatively, many of which are used concurrently.
- Opioid analgesics are used during the induction phase of anaesthesia and during surgical procedures, these include *morphine sulphate*, *fentanyl*, *remifentanil*, and *tramadol hydrochloride*.
- NSAIDs are effective analgesics, but are contraindicated in patients with gastric ulceration, respiratory disease, and can cause renal failure with prolonged use. These drugs include *ibuprofen* and *diclofenac*.
- The use of the above-mentioned drugs in combination with IV paracetamol has been shown to reduce postoperative opioid need.

## Muscle relaxants

- These drugs form the final part of the triad of anaesthesia and affect the neuromuscular synapse thus producing muscle relaxation.
- Their use enables intubation by relaxing the larynx and also facilitating surgery by relaxing skeletal muscle thus easing access to the surgical field.

- Mechanical ventilation is required in patients who have had muscle relaxants.
- These drugs are classed into two groups: depolarizing and non-depolarizing muscle relaxants.
- Depolarizing muscle relaxants such as *suxamethonium* have a rapid onset of action, and acts by binding to acetylcholine receptors on the motor end plate, thus maintaining a state of depolarization. Therefore, the muscle cannot repolarize.
- This process causes muscle spasms (fasciculations) which can cause postoperative muscle pain.
- Non-depolarizing muscle relaxants include *atracurium*, *pancuronium*, *rocuronium*, and *cisatracurium*. These muscle relaxants compete with acetylcholine for acetylcholine receptors at the motor end plate; their longer half-life means they occupy these receptors, thus causing muscle relaxation.

### Reversal agents

- These drugs are used to reverse muscle relaxation from non-depolarizing muscle relaxants.
- *Neostigmine* acts by inhibiting acetylcholinesterase, which usually breaks down acetylcholine, therefore more acetylcholine is available in the neuromuscular synapse.
- *Neostigmine* can cause bradycardia, therefore it is given with *glycopyrronium bromide* to counter this effect.
- *Neostigmine* also causes increased salivation which can be a hindrance during extubation.

### Antiemetics

- Nausea and vomiting is a common side effect bought about by GA or opioid administration, therefore prophylactic antiemetics are commonplace in the perioperative environment.
- Surgical procedures can also induce nausea and vomiting, for example, laparoscopic procedures, particularly with incomplete abdominal decompression.
- Examples of antiemetics are *ondansetron*, *metoclopramide*, and *cyclizine*.

### Emergency drugs

- Due to the risk of patient instability during anaesthesia and surgery, emergency drugs must be prepared prior to anaesthesia and be available throughout the procedure.
- Vasopressors cause vasoconstriction, countering the vasodilatory effects of anaesthetic agents. Vasopressors include *metaraminol* and *ephedrine* (also causes increased heart rate and force of contraction).
- If the vagus nerve is stimulated during laryngoscopy or tracheal intubation, the patient may well become bradycardic, therefore *atropine* must be available. *Atropine* blocks the vagus nerve, resulting in the sinoatrial node's intrinsic rate controlling heart rate (approximately 100 bpm).
- *Suxamethonium* must also be available in case the patient requires emergency endotracheal intubation.

## Further reading

Freedman R, Herbert L, O'Donnell A, et al. (eds) (2022). Oxford handbook of anaesthesia (5th ed). Oxford: Oxford University Press.

Joint Formulary Committee (2022). British national formulary. Available at: ℬ https://bnf.nice.org.uk/

Maund E, McDaid C, Rice S, et al. (2011). Paracetamol and selective and non-selective non-steroidal anti-inflammatory drugs for the reduction in morphine-related side-effects after major surgery: a systematic review. British Journal of Anaesthesia, 106(3):292–297.

Scarth E, Smith S (2016). Drugs in anaesthesia and intensive care (5th ed). Oxford: Oxford University Press.

# Oxygen therapy

## Definition

- The administration of $O_2$ at a concentration greater than that of ambient air.
- Effective delivery of $O_2$ is predicated on the maintenance of a patent airway.

## Indications

- Cardiac or respiratory arrest.
- Acute hypotension.
- Carbon monoxide poisoning.
- Major head injury.
- Major trauma, shock, sepsis.
- Anaphylaxis.
- Pulmonary haemorrhage.
- Epileptic seizure.
- Exacerbation of cystic fibrosis.
- Post-anaesthesia recovery.
- Use of opiates or other respiratory depressant drugs.
- Low cardiac output and metabolic acidosis (bicarbonate <18 mmol/L).
- Respiratory distress (respiratory rate >24 breaths per minute).
- Respiratory acidosis.
- Cluster headache.

*In cardiac or respiratory arrest, the absence of $O_2$ will be fatal!*

## Equipment

Two basic types of devices are used for delivery of $O_2$ (Table 23.1):
- Variable flow devices: deliver a variable concentration of $O_2$ which is dependent on the patient's respiratory rate, for example, nasal specula, Hudson oxygen mask, simple mask with reservoir bag (non-rebreather).
- Fixed flow devices: deliver a fixed concentration of $O_2$ independent of the patient's respiratory rate, for example, Venturi masks (Table 23.2).

**Table 23.1** $O_2$ delivery devices

| Devices | % $O_2$ delivered | Uses |
|---|---|---|
| Nasal cannulae | Variable—flow rate dependent<br>Maximum 40% | Postoperative recovery when maintaining patent airway unassisted<br>Procedures under LA<br>Endoscopy<br>Long-term home $O_2$ therapy |
| Hudson/MC mask | Variable—flow rate dependent<br>Maximum 50% at 15 L/min | Severe asthma<br>Left acute ventricular failure<br>Trauma |
| Simple mask with reservoir bag (non-rebreather) | Variable—flow rate dependent<br>Maximum 60–70% | Severe sepsis<br>NB: minimum flow rate 5 L/min |
| Venturi mask | Fixed variable (see Table 23.2 for details; 24–60%) | Controlled treatment of chronic respiratory failure |

## Risks associated with oxygen therapy

*$O_2$ therapy in COPD*

Caution should be exercised as high concentrations of $O_2$ reduce the hypoxic drive to breathe. This in turn causes $CO_2$ retention that can result in potentially fatal respiratory acidosis.

**Table 23.2** Fixed concentration (Venturi) masks

| Colour | Flow rate (L/min) | % $O_2$ delivered |
| --- | --- | --- |
| Blue | 2–3 | 24 |
| White | 4–6 | 28 |
| Yellow | 8–12 | 35 |
| Red | 10–15 | 40 |
| Green | 12–15 | 60 |

Administration of an inappropriate concentration of $O_2$ can have serious or even fatal consequences.[1]

## Oxygen toxicity

When high concentrations of $O_2$ (>60%) have been inhaled for >48 hours, damage to the alveolar membrane can occur resulting in adult respiratory distress syndrome.

## Oxygen therapy in neonates

- Prolonged exposure to high concentrations of $O_2$ can result in retinopathy of prematurity (formerly known as retrolental fibroplasia).
- Supplemental $O_2$ should only be used when explicitly indicated (e.g. respiratory distress or cyanosis).
- As with COPD, in emergencies $O_2$ should be used without restriction as *hypoxia will kill*.

## Long-term oxygen therapy

When administered for a minimum of 15 hours daily prolongs survival in some patients with chronic obstructive pulmonary disease.

*Intermittent $O_2$ therapy*

- Episodes of breathlessness not relieved by other treatment.
- In patients with severe COPD.
- Interstitial lung disease.
- Heart failure.
- Palliative care.

## Reference

1. National Institute of Health Research (2018). A reminder that too much oxygen increases mortality in acutely ill adults. Available at: ℛ https://evidence.nihr.ac.uk/alert/a-reminder-that-too-much-oxygen-increases-mortality-in-acutely-ill-adults/

## Further reading

Cross ME, Plunkett EVE (2014). Physics, pharmacology and physiology for anaesthetists (2nd ed). Cambridge: Cambridge University Press.

Freedman R, Herbert L, O'Donnell A, et al. (eds) (2022). Oxford handbook of anaesthesia (5th ed). Oxford: Oxford University Press.

National Institute for Health and Care Excellence (2018). Oxygen. Available at: ℜ https://bnf.nice. org.uk/treatment-summary/oxygen.html

O'Driscoll BR, Howard LS, Earis J, et al. (2017). BTS guideline for oxygen use in adults in healthcare and emergency settings. Thorax, 72(Suppl 1):i1–i90.

Scarth E, Smith S (2016). Drugs in anaesthesia and intensive care (5th ed). Oxford: Oxford University Press

# Perioperative drugs

See Tables 23.3–23.23.

**Table 23.3** Anaesthetic induction agents

| Drug | Indication | Contraindications/cautions | Side effects | Drug route | Perioperative drug dose |
|---|---|---|---|---|---|
| Propofol | Induction of anaesthesia<br>Maintenance of anaesthesia<br>Total IV anaesthesia<br>Sedation and maintenance of sedation<br>Refractory nausea and vomiting during end of life care<br>To treat nausea in chemotherapy<br>Treatment of status epilepticus in repeated fits with no return of consciousness | Not to be used for the sedation of ventilated children and adolescents <16 years old due to risk of potentially fatal effects, e.g. metabolic acidosis, cardiac failure<br>Caesarean section<br>Shock<br>Cardiac and respiratory impairment<br>Hypotension<br>Hypovolaemia<br>Raised ICP<br>Allergy to eggs, soya, soybean oil, and peanuts<br>Reduce dose for older people or haemodynamically unstable patients<br>A bolus injection can cause significant respiratory depression and bronchodilation<br>IV infusion can cause a reduction in tidal volume | **Common**<br>Headache, hypotension, apnoea, tachycardia<br>Pain on injection<br>Bradycardia<br>**Uncommon**<br>Phlebitis, thrombosis<br>**Rare**<br>Pancreatitis, anaphylaxis, convulsions, arrhythmia, euphoria, discoloration of hair and urine, pulmonary oedema, delayed recovery from anaesthesia | IV injection<br>IV infusion | **Adult dose: 18–54 years**<br>IV injection 0.5% or 1%<br>1.5–2.5 mg/kg (20–40 mg every 10 seconds)<br>**Older adult dose:**<br>**>55 years**<br>IV injection 0.5% or 1%<br>1–1.5 mg/kg (20 mg every 10 seconds)<br>**Paediatric dose:**<br>**1 month–16 years**<br>IV injection 0.5% or 1%<br>2.5 mg/kg (titrated according to age, weight, response)<br>**Paediatric dose:**<br>**17 years**<br>IV injection 0.5% or 1%<br>1.5–2.5 mg/kg (20–40 mg every 10 seconds) |

| Thiopental | Induction of anaesthesia of short duration | Myotonic dystrophy | IV injection | **Frequency unknown** | **Adult dose: 2.5%** |
|---|---|---|---|---|---|
| | Anticonvulsant | Acute porphyrias | | Arrhythmia, myocardial depression, injection site reaction, laryngeal spasm, hypotension, coughs and sneezing, hypersensitivity reaction (rash) | Slow IV injection 100–150 mg over 10–15 seconds |
| | Hypnotic | Hepatic impairment | | | **Paediatric dose: neonate** |
| | | Shock | | **Rare** | Slow IV injection |
| | | Cardiovascular disease | | Severe anaphylactic reaction | 2 mg/kg, followed by 1 mg/kg (maximum 4 mg/kg per dose) |
| | | Hypovolaemia | | Necrosis if injected intra-arterial | **Paediatric dose: child** |
| | | Avoid intra-arterial injection | | | Slow IV injection |
| | | Extravasation causes severe pain | | | 4 mg/kg, followed by 1 mg/kg (maximum 7 mg/kg per dose) |
| | | Sedative effects may persist up to 24 hours | | | |

(continued)

**Table 23.3 (Contd.)**

| Drug | Indication | Contraindications/cautions | Side effects | Drug route | Perioperative drug dose |
|---|---|---|---|---|---|
| Etomidate | Induction of anaesthesia | Avoid in acute porphyrias | **Common** | IV injection | **Adult dose** |
| | Treatment of Cushing's syndrome prior to surgery | Shock | Hyperventilation, nausea, rash, vomiting, stridor, apnoea, hypotension | | 150–300 mcg/kg slowly over 30–60 seconds |
| | | Adrenal insufficiency | **Uncommon** | | **Older adult dose** |
| | | Cardiovascular disease | Arrhythmias, hiccups, cough, hypertension, increased salivary function, phlebitis | | 150–200 mcg/kg slowly over 30–60 seconds |
| | Considered to be cardiovascularly stable | Hypovolaemia | **Rare** | | **Paediatric dose: 1 month–14 years** |
| | | Pregnancy | Pain on induction (can be reduced with lidocaine) | | Slow IV injection |
| | | Breastfeeding | Decreased respiratory rate and tidal volume | | 150–300 mcg/kg over 30–60 seconds |
| | | Hepatic impairment | Venous thrombosis | | **Paediatric dose: child 15–17 years** |
| | | | Thrombophlebitis if injected into small vein | | Slow IV injection |
| | | | Involuntary muscle movements may occur on induction | | 1.5–2.5 mg/kg (20–40 mg every 10 seconds) |
| | | | May suppress adrenocortical function | | |

## Further reading

Joint Formulary Committee (2022). British national formulary. Available at: ℗ https://bnf.nice.org.uk/

Joint Formulary Committee (2022). British national formulary for children. Available at: ℗ https://bnfc.nice.org.uk/

Scarth E, Smith S (2016). Drugs in anaesthesia and intensive care (5th ed.). Oxford: Oxford University Press.

**Table 23.4** Analgesic drugs: opiates

| Drug | Indication | Contraindications/cautions | Side effects | Drug route | Perioperative drug dose |
|---|---|---|---|---|---|
| **Morphine** | Pain and intraoperatively to augment GA, postoperative pain control. | Acute abdomen, hypotension, bradypnoea, delayed gastric emptying, cor pulmonale, head injury, comatose patients, raised ICP, paralytic ileus, adrenocortical insufficiency, convulsive disorders, pheochromocytoma, myasthenia gravis | **Common** Respiratory depression, bradycardia, tachycardia, nausea & vomiting, flushing & itching, drowsiness, dizziness, constipation, micturition difficulties/urinary retention, headache, hallucinations **Frequency unknown** Adrenal insufficiency, hyperanalgesia, biliary spasm, hypotension | IV injection IV infusion IM injection SC injection Epidural Oral solution Modified-release tablets Modified-release granules Rectal | **Adult dose** IV injection 10 mg every 4 hours, titrated for effect **Older adult dose** Slow IV injection 5 mg every 4 hours, titrated for effect **Paediatric dose: 12–17 years** Slow IV injection 5 mg every 4 hours **Paediatric dose: 6 months–11 years** Slow IV injection 100 mcg/kg every 4 hours **Paediatric dose: 1–5 months** Slow IV injection 100 mcg/kg every 6 hours. |

(continued)

**Table 23.4 (Contd.)**

| Drug | Indication | Contraindications/cautions | Side effects | Drug route | Perioperative drug dose |
|------|-----------|---------------------------|--------------|-----------|------------------------|
| Diamorphine | Acute pain | CNS depression, cor pulmonale, diarrhoea, psychosis, respiratory depression, head injury, comatose patients, raised ICP, paralytic ileus, adrenocortical insufficiency, convulsive disorders, pheochromocytoma, myasthenia gravis | **Common** <br> Respiratory depression, bradycardia, tachycardia, nausea & vomiting, flushing & itching, drowsiness, dizziness, constipation, micturition difficulties/urinary retention, headache, hallucinations <br> **Frequency unknown** <br> Adrenal insufficiency, hyperanalgesia, biliary spasm, hypotension | IV injection <br> IV infusion <br> IM injection <br> SC injection | **Adult dose** <br> Slow IV injection: 1.25–2.5 mg every 4 hours, titrated for effect <br> Slow IV infusion: 2.5–5 mg every 4 hours, if required <br> **Paediatric dose: slow IV injection** <br> Adjusted according to effect <br> Child 1–2 months: 20 mcg/kg every 4 hours <br> Child 3–5 months: 20–25 mcg/kg every 6 hours <br> Child 6–11 months: 75 mcg/kg every 4 hours <br> Child 1–11 years: 75–100 mcg/kg every 4 hours <br> Child 12–17 years: 2.5–5 mg/kg every 4 hours |

| Fentanyl | Pain and intraoperatively to augment GA | Diabetes mellitus, cerebral tumour, impaired consciousness, hypotension, bradypnoea, head injury, comatose patients, raised ICP, paralytic ileus, adrenocortical insufficiency, convulsive disorders, myasthenia gravis | **Common**<br>Abdominal pain, asthenia, diarrhoea, dyspepsia, anxiety, tachycardia, constipation, tremor, bradycardia, hypotension, hypertension, dyspnoea, paraesthesia, respiratory depression, nausea & vomiting, flushing & itching, drowsiness, dizziness, micturition difficulties/urinary retention, biliary spasm, headache, hallucinations<br>**Uncommon**<br>Laryngospasm, amnesia, seizures, thirst, pyrexia<br>**Rare**<br>Hiccups, ataxia, delusions, apnoea, arrhythmia, insomnia<br>**Frequency unknown**<br>Adrenal insufficiency, hyperanalgesia, hypotension | IV injection<br>IV infusion<br>Sublingual<br>Oral tablet<br>Transdermal<br>Buccal<br>Epidural<br>Intrathecal | **Adult dose: spontaneous respiration for short surgery**<br>Slow IV injection<br>Up to 500 mcg over 30 seconds<br>**Adult dose: assisted respiration for short surgery**<br>Slow IV injection<br>30–500 mcg<br>**Adult dose: assisted respiration for longer surgery**<br>50–100 mcg/kg over 10 minutes<br>Enhancement of anaesthesia via IV injection<br>300–3500 mcg<br>**Paediatric dose: spontaneous respiration via IV injection**<br>1 month–11 years: 1–3 mcg/kg over 30 seconds<br>12–17 years: 50–100 mcg over 30 seconds<br>**Paediatric dose: assisted ventilation via IV injection**<br>Neonate: 1–5 mcg/kg over 30 seconds<br>1 month–11 years: 1–5 mcg/kg over 30 seconds<br>12–17 years: 1–5 mcg over 30 seconds |

(continued)

**Table 23.4 (Contd.)**

| Drug | Indication | Contraindications/cautions | Side effects | Drug route | Perioperative drug dose |
|---|---|---|---|---|---|
| **Alfentanil** | Intraoperative analgesia and to augment GA | Diabetes mellitus, impaired consciousness, hypotension, bradypnoea, head injury, comatose patients, raised ICP, paralytic ileus, adrenocortical insufficiency, convulsive disorders, myasthenia gravis | **Common** Tachycardia, constipation, bradycardia, dry mouth, euphoria, hypertension, dyspnoea, respiratory depression, nausea & vomiting, flushing & itching, drowsiness, dizziness, micturition difficulties/urinary retention, biliary spasm, headache, hallucinations **Uncommon** Laryngospasm, hiccups, arrhythmia **Rare** Epistaxis **Frequency unknown** Cardiac arrest, convulsions, adrenal insufficiency, cough, pyrexia, hyperanalgesia, hypotension | IV injection IV infusion | **Adult dose: spontaneous respiration for short surgery** IV injection 500 mcg over 30 seconds **Adult dose: assisted respiration for short surgery** IV injection 30–50 mcg/kg **Adult dose: assisted respiration via IV infusion** 50–100 mcg/kg over 10 minutes **Paediatric dose: assisted respiration for short surgery** Slow IV injection Neonate: 5–20 mcg/kg over 30 seconds Child: 10–20 mcg/kg over 30 seconds **Paediatric dose: assisted respiration via IV infusion** Neonate: 10–50 mcg/kg over 10 minutes Child: 50–100 mcg/kg over 10 minutes |

| Remifentanil | Intraoperative analgesia and to augment GA | Analgesia for conscious patients, impaired consciousness, hypotension, bradypnoea, head injury, comatose patients, raised ICP, paralytic ileus, adrenocortical insufficiency, convulsive disorders, myasthenia gravis | **Common**<br>Tachycardia, constipation, bradycardia, dry mouth, euphoria, hypertension, dyspnoea, respiratory depression, nausea & vomiting, flushing & itching, drowsiness, dizziness, micturition difficulties/urinary retention, biliary spasm, headache, hallucinations<br>**Uncommon**<br>Hypoxia<br>**Rare**<br>Asystole<br>**Frequency unknown**<br>Convulsions, AV block | IV injection<br>IV infusion | **Adult dose: induction of anaesthesia**<br>IV injection<br>0.25–1 mcg/kg over 30 seconds<br>**Adult dose: assisted respiration during anaesthesia**<br>IV infusion<br>3–100 mcg/kg/hour<br>**Adult dose: spontaneous respiration during anaesthesia**<br>IV infusion<br>2.4 mcg/kg/hour<br>**Paediatric dose: induction of anaesthesia**<br>Slow IV injection<br>Child 12–17 years: 0.25–1 mcg/kg over 30 seconds<br>**Paediatric dose: assisted respiration during anaesthesia**<br>IV injection<br>1 month–11 years: 0.1–1 mcg/kg over 30 seconds<br>12–17 years: 0.1–1 mcg/kg over 30 seconds |

*(continued)*

**Table 23.4 (Contd.)**

| Drug | Indication | Contraindications/cautions | Side effects | Drug route | Perioperative drug dose |
|---|---|---|---|---|---|
| Pethidine | Postoperative pain<br>Acute pain<br>Obstetric analgesia | Acute abdomen, hypotension, bradypnoea, delayed gastric emptying, cor pulmonale, head injury, comatose patients, raised ICP, paralytic ileus, adrenocortical insufficiency, convulsive disorders, pheochromocytoma, myasthenia gravis, arrhythmias | **Common**<br>Tachycardia, constipation, bradycardia, dry mouth, euphoria, hypertension, dyspnoea, respiratory depression, nausea & vomiting, flushing & itching, drowsiness, dizziness, micturition difficulties/urinary retention, biliary spasm, headache, hallucinations<br>**Frequency unknown**<br>Adrenal insufficiency, hyperanalgesia, hypothermia, restlessness, tremor | IV injection<br>IM injection<br>SC injection<br>Oral solution | **Adult dose**<br>Slow IV injection<br>25–50 mg every 4 hours, titrated for effect<br>IM or SC injection (postoperative pain)<br>25–100 mg every 2–3 hours<br>**Older adult dose**<br>Slow IV injection<br>25 mg every 4 hours, titrated for effect<br>IM or SC injection (postoperative pain)<br>25 mg every 2–3 hours<br>**Paediatric dose: 12–17 years**<br>IM or SC injection<br>1 mg/kg every 3 hours<br>**Obstetric analgesia**<br>IM or SC injection<br>50–100 mg every 3 hours as required |

| Tramadol | Moderate pain<br>Postoperative pain | Excess bronchial secretions, epilepsy, seizure-related conditions, head injury, comatose patients, raised ICP | **Common**<br>Tachycardia, constipation, bradycardia, dry mouth, euphoria, hypertension, dyspnoea, respiratory depression, nausea & vomiting, flushing & itching, drowsiness, dizziness, micturition difficulties/ urinary retention, biliary spasm, headache, hallucinations, malaise<br><br>**Uncommon**<br>Diarrhoea, retching, gastritis, flatulence<br><br>**Rare**<br>Anxiety, bronchospasm, seizures, nightmares, tremor, syncope, wheeziness, dyspnoea, delirium<br><br>**Frequency unknown**<br>Adrenal insufficiency, hyperanalgesia, hypothermia, restlessness, tremor | IV injection<br>IV infusion<br>IM injection<br>Oral | **Adult dose (postoperative pain)**<br>Slow IV injection over 2–3 minutes<br>100 mg initial dose then 50 mg every 10–20 minutes (maximum 250 mg during first hour); 50–100 mg every 4–6 hours<br>**Paediatric dose: 12–17 years**<br>Slow IV injection over 2–3 minutes<br>100 mg initial dose then 50 mg every 10–20 minutes (maximum 250 mg during first hour); 50–100 mg every 4–6 hours |

*(continued)*

**Table 23.4 (Contd.)**

| Drug | Indication | Contraindications/ cautions | Side effects | Drug route | Perioperative drug dose |
|---|---|---|---|---|---|
| Codeine | Mild to moderate pain<br>Postoperative analgesia<br>Cough suppression<br>Acute diarrhoea | Acute abdomen, gallstones, arrhythmias, acute ulcerative colitis, hypotension, bradypnoea, head injury, comatose patients, raised ICP, paralytic ileus, adrenocortical insufficiency, convulsive disorders, myasthenia gravis, breastfeeding<br>Restricted use in children due to morphine toxicity<br>Contraindicated in adolescents aged 12–18 years with breathing difficulties | **Common**<br>Tachycardia, constipation, bradycardia, dry mouth, euphoria, hypertension, dyspnoea, respiratory depression, nausea & vomiting, flushing & itching, drowsiness, dizziness, micturition difficulties/urinary retention, biliary spasm, headache, hallucinations, malaise<br>**Frequency unknown**<br>Adrenal insufficiency, hyperanalgesia, abdominal pain, anorexia, hypothermia, seizures | IM injection<br>Oral | **Adult dose**<br>IM injection for mild to moderate pain<br>30–60 mg every 4 hours<br>**Paediatric dose: short-term treatment of acute moderate pain**<br>IV injection or oral<br>12–17 years: 30–60 mg every 6 hours (maximum use = 3 days) |

# Further reading

Joint Formulary Committee (2022). British national formulary. Available at: ℗ https://bnf.nice.org.uk/

Joint Formulary Committee (2022). British national formulary for children. Available at: ℗ https://bnfc.nice.org.uk/

Scarth E. Smith S (2016). Drugs in anaesthesia and intensive care (5th ed). Oxford: Oxford University Press.

Table 23.5 Analgesia drugs: non-opiate and NSAIDs

| Drug | Indication | Contraindications/cautions | Side effects | Drug route | Perioperative drug dose |
|---|---|---|---|---|---|
| **Paracetamol** | Mild to moderate pain<br><br>Pyrexia | Hepatotoxicity with low BMI<br>Malnutrition<br>Dehydration<br>Chronic alcohol abuse<br>Liver disease | **Common**<br>Liver damage with overdose<br>Rash<br>Blood disorders<br>IV infusion: tachycardia, hypotension, flushing<br>**Rare**<br>Skin reactions, malaise<br>**Unknown frequency**<br>Thrombocytopenia, leucopenia; neutropenia | IV infusion<br>PR<br>Oral | **Adult dose**<br>IV infusion, PR, oral<br>0.5–1 g: 4–6-hourly, maximum 4 g/day<br>**Paediatric dose: postoperative pain**<br>PR<br>1–2 months: 30 mg/kg for one dose (then 15–20 mg every 4–6 hours)<br>3 months–5 years: 30–40 mg/kg for one dose (then 15–20 mg every 4–6 hours)<br>6–11 years: 30–40 mg/kg for one dose (then 15–20 mg every 4–6 hours)<br>12–17 years: 1 g every 4–6 hours |

(continued)

**Table 23.5 (Contd.)**

| Drug | Indication | Contraindications/cautions | Side effects | Drug route | Perioperative drug dose |
|------|-----------|---------------------------|--------------|-----------|------------------------|
| **Ibuprofen (NSAID)** | Postoperative analgesia | GI ulceration and/or bleeding<br>Infection in neonates<br>Pulmonary hypertension in neonates<br>Heart failure<br>Asthma<br>Coagulopathies<br>Cerebrovascular bleeding<br>Connective tissue disease<br>Crohn's disease<br>Ulcerative colitis | **Common**<br>Exacerbation of asthma<br>GI irritation: bleeding, ulceration<br>Hypersensitivity reactions<br>**Rare**<br>Hepatic damage, visual disturbances, pancreatitis<br>**Unknown frequency**<br>Hypoxaemia in neonates, colitis, bronchospasm, fluid retention, depression, nausea | Oral<br>Gel | **Adult dose**<br>Oral<br>300–400 mg × 3–4 daily<br>**Paediatric dose**<br>Oral<br>12–17 years: 300–400 mg × 3–4 daily |
| **Diclofenac (NSAID)** | Postoperative pain and inflammatory conditions | GI bleeding<br>Asthma<br>Renal disease<br>Heart failure<br>Peripheral artery disease<br>Connective tissue disease<br>Crohn's disease<br>Ulcerative colitis | Aseptic meningitis, gastric ulceration, renal impairment, hepatic damage, pancreatitis bronchospasm<br>**Unknown frequency**<br>Hypoxaemia in neonates, colitis, bronchospasm, fluid retention, depression, nausea | IV infusion<br>IM injection<br>Oral<br>PR | **Adult dose**<br>IV infusion: 75 mg 4–6 hours, maximum 150 mg day<br>IM: 75 mg 1–2 times a day<br>Rectal: 75–150 mg/day divided doses<br>Oral: 75–150 mg daily in 2–3 doses |

| Ketorolac (NSAID) | Short-term management of moderate to severe postoperative pain | GI bleeding | Exacerbation of asthma | IV injection | Adult dose |
|---|---|---|---|---|---|
| | | Asthma | GI irritation: bleeding, ulceration | IM injection | IV/IM injection |
| | | Renal disease | Hypersensitivity reactions | | 10 mg, then 10–30 mg 4–6 hourly, maximum 90 mg/day (maximum 60 mg/day for older adults) |
| | | Surgery with high risk of haemorrhage | **Rare** | | **Paediatric dose** |
| | | Suspected cerebrovascular bleeding | Renal failure, pancreatitis, hepatic damage | | IV/IM injection |
| | | Peripheral artery disease | **Unknown frequency** | | 16–17 years: 10 mg, then 10–30 mg 4–6 hourly, maximum 90 mg/day (maximum 60 mg/day for body weight up to 50 kg) |
| | | Cardiovascular disease | Hypoxaemia in neonates, colitis, bronchospasm, fluid retention, depression, nausea, headache, bradycardia, confusion, convulsions | | IV injection |
| | | Heart failure | | | 6 months–15 years: 0.5–1 mg/kg, then 500 mcg/kg every 6 hours (mx 60 kg/day) |
| | | Dehydration | | | |
| | | Hypovolaemia | | | |
| | | Peripheral artery disease | | | |
| | | Connective tissue disease | | | |
| | | Crohn's disease | | | |
| | | Ulcerative colitis | | | |

(continued)

**Table 23.5 (Contd.)**

| Drug | Indication | Contraindications/cautions | Drug route | Perioperative drug dose |
|------|-----------|---------------------------|-----------|------------------------|
| Parecoxib (NSAID) | Short-term management of postoperative pain | Hypersensitivity to aspirin or NSAIDs<br>GI ulceration and/or bleeding<br>Heart failure<br>Ischaemic heart disease<br>Dehydration<br>Post-CABG<br>Asthma<br>Coagulopathies<br>Cerebrovascular bleeding<br>Connective tissue disease<br>Crohn's disease<br>Ulcerative colitis<br>Efficacy and safety of parecoxib in children remain unclear | IV injection<br>IM injection | **Adult dose**<br>IV/IM injection<br>40 mg, then 20–40 mg 6–12 hourly, (maximum 80 mg/day)<br>**Older adult dose**<br>IV/IM injection<br>20 mg (maximum 40 mg/day) |

Side effects:

**Common**
Alveolar osteitis, flatulence, hypokalaemia, hypotension, sweating, hypoaesthesia

**Uncommon**
Malaise, PE, bradycardia, anorexia, hyperglycaemia

**Rare**
Aseptic meningitis, renal impairment, hepatic damage

**Unknown frequency**
Bronchospasm, colitis, haematuria, headache, hearing disturbances, vertigo, tinnitus, nausea, diarrhoea, rash, tachycardia

## Further reading

Joint Formulary Committee (2022). British national formulary. Available at: ℘ https://bnf.nice.org.uk/
Joint Formulary Committee (2022). British national formulary for children. Available at: ℘ https://bnfc.nice.org.uk/
Scarth E, Smith S (2016). Drugs in anaesthesia and intensive care (5th ed). Oxford: Oxford University Press.

**Table 23.6** Muscle relaxants/neuromuscular drugs

| Drug | Indication | Contraindications/cautions | Side effects | Drug route | Perioperative drug dose |
|---|---|---|---|---|---|
| **Suxamethonium** | Depolarizing muscle relaxant<br>To facilitate endotracheal intubation when rapid neuromuscular block is required | Avoid use if patient has a family history of MH; hyperkalaemia; major trauma; severe burns; major muscle wasting and immobilization; congenital myotonic disease, sepsis, and muscular dystrophy<br>Caution is advised for patients who are known to have an atypical pseudocholinesterase enzyme, which has very little ability to break down the drug, thus prolonging its effect (suxamethonium (Scoline®) apnoea) | **Common**<br>Rash and flushing, skeletal muscle pain, rise in intraocular pressure, hyperkalaemia<br>**Rare**<br>Bronchospasm, apnoea, arrhythmias, prolonged respiratory depression, cardiac arrest, severe anaphylaxis, MH<br>**Unknown frequency**<br>Bradycardia, tachycardia, hypertension, hypotension | IV injection<br>IM injection | **Adult dose**<br>IV injection<br>1–1.5 mg/kg<br>**Paediatric dose: IV injection**<br>Neonate: 2 mg/kg<br>1–11 months: 2 mg/kg<br>1–17 years: 1 mg/kg<br>**Paediatric dose: IM injection**<br>Neonate: up to 4 mg/kg<br>1–11 months: up to 5 mg/kg<br>1–11 years: up to 4 mg/kg (maximum 150 mg per dose) |
| **Atracurium** | Non-depolarizing muscle relaxant<br>Muscle relaxation for surgery of short to intermediate duration | Pregnancy, breastfeeding, hypothermia, burns<br>Avoid excessive dosages in obese patients<br>The activity of the drug is prolonged in patients with myasthenia gravis | **Common**<br>Histamine release<br>**Rare**<br>Anaphylaxis<br>**Unknown frequency**<br>Tachycardia, myopathy, hypotension, bronchospasm, seizures | IV injection<br>IV infusion | **Adult dose: 2.5%**<br>Slow IV injection<br>300–600 mcg/kg, then 100–200 mcg/kg as required<br>**Paediatric dose: neonate**<br>Slow IV injection<br>300–500 mcg/kg, then by 100–200 mcg/kg<br>**Paediatric dose: child**<br>Slow IV injection<br>300–600 mcg/kg, then 100–200 mcg/kg as required |

(continued)

**Table 23.6 (Contd.)**

| Drug | Indication | Contraindications/cautions | Side effects | Drug route | Perioperative drug dose |
|---|---|---|---|---|---|
| Miva-curium | Non-depolarizing muscle relaxant  Muscle relaxation for surgery of short duration | Patients with hepatic impairment, renal impairment, and older adults  The activity of the drug is prolonged in patients with myasthenia gravis | **Rare**  Anaphylaxis  **Unknown frequency**  Tachycardia, skin flushing, hypotension, bronchospasm | IV injection | **Adult dose**  70–250 mcg/kg; maintenance of 100 mcg/kg every 15 minutes  **Paediatric dose: 2–5 months**  Slow IV injection  150 mcg/kg; maintenance of 100 mcg/kg every 6–9 minutes  **Paediatric dose: 6 months–11 years**  Slow IV injection  200 mcg/kg; maintenance of 100 mcg/kg every 6–9 minutes  **Paediatric dose: child 12–17 years**  Slow IV injection  70–250 mcg/kg; maintenance of 100 mcg/kg every 15 minutes |
| Vecuro-nium | Non-depolarizing muscle relaxant  Muscle relaxation for surgery of intermediate duration | The activity of the drug is prolonged in patients with myasthenia gravis, and in neonates and infants, requiring a longer recovery period | **Rare**  Anaphylaxis  **Unknown frequency**  Tachycardia, myopathy, hypotension, bronchospasm, skin flushing | IV injection | **Adult dose**  80–100 mcg/kg; maintenance of 20–30 mcg/kg titrated according to response  **Paediatric dose: neonate**  Slow IV injection  80 mcg/kg; maintenance of 30–50 mcg/kg titrated according to response  **Paediatric dose: child**  Slow IV injection  80–100 mcg/kg; maintenance of 20–30 mcg/kg titrated according to response |

| | | | | |
|---|---|---|---|---|
| **Pancuronium** | Non-depolarizing muscle relaxant<br><br>Muscle relaxation for surgery of long duration | Patients with hepatic impairment, renal impairment, and pregnancy<br><br>The activity of the drug is prolonged in patients with myasthenia gravis | **Unknown frequency**<br>Tachycardia, myopathy, hypotension | IV injection | **Adult dose**<br>100 mcg/kg; then 20 mcg/kg as required<br>**Paediatric dose: neonate**<br>Slow IV injection<br>100 mcg/kg; then 50 mcg/kg as required<br>**Paediatric dose: child**<br>Slow IV injection<br>100 mcg/kg; then 20 mcg/kg as required |
| **Rocuronium** | Non-depolarizing muscle relaxant<br><br>Muscle relaxation of moderate duration of action to facilitate surgery | Fatal anaphylactoid reactions to Rrocuronium have been reported<br><br>The activity of the drug is prolonged in patients with myasthenia gravis<br><br>Caution advised for patients with hepatic and renal impairment<br><br>Pregnancy<br><br>Breastfeeding | **Rare**<br>Anaphylaxis<br>**Unknown frequency**<br>Tachycardia, myopathy, hypotension, bronchospasm, skin flushing | | **Adult dose**<br>600 mcg/kg; maintenance of 150 mcg/kg, titrated according to response<br>**Older adult dose**<br>600 mcg/kg; maintenance of 75–100 mcg/kg, titrated according to response<br>**Paediatric dose: neonate**<br>Slow IV injection<br>600 mcg/kg; then 150 mcg/kg as required<br>**Paediatric dose: child**<br>Slow IV injection<br>600 mcg/kg; then 150 mcg/kg as required |

(continued)

**Table 23.6 (Contd.)**

| Drug | Indication | Contraindications/cautions | Side effects | Drug route | Perioperative drug dose |
|------|-----------|---------------------------|--------------|-----------|------------------------|
| Cisatracurium | Non-depolarizing muscle relaxant<br><br>Muscle relaxation for surgery of intermediate duration | Cardiovascular disease, burns, fluid and electrolyte disturbances, hypothermia, neuromuscular disorders.<br><br>The activity of the drug is prolonged in patients with myasthenia gravis | **Unknown frequency**<br>Bradycardia, myopathy | IV injection | **Adult dose**<br>150 mcg/kg; maintenance of 30 mcg/kg, titrated according to response<br><br>**Paediatric dose: 1 month–1 year**<br>Slow IV injection<br>150 mcg/kg; then 130 mcg/kg every 20 minutes<br><br>**Paediatric dose: 2–11 years**<br>Slow IV injection<br>150 mcg/kg; then 20 mcg/kg every 10 minutes<br><br>**Paediatric dose: 12–17 years**<br>Slow IV injection<br>150 mcg/kg; then 30 mcg/kg every 20 minutes |
| Dantrolene sodium | Malignant hyperthermia | Avoid extravasation due to risk of tissue necrosis<br><br>Hepatic disease | **Unknown frequency**<br>Pulmonary oedema, rash, swelling, weakness, dizziness, erythema, injection site reaction, hepatotoxicity, thrombophlebitis | Rapid IV injection | **Adult dose**<br>2–3 mg/kg; then 1 mg/kg repeated if necessary. Maximum dose 10 mg/kg<br><br>**Paediatric dose (unlicensed)**<br>2–3 mg/kg; then 1 mg/kg repeated if necessary. Maximum dose 10 mg/kg |

## Further reading

Joint Formulary Committee (2022). British national formulary. Available at: ⊗ https://bnf.nice.org.uk/

Joint Formulary Committee (2022). British national formulary for children. Available at: ⊗ https://bnfc.nice.org.uk/

Scarth E, Smith S (2016). Drugs in anaesthesia and intensive care (5th ed). Oxford: Oxford University Press.

**Table 23.7** Anticoagulant drugs

| Drug | Indication | Contraindications/cautions | Side effects | Drug route | Perioperative drug dose |
|------|-----------|---------------------------|--------------|-----------|------------------------|
| **Heparin** | Prophylactic prevention of venous thromboembolic disease with LMWH<br><br>Treatment of DVT, fat embolus, pulmonary embolus, DIC | Spinal and epidural anaesthesia with treatment doses of heparin<br>Thrombocytopenia<br>Haemophilia<br>Acute bacterial endocarditis<br>Hypertension<br>Cerebral haemorrhage<br>Hepatic impairment<br>Renal impairment<br>Pregnancy: older adults | **Rare**<br>Injection site reactions, skin necrosis, priapism, hyperkalaemia, osteoporosis, hypersensitivity reactions<br>**Frequency unknown**<br>Haemorrhage, thrombocytopenia | IV injection<br>IV infusion<br>SC injection | **Adult dose**<br>SC injection<br>5000 units for one dose, 2 hours prior to surgery. Then 5000 units every 8–12 hours |
| **Fondaparinux sodium** | Prophylaxis of VTE in patients following abdominal surgery or major orthopaedic surgery of the hip or leg | Bleeding disorders, bacterial endocarditis<br>Older adults, low body weight, spinal or epidural anaesthesia, spinal surgery, bleeding disorders, brain surgery, recent intracranial haemorrhage, ophthalmic surgery, active GI ulcer disease | **Common**<br>Bleeding, anaemia, purpura<br>**Uncommon**<br>Oedema, pruritus, rash, dyspnoea, chest pain, GI disturbances, hepatic impairment, thrombocytopenia<br>**Rare**<br>Flushing, headache, vertigo, anxiety, drowsiness, hypotension, injection-site reaction, confusion, cough<br>**Frequency unknown**<br>Tachycardia, pyrexia, atrial fibrillation | SC injection | **Adult dose**<br>SC injection<br>2.5 mg, 6 hours postoperatively. Then 2.5 mg daily |

(continued)

**Table 23.7 (Contd.)**

| Drug | Indication | Contraindications/cautions | Side effects | Drug route | Perioperative drug dose |
|------|-----------|---------------------------|--------------|-----------|------------------------|
| **Tinzaparin** | Prophylactic prevention of venous thromboembolic disease with LMWH<br><br>Treatment of DVT, fat embolus, pulmonary embolism, unstable angina, and acute peripheral arterial occlusion | Spinal and epidural anaesthesia with treatment doses of heparin<br>Thrombocytopenia<br>Haemophilia<br>Acute bacterial endocarditis<br>Hypertension<br>Cerebral haemorrhage<br>Hepatic impairment<br>Renal impairment<br>Pregnancy; breastfeeding; elderly | **Rare**<br>Injection site reactions, skin necrosis, priapism, hyperkalaemia, osteoporosis, hypersensitivity reactions<br>**Frequency unknown**<br>Haemorrhage, thrombocytopenia | SC injection | **Adult dose (prior to general surgery)**<br>SC injection<br>3500 units for one dose, 2 hours prior to surgery. Then 3500 units every 24 hours<br>**Adult dose (prior to orthopaedic surgery)**<br>SC injection<br>50 units/kg for one dose, 2 hours prior to surgery. Then 50 units/kg every 24 hours<br>**Paediatric dose: child**<br>SC injection<br>50 units/kg daily |

# Further reading

Joint Formulary Committee (2022). British national formulary. Available at: ℗ https://bnf.nice.org.uk/

Joint Formulary Committee (2022). British national formulary for children. Available at: ℗ https://bnfc.nice.org.uk/

National Institute for Health and Care Excellence (2018). Venous thromboembolism in over 16s: reducing the risk of hospital-acquired deep vein thrombosis or pulmonary embolism. NICE guideline [NG89]. Available at: ℗ https://www.nice.org.uk/guidance/ng89

Scarth E, Smith S (2016). Drugs in anaesthesia and intensive care (5th ed). Oxford: Oxford University Press.

**Table 23.8** Obstetric drugs

| Drug | Indication | Contraindications/cautions | Side effects | Drug route | Perioperative drug dose |
|------|------------|---------------------------|--------------|------------|------------------------|
| Nitrous oxide | Maintenance of anaesthesia in conjunction with other anaesthetic agents<br><br>Analgesia used in obstetrics (as Entonox 50% $N_2O$: 50% $O_2$) | Susceptibility to MH<br><br>Can significantly increase the size of a pneumothorax<br><br>Renal impairment<br><br>Presence of intracranial air after head injury; recent intra-ocular gas injection | **Frequency unknown**<br>Diffusion hypoxia, megaloblastic anaemia, neurological toxic effects, can cause neonatal respiratory depression in third trimester of pregnancy | Inhalation | **Anaesthesia**<br>50–66% administered using appropriate anaesthetic apparatus in $O_2$<br><br>**Analgesia**<br>Up to 50% self-administered using appropriate anaesthetic apparatus in $O_2$ |
| Oxytocin | Induction of labour<br><br>To reduce postpartum haemorrhage<br><br>Aid expulsion of the placenta following delivery and evacuation of retained products of conception<br><br>To promote lactation<br><br>Missed and incomplete abortion | Pregnancy induced hypertension or cardiac disease<br><br>Fetal distress<br><br>Pre-eclampsia<br><br>Cardiovascular disease<br><br>Monitor for DIC<br><br>Caudal anaesthesia | **Common**<br>Nausea, vomiting, headache, arrhythmia<br><br>**Rare**<br>Uterine spasm and/or hyperstimulation, anaphylactic reactions (with shock, dyspnoea, hypotension), DIC; hyponatraemia with high doses, rash | IV injection<br>IV infusion<br>IM injection | **Adult dose**<br>Slow IV injection<br><br>5 units after delivery (can be repeated in the case of postpartum haemorrhage) |

(continued)

**Table 23.8 (Contd.)**

| Drug | Indication | Contraindications/cautions | Side effects | Drug route | Perioperative drug dose |
|---|---|---|---|---|---|
| **Ergometrine maleate** | To control haemorrhage | Hypertension<br>Cardiac disease<br>Vascular disease<br>Severe hepatic impairment<br>Severe renal impairment<br>Sepsis<br>Eclampsia<br>Multiple pregnancy | **Common**<br>Nausea, vomiting, abdominal pain, dizziness, hypertension, rash, pulmonary oedema, arrhythmias, palpitation, bradycardia, chest pain, headache, dyspnoea, vasoconstriction, tinnitus<br>**Rare**<br>MI | IV injection<br>IM injection | **Adult dose**<br>Slow IV injection<br>250–500 mcg for postpartum haemorrhage |
| **Anti-D immunoglobulin** | To prevent rhesus-negative mother from forming antibodies to fetal rhesus-positive cells<br>Should be administered following birth, miscarriage, and abortion within 72 hours | Treatment of idiopathic thrombocytopenia purpura in rhesus-negative patients; treatment of idiopathic thrombocytopenia purpura following splenectomy<br>Immunoglobulin A deficiency, live virus vaccines<br>**Store in a refrigerator** | **Rare**<br>Anaphylaxis, tachycardia, hypotension, dyspnoea<br>**Frequency unknown**<br>Nausea, vomiting, abdominal pain, diarrhoea, drowsiness, dizziness, headache, hypertension, rash, pruritus, malaise, arthralgia, asthenia, back pain, fever, injection site pain, myalgia, sweating<br>**Frequency unknown with IV use**<br>MI, PE, DVT, stroke, abdominal distension, haemolytic anaemia; BP instability, injection site reactions | IM injection | **Antenatal prophylaxis**<br>500 units at 28 weeks' gestation and 34 weeks' gestation<br>500 units immediately following birth<br>250 units following abortion up until 20 weeks' gestation<br>500 units after 20 weeks' gestation |

| | | | | | |
|---|---|---|---|---|---|
| Sodium citrate | To reduce gastric acidity<br>To reduce the risk of acid aspiration (Mendelson's syndrome) in women undergoing operative procedures | Renal impairment<br>Cardiac disease<br>Hypertension<br>Caution advised with toxaemia in pregnancy | **Uncommon**<br>Metabolic alkalosis may occur in patients with renal dysfunction | Orally<br>**Draw up fresh as shelf-life is short** | **Adult dose**<br>30 mL of 0.3 molar solution prior to induction of GA |
| Ranitidine | To reduce gastric acidity<br>To reduce the risk of acid aspiration (Mendelson's syndrome) | Renal impairment<br>Breastfeeding<br>Porphyria | **Common**<br>Diarrhoea, dizziness, headache<br>**Uncommon**<br>Rash<br>**Rare**<br>GI disturbances, tachycardia, visual disturbance<br>**Frequency unknown**<br>Alopecia | IV injection<br>IV infusion<br>IM injection<br>Orally | **Adult dose**<br>150 mg orally (onset of labour)<br>**General anaesthesia**<br>45–60 minutes before induction via IM injection or slow IV injection diluted to 20 mL |

## Further reading

Clark V, Van de Velde M, Fernando R (eds) (2016). Oxford textbook of obstetric anaesthesia. Oxford: Oxford University Press.

Joint Formulary Committee (2022). British national formulary. Available at: ℅ https://bnf.nice.org.uk/

National Institute for Health and Care Excellence (2008). Routine antenatal anti-D prophylaxis for women who are rhesus D negative. Technology appraisal guidance [TA156]. Available at: ℅ https://www.nice.org.uk/guidance/TA156

Scarth E, Smith S (2016). Drugs in anaesthesia and intensive care (5th ed). Oxford: Oxford University Press.

Yentis S, Malhotra S (2013). Analgesia, anaesthesia and pregnancy: a practical guide (3rd ed). Cambridge: Cambridge University Press.

**Table 23.9** Inhalational drugs

| Drug | Indication | Contraindications/ cautions | Side effects | Drug route | Perioperative drug dose |
|------|-----------|----------------------------|-------------|-----------|------------------------|
| Isoflurane | Mainly used for the maintenance of anaesthesia during surgery It has been used as sedation during intensive care | Susceptibility to MH Can cause hepatotoxicity sensitive patients Can cause neonatal respiratory depression in third trimester of pregnancy Can cause raised ICP | **Common** Cardiorespiratory depression, arrhythmias, hypotension **Unknown frequency** Convulsions, mood change, laryngospasm, breath-holding, cough, irritation of mucous membrane | By inhalation via a calibrated vaporizer | **Adult dose** Induction of anaesthesia: 0.5%, increased to 3%, adjusted according to response Maintenance of anaesthesia: 1–2.5%, additional 0.5–1% may be required when given with $O_2$ alone Maintenance of anaesthesia in caesarean section: 0.5–0.75% **Paediatric dose (induction)** Neonate: 0.5%, increased to 3%, adjusted according to response Child: 0.5%, increased to 3%, adjusted according to response **Paediatric dose (maintenance)** Neonate: 1–2.5%, additional 0.5–1% may be required when given with $O_2$ alone Child: 1–2.5%, additional 0.5–1% may be required when given with $O_2$ alone |

| Sevo-flurane | Mainly used for the maintenance of anaesthesia during surgery It can be used for the induction of anaesthesia | Susceptibility to MH Susceptibility to prolonged QT-interval Manufacturer recommends caution in cases of renal impairment Can cause neonatal respiratory depression in third trimester of pregnancy | **Common** Cardiorespiratory depression, arrhythmias, hypotension **Unknown frequency** Convulsions, mood change, torsade de pointes (ventricular tachycardia), cardiac arrest, dystonia, leucopenia, urinary retention | By inhalation via a calibrated vaporizer | **Adult dose** Induction of anaesthesia: 0.5–1%, increased to 8%, adjusted according to response Maintenance of anaesthesia: 0.5–3%, adjusted according to response **Paediatric dose (induction)** Neonate: up to 4%, adjusted according to response Child: 0.5–1%, increased to 8%, adjusted according to response **Paediatric dose (maintenance)** Neonate: 0.5–2%, adjusted according to response Child: 0.5–3%, adjusted according to response |
| Des-flurane | Mainly used for the maintenance of anaesthesia during surgery Not recommended for induction of anaesthesia | Susceptibility to MH Can cause neonatal respiratory depression in third trimester of pregnancy | **Common** Cardiorespiratory depression, arrhythmias, hypotension **Unknown frequency** Convulsions, mood change, apnoea, laryngospasm, cough, breath holding, increased secretions | By inhalation via a calibrated vaporizer | **Adult dose** Maintenance of anaesthesia: 2–6% **Paediatric dose (maintenance)** Neonate: 2–6%, adjusted according to response Child: 2–6%, adjusted according to response |

(continued)

**Table 23.9 (Contd.)**

| Drug | Indication | Contraindications/ cautions | Side effects | Drug route | Perioperative drug dose |
|------|-----------|----------------------------|--------------|-----------|------------------------|
| Nitrous oxide | Mainly used for the maintenance of anaesthesia during surgery<br><br>Can be used for pain relief during labour | Can significantly increase the size of a pneumothorax<br><br>Manufacturer recommends caution in cases of renal impairment<br><br>Can cause neonatal respiratory depression in third trimester of pregnancy<br><br>May increase gas embolus size, e.g. with neurosurgery<br><br>Avoid in patients following recent intraocular gas injection | **Unknown frequency**<br>Hypoxia, depression of white cell formation, megaloblastic anaemia, neurological toxicity | By inhalation via suitable anaesthesia apparatus in oxygen | **Adult dose**<br>Maintenance of anaesthesia: 50–66%<br>Analgesia: up to 50%, adjusted according to response<br>**Paediatric dose (maintenance)**<br>Neonate: 50–66%<br>Child: 50–66%<br>**Paediatric dose (analgesia)**<br>Neonate: up to 50%, adjusted according to response<br>Child: up to 50%, adjusted according to response |

## Further reading

Joint Formulary Committee (2022). British national formulary. Available at: ℜ https://bnf.nice.org.uk/
Joint Formulary Committee (2022). British national formulary for children. Available at: ℜ https://bnfc.nice.org.uk/
Scarth E, Smith S (2016). Drugs in anaesthesia and intensive care (5th ed). Oxford: Oxford University Press.

**Table 23.10** Antimuscarinic drugs

| Drug | Indication | Contraindications/cautions | Side effects | Drug route | Perioperative drug dose |
|------|-----------|---------------------------|--------------|------------|------------------------|
| **Atropine** | Reduces salivary function Reversal of bradycardia With anticholinesterase, reversal of non-depolarizing neuromuscular block | Myasthenia gravis, paralytic ileus, prostate enlargement, pyloric stenosis, cardiovascular disease, children <3 months and older people, Down syndrome, severe ulcerative colitis, toxic megacolon, urinary retention | **Common** Constipation, skin flushing, bradycardia, photophobia, dry mouth, urinary retention, urinary urgency **Uncommon** Nausea, vomiting, confusion, giddiness **Rare** Glaucoma **Frequency unknown** Hallucinations, rash, blurred vision, headache, convulsion, drowsiness, diarrhoea, difficulty in micturition, flatulence, fatigue, disorientation, dry eyes, taste disturbances, euphoria, impaired memory, palpitation | IV injection | **For intraoperative bradycardia** Adult dose 300–600 mcg Paediatric dose Unlicensed in children <12 years Child (12–17 years): 300–600 mcg |

(continued)

**Table 23.10 (Contd.)**

| Drug | Indication | Contraindications/cautions | Side effects | Drug route | Perioperative drug dose |
|---|---|---|---|---|---|
| Glycopyrronium bromide | Reversal of bradycardia Drying secretions Reversal of non-depolarizing neuromuscular block with neostigmine **Glycopyrronium bromide is incompatible with thiopentone, diazepam, and methohexitone** | Myasthenia gravis, paralytic ileus, prostate enlargement, pyloric stenosis, cardiovascular disease, children <3 months and older people, Down syndrome, severe ulcerative colitis, toxic megacolon, urinary retention | **Common** Constipation, skin flushing, bradycardia, photophobia, dry mouth, urinary retention, urinary urgency **Uncommon** Nausea, vomiting, confusion, giddiness **Rare** Glaucoma **Frequency unknown** Hallucinations, rash, blurred vision, headache, convulsion, drowsiness, diarrhoea, difficulty in micturition, flatulence, fatigue, disorientation, dry eyes, taste disturbances, euphoria, impaired memory, palpitation | IV injection | **For intraoperative bradycardia** Adult dose 200–400 mcg Paediatric dose Neonate: 10 mcg/kg Child: 4–8 mcg/kg **Control of side effects of neostigmine** Adult dose 10–15 mcg/kg Paediatric dose Neonate: 10 mcg/kg Child (1 month–11 years): 10 mcg/kg Child (12–17 years): 10–15 mcg/kg |

## Further reading

Joint Formulary Committee (2022). British national formulary. Available at: ⊕ https://bnf.nice.org.uk/

Joint Formulary Committee (2022). British national formulary for children. Available at: ⊕ https://bnfc.nice.org.uk/

Scarth E, Smith S (2016). Drugs in anaesthesia and intensive care (5th ed). Oxford: Oxford University Press.

**Table 23.11** Anticholinesterase drugs

| Drug | Indication | Contraindications/cautions | Side effects | Drug route | Perioperative drug dose |
|------|-----------|---------------------------|--------------|-----------|------------------------|
| Neostigmine | Reversal of non-depolarizing neuromuscular blockade Myasthenia gravis **Neostigmine has a longer duration of action than edrophonium** | Intestinal or urinary obstruction Asthma, arrhythmias, recent MI, bradycardia, hypotension, epilepsy, pregnancy, breastfeeding | **Frequency unknown** Nausea, vomiting, diarrhoea, increased salivary function, abdominal cramps **Overdose** includes lacrimation, increased bronchial secretions, excessive sweating, heart block, hypotension | IV injection over 1 minute duration | **Reversal of neuromuscular blockade** <u>Adult dose</u> 2.5 mg (maximum dose 5 mg) <u>Paediatric dose</u> Neonate: 50 mcg/kg Child (1 month–11 years): 50 mcg/kg Child (12–17 years): 50 mcg/kg |
| Sugammadex | Routine reversal of neuromuscular blockade induced by vecuronium or rocuronium in adults. Immediate reversal of neuromuscular blockade induced by rocuronium in adults Routine reversal of neuromuscular blockade induced by rocuronium in children | Recurrence of neuromuscular blockade Potential delayed recovery in older people and those with cardiovascular disease Pre-existing coagulation disorders Use of anticoagulant therapy Pregnancy Renal impairment | **Frequency unknown** Hypersensitivity, bradycardia, cardiac arrest, bronchospasm | IV injection | **Routine reversal induced by vecuronium/rocuronium** <u>Adult dose</u> 2–4 mg/kg, then 4 mg/kg if required **Immediate reversal of rocuronium** <u>Adult dose</u> 16 mg/kg **Routine reversal induced by rocuronium** <u>Paediatric dose</u> Child (2–17 years): 2 mg/kg |

# Further reading

Joint Formulary Committee (2022). British national formulary. Available at: ℗ https://bnf.nice.org.uk/
Joint Formulary Committee (2022). British national formulary for children. Available at: ℗ https://bnfc.nice.org.uk/
Scarth E, Smith S (2016). Drugs in anaesthesia and intensive care (5th ed). Oxford: Oxford University Press.

**Table 23.12** Anxiolytic benzodiazepine drugs

| Drug | Indication | Contraindications/cautions | Side effects | Drug route | Perioperative drug dose |
|------|-----------|---------------------------|-------------|-----------|------------------------|
| **Diazepam** | Premedication<br>Sedation with amnesia and LA<br>Short-term use in anxiety or insomnia<br>Status epilepticus<br>Febrile convulsions | Respiratory depression<br>Neuromuscular weakness<br>Sleep apnoea<br>Severe hepatic impairment<br>Second period of drowsiness can occur several hours after<br>Hepatic impairment<br>Renal impairment<br>Pregnancy<br>Breastfeeding | **Common**<br>Amnesia, drowsiness and light-headedness the following day, muscle weakness, confusion, ataxia<br>**Uncommon**<br>GI disturbances, hypotension, tremor, visual disturbances, vertigo<br>**Rare**<br>Respiratory depression, jaundice, skin reactions, apnoea, blood disorders<br>**Frequency unknown**<br>Hypotonia, pain, thrombophlebitis | IV injection<br>IM injection<br>Orally<br>Rectal | **Premedication**<br>Adult dose<br>5–10 mg (1–2 hours prior to surgery)<br>2.5–5 mg (older/debilitated patients)<br>**Conscious sedation**<br>Adult dose<br>10–20 mg (slow IV) over 2–4 minutes<br>Paediatric dose<br>Unlicensed for perioperative interventions |

| Midazolam | Sedation with amnesia | Neuromuscular respiratory weakness including unstable myasthenia gravis | **Frequency unknown** | IV injection | **Conscious sedation** |
|---|---|---|---|---|---|
| | Sedation in intensive care | Severe respiratory depression | Anaphylaxis, amnesia, bronchospasm, confusion, | Buccal, oral, rectal and IV for paediatric patients | Adult dose<br>2–2.5 mg—slow IV |
| | Premedication | Acute pulmonary insufficiency | headache, vertigo, dizziness, laryngospasm, vertigo, visual | | (5–10 minutes prior to intervention), |
| | Induction of anaesthesia (rare) | Cardiac disease | disturbances, respiratory depression/arrest, GI | | maximum 7 mg<br>Older patients: |
| | Status epilepticus | Respiratory disease | disturbances, restlessness, hiccups, jaundice | | 0.5–1 mg—slow IV<br>(5–10 minutes prior |
| | **The effects of midazolam can** | Myasthenia gravis | | | to intervention), maximum 3.5 mg |
| | **be reversed with flumazenil,** | Neonates & children | | | Paediatric dose (slow IV) |
| | **glycopyrronium, and** | History of drug or alcohol abuse | | | Child (1 month– 5 years): 25–50 mcg/kg, |
| | **physostigmine** | Reduce dose in elderly and debilitated | | | maximum 6 mg dose |
| | | | | | Child (6–11 years): 25–50 mcg/kg, maximum 10 mg dose |
| | | | | | Child (12–17 years): 25–50 mcg/kg, maximum 7.5 mg dose |

(continued)

**Table 23.12 (Contd.)**

| Drug | Indication | Contraindications/cautions | Side effects | Drug route | Perioperative drug dose |
|------|-----------|---------------------------|--------------|-----------|------------------------|
| Loraze pam | Premedication<br>Sedation with amnesia and LA<br>Short-term use in anxiety and/or insomnia<br>Status epilepticus<br>Febrile convulsions<br>Acute panic attacks | Neuromuscular respiratory weakness, sleep apnoea syndrome, acute pulmonary insufficiency, unstable myasthenia gravis<br>Respiratory depression, CNS depression, compromised airway, avoid injections containing benzyl alcohol in neonates; chronic psychosis (in adults); organic brain changes | **Common**<br>Amnesia, drowsiness and light-headedness the following day<br>Muscle weakness, confusion ataxia<br>**Uncommon**<br>GI disturbances, hypotension, tremor; visual disturbances, vertigo<br>**Rare**<br>Respiratory depression, jaundice, skin reactions, apnoea, blood disorders<br>**Frequency unknown**<br>Hypotonia, pain, thrombophlebitis; delusions, excitement, and hallucinations in children | Oral<br><br>IV injection | **Premedication**<br>Adult dose (oral)<br>2–3 mg (night prior to surgery); 2–4 mg (1–2 hours prior to surgery)<br>Paediatric dose (oral)<br>Child (1 month–11 years): 50–100 mcg/kg (1 hour before surgery)<br>Child (12–17 years): 1–4 mg (1 hour before procedure)<br>**Conscious sedation**<br>Adult dose<br>50 mcg/kg (slow IV) 30–45 minutes before surgery |

| | | | Common | Premedication |
|---|---|---|---|---|
| Temazepam | Preoperative medication | Respiratory depression | Amnesia, drowsiness, and light-headedness the following day | Adult dose (oral) 10–20 mg (1–2 hours prior to surgery) |
| | Anxiety | Neuromuscular weakness | Muscle weakness, confusion, ataxia, dependence | Older patients: 10 mg (1–2 hours before surgery) |
| | Hypnotic | Sleep apnoea, compromised airway, phobic state | **Uncommon** | Paediatric dose (oral) |
| | **Temazepam has controlled drug status** | Severe hepatic impairment: second period of drowsiness can occur several hours after | GI disturbances, hypotension, tremor, visual disturbances, vertigo, urinary retention, slurred speech, incontinence, tremor, hypotension | Child (12–17 years): 10–20 mg (1 hour before procedure) |
| | | | **Rare** | |
| | | | Respiratory depression, jaundice, skin reactions, apnoea, blood disorders | |
| | | | **Frequency unknown** | |
| | | | Respiratory depression | |

Orally

## Further reading

Joint Formulary Committee (2022). British national formulary. Available at: ℗ https://bnf.nice.org.uk/
Joint Formulary Committee (2022). British national formulary for children. Available at: ℗ https://bnfc.nice.org.uk/
Scarth E, Smith S (2016). Drugs in anaesthesia and intensive care (5th ed). Oxford: Oxford University Press.

**Table 23.13** Antagonists for central and respiratory depression/respiratory stimulants

| Drug | Indication | Contraindications/ cautions | Side effects | Drug route | Perioperative drug dose |
|---|---|---|---|---|---|
| Naloxone (Narcan[9]) | Reversal of opiate-induced respiratory depression Overdose of opiate drugs Reversal of neonatal respiratory depression following opiate administration to mother during labour | Cardiovascular disease Opiate dependence | **Common** Reverses effects of analgesia, hypotension, nausea, vomiting, dyspnoea, hypertension **Uncommon** Diarrhoea, bradycardia, tremor, sweating, hyperventilation **Rare** Seizures, cardiac arrest, anaphylaxis, pulmonary oedema, ventricular tachycardia & fibrillation **Frequency unknown** Agitation | IV injection SC or IM injection in the absence of IV access **Short duration of action so repeated doses may be necessary** | **Overdose with opiates** Adult dose 400 mcg, then 800 mcg for up to 2 doses at 1-minute intervals until desired effect Paediatric dose Neonate: 100 mcg/kg, review and repeat as per policy Child (1 month–11 years): 100 mcg/kg (maximum per dose 2 mg), review and repeat as per policy Child (12–17 years): 400 mcg, review and repeat as per policy **Reversal of postoperative respiratory depression** Adult dose 100–200 mcg until desired effect Paediatric dose Neonate: 1 mcg/kg, review and repeat as per policy Child (1 month–11 years): 1 mcg/kg, review and repeat as per policy Child (12–17 years): 100–200 mcg, review and repeat as per policy |

| Flumazenil (Anexate®) | Reversal of sedative effects of benzodiazepines in anaesthesia. To reverse sedative effects in intensive care and endoscopy During 'wake-up' test for scoliosis surgery Reduces postoperative shivering | Raised ICP, status epilepticus Any life-threatening condition controlled by benzodiazepine drugs Benzodiazepine dependence Prolonged benzodiazepine therapy for epilepsy History of panic disorders, hepatic impairment, head injury, older people, children, breastfeeding | **Common** Nausea, vomiting **Uncommon** Palpitations, fear, anxiety **Frequency unknown** Flushing, dizziness, chills, agitation, tachycardia, sweating, transient hypertension | IV injection **Short duration of action so repeated doses may be necessary** | **Reversal of sedative effects of benzodiazepines** <u>Adult dose</u> 200 mcg—slow IV (maximum 1 mg) <u>Paediatric dose (slow IV)</u> Neonate: 10 mcg/kg every 1 minute Child: 10 mcg/kg every 1 minute maximum 1 mg dose |

*(continued)*

**Table 23.13 (Contd.)**

| Drug | Indication | Contraindications/cautions | Drug route | Perioperative drug dose |
|------|-----------|---------------------------|-----------|------------------------|
| **Doxapram (Dopram®)** | Postoperative respiratory depression<br>Acute respiratory failure<br>Postoperative shivering | Severe hypertension<br>Status asthmaticus<br>Coronary artery disease<br>Epilepsy<br>Thyrotoxicosis<br>Give O₂ in severe irreversible airway obstruction<br>Hypertension<br>Hepatic impairment<br>Pregnancy | IV injection | **Postoperative respiratory depression**<br><u>Adult dose (oral)</u><br>1–1.5 mg/kg over 30 seconds (repeat according to response)<br><u>Paediatric dose</u><br>Not licensed |

Side effects: **Frequency unknown** Perineal warmth, dizziness, restlessness, excessive sweating, slight increase in BP and heart rate. During postoperative period, muscle fasciculations, confusion, hallucinations, laryngospasm, bronchospasm, sinus tachycardia, bradycardia, nausea, vomiting, salivation

# Further reading

Joint Formulary Committee (2022). British national formulary. Available at: ℗ https://bnf.nice.org.uk/
Joint Formulary Committee (2022). British national formulary for children. Available at: ℗ https://bnfc.nice.org.uk/
Scarth E, Smith S (2016). Drugs in anaesthesia and intensive care (5th ed). Oxford: Oxford University Press.

Table 23.14 Antiemetic drugs

| Drug | Indication | Contraindications/cautions | Side effects | Drug route | Perioperative drug dose |
|------|-----------|---------------------------|--------------|-----------|------------------------|
| Prochlorperazine (Stemetil®) | Nausea & vomiting<br>Vertigo<br>Labyrinthitis<br>Cytotoxic therapy<br>Radiotherapy<br>Emesis caused by opiates and GA<br>Psychosis | Hypotension likely after IM injection<br>Elderly<br>Comatose state<br>Hepatic impairment<br>Renal impairment<br>Epilepsy<br>Parkinson's disease | **Rare**<br>Glaucoma<br>**Frequency unknown**<br>Extra-pyramidal symptoms, rash, jaundice, respiratory depression, confusion, dry mouth, blurred vision, constipation, dystonic reactions | IV injection<br>IM injection<br>Orally<br>Rectal | **Acute nausea & vomiting**<br><u>Adult dose</u><br>12.5 mg (IM)<br><u>Paediatric dose (IM)</u><br>Child (2–4 years): 1.25–2.5 mg<br>Child (5–7 years): 5–6.25 mg<br>Child (12–17 years): 12.5 mg |
| Metaclopramide (Maxolon®) | Prevention of PONV<br>Cytotoxic therapy<br>Radiotherapy<br>**Should only be prescribed for 5 days maximum** | GI surgery/obstruction<br>Haemorrhage, breastfeeding, hepatic disease, renal impairment, epilepsy, pregnancy, older people, children | **Common**<br>Extra-pyramidal symptoms, menstrual changes, galactorrhoea<br>**Rare**<br>Depression, neuroleptic malignant syndrome<br>**Frequency unknown**<br>Restlessness, drowsiness, rash, diarrhoea, pruritus, tremor, oedema, visual disturbances, anxiety, confusion | IV injection<br>IM injection<br>Orally | **Prevention of nausea & vomiting**<br><u>Adult dose</u><br>Body weight <60 kg: 500 mcg/kg (slow IV)<br>Body weight >60 kg: 10 mg (slow IV)<br><u>Paediatric dose (slow IV)</u><br>Child: 100–150 mcg/kg (maximum 10 mg) |

(continued)

**Table 23.14 (Contd.)**

| Drug | Indication | Contraindications/cautions | Side effects | Drug route | Perioperative drug dose |
|---|---|---|---|---|---|
| **Cyclizine** (Valoid®) | Nausea; vomiting Labyrinthitis; vertigo Motion sickness Radiation sickness | Ischaemic heart disease, severe heart failure, older patients, and neonates Prostatic hypertrophy, hepatic disease, renal impairment, urinary retention Susceptibility to angle-closure glaucoma Pyloroduodenal obstruction May counteract haemodynamic benefits of opioids | **Common** Drowsiness **Rare** Tachycardia, dysrhythmias, psychomotor impairment, hypotension, rash, tremor Less sedating effect **Frequency unknown** Headache, dry mouth, blurred vision, antimuscarinic effects such as urinary retention GI disturbances | Oral IV injection IM injection | **Nausea & vomiting** <u>Adult dose</u> 50 mg (IV or IM) up to 3 times daily <u>Paediatric dose (slow IV)</u> Child (1 month–6 years): 0.5–1 mg/kg (maximum dose 25 mg) Child (6–11 years): 25 mg Child (12–17 years): 50 mg |

| Ondansetron (Zofran®) | Prophylactically for PONV<br>Treatment of PONV<br>Prophylactically before cytotoxic therapy<br>**Ondansetron has been known to reduce the incidence of postoperative shivering** | Hepatic impairment<br>Pregnancy<br>Breastfeeding<br>**Should not be used in patients with or at risk of QT interval prolongation** | **Common**<br>Headache, flushing constipation, reactions at injection site<br>**Uncommon**<br>Hypotension, movement disorders, seizures, hiccups, chest pain, bradycardia<br>**Rare**<br>Dizziness, transient visual disturbances, suppositories may cause rectal irritation | IV injection<br>IM injection<br>Oral<br>Rectal | **Prevention of PONV**<br>Adult dose<br>4 mg via slow IV injection on induction of anaesthesia<br>Paediatric dose<br>100 mcg/kg via slow IV on induction of anaesthesia (maximum dose 4 mg)<br>**Treatment of PONV**<br>Adult dose<br>4 mg via IM or slow IV injection<br>Paediatric dose<br>100 mcg/kg via slow IV injection (maximum dose 4 mg) |

# Further reading

Joint Formulary Committee (2022). British national formulary. Available at: ℞ https://bnf.nice.org.uk/
Joint Formulary Committee (2022). British national formulary for children. Available at: ℞ https://bnfc.nice.org.uk/
Medicines and Healthcare products Regulatory Agency (2013). Metoclopramide: risk of neurological adverse effects. London: Department of Health.
Scarth E, Smith S (2016). Drugs in anaesthesia and intensive care (5th ed). Oxford: Oxford University Press.

**Table 23.15** Local anaesthetic drugs

| Drug | Indication | Contraindications/cautions | Side effects | Drug route | Perioperative drug dose |
|------|-----------|---------------------------|--------------|------------|------------------------|
| Lidocaine | LA of low toxicity<br>Local infiltration<br>Postoperative analgesia<br>Ventricular arrhythmias<br>Dental procedures with adrenaline | Hypovolaemia, complete heart block, respiratory impairment, impaired cardiac conduction, epilepsy, bradycardia, porphyria, severe shock, myasthenia gravis, older or debilitated patients, hepatic impairment, renal impairment, pregnancy | **Common**<br>Drowsiness, paraesthesia<br>**Rare**<br>Hypersensitivity<br>**With IV use**<br>Respiratory depression, confusion<br>Convulsions, hypotension, and bradycardia | SC injection | **Infiltration anaesthesia**<br>_Adult dose_<br>Doses given according to weight and procedure; maximum dose 200 mg<br>**Local infiltration**<br>_Paediatric dose_<br>Doses given according to weight and procedure; should not be repeated less than every 4 hours |
| Bupivacaine | Peripheral nerve block<br>Local infiltration<br>Epidural anaesthesia<br>Sympathetic block<br>Intrathecal anaesthesia (slow onset, longer acting) | Hypovolaemia, complete heart block, respiratory impairment, impaired cardiac conduction, epilepsy, bradycardia, porphyria, severe shock, myasthenia gravis, older or debilitated patients, hepatic impairment, renal impairment, pregnancy | **Frequency unknown**<br>Arrhythmias, cardiac arrest, tinnitus, blurred vision, drowsiness, feeling of inebriation, sweating, headache, tremors, muscle twitching, hypotension and bradycardia, paraesthesia, pyrexia, restlessness, transient excitation | Intrathecal injection<br>Epidural injection | **Surgical anaesthesia**<br>_Adult dose_<br>Lumbar epidural block: 75–150 mg<br>Caudal epidural block: 50–150 mg<br>Thoracic epidural block: 12.5–50 mg<br>Intrathecal anaesthesia<br>Heavy Marcaine® 10–20 mg<br>_Paediatric dose_<br>Doses adjusted according to product literature and local policy |

| | | | | Surgical anaesthesia |
|---|---|---|---|---|
| **Levobupivacaine** | Peripheral nerve block<br>Local infiltration<br>Epidural anaesthesia<br>Intrathecal anaesthesia<br>(slow onset, longer acting) | Hypovolaemia, complete heart block, respiratory impairment, impaired cardiac conduction, epilepsy, bradycardia, porphyria, severe shock, myasthenia gravis, older or debilitated patients, hepatic impairment, renal impairment, pregnancy<br>Avoid regional anaesthesia if preparation contains preservatives | **Frequency unknown**<br>Cardiac arrest, convulsions, dizziness, nausea, vomiting, anaemia, numbness of the tongue and perioral region, arrhythmias, tinnitus, blurred vision, drowsiness, feeling of inebriation, sweating, headache, tremors, muscle twitching, hypotension and bradycardia, paraesthesia, pyrexia, restlessness, transient excitation | Intrathecal injection<br>Epidural injection | **Adult dose**<br>Adult (lumbar epidural): 50–150 mg given over 5 minutes, dose administered using a 5 mg/mL (0.5%) or 7.5 mg/mL (0.75%) solution<br>Adult (intrathecal injection): 15 mg, dose administered using a 5 mg/mL (0.5%) solution<br>Adult (local infiltration): 2.5–150 mg, dose administered using a 2.5 mg/mL (0.25%) solution<br>**Paediatric dose**<br>Doses adjusted according to product literature and local policy |

*(continued)*

**Table 23.15 (Contd.)**

| Drug | Indication | Contraindications/cautions | Side effects | Drug route | Perioperative drug dose |
|---|---|---|---|---|---|
| **Prilocaine** | LA of low toxicity<br>Intrathecal anaesthesia<br>Nerve block<br>Infiltration anaesthesia | Hypovolaemia, complete heart block<br>Severe or untreated hypertension, severe heart disease, older or debilitated patients, pregnancy, respiratory impairment, impaired cardiac conduction, epilepsy, bradycardia, porphyria, shock, myasthenia gravis, older or debilitated patients, hepatic impairment, renal impairment, pregnancy | **Frequency unknown**<br>Arrhythmias, cardiac arrest, tinnitus, blurred vision, drowsiness, feeling of inebriation, sweating, headache, tremors, muscle twitching, hypotension and bradycardia, paraesthesia, pyrexia, restlessness, transient excitation | Intrathecal injection<br>Regional injection | **Infiltration anaesthesia, nerve block**<br><u>Adult dose</u><br>100–200 mg/min (maximum 400 mg)<br>Intrathecal injection<br>40–60 mg (maximum 80 mg)<br><u>Paediatric dose</u><br>Child (6 months–11 years): Up to 5 mg/kg (maximum of 400 mg)<br>Child (12–17 years): 100–200 mg (maximum of 400 mg) |
| **Ropivacaine** | Surgical anaesthesia<br>Surface anaesthesia<br>Postoperative pain<br>**Less cardiotoxic and less potent than bupivacaine** | Hypovolaemia, complete heart block<br>Severe or untreated hypertension, severe heart disease, older or debilitated patients, pregnancy, respiratory impairment, impaired cardiac conduction, epilepsy, porphyria, bradycardia, shock, myasthenia gravis, older or debilitated patients, hepatic impairment, renal impairment, pregnancy | **Common**<br>Hypertension, pyrexia<br>**Uncommon**<br>Hypothermia, syncope<br>**Frequency unknown**<br>Arrhythmias, cardiac arrest, tinnitus, blurred vision, drowsiness, feeling of inebriation, sweating, headache, tremors, muscle twitching, hypotension and bradycardia, paraesthesia, pyrexia, restlessness, transient excitation | Epidural injection<br>Epidural infusion<br>Regional injection | **Surgical anaesthesia**<br><u>Adult dose</u><br>7.5–225 mg by regional injection<br>**Postoperative pain**<br><u>Adult dose</u><br>Up to 28 mg/hour by epidural infusion<br>**Surgical anaesthesia**<br><u>Paediatric dose</u><br>Doses adjusted according to physical status and nature of procedure. Refer to product literature and local policy |

| Tetracaine | LA for topical application: venepuncture and cannulation | Damaged skin | **Frequency unknown**<br>Localized skin reactions | Topical | **Venepuncture and cannulation**<br>*Paediatric dose*<br>Neonate: apply contents of tube (or appropriate proportion) to site of venepuncture or cannulation; remove after 30 minutes for venepuncture and after 45 minutes for venous cannulation<br>Child (1 month–4 years): apply contents of up to 1 tube (or appropriate proportion) to site of venepuncture or venous cannulation; remove after 30 minutes for venepuncture and after 45 minutes for venous cannulation<br>Child (5–17 years): apply up to 5 tubes (applied at separate sites at a single time or appropriate proportion) to site of venepuncture or cannulation; remove gel and dressing after 30 minutes for venepuncture and after 45 minutes for venous cannulation |

*(continued)*

**Table 23.15 (Contd.)**

| Drug | Indication | Contraindications/cautions | Side effects | Drug route | Perioperative drug dose |
|------|-----------|---------------------------|--------------|------------|------------------------|
| EMLA | LA (lidocaine and prilocaine) for topical application venepuncture and cannulation | Cardiac disorders, epilepsy, methaemoglobinaemia<br><br>Caution advised with atopic dermatitis<br><br>Should only be applied to intact skin | **Common**<br>Transient local skin reactions, mild sensation of burning, itching or warmth at the treated area during treatment of genital mucosa or leg ulcers<br><br>**Uncommon**<br>Irritation of the treated skin<br><br>**Rare**<br>Allergic reactions, methaemoglobinaemia, dot-shaped bleeding on the treated area (particularly on children) | Topical | **Venepuncture and cannulation**<br>*Paediatric dose*<br>Neonates (up to 2 months) up to 1 g of cream on a skin area not larger than 10 cm². Application time: 1 hour maximum. Maximum of one single dose in any 24-hour period<br>Infants (3–11 months): up to 2 g of cream on skin area not larger than 20 cm². Application time: 1 hour, maximum of 4 hours<br>Children (1–5 years): up to 10 g of cream on skin area not larger than 100 cm². Application time: 1 hour, maximum of 5 hours<br>Children (6–11 years): up to 20 g of cream on skin area not larger than 200 cm². Application time: 1 hour, maximum of 5 hours |

## Further reading

Electronic Medicines Compendium (2018). Emla cream 5%. Available at: ℘ https://www.medicines.org.uk/emc/product/871/pil
Joint Formulary Committee (2022). British national formulary. Available at: ℘ https://bnf.nice.org.uk/
Joint Formulary Committee (2022). British national formulary for children. Available at: ℘ https://bnfc.nice.org.uk/
Scarth E, Smith S (2016). Drugs in anaesthesia and intensive care (5th ed.). Oxford: Oxford University Press.

**Table 23.16** Antibacterial drugs

| Drug | Indication | Contraindications/cautions | Side effects | Drug route | Perioperative drug dose |
|------|-----------|---------------------------|--------------|-----------|------------------------|
| **Penicillin** | | | | | |
| **Amoxicillin** | Broad-spectrum antibiotic for Gram-positive and Gram-negative bacteria<br><br>Susceptible infections—urinary tract infections, otitis media, sinusitis, uncomplicated community acquired pneumonia, salmonellosis, oral infections | Renal impairment; penicillin hypersensitivity; history of allergic reactions; acute lymphocytic leukaemia; chronic lymphocytic leukaemia; cytomegalovirus infection; glandular fever; maintain adequate hydration with high doses | Nausea; vomiting; anaphylaxis; angioedema; diarrhoea; fever; hypersensitivity reactions; joint pains; rashes; serum sickness-like reaction; urticaria<br><br>**Rare**<br>Cerebral irritation; CNS toxicity | IV injection<br>IV infusion<br>IM injection<br>Oral | Child dose: 125–250 mg 3 times a day<br>Adult dose: 500–1000 mg every 8 hours |
| **Ampicillin** | Broad-spectrum antibiotic for Gram-positive and Gram-negative bacteria<br><br>Susceptible infections—bronchitis, urinary tract infections, otitis media, sinusitis, uncomplicated community-acquired pneumonia, salmonellosis. | Renal impairment; penicillin hypersensitivity; history of allergic reactions; acute lymphocytic leukaemia; chronic lymphocytic leukaemia; cytomegalovirus infection; glandular fever | Nausea; vomiting; anaphylaxis; angioedema; diarrhoea; fever; hypersensitivity reactions; joint pains; rashes; serum sickness-like reaction; urticaria<br><br>**Rare**<br>Cerebral irritation; CNS toxicity | IV injection<br>IV infusion<br>IM injection<br>Oral | Child dose: 125–500 mg 4 times a day<br>Adult dose: 0.5–1 g every 6 hours |

(continued)

**Table 23.16 (Contd.)**

| Drug | Indication | Contraindications/cautions | Side effects | Drug route | Perioperative drug dose |
|---|---|---|---|---|---|
| **Benzylpenicillin sodium** | Broad-spectrum antibiotic for Gram-positive and Gram-negative bacteria Susceptible infections—throat infections, otitis media cellulitis, pneumonia, endocarditis, anthrax, meningitis | Renal impairment; penicillin hypersensitivity; history of allergic reactions; acenocoumarol, methotrexate, phenindione, warfarin | Nausea; vomiting; anaphylaxis; angioedema; diarrhoea; fever; hypersensitivity reactions; joint pains; rashes; serum sickness-like reaction; urticaria **Rare** Cerebral irritation; CNS toxicity | IV injection IV infusion IM injection | Child dose: 50 mg/kg every 4–12 hours Adult dose: 0.6–1.2 g every 6 hours |
| **Co-amoxiclav** | Broad-spectrum antibiotic for Gram-positive and Gram-negative bacteria Infections due to beta-lactamase-producing strains (where amoxicillin alone not appropriate), including respiratory tract infections, bone and joint infections, genitourinary and abdominal infections, cellulitis, and animal bites | Renal impairment; hepatic impairment; penicillin hypersensitivity; history of allergic reactions; acute lymphocytic leukaemia; chronic lymphocytic leukaemia; cytomegalovirus infection; glandular fever; maintain adequate hydration with high doses; acenocoumarol, methotrexate, phenindione, warfarin | Nausea; vomiting; anaphylaxis; angioedema; diarrhoea; fever; hypersensitivity reactions; joint pains; rashes; serum sickness-like reaction; urticaria **Rare** Cerebral irritation; CNS toxicity | IV injection IV infusion Oral | **IV injection or infusion** Child dose: 30 mg/kg every 8–12 hours Adult dose: 1.2 g every 8 hours **Oral** Child and adult dose: 125–250 mg dependent on infection |

| Drug | Indication | Cautions | Side effects | Routes | Dose |
|---|---|---|---|---|---|
| Co-fluampicil | Broad-spectrum antibiotic for Gram-positive and Gram-negative bacteria. Mixed/severe infections involving beta-lactamase-producing staphylococci | Renal impairment; hepatic impairment; penicillin hypersensitivity; acute lymphocytic leukaemia; chronic lymphocytic leukaemia; cytomegalovirus infection; glandular fever | Nausea; vomiting; anaphylaxis; angioedema; diarrhoea; fever; hypersensitivity reactions; joint pains; rashes; serum sickness-like reaction; urticaria; GI disturbances **Rare** Cerebral irritation; CNS toxicity | IV injection<br>IV infusion<br>IM injection<br>Oral | Child dose: 125–250 mg every 6 hour. Adult dose: 250 mg every 6 hours |
| Flucloxacillin | Narrow-spectrum antibiotic for Gram-positive bacteria. Infections due to beta-lactamase-producing staphylococci including otitis externa, adjunct in pneumonia, adjunct in impetigo, adjunct in cellulitis, surgical prophylaxis | Renal impairment; hepatic impairment; penicillin hypersensitivity | Anaphylaxis; angioedema; diarrhoea; fever; hypersensitivity reactions; joint pains; rashes; serum sickness-like reaction; urticaria; GI disturbances **Rare** Cerebral irritation; CNS toxicity, hepatitis | IV injection<br>IV infusion<br>IM injection<br>Oral | **Oral**<br>Child dose: 62.5–250 mg 4 times a day<br>Adult dose: 250–500 mg 4 times a day<br>**IM injection**<br>Adult dose: 250–500 mg every 6 hours<br>**IV injection or infusion**<br>Adult dose 0.25–2 g every 6 hours |

(continued)

**Table 23.16 (Contd.)**

| Drug | Indication | Contraindications/cautions | Side effects | Drug route | Perioperative drug dose |
|------|-----------|---------------------------|--------------|-----------|------------------------|
| **Phenoxymethyl-penicillin** | Oral infections, tonsillitis, otitis media, erysipelas, cellulitis. Prevention of reoccurrence of rheumatic fever, streptococcal infection | Acenocoumarol, methotrexate, phenindione, warfarin | Anaphylaxis; angioedema; diarrhoea; fever; hypersensitivity reactions; joint pains; rashes; serum sickness-like reaction; urticaria **Rare** Cerebral irritation; CNS toxicity | Oral | **Oral** Child dose: 62.5–500 mg 4 times a day Adult dose: 500 mg–1 g every 6 hours |
| **Piperacillin (with tazobactam)** | Broad-spectrum antibiotic for Gram-positive and Gram-negative bacteria used for pneumonia, septicaemia, complicated urinary tract infection/skin/soft tissue infections, neutropenic patients | Renal impairment, penicillin hypersensitivity, pregnancy, breastfeeding | Nausea, vomiting, diarrhoea Sore throat; rash; joint pains; urticaria Rarely hepatitis, abdominal pain, constipation, jaundice **Rare** Abdominal pain; eosinophilia; hepatitis | IV infusion | Adult dose: 4.5 g every 6–8 hours |

| | | | |
|---|---|---|---|
| **Ticarcillin (with clavulanic acid)** | Infections due to *Pseudomonas* and *Proteus* spp. | Renal impairment; penicillin hypersensitivity; hepatic impairment, history of allergic reactions; acute lymphocytic leukaemia; chronic lymphocytic leukaemia; cytomegalovirus infection; glandular fever | Anaphylaxis; angioedema; diarrhoea; fever; hypersensitivity reactions; joint pains; rashes; serum sickness-like reaction; urticaria<br><br>**Rare**<br>Cerebral irritation; CNS toxicity | IV infusion | Adult dose: 3.2 g every 6–8 hours |
| *Cephalosporins and beta-lactam antibiotics* | | | | | |
| **Ceftazidime** | Antibacterials that attach to penicillin binding proteins to interrupt cell wall biosynthesis. Infections due to sensitive Gram-positive and Gram-negative bacteria UTI, septicaemia, pneumonia, meningitis, surgical prophylaxis | Cephalosporin hypersensitivity; renal impairment; pregnancy; breastfeeding; hepatic impairment. | Nausea and vomiting; abdominal discomfort; diarrhoea; headache; pruritus; rash, urticaria, anaphylaxis; jaundice; thrombocytopenia sleep disturbances, confusion, hallucinations, hypertonia, dizziness<br><br>**Rare**<br>Acute kidney injury | IV injection<br>IV infusion<br>IM injection | Surgical prophylaxis<br>Adult dose: 1 g by IV injection on induction of anaesthesia. |

(continued)

**Table 23.16** (Contd.)

| Drug | Indication | Contraindications/cautions | Side effects | Drug route | Perioperative drug dose |
|---|---|---|---|---|---|
| **Cefuroxime** | Antibacterials that attach to penicillin binding proteins to interrupt cell wall biosynthesis. Surgical prophylaxis<br><br>Infections due to sensitive Gram-positive and Gram-negative bacteria<br><br>Lyme disease, urinary tract infection, pyelonephritis, surgical prophylaxis | Cephalosporin hypersensitivity; renal impairment; breastfeeding | Nausea and vomiting; abdominal discomfort; diarrhoea; headache; pruritus; rash; urticaria, anaphylaxis; jaundice; thrombocytopenia<br><br>Sleep disturbances, confusion, hallucinations, hypertonia, dizziness | IV injection<br><br>IV infusion<br><br>IM injection<br><br>Oral | Oral<br>Child dose: 10 mg/kg–250 mg (twice a day)<br>Adult dose: 250 mg twice a day<br>IV infusion/injection or IM injection<br>Child dose: 20 mg/kg every 8 hours<br>Adult dose: 750 mg–1.5 mg every 6–8 hours. |
| **Imipenem (with cilastatin)** | Infections due to sensitive Aerobic and anaerobic Gram-positive and Gram-negative bacteria<br><br>Hospital-acquired septicaemia, pseudomonas infections | Cephalosporin hypersensitivity; renal impairment; pregnancy; breastfeeding; CNS disorders; epilepsy. | Diarrhoea; eosinophilia; nausea; rash; vomiting<br>**Rare**<br>Confusion; dizziness; drowsiness; hallucinations; hypotension; leucopenia; myoclonic activity; seizures; thrombocytopenia; thrombocytosis | IV infusion | Adult dose: 500 mg every 6 hours |

**Tetracyclines**

| | | | |
|---|---|---|---|
| **Tetracycline** | Broad-spectrum antibiotic. Susceptible infections—chlamydia, rickettsia, mycoplasma, rosacea, acne | Hepatic impairment; myasthenia gravis; history of allergic reactions; breastfeeding | Nausea, vomiting, diarrhoea; renal impairment; hepatic impairment; dysphagia; oesophageal irritation; urticaria; rash; headache; tooth staining; increased ICP | Oral | Child dose: 250 mg 4 times a day Adult dose: 250–500 mg 4 times a day |

**Aminoglycosides**

| | | | | |
|---|---|---|---|---|
| **Gentamicin** | Bacterial eye infection, bacterial infection in otitis externa, septicaemia, meningitis, and other CNS infections | Renal impairment Pregnancy; elderly; neonates and infants Myasthenia gravis May prolong the effect of non-depolarizing muscle relaxants Should be administered by injection for systemic infection | Nephrotoxicity; vestibular and auditory damage; blood disorders Nausea; vomiting; rash; headache; colitis Altered liver function | IV injection IV infusion IM injection Drops to eye and ear Intrathecal injection | Drops (eye)—1 drop every 2 hours Drops (ear) 2–3 drops 4/5 times a day IM injection 1 mg/kg every 12 hours IV infusion 3–5 mg/kg dived into 3 doses |

(continued)

**Table 23.16 (Contd.)**

| Drug | Indication | Contraindications/cautions | Side effects | Drug route | Perioperative drug dose |
|---|---|---|---|---|---|
| *Macrolides* | | | | | |
| **Erythromycin** | Susceptible infections in patients with penicillin hypersensitivity—respiratory tract infections, skin and oral infections, and *Campylobacter* enteritis. Also lime disease, early syphilis, uncomplicated genital chlamydia | Hepatic impairment; renal impairment Breastfeeding; porphyria; neonates May potentiate the action of midazolam, warfarin, digoxin | Abdominal discomfort; diarrhoea; nausea; vomiting. GI side effects. | IV infusion Oral | **Oral** Child dose: 125–500 mg 4 times a day Adult dose: 250–500 mg 4 times a day **IV infusion** Child dose: 12.5 mg/kg every 6 hours Adult dose: 6.25 mg/kg every 6 hours |
| **Clarithromycin** | Infections associated with the respiratory tract; skin and tissue infections; otitis media *Helicobacter pylori* | Hepatic impairment; renal impairment Breastfeeding; porphyria; neonates May potentiate the action of midazolam, warfarin, digoxin | Nausea, vomiting, diarrhoea, hepatitis, dyspepsia, headache, smell and taste disturbances, glossitis Rarely hearing loss, jaundice, pancreatitis, chest pain, arrhythmias | IV infusion Oral | **Oral** Child dose: 62.5–250 mg twice a day Adult dose: 250–500 mg twice a day |

**Quinolones**

| | | | | |
|---|---|---|---|---|
| **Ciprofloxacin** | Infections associated with the respiratory, urinary and GI tract; skin, joint, eye, ear, nose, throat; septicaemia; pelvic and intra-abdominal infection | Myasthenia gravis; pregnancy; breastfeeding; epilepsy; renal impairment; children | Nausea, vomiting, diarrhoea, abdominal pain; rash; headache<br>Rarely anorexia; confusion; drowsiness; restlessness; anxiety<br>Rarely convulsions when taking NSAIDs | IV infusion; Oral | 200–400 mg daily via IV infusion |
| **Metronidazole** | Anaerobic bacteria infections and protozoa<br>Surgical prophylaxis, anaerobic infections, *Helicobacter* infection, alternative to penicillin, fistulating Crohn's disease, leg ulcers and pressure sores, bacterial vaginosis | Hepatic impairment; pregnancy; breastfeeding; porphyria; alcohol<br>May prolong the effect of vecuronium | Nausea, vomiting, diarrhoea, anorexia, taste alterations, rash, darkening of urine<br>Rarely hepatitis, pancreatitis, jaundice, dizziness, headache, drowsiness, ataxia | IV Infusion; Oral; PR | **Oral**<br>Child dose: 7.5 mg/kg every 12 hours<br>Adult dose: 400 mg every 8 hours<br>**PR**<br>Child dose: 125 mg–1 g 3 times a day<br>Adult dose: 1 g 3 times a day<br>**IV infusion**<br>Adult dose: 500 mg every 8 hours |

## Further reading

Joint Formulary Committee (2022). British national formulary. Available at: ℗ https://bnf.nice.org.uk/

Joint Formulary Committee (2022). British national formulary for children. Available at: ℗ https://bnf.nice.org.uk/

Scarth E, Smith S (2016). Drugs in anaesthesia and intensive care (5th ed). Oxford: Oxford University Press.

**Table 23.17** Corticosteroid drugs

| Drug | Indication | Contraindications/cautions | Side effects | Drug route | Common dose |
|------|-----------|---------------------------|-------------|-----------|------------|
| **Predni solone** | Acute exacerbation of COPD, severe or mild croup that might cause complications (before transfer to hospital), mild to moderate acute asthma, severe or life-threatening acute asthma, local treatment of inflammation, suppression of inflammatory and allergic disorders, idiopathic thrombocytopenic purpura, eczematous inflammation in otitis externa, ulcerative colitis, Crohn's disease, neuritic pain or weakness heralding rapid onset of permanent nerve damage (during reversal reactions multibacillary leprosy). | Congestive heart failure; diabetes mellitus; diverticulitis; epilepsy; glaucoma; history of steroid myopathy; history of TB or X-ray changes; hypertension; hypothyroidism; infection (particularly untreated); long-term use; myasthenia gravis; ocular herpes simplex (risk of corneal perforation); osteoporosis (in children); osteoporosis (post-menopausal women and the elderly at risk) (in adults); peptic ulcer; psychiatric reactions; recent intestinal anastomoses; recent MI (rupture reported); severe affective disorders (particularly if history of steroid-induced psychosis); thromboembolic disorders; ulcerative colitis | **Common or very common** Anxiety; behaviour abnormal; cataract subcapsular; cognitive impairment; Cushing's syndrome; electrolyte imbalance; fatigue; fluid retention; GI discomfort; headache; healing impaired; hirsutism; hypertension; increased risk of infection; menstrual cycle irregularities; mood altered; nausea; osteoporosis; peptic ulcer; psychotic disorder; skin reactions; sleep disorders; weight increased **Uncommon** Adrenal suppression: alkalosis hypokalaemic; appetite increased; bone fractures; diabetic control impaired; eye disorders; glaucoma: haemorrhage; heart failure; hyperhidrosis; hypotension; leucocytosis; myopathy; osteonecrosis; pancreatitis; papilloedema; seizure; thromboembolism; TB reactivation; vertigo; vision blurred | Oral suspension, oral solution, ear drops, eye drops, enema | Adult by mouth 2.5–30 mg (for suppression of inflammatory and allergic disorders) Child by mouth 1–2 mg/kg IM injection for adult 25–100 mg 1–2 times a week for inflammatory suppression |

| Dexa metha sone | Suppression of inflammatory and allergic disorders, local treatment of inflammation, mild/ severe croup, congenital adrenal hyperplasia, adjunctive treatment of bacterial meningitis, symptom control of anorexia in palliative care | Congestive heart failure; diabetes mellitus; diverticulitis; epilepsy; glaucoma (including a family history of or susceptibility to); history of steroid myopathy; history of TB or X-ray changes; hypertension; hypothyroidism; infection, long-term use; myasthenia gravis; ocular herpes simplex (risk of corneal perforation); osteoporosis (in children); osteoporosis (post-menopausal women and the elderly at risk) (in adults); peptic ulcer; psychiatric reactions; recent intestinal anastomoses; recent MI (rupture reported) severe affective disorders (particularly if history of steroid-induced psychosis); thromboembolic disorders; ulcerative colitis | **Common or very common** Anxiety; behaviour abnormal; cataract subcapsular; cognitive impairment; Cushing's syndrome; electrolyte imbalance; fatigue; fluid retention; GI discomfort; headache; healing impaired; hirsutism; hypertension; increased risk of infection; menstrual cycle irregularities; mood altered; nausea; osteoporosis; peptic ulcer; psychotic disorder; skin reactions; sleep disorders; weight increased **Uncommon** Adrenal suppression; alkalosis hypokalaemic; appetite increased; bone fractures; diabetic control impaired; eye disorders; glaucoma; haemorrhage; heart failure; hyperhidrosis; hypotension; leucocytosis; myopathy; osteonecrosis; pancreatitis; papilloedema; seizure; thromboembolism; TB reactivation; vertigo; vision blurred | Capsule, oral suspension, oral solution, eye drops | **Suppression of inflammatory and allergic disorders** By mouth for adult: 0.5–10 mg daily **Local inflammation of joints** By intra-articular injection for adult: 0.3–3.3 mg, where appropriate **Mild croup** By mouth for child: 150 mcg/kg for 1 dose |

(continued)

**Table 23.17 (Contd.)**

| Drug | Indication | Contraindications/cautions | Side effects | Drug route | Common dose |
|---|---|---|---|---|---|
| **Hydro cortisone** | Thyrotoxic crisis, adrenocortical insufficiency resulting from septic shock, acute hypersensitivity reactions such as angioedema of the upper respiratory tract and anaphylaxis, corticosteroid replacement, in patients who have taken >10 mg prednisolone daily (or equivalent) within 3 months of minor surgery under GA/moderate or major surgery, adrenocortical insufficiency | Congestive heart failure; diabetes mellitus; diverticulitis; epilepsy; glaucoma; history of steroid myopathy; history of TB or X-ray changes; hypertension; hypothyroidism; infection; long-term use; myasthenia gravis; ocular herpes simplex (risk of corneal perforation); osteoporosis (in children); osteoporosis (post-menopausal women and the elderly at risk) (in adults); peptic ulcer; psychiatric reactions; recent intestinal anastomoses; recent MI (rupture reported); severe affective disorders (particularly if history of steroid-induced psychosis); thromboembolic disorders; ulcerative colitis | Anxiety; behaviour abnormal; cataract subcapsular; cognitive impairment; Cushing's syndrome; electrolyte imbalance; fatigue; fluid retention; GI discomfort; headache; healing impaired; hirsutism; hypertension; increased risk of infection; menstrual cycle irregularities; mood altered; nausea; osteoporosis; peptic ulcer; psychotic disorder; skin reactions; sleep disorders; weight increased  Adrenal suppression; alkalosis hypokalaemic; appetite increased; bone fractures; diabetic control impaired; eye disorders; glaucoma; haemorrhage; heart failure; hyperhidrosis; hypotension; leucocytosis; myopathy; osteonecrosis; pancreatitis; papilloedema; seizure; thromboembolism; TB reactivation; vertigo; vision blurred | Capsule, oral suspension, oral solution, liquid, cream, ointment | **Corticosteroid replacement, in patients who have taken >10 mg prednisolone daily (or equivalent) within 3 months of minor surgery under general anaesthesia**  By IV injection, or by IV infusion  For adult: initially 25–50 mg, to be administered at induction of surgery, the patient's usual oral corticosteroid dose is recommended after surgery |

| Fludro cortisone | Neuropathic postural hypotension, Mineralocorticoid replacement in adrenocortical insufficiency, Adrenocortical insufficiency resulting from septic shock (in combination with hydrocortisone) | Avoid injections containing benzyl alcohol in neonates (in neonates); avoid live virus vaccines in those receiving immunosuppressive doses (serum antibody response diminished); systemic infection (unless specific therapy given); congestive heart failure; diabetes mellitus (including a family history of); diverticulitis; epilepsy; glaucoma | Anxiety; behaviour abnormal; cataract subcapsular; cognitive impairment; Cushing's syndrome; electrolyte imbalance; fatigue; fluid retention; GI discomfort; headache; healing impaired; hirsutism; hypertension; increased risk of infection; menstrual cycle irregularities; mood altered; nausea; osteoporosis; peptic ulcer; psychotic disorder; skin reactions; sleep disorders; weight increased | Tablet, capsule, oral suspension | **Neuropathic postural hypotension** By mouth for adult: 100–400 mcg daily **Mineralocorticoid replacement in adrenocortical insufficiency by mouth** For adult: 50–300 mcg once daily |
|---|---|---|---|---|---|

## Further reading

Joint Formulary Committee (2022). British national formulary. Available at: ℗ https://bnf.nice.org.uk/

Joint Formulary Committee (2022). British national formulary for children. Available at: ℗ https://bnfc.nice.org.uk/

Scarth E, Smith S (2016). Drugs in anaesthesia and intensive care (5th ed.). Oxford: Oxford University Press.

**Table 23.18** Bronchodilating drugs

| Drug | Indication | Contraindications/ cautions | Side effects | Drug route | Perioperative drug dose |
|------|-----------|----------------------------|--------------|-----------|------------------------|
| **Aminophylline (Phyllocontin®)** | Severe acute asthma; acute COPD; chronic asthma; reversible airway obstruction | Cardiac disease; epilepsy; fever; hypertension; hyperthyroidism | GI disturbances Nausea Headache Insomnia Tachycardia Palpitation Arrhythmias Convulsions if given rapidly by IV injection | IV injection IV infusion Oral | **Adult dose** 5 mg/kg (250–500 mg) by slow IV injection **Child dose** 250 mg/kg by slow IV injection |
| **Salbutamol (Ventolin®)** | Asthma; prophylaxis of allergen or exercise-induced bronchospasm; acute asthma; chronic asthma **There is a possibility that salbutamol potentiates non-depolarizing muscle relaxing drugs** | Arrhythmias, cardiovascular disease, diabetes, hypertension, hyperthyroidism, hypokalaemia | Angioedema, arrhythmias, behavioural disturbances, collapse, fine tremor, headache, muscle cramps, myocardial ischaemia, palpitation, rash, sleep disturbance, tachycardia, urticaria, nausea | SC injection IM injection IV injection IV infusion Inhalation of aerosol | **Adult dose (acute bronchospasm)** 200 mcg via inhalational **Child dose (severe asthma)** By inhalation of nebulized solution Child 1 month–4 years: 2.5 mg, every 20–30 minutes or when required Child 5–11 years: 2.5–5 mg, repeat every 20–30 minutes or when required Child 12–17 years: 5 mg, repeat every 20–30 minutes or when required |

| | | | |
|---|---|---|---|
| **Salmeterol** | For patients requiring long-term bronchodilator therapy<br><br>Reversible airway obstruction, nocturnal asthma, prevention of exercise-induced bronchospasm, chronic asthma | Severe pre-eclampsia, arrhythmias, cardiovascular disease<br><br>Diabetes, hypertension, hyperthyroidism, hypokalaemia, susceptibility to QT-interval prolongation. | Angioedema, arrhythmias, behavioural disturbance, collapse, fine tremor, headache, hyperglycaemia, hypersensitivity reaction, ketoacidosis, muscle cramps, myocardial ischaemia, palpitations | Inhalation of aerosol or powder | 50–100 mcg twice a day |
| **Theophylline** | Chronic asthma; reversible airway obstruction; severe acute asthma | Cardiac arrhythmias; cardiac disease; elderly; epilepsy; hyperthyroidism; peptic ulcer; risk of hypokalaemia | Arrhythmias, CNS stimulation, convulsion, diarrhoea, gastric irritation, headache, insomnia, nausea, palpitation, tachycardia, vomiting, hepatic impairment | Oral | **Child dose**<br>60–500 mg every 12 hours<br>**Adult dose**<br>250–500 mg every 12 hours |

(continued)

**Table 23.18 (Contd.)**

| Drug | Indication | Contraindications/cautions | Side effects | Drug route | Perioperative drug dose |
|------|-----------|---------------------------|--------------|-----------|------------------------|
| **Ipratropium bromide** | Reversible airway obstruction; COPD; acute bronchospasm; acute asthma; rhinorrhoea-associated with allergic and non-allergic rhinitis | Bladder outflow obstruction, paradoxical bronchospasm, prostatic hyperplasia | Constipation, cough, diarrhoea, dry mouth, GI motility disorder, headache, sinusitis, nasal dryness, epistaxis, nasal irritation | Aerosol inhalation Nebulized inhalation | **Aerosol inhalation** Child dose: 20–40 mcg 3 times a day Adult dose: 20–40 mcg 3–4 times a day **Nebulized inhalation** Adult dose: 250–500 mcg 3–4 times a day |

## Further reading

Joint Formulary Committee (2022). British national formulary. Available at: ᐩ https://bnf.nice.org.uk/
Joint Formulary Committee (2022). British national formulary for children. Available at: ᐩ https://bnfc.nice.org.uk/
Scarth E, Smith S (2016). Drugs in anaesthesia and intensive care (5th ed). Oxford: Oxford University Press.

**Table 23.19** Nitrates

| Drug | Indication | Contraindications/cautions | Side effects | Drug route | Perioperative drug dose |
|------|-----------|----------------------------|--------------|------------|--------------------------|
| **Glyceryl trinitrate** | Prophylaxis and treatment of angina | Hypotension<br>Hypovolaemia<br>Obstructive heart failure<br>Cardiomyopathy<br>Aortic stenosis<br>Mitral stenosis<br>Cardiac tamponade<br>Raised ICP<br>Hypothermia<br>Hypoxaemia | Postural hypotension<br>Dizziness<br>Syncope<br>Tachycardia<br>Headache | Sublingual tablet<br>Sublingual spray<br>IV infusion<br>Transdermal | **Adult (sublingual tablet)**<br>0.3–1 mg<br>**Adult (sublingual spray)**<br>1–2 sprays<br>**Adult (IV infusion)**<br>10–200 mcg/min |

(continued)

**Table 23.19 (Contd.)**

| Drug | Indication | Contraindications/cautions | Side effects | Drug route | Perioperative drug dose |
|---|---|---|---|---|---|
| **Isosorbide dinitrate** | Prophylaxis and treatment of angina | Hypotension<br>Hypovolaemia<br>Obstructive heart failure<br>Cardiomyopathy<br>Aortic stenosis<br>Mitral stenosis<br>Cardiac tamponade<br>Raised ICP<br>Hypothermia<br>Hypoxaemia | Postural hypotension<br>Dizziness<br>Syncope<br>Tachycardia<br>Headache | Oral tablet<br>Sublingual spray<br>IV infusion | **Adult (oral)**<br>30–120 mg daily divided into doses<br>**Adult (sublingual spray)**<br>1–3 sprays<br>**Adult (IV infusion)**<br>2–10 mg/hour |

## Further reading

Joint Formulary Committee (2022). British national formulary. Available at: ⅋ https://bnf.nice.org.uk/
Joint Formulary Committee (2022). British national formulary for children. Available at: ⅋ https://bnfc.nice.org.uk/
Scarth E, Smith S (2016). Drugs in anaesthesia and intensive care (5th ed). Oxford: Oxford University Press.

**Table 23.20** Calcium channel blockers

| Drug | Indication | Contraindications/cautions | Side effects | Drug route | Perioperative drug dose |
|------|-----------|---------------------------|--------------|-----------|------------------------|
| **Amlodipine** | Hypertension Prophylaxis of angina | Aortic stenosis Unstable angina Cardiogenic shock | Dizziness Abdominal pain Headache Fatigue Palpitations Nausea Sleep disturbances GI disturbances Dry mouth | Oral tablet | **Adult (oral)** 5 mg twice daily, maximum 10 mg/day |
| **Nimodipine** | Treating ischaemic neurological issues following haemorrhagic CVA | Unstable angina MI in last month Hypotension Raised ICP Cerebral oedema | Nausea & vomiting Dizziness Confusion Agitation | IV infusion Oral tablet | **Adult (IV infusion)** 1 mg/hour for first hour; if no severe BP drop, increased to 2 mg/hour **Adult (oral)** 60 mg 4-hourly |

(continued)

**Table 23.20 (Contd.)**

| Drug | Indication | Contraindications/cautions | Side effects | Drug route | Perioperative drug dose |
|------|-----------|---------------------------|--------------|-----------|------------------------|
| **Verapamil** | Hypertension<br>Prophylaxis of angina<br>Supraventricular tachycardia | Acute porphyrias<br>Atrial fibrillation or flutter<br>Acute phase MI<br>Heart failure<br>Wolff–Parkinson–White syndrome<br>Bradycardia<br>Cardiogenic shock<br>Hypotension<br>Second- and third-degree AV block | Constipation<br>Dizziness<br>Abdominal pain<br>Headache<br>Fatigue<br>Palpitations<br>Nausea & vomiting<br>Sleep disturbances<br>GI disturbances<br>Dry mouth | IV injection<br>Oral | **Adult (IV)**<br>5–10 mg over 2 minutes |

# Further reading

Joint Formulary Committee (2022). British national formulary. Available at: Ⓜ https://bnf.nice.org.uk/
Ritter JM, Flower RJ, Henderson G, et al. (2015). Rang & Dale's pharmacology (8th ed.). Edinburgh: Churchill Livingstone.
Scarth E, Smith S (2016). Drugs in anaesthesia and intensive care (5th ed.). Oxford: Oxford University Press.

**Table 23.21** Inotropic sympathomimetics

| Drug | Indication | Contraindications/cautions | Side effects | Drug route | Perioperative drug dose |
|------|-----------|---------------------------|-------------|-----------|------------------------|
| **Adrenaline** | Acute anaphylaxis<br>Cardiac arrest | Cor pulmonale<br>Arteriosclerosis<br>Cerebrovascular disease<br>Diabetes mellitus<br>Arrhythmias<br>Obstructive cardiomyopathy<br>Ischaemic heart disease<br>Hypercalcaemia<br>Hypokalaemia | Angina<br>Cold peripheries<br>Anxiety<br>Confusion<br>Arrhythmias<br>Dyspnoea<br>Dizziness<br>Dry mouth | IV infusion<br>IV injection<br>IM injection | **Adult (IV infusion for anaphylaxis)**<br>50 mcg (1 in 10,000)<br>**Adult (IV for cardiac arrest)**<br>1 mg every 3–5 minutes |
| **Dobutamine** | Inotropic support in sepsis<br>During cardiac surgery<br>Post MI<br>Cardiogenic shock | Hypercapnia<br>Hypovolaemia<br>Phaeochromocytoma<br>Ischaemic heart failure<br>Acute heart failure<br>Arrhythmias<br>Acute phase MI | Arrhythmias<br>Anxiety<br>Hypertension<br>Chest pain<br>Bronchospasm<br>Phlebitis<br>Tachycardia | IV infusion | **Adult (IV infusion)**<br>2.5–10 mcg/kg/min titrated for response |

(continued)

**Table 23.21 (Contd.)**

| Drug | Indication | Contraindications/cautions | Side effects | Drug route | Perioperative drug dose |
|---|---|---|---|---|---|
| **Dopamine** | Cardiogenic shock post MI<br>Cardiac surgery | Hypertension<br>Correct hypovolaemia<br>Hyperthyroidism<br>Keep dose low in shock due to MI | Dyspnoea<br>Headache<br>Chest pain<br>Tachycardia<br>Hypotension<br>Nausea & vomiting<br>Palpitation | IV infusion | **Adult (IV infusion)**<br>2–5 mcg/kg/min |
| **Dopexamine** | Cardiac surgery associated heart failure<br>Exacerbations of chronic heart failure | Aortic stenosis<br>Cardiomyopathy<br>Thrombocytopenia<br>Phaeochromocytoma<br>Hypertension<br>Correct hypovolaemia<br>Hyperthyroidism<br>Hyperglycaemia<br>Hypokalaemia<br>Angina<br>MI | Arrhythmias<br>Angina<br>Dyspnoea<br>Bradycardia<br>MI<br>Nausea & vomiting<br>Sweating<br>Tachycardia<br>Headache<br>Reversible thrombocytopenia | IV infusion | **Adult (IV infusion)**<br>0.5–6 mcg/kg/min in 0.5–1.0 mcg/kg/min increments |

## Further reading

Joint Formulary Committee (2022). British national formulary. Available at: ℜ https://bnf.nice.org.uk/
Ritter JM, Flower RJ, Henderson G, et al. (2015). Rang & Dale's pharmacology (8th ed.). Edinburgh: Churchill Livingstone.
Scarth E, Smith S (2016). Drugs in anaesthesia and intensive care (5th ed.). Oxford: Oxford University Press.

**Table 23.22** Vasoconstrictor sympathomimetic drugs

| Drug | Indication | Contraindications/ cautions | Side effects | Drug route | Perioperative drug dose |
|---|---|---|---|---|---|
| **Ephedrine** | Reversal of hypotension from general, spinal, or epidural anaesthesia<br>Narcolepsy<br>Hiccups<br>Nasal decongestant | Breastfeeding, diabetes mellitus<br>Ischaemic heart disease, hyperthyroidism, hypertension, older patients, pregnancy, susceptibility to angle-closure glaucoma, acute urine retention in prostatic hypertrophy, renal impairment | **Common**<br>Headache, nausea, anorexia, anginal pain, hypersalivation, dyspnoea, dizziness and flushing, sweating, psychoses, urine retention, vomiting, vasoconstriction with hypertension and hypotension, difficulty in micturition, confusion, anxiety, arrhythmias, tremor, tachycardia, restlessness<br>**Rare**<br>Angle-closure glaucoma<br>**Frequency unknown**<br>Bradycardia | Slow IV injection, Intranasal<br>Oral | **Adult dose (slow IV injection)**<br>Reversal of hypotension 3–6 mg (according to response) every 3–4 minutes (maximum 9 mg per dose). Maximum course dose 30 mg<br>**Paediatric dose (slow IV injection)**<br>Child 1–11 years: 500–750 mcg/kg every 3–4 minutes (according to response). Maximum course dose 30 mg<br>Child 12–17 years: 3–7.5 mg (according to response) every 3–4 minutes (maximum 9 mg per dose). Maximum course dose 30 mg |

(continued)

**Table 23.22 (Contd.)**

| Drug | Indication | Contraindications/ cautions | Side effects | Drug route | Perioperative drug dose |
|------|------------|------------------------------|--------------|------------|--------------------------|
| Metaraminol | Acute hypotension during general/ spinal anaesthesia<br><br>Hypotension during cardiopulmonary bypass surgery<br><br>Priapism<br><br>**Tissue necrosis may occur following extravascular injection** | Hypertension, pregnancy<br><br>Coronary, mesenteric, or peripheral vascular thrombosis, cirrhosis, older patients, hypoxia, hypercapnia, breastfeeding<br><br>**Extravasation at injection site may cause necrosis** | **Frequency unknown**<br>Tachycardia, arrhythmias, hypertension, headache, dizziness, bradycardia, peripheral ischaemia, nausea, palpitation, anxiety, anorexia, tremor, vomiting, weakness<br><br>Excessive vasopressor response may cause a prolonged rise in BP | IV injection<br>IV infusion<br>Intraca vermosal injection | **Adult dose**<br><u>Acute hypotension</u><br>15–100 mg via IV infusion (according to response)<br><u>Emergency treatment of acute hypotension</u><br>0.5–5 mg via IV injection; then 15–100 mg via IV infusion according to response<br>**Paediatric dose**<br><u>Acute hypotension</u><br>Child 12–17 years: 15–100 mg via IV infusion (according to response)<br><u>Emergency treatment of acute hypotension</u><br>Child 12–17 years: 0.5–5 mg via IV injection; then 15–100 mg via IV infusion (according to response) |

| Noradrenaline | Acute hypotension Septic shock | Hypertension, pregnancy Coronary, mesenteric, or peripheral vascular thrombosis, uncorrected hypovolaemia, older patients Extravasation at injection site may cause necrosis | **Frequency unknown** Hypertension, headache, arrhythmias, bradycardia, peripheral ischaemia, nausea, tremor, palpitations, hypoxia, vomiting, weakness, dyspnoea, confusion, urinary retention | IV injection IV infusion Intracardiac injection | **Adult dose** <u>Acute hypotension</u> 0.16–0.33 mL/min via IV infusion, according to response; dose applies to a solution containing noradrenaline 40 mcg/mL only; refer to product literature **Paediatric dose** <u>Acute hypotension/septic shock</u> Neonate: 20–100 ng/kg/min (maximum dose 1 mcg/kg/min), according to response; refer to product literature Child: 20–100 ng/kg/min (maximum dose 1 mcg/kg/min), according to response; refer to product literature |

# Further reading

Joint Formulary Committee (2022). British national formulary. Available at: ⊗ https://bnf.nice.org.uk/

Joint Formulary Committee (2022). British national formulary for children. Available at: ⊗ https://bnfc.nice.org.uk/

Scarth E, Smith S (2016). Drugs in anaesthesia and intensive care (5th ed). Oxford: Oxford University Press.

# Chapter 24

# Fluid therapy and replacement

# Fluid therapy

Fluid compartment equilibrium may be disrupted by anaesthesia, surgery, and illness.[1]

## Perioperative considerations
- Patients undergoing surgery may need IV fluid to replace abnormal losses of fluid from bleeding or 'third-space' loss. This usually amounts to approximately 10 mL/kg/hour of surgery.
- Third-space loss refers to fluid lost from the circulation during surgery:
  - Some of this fluid forms oedema in the area of the operation.
  - Some fluid may be lost into the bowel.
  - Fluid loss can also occur from evaporation.
- A general rule is that more replacement fluid will be required for major surgery.
- Measurement of pulse rate, CVP, and urine output will help to guide fluid therapy intraoperatively.
- These losses are usually replaced by balanced salt solutions (e.g. Hartmann's solution).
- Preoperative fasting does not necessitate fluid replacement unless fasting has been prolonged.
- Perioperative hypovolaemia and dehydration are associated with morbidity.
- Warming fluid perioperatively can help to regulate temperature, particularly for infants and neonates.

## Indications of fluid therapy
- Replacement and expansion of circulating volume.
- Replace existing fluid and electrolyte deficits.
- Maintain fluid and electrolyte balance.
- Replace surgical fluid and electrolyte losses.

## General complications/side effects
- Fluid overload leading to oedema.
- Electrolyte imbalances.
- Coagulopathies.
- DVT.
- Patient discomfort.
- Infection.
- Air embolism.

## Types of fluids
- *Colloids*: large-molecule fluids used primarily for short-term fluid expansion.
- *Crystalloids*: smaller-molecule fluids used for fluid (i.e. water) and electrolyte replacement.
- *Blood and blood products*: for long-term circulating volume and red cell replacement and treatment of coagulopathies.

## Fluids after surgery

While it is often indicated that caution should be exercised in the use of crystalloid fluids containing sodium in the immediate postoperative period, all fluid (and associated electrolyte) replacement should be determined on the basis of individual patient requirements.

## Reference

1. Freedman R, Herbert L, O'Donnell A, et al. (eds) (2022). Oxford handbook of anaesthesia (5th ed). Oxford: Oxford University Press.

## Further reading

Joint Formulary Committee (2022). British national formulary. Available at: ℘ https://bnf.nice.org.uk/

Joint Formulary Committee (2022). British national formulary for children. Available at: ℘ https://bnfc.nice.org.uk/

# Crystalloids

Crystalloids are fluids comprising of water with either electrolytes and/or glucose used in the treatment or prevention of fluid, electrolyte, and small-scale calorific deficits. They are effective with few adverse side effects.[1]

### Indications—general

For surgical patients in all perioperative phases:
- To meet normal fluid and electrolyte requirements.
- To replenish substantial deficits, for example, from preoperative fasting, or continuing losses through surgical trauma.
- When adequate oral intake is not possible, for example, nausea and vomiting.

When IV administration is not possible, fluid can be administered by SC infusion (hypodermoclysis), though this route is highly unlikely to be used in a perioperative setting. See Box 24.1 for 24-hour fluid replacements.

> **Box 24.1 Formula for 24-hour fluid requirements**
> The following formula is commonly used to calculate the maintenance fluid requirements for a 24-hour period in adults:
>
> 1500 mL for the first 20 kg of body weight + 20 mL/kg
>
> for each additional kg

*The individual circumstances of each patient should be considered but as a general guide*
- Replace ECF depletion with saline.
- Rehydrate with glucose.

### Perioperative considerations

See Table 24.1.
- Balanced salt solutions (Hartmann's solution) are usually the first-line fluid replacement therapy within the perioperative period.
- Saline 0.9% is used for electrolyte replacement.
- Saline 0.9% is also used for hypovolaemic resuscitation.
- Glucose 5% is used for restore dehydration.
- Glucose 10%, 20%, and 50% can be used to promote normoglycaemia.[1]

### Reference

1. Freedman R, Herbert L, O'Donnell A, et al. (eds) (2022). Oxford handbook of anaesthesia (5th ed). Oxford: Oxford University Press.

**Table 24.1** Serum and crystalloid electrolyte composition

| | | $Na^+$ | $K^+$ | $Ca^{2+}$ | $Cl^-$ | $HCO_3^-$ | pH |
|---|---|---|---|---|---|---|---|
| **Serum value** | | 135–145 mmol/L | 3.1–5.1 mmol/L | 4.5–5.8 mmol/L | 95–105 mmol/L | 22–26 mmol/L | 7.35–7.45 |
| **Fluid** | **Indications** | | | | | | |
| Hartmann's | In place of NaCl during surgery | 131 | 5 | 4 | 112 | 129 | 6.5 |
| 0.9% saline | Sodium depletion | 154 | 0 | 0 | 154 | 0 | 5.5 |
| Dextrose-saline | Water and sodium depletion | 31 | 0 | 0 | 31 | 0 | 4.5 |
| 5% glucose | Water depletion emergency treatment of hyper kalaemia[a] Treatment of diabetic ketoacidosis[b] | | 0 | 0 | 0 | 0 | 4.1 |

[a] As part of a treatment regimen with calcium, bicarbonate, and insulin.

[b] Following correction of hyperglycaemia and must be accompanied by an ongoing insulin infusion.

## Further reading

Joint Formulary Committee (2022). British national formulary. Available at: ℘ https://bnf.nice.org.uk/

Joint Formulary Committee (2022). British national formulary for children. Available at: ℘ https://bnfc.nice.org.uk/

National Institute for Health and Care Excellence (2020). Intravenous fluid therapy in children and young people in hospital. NICE guideline [NG29]. Available at: ℘ https://www.nice.org.uk/guidance/ng29

Norfolk D (2013). Transfusion ten commandments. In: Handbook of transfusion medicine (5th ed). Joint United Kingdom (UK) Blood Transfusion and Tissue Transplantation Services. Sheffield: The Stationary Office.

Royal College of Anaesthetists (2019). Chapter 3: guidelines for the provision of anaesthesia services for intraoperative care. London: Royal College of Anaesthetists.

Royal College of Anaesthetists (2019). Chapter 4: guidelines for the provision of postoperative care. London: Royal College of Anaesthetists.

Royal College of Anaesthetists (2020). Chapter 5: guidelines for the provision of emergency anaesthesia. London: Royal College of Anaesthetists.

# Colloids

Colloids are fluids that, because of their large molecular weight, remain within the vascular fluid compartment for extended periods of time and thus expand and maintain circulating volume. The duration of action of colloids is determined by physiochemical properties, integrity of capillary membrane, and by metabolic and clearance pharmacokinetics.[1] Colloid solutions are sometimes used when losses are heavy.

### Indications
- Immediate, short-term treatment of non-haemorrhagic hypovolaemia and shock.

### Contraindications
- Long-term maintenance of plasma volume in burns or peritonitis.
- Known hypersensitivity to any constituents.

### Cautions
- Cardiac disease.
- Liver disease.
- Renal impairment.
- Monitoring of urine output required.

### Side effects
- Hypersensitivity reactions.
- Anaphylactoid reactions.
- Increased bleed times—transient.

### Types of colloids
See Table 24.2.

Colloids in general use fall into one of three groups:

*Dextrans*
- Hypertonic fluids exerting powerful osmotic effect.
- Can interfere with cross-matching—blood samples should be taken before starting dextran infusions.

*Gelatins*
- Isotonic.
- Circulatory half-life of 2–3 hours.
- Associated with anaphylactoid reactions.

*Starches*
- Hypertonic.
- Expand volume on approximate 1:1 ratio.
- Improved haemodynamic status for up to 24 hours.

### Reference
1. Freedman R, Herbert L, O'Donnell A, et al. (eds) (2022). Oxford handbook of anaesthesia (5th ed). Oxford: Oxford University Press.

**Table 24.2** Colloid fluids overview

| Fluid | Molecular weight | Dose |
|---|---|---|
| **Dextrans** | | |
| Dextran 40® | 40,000 | Initially 500–1000 mL |
| Dextran 70® | 70,000 | Initially 500–1000 mL rapidly, followed by 500 mL if necessary to a maximum total dosage of 20 mL/kg during initial 24 hours |
| **Gelatins** | | |
| e.g. Gelofusine®, Haemaccel® | 30,000–35,000 | 3.5–4% 500–1000 mL |
| **Starches** | | |
| Hetastarch | 450,000 | 1500 mL (max. 24 hours) |
| Pentastrach | 200,000 | 6% 2500 mL (max. 24 hours) 10% 1500 mL (max. 24 hours) |
| Tetrastarch e.g. Venofundin®, Voluven® | 130,000 | 50 mg/kg |

# Further reading

Joint Formulary Committee (2022). British national formulary. Available at: ✍ https://bnf.nice.org.uk/

Joint Formulary Committee (2022). British national formulary for children. Available at: ✍ https://bnfc.nice.org.uk/

National Institute for Health and Care Excellence (2020). Intravenous fluid therapy in children and young people in hospital. NICE guideline [NG29]. Available at: ✍ https://www.nice.org.uk/guidance/ng29

Norfolk D (2013). Transfusion ten commandments. In: Handbook of transfusion medicine (5th ed). Joint United Kingdom (UK) Blood Transfusion and Tissue Transplantation Services. Sheffield: The Stationary Office.

Royal College of Anaesthetists (2019). Chapter 3: guidelines for the provision of anaesthesia services for intraoperative care. London: Royal College of Anaesthetists.

Royal College of Anaesthetists (2019). Chapter 4: guidelines for the provision of postoperative care. London: Royal College of Anaesthetists.

Royal College of Anaesthetists (2020). Chapter 5: guidelines for the provision of emergency anaesthesia. London: Royal College of Anaesthetists.

# Blood

- Blood is a fluid, connective tissue comprising of cells and cell fragments—approximately 45% blood volume suspended in a fluid medium (plasma approximately 55% blood volume).
- The primary purpose of blood is to ensure adequate oxygenation of tissue. Failure to perfuse tissue results in shock.

### General indications for transfusion

- Restoration of circulating volume when a loss >30% of circulating blood volume has occurred—class 3 and class 4 shock.
- Where patients are symptomatic following blood loss of <30% and/or further blood loss is expected.
- Chronic anaemia.

> Crystalloid and colloid administration should be avoided during uncontrolled haemorrhage, unless there is profound hypotension and no imminent availability of blood products.[1]

### Adverse effects

- Transfusion reactions.
- Haemolytic transfusion reaction—caused by ABO incompatibility.
- Delayed extravascular haemolysis—caused by Rh or non-ABO reactions.
- Non-haemolytic febrile reaction.
- Anaphylactoid reaction—caused by recipient reaction to plasma proteins in donor blood.
- Anaphylactic reaction—rare.
- Transmission of infection.
- Transfusion-related acute lung injury (TRALI).
- With massive transfusions, that is, transfusion of entire circulating volume within 24 hours:
- Hyperkalaemia and acidosis.
- Coagulopathies including disseminated intravascular coagulation (DIC).
- Citrate toxicity ± citrate toxicity.
- Impaired tissue $O_2$ delivery.

### Autologous transfusion

The re-transfusion of the patients own blood/blood products is collected in one of four ways:

- *Preoperative autologous donation (PAD)*:
  - Blood donated in the weeks leading up to surgery.
  - Tested and stored as with allogenic blood, but is reserved for that patient alone.
  - Reinfused with the same safeguards for prescribed allogenic blood/products.

- *Acute normovolaemic haemodilution (ANH):*
  - Whole blood is taken from the patient (1–3 units) prior to the start of surgery (often post induction).
  - Blood volume restored with acellular fluid.
  - Blood is reinfused to the patient when needed or at the end of surgery.
- *Intraoperative cell salvage (ICS)* (➔ see Intraoperative cell salvage, p. 732):
  - Blood lost during surgery is collected, red blood cells (RBCs) are separated from the whole blood and washed (with saline).
  - Resulting RBCs suspended in saline reinfused to the patient when needed or at the end of surgery.
- *Postoperative cell salvage (PCS)* (➔ see Postoperative cell salvage, p. 736):
  - Postoperative blood loss is collected.
  - Depending on the system in use, salvaged blood is either filtered (unwashed system) or RBCs are separated out and washed as with ICS (washed system).
  - Resulting product reinfused as required.

### Indications
- A clean operative field.
- Anticipated blood loss >1000 mL or >20% Epstein–Barr virus[1] (ICS).
- Anticipated postoperative blood loss >500 mL for PCS.
- Low Hb/risk factors for bleeding.
- Rare blood type/multiple antibodies.
- Patients with objections to receiving allogenic blood.

### Contraindications
- Contamination within the surgical field.
- Malignancy within the surgical field (where is no indication of metastatic spread).
- Non-IV materials should not be present within the surgical site.
- Sickle cell anaemia.

### Cautions
- Use of leuco-depletion filters is recommended in obstetrics and malignancy.

## Reference

1. Association of Anaesthetists of Great Britain and Ireland (2016). AAGBI guidelines: the use of blood components and their alternatives. *Anaesthesia*, 71(7):829-842.

## Further reading

National Institute for Health and Care Excellence (2015). Blood transfusion. NICE guideline [NG24]. Available at: ⚘ https://www.nice.org.uk/Guidance/NG24

# Patient blood management

Preoperative anaemia and perioperative RBC transfusion carry significant consequences when it comes to surgical outcomes.[1] The three pillars of patient blood management (PBM) are aimed at reducing the use of blood transfusion and improving the patient's clinical outcome and safety. PBM focuses on the timely and appropriate management of anaemia, prevention of blood loss, and restrictive transfusion where appropriate.

PBM is paramount to reduce the risks posed by perioperative anaemia and blood transfusions, which have been associated with increased morbidity and mortality in surgical patients. The systematic application of a PBM programme in the perioperative period has been consistently found to improve patients' clinical outcomes following surgery.[2]

> Although PBM usually refers to surgical patients, its clinical use has gradually evolved and now also refers to medical conditions.

The principles of PBM help structure the interventions and decisions relating to anaemia and blood transfusion, and represent a paradigm shift towards a more considered approach to blood transfusion, recognizing its risks, preventatives, and alternatives. Box 24.2 outlines the measures that should be taken in patients at risk of bleeding perioperatively.

> **Box 24.2 Action points for patients who are expected to bleed during surgery**
>
> *Preoperative*
> - Preoperative Hb should be measured, recorded, and optimized as required.
> - Elective surgery should be postponed in patients with untreated anaemia.
> - Review and consider stopping antiplatelet and anticoagulant medication 7 days prior to surgery.
> - The use of minimally invasive or laparoscopic surgical technique should be considered.
>
> *Intraoperative*
> - Position patient carefully to maintain venous drainage.
> - Maintain patient temperature >36°C.
> - Consider cell salvage if anticipated blood loss >500 mL.
> - Consider tranexamic acid 1 g if anticipated blood loss >500 mL.
> - Apply restrictive transfusion threshold (Hb 70–80 g/L depending on patient characteristics and haemodynamics).
> - Consider use of topical haemostatic agents.
>
> *Postoperative*
> - Maintain $O_2$ delivery, targeting $O_2$ saturation levels >95%.
> - Single unit blood transfusion policy—reassess Hb and clinical need between units.
> - Postoperative drains or cell salvage.
>
> *Source:* data from Association of Anaesthetists of Great Britain and Ireland (2016). AAGBI guidelines: the use of blood components and their alternatives. Anaesthesia, 71:829–842.

## Patient information

Patients who may have or who have received a transfusion and their family members or carers must be offered verbal and written information explaining the points in Box 24.3.

> **Box 24.3 Information for patients**
> - The reason for the transfusion.
> - The risks and benefits.
> - The transfusion process.
> - Any transfusion needs specific to them.
> - Any alternatives that are available, and how they might reduce their need for a transfusion.
> - That they are no longer eligible to donate blood.
> - That they are encouraged to ask questions.
>
> Source: data from NICE (2015) Blood transfusion. Available at: ℅ https://www.nice.org.uk/Guidance/NG24

Norfolk[3] outlines the 'Transfusion ten commandments' that underpin safe and effective transfusion practice:

1. Blood transfusion should only be used when the benefits outweigh the risks and there are no appropriate alternatives.
2. Results of laboratory tests are not the sole deciding factor for transfusion.
3. Transfusion decisions should be based on clinical assessment supported by evidence-based clinical guidelines.
4. Not all anaemic patients need transfusion.
5. The patient must be informed of the risks, benefits, and alternatives to transfusion and provide informed consent.
6. The reason for transfusion should be documented in the patient's clinical record.
7. Timely provision of blood component support in major haemorrhage can improve outcome so communication and team work are essential.
8. *Failure to check patient identity can be fatal*. Patients must wear an ID band with name, date of birth, and ID number. Patient identity must be confirmed at every stage of the transfusion process. Patient identifiers on the ID band and blood pack must be identical. If there is any discrepancy, *DO NOT TRANSFUSE*.
9. The patient must be monitored during the transfusion.
10. Education and training underpin safe transfusion practice.

## References

1. Butcher A, Richards T (2017). Cornerstones of patient blood management in surgery. Transfusion Medicine, 28(2):150–157.
2. Franchini M, Marano G, Veropalumbo E, et al. (2019). Patient blood management: a revolutionary approach to transfusion medicine. Blood Transfusion, 17(3):191–195.
3. Norfolk D (2013). Transfusion ten commandments. In: Handbook of transfusion medicine (5th ed). Joint United Kingdom (UK) Blood Transfusion and Tissue Transplantation Services. Sheffield: The Stationary Office.

## Further reading

Association of Anaesthetists of Great Britain and Ireland (2016). AAGBI guidelines: the use of blood components and their alternatives. Anaesthesia, 71(7):829–842.
National Institute for Health and Care Excellence (2015). Blood transfusion. NICE guideline [NG24]. Available at: ℅ https://www.nice.org.uk/Guidance/NG24

# Managing patients who refuse blood transfusion

Every patient has the right to be treated with respect and staff must be sensitive to their individual needs, acknowledging their values, beliefs, and cultural background.[1] Many patients are anxious about the risks associated with blood transfusion whereas others decline a transfusion based on their religious beliefs.

> A patient does not need to give a reason for refusing consent, but where refusal may lead to a loss of life or serious harm, it is good practice to ensure that there is specific documentation, both of the fact of refusal and of the patient's awareness of its potential consequences.[2]

Jehovah's Witnesses regard blood as sacred and decline treatment with allogeneic (donor) blood (red cells, white cells, platelets, and plasma).

Many carry an advance directive prohibiting blood transfusion, which is legally binding. When confronted with such patients, blood-free major surgery will be a great challenge to both the anaesthetic and surgical teams. It is important to explain all the available options to patients who refuse blood and blood products. This might also include a decision regarding available blood conservation measures, for example, ICS and PCS.

Other procedures that are usually acceptable to Jehovah's Witness patients might include:

- Cell salvage, either during surgery or postoperatively
- Renal replacement therapy with haemodialysis or haemofiltration
- Cardiopulmonary bypass
- Extracorporeal membrane oxygenation.

Jehovah's Witness patients who accept cell salvage may specifically request that the system be set up to allow for continuous connectivity.[3]

The children of Jehovah's Witnesses requiring blood transfusion present the most difficult management problem. The well-being of the child is paramount and if, after full parental consultation, blood is refused, the surgeon should make use of the law to protect the child's interests:

- If a child needs blood in an emergency, despite the surgeon's best efforts to contain haemorrhage, it should be given.
- Children aged 16 or 17 can give legally valid consent for medical treatment whereas children under this age can give consent if they are deemed to *Gillick competent*.
- The High Court is the most appropriate forum to achieve a fair and impartial hearing when conflict arises between religious, medical, and ethical opinions.

All effort should be made to avoid the use of blood products where refused. Alternatives to consider include:

- Minimize blood sampling
- Maintain normothermia
- Tranexamic acid
- Acute normovolaemic haemodilution if patient suitable.

For management see Box 24.4.

### Box 24.4  Managing patients who refuse blood

- Respect the values, beliefs, and cultural backgrounds of all patients.
- Anxiety about the risks of transfusion can be allayed by candid discussion.
- Blood Transfusion Services provide a range of quality assured information resources for patients, parents, and their families.
- Jehovah's Witnesses decline transfusion of specific blood products so it is essential to clearly establish the preference of each patient.
- Advance decisions/lasting power of attorney for health and welfare must be respected.
- No one can give consent on behalf of a patient with mental capacity.
- Emergency or critically ill patients with temporary incapacity must be given life-saving transfusion unless there is clear evidence of prior refusal such as a valid advance decision/lasting power of attorney.
- Where the parents or legal guardians of a child <16 years refuse essential blood transfusion, a Specific Issue Order (or national equivalent) can be rapidly obtained from a High Court.

*Source:* data from Norfolk D (2013) Transfusion Ten Commandments. Handbook of Transfusion Medicine (5th Ed). Joint United Kingdom (UK) Blood Transfusion and Tissue Transplantation Services; The Stationary Office: Sheffield

## References

1. Norfolk D (2013). Transfusion ten commandments. In: Handbook of transfusion medicine (5th ed). Joint United Kingdom (UK) Blood Transfusion and Tissue Transplantation Services. Sheffield: The Stationary Office.
2. Association of Anaesthetists of Great Britain and Ireland (2018). Anaesthesia and peri-operative care for Jehovah's Witnesses and patients who refuse blood. Available at: ℘ https://onlinelibrary.wiley.com/doi/full/10.1111/anae.14441
3. UK Cell Salvage Action Group (2018). Intraoperative cell salvage education workbook (2nd ed). Available at: ℘ https://www.transfusionguidelines.org/transfusion-practice/uk-cell-salvage-action-group/cell-salvage-competency-workbooks

## Further reading

Association of Anaesthetists of Great Britain and Ireland (2018). Cell salvage for peri-operative blood conservation. Available at: ℘ https://onlinelibrary.wiley.com/doi/full/10.1111/anae.14331
Association of Anaesthetists of Great Britain and Ireland (2016). AAGBI guidelines: the use of blood components and their alternatives. Anaesthesia, 71(7):829–842.
Franchini M, Marano G, Veropalumbo E, et al. (2019). Patient blood management: a revolutionary approach to transfusion medicine. Blood Transfusion, 17(3):191–195.
Joint Formulary Committee (2022). British national formulary. Available at: ℘ https://bnf.nice.org.uk/
National Institute for Health and Care Excellence (2015). Blood transfusion. NICE guideline [NG24]. Available at: ℘ https://www.nice.org.uk/Guidance/NG24
Royal College of Surgeons (2018). Caring for patients who refuse blood. London: Royal College of Surgeons.

# Intraoperative cell salvage

ICS is a technique whereby blood lost during a surgical procedure is collected and processed to produce autologous (the patient's own) RBCs for reinfusion. ICS can greatly reduce the need to transfuse allogeneic (donor) RBCs.

ICS is effective (and may be life-saving) in elective or emergency high blood loss surgery and management of major haemorrhage.

## Indications

- Elective and emergency surgical procedures.
- Where there is a 'clean' surgical field.
- Anticipated blood loss of >1000 mL or 20% of the patients' estimated total blood volume.

ICS may also be considered when the patient has:
- A low preoperative Hb level
- Risk factors for bleeding (e.g. factor deficiencies)
- Rare blood groups or multiple antibodies
- Objections to receiving allogeneic blood (and has consented to ICS).

Alternatives and adjuncts to blood transfusion are most effective when used in combination and as part of a comprehensive PBM programme.[1]

## Contraindications

- Contaminated surgical field (e.g. bowel content).
- Non-IV substances within the surgical field (discontinue ICS and irrigate the wound with IV saline before resuming).
- Heparin-induced thrombocytopenia when heparin is the anticoagulant (acid citrate dextrose may be used as an alternative).

## Warnings

The following have been identified as areas of concern when using ICS:
- The presence of the following contaminants within the surgical field:
  - Infection
  - Gastric/pancreatic secretions
  - Pleural effusions
  - Amniotic fluid.
- Malignant disease (within the surgical field).
- Abnormal RBC disorders (e.g. sickle cell disease).

In these circumstances, ICS should be carried out with caution, avoiding the aspiration of contaminants and at the direction of the lead clinician.

## Equipment

In addition to the ICS machine, the equipment required for ICS includes:
- Anticoagulant: 30,000 IU heparin/1000 mL IV saline or acid citrate dextrose

- Aspiration and anticoagulation line
- Collection reservoir
- Processing set
- Blood giving set/filter (appropriate for the type of surgery).

The procedure also requires a vacuum (some ICS machines have an onboard vacuum) and other equipment generally available within the operating theatre department (e.g. a wide-bore plastic suction tip).

## Procedure

The reinfusion bag should be labelled with an autologous transfusion label that includes handwritten patient details and the expiry time of the ICS blood (see local policy). Throughout the procedure it is important to:
- Maintain a low vacuum (−100 to −200 mmHg) to minimize RBC damage (the vacuum may be increased during excessive bleeding)
- Ensure sufficient anticoagulant is flowing to prevent coagulation
- Avoid aspirating non-IV substances into the system.

The ICS procedure can be divided into four main steps:

### Collection
Blood is aspirated from the surgical field, anticoagulated, and filtered (in the collection reservoir) to remove large debris (e.g. bone fragments).

### Separation
RBCs are separated from whole blood and waste products (e.g. anticoagulant) and concentrated to produce a high haematocrit (>50%).

### Washing
The RBCs are washed with IV saline to remove residual waste products.

> To prevent the reinfusion of potentially harmful contaminants, the minimum wash volume specified by the manufacturer should be used.

### Reinfusion
The RBCs are pumped to a reinfusion bag. Upon reinfusion:
- Check the ICS blood has been prescribed by a clinician.
- Check the patient's identification against the label on the reinfusion bag.
- Check the expiry time of the blood—refer to local policy.
- Use a filter appropriate to the surgical procedure—refer to local policy.
- Monitor the patient for signs of reaction.
- Record the volume/time of the reinfusion in the patient's clinical record.

> ICS blood should not be reinfused under pressure due to the presence of air in the reinfusion bag.

### Drugs that decrease blood loss
- Tranexamic acid is a synthetic derivative of the amino acid lysine that inhibits plasminogen activation, thus preventing impairment of fibrinolysis. There is increased evidence that its use may reduce bleeding in trauma, cardiac surgery, and other major surgery.

- It is contraindicated in fibrinolytic conditions following DIC (unless predominant activation of fibrinolytic system with severe bleeding); history of convulsions; thromboembolic disease.[2,3]
- The use of intraoperative cell salvage and tranexamic acid administration should be considered in all non-obstetric patients where blood loss >500 mL is possible and in traumatic and obstetric major haemorrhage.[3]

### For consideration

- Staff should undergo appropriate training prior to using ICS (a UK ICS competency assessment framework is available).
- ICS should, where possible, be discussed with the patient prior to use.
- ICS only returns RBCs to the patient when massive blood loss occurs, it may also be necessary to transfuse allogeneic blood components.
- Local policy and manufacturers' guidelines should be adhered to.
- Some machines are designed to continue the cell salvage process by salvaging blood lost from the wound postoperatively.

ICS and PCS are usually acceptable to Jehovah's Witness patients.

### References

1. Norfolk D (2013). Transfusion ten commandments. In: Handbook of transfusion medicine (5th ed). Joint United Kingdom (UK) Blood Transfusion and Tissue Transplantation Services. Sheffield: The Stationery Office.
2. National Institute for Health and Care Excellence (2015). Blood transfusion. NICE guideline [NG24]. Available at: ⅍ https://www.nice.org.uk/Guidance/NG24
3. Association of Anaesthetists of Great Britain and Ireland (2016). AAGBI guidelines: the use of blood components and their alternatives. Anaesthesia, 71(7):829–842.

### Further reading

Association of Anaesthetists of Great Britain and Ireland (2018). Cell salvage for peri-operative blood conservation. Available at: ⅍ https://onlinelibrary.wiley.com/doi/full/10.1111/anae.14331
Butcher A, Richards T (2017). Cornerstones of patient blood management in surgery. Transfusion Medicine, 28(2):150–157.
Franchini M, Marano G, Veropalumbo E, et al. (2019). Patient blood management: a revolutionary approach to transfusion medicine. Blood Transfusion, 17(3):191–195.
Joint Formulary Committee (2022). British national formulary. Available at: ⅍ https://bnf.nice.org.uk/
UK Cell Salvage Action Group (2018). Intraoperative cell salvage education workbook (2nd ed). Available at: ⅍ https://www.transfusionguidelines.org/transfusion-practice/uk-cell-salvage-action-group/cell-salvage-competency-workbooks

# Postoperative cell salvage

PCS is a technique whereby blood lost from the wound postoperatively is collected and reinfused. PCS involves either washed systems, which use a machine to produce autologous RBCs, or unwashed systems, which use an autologous wound drain to produce filtered autologous blood. This section relates to the use of unwashed systems (however, the indications and contraindication are the same for washed systems). PCS can reduce the need to transfuse allogeneic RBCs.

### Indications

- Elective and emergency orthopaedic surgical procedures.
- An uncontaminated wound.
- Anticipated postoperative blood loss of 500–1000 mL.

PCS may also be considered when the patient has:
- A low preoperative Hb level
- Risk factors for bleeding (e.g. factor deficiencies)
- Rare blood groups or multiple antibodies
- Objections to receiving allogeneic blood (and has consented to PCS).

### Contraindications

- A contaminated wound (e.g. infection or malignancy).
- Non-IV substances within the wound (e.g. antibiotics not licensed for IV use).

As with ICS, the use of PCS in patients with abnormal RBC disorders, such as sickle cell disease, should be carried out with caution at the direction of the lead clinician.

### Equipment

The PCS system (autologous wound drain) normally comprises:
- Trocar and wound drain tubing
- Collection set—including vacuum system and may include filters
- Reinfusion set—this may be integral to the collection set or a separate reinfusion bag and normally includes filters.

Because PCS systems vary significantly, it is vital that all staff involved in the process have received appropriate training and are competency assessed for each of the devices they use.

### Procedure

The PCS system (and where appropriate the reinfusion bag) should be labelled with an autologous transfusion label that includes handwritten patient details and the expiry time of the PCS blood (see local policy).

The PCS procedure begins within the operating theatre and continues into the recovery area and often onto the ward. The PCS system should be monitored throughout.

The PCS procedure can be divided into three main steps:

*Insertion of the wound drain (within sterile field)*

Prior to insertion of the drain, the surgical site should be irrigated with IV saline. The autologous drain is inserted prior to skin closure using the trocar and the collection set is attached to the drain. Most manufacturers recommend that the drain remain closed (clamped) for 20 minutes following skin closure (especially if a tourniquet has been used).

*Collection*

Following the release of the clamp, blood collects into the PCS system. Because clotting occurs within the wound, the blood that collects in the drain is defibrinated (i.e. depleted of fibrinogen). The lack of fibrinogen in the collected blood prevents coagulation; therefore, anticoagulant is not required for PCS. In some PCS systems, the blood is filtered in the collection set.

During the collection phase it may be necessary to:
• Reprime the vacuum on systems with an intermittent vacuum
• Transfer the collected blood into the reinfusion bag on systems where the reinfusion set is not integral to the collection set.

Staff should be alert to large blood loss and contact the surgeon and/or anaesthetist under these circumstances.

*Reinfusion*

The collected blood is filtered prior to reinfusion. Depending on the system used, the individual responsible for the PCS system may need to attach a filter to the reinfusion set. Upon reinfusion:
• Check the PCS blood has been prescribed by a clinician.
• Check the patient's identification against the label on the PCS system.
• Check the expiry time of the blood (refer to local policy).
• Use the filter specified by the manufacturer.
• Monitor the patient for signs of reaction.
• Record the volume/time of the reinfusion in the patient's clinical record.

PCS blood should not be reinfused under pressure due to the presence of air in the reinfusion bag.

## For consideration

• Staff should undergo appropriate training and be assessed as competent before using PCS.
• PCS should, where possible, be discussed with the patient prior to use.
• When massive blood loss occurs, it may also be necessary to transfuse allogeneic blood components.
• Local policy and manufacturers guidelines should be adhered to.

## Further reading

Association of Anaesthetists of Great Britain and Ireland (2016). AAGBI guidelines: the use of blood components and their alternatives. Anaesthesia, 71(7):829–842.

Association of Anaesthetists of Great Britain and Ireland (2018). Cell salvage for peri-operative blood conservation. Available at: ℘ https://onlinelibrary.wiley.com/doi/full/10.1111/anae.14331

Butcher A, Richards T (2017). Cornerstones of patient blood management in surgery. Transfusion Medicine, 28(2):150–157.

Franchini M, Marano G, Veropalumbo E, et al. (2019). Patient blood management: a revolutionary approach to transfusion medicine. Blood Transfusion, 17(3):191–195.

Joint Formulary Committee (2022). British national formulary. Available at: ℘ https://bnf.nice.org.uk/

National Institute for Health and Care Excellence (2015). Blood transfusion. NICE guideline [NG24]. Available at: ℘ https://www.nice.org.uk/guidance/ng24

Norfolk D (2013). Transfusion ten commandments. In: Handbook of transfusion medicine (5th ed). Joint United Kingdom (UK) Blood Transfusion and Tissue Transplantation Services. Sheffield: The Stationary Office.

UK Cell Salvage Action Group (2018). Intraoperative cell salvage education workbook (2nd ed). Available at: ℘ https://www.transfusionguidelines.org/transfusion-practice/uk-cell-salvage-action-group/cell-salvage-competency-workbooks

# Emergency care

# Principles of emergency care

*Prevention is better than cure.* It is widely accepted that, in a large number of in-hospital emergencies, critically ill patients have presented with a history of physiological deterioration during the preceding hours.[1]

- Deterioration may be prevented by regular assessment and appropriate and timely interventions by suitably trained personnel.
- The introduction of track and trigger systems, such as the NEWS scoring system[2] can help individual practitioners to identify the deteriorating patient.

> If you have doubts about your patient's condition, inform senior staff of your concerns immediately, ensure the patient has patent venous access, administer high-flow $O_2$, and observe continuously for changes to his/her condition.

The **ABCDE** approach to assessment is now recommended to '*treat first that which kills first*' in all critically ill and emergency patients. Each stage of this approach must be assessed, treated as necessary, and re-evaluated before moving on to the next stage. If, during the course of treatment, any unexpected change occurs in the patient's condition, then assessment must begin again at 'A'.

## Initial approach

Is it safe to approach the patient? Do not forget personal safety!

The best immediate assessment of a patient is by talking with him/her. If the patient is unresponsive to voice or touch and not (for example) intubated and ventilated, call for help immediately and begin **ABCDE** assessment:

### Airway

Is the patient's breathing normal/noisy/silent? Noise on inspiration generally indicates partial *upper airway obstruction* (including laryngospasm), wheezing noise on expiration may indicate bronchospasm/partial lower airway obstruction; silence may indicate complete airway obstruction! Check patient's mouth is clear of visible obstruction (e.g. vomit, secretions, foreign bodies, etc.). Remove any secretions or foreign bodies safely (NB: well-fitting dentures should not be removed as they may enable effective airway maintenance). Apply basic manoeuvres to open airway: head tilt/chin lift or jaw thrust; (jaw thrust preferable in infants and trauma victims); place own fingers *only* on bony parts of patient's face or jaw—pressing soft tissues may exacerbate airway obstruction. Reassess. If patient is unconscious (see below) or judged incapable of maintaining own airway, endotracheal intubation utilizing *RSI* (q.v.) should be considered.

### Breathing

*Tachypnoea and dyspnoea are important signs of physiological disturbance and may indicate serious deterioration in the patient's condition.*

Assess patient's respiratory rate, $O_2$ saturation, $ETCO_2$ monitoring (where available), depth, symmetry and equal, bilateral air entry (left:right) when listened to with a stethoscope. Chest/abdominal movement should be observed during respiration—'see-saw' (paradoxical) respiration may indicate complete airway obstruction—and check for central cyanosis/pallor. NB: the presence, or lack of, cyanosis is not always a reliable indicator of hypoxaemia.

- If atypical clinical signs or physiological measurements present, supportive interventions should be considered *urgently*, for example, administer high-flow $O_2$ via non-rebreathing face mask if rate and depth sufficient, if not, assist ventilations using face mask with self-inflating resuscitator bag or Waters circuit (Mapleson C; q.v.).
- If intubated patient exhibits adverse signs, also exclude *DOPES*: (Displaced ETT, Oesophageal intubation, Pneumothorax, Equipment malfunction, Stomach insufflation) and treat as required.
- If tension pneumothorax suspected (asymmetric respiration, unilateral air entry, hyper-resonance and decreasing BP) consider *needle decompression* of the affected side of the chest (see below).
- Reassess the patient following all interventions. If at this stage the patient is not breathing or exhibiting other signs of life (e.g. choking, coughing, moving limbs etc.), the *cardiac arrest team* should be called immediately and treatment protocols for adult or paediatric life support (q.v.) followed.

*Needle decompression*: emergency treatment of tension pneumothorax involving insertion of wide-bore cannula above third rib in midclavicular line into intrapleural space of affected side. Chest drain to be inserted aseptically following resuscitation, and chest X-rays taken.

## Circulation

Assess the patient's pulse, BP, perfusion, urine output, and temperature. Homeostatic mechanisms normally maintain sufficient perfusion of tissues with $O_2$ and nutrients and the removal of waste products. This balance may be affected and hypoperfusion (shock, see Box 25.1) occurs when circulating fluid volume is lost or when mechanical failure or obstruction impedes circulation. *Tachycardia* is a valuable sign of cardiovascular compensation for fluid volume loss but may also be caused by pain, anxiety, exercise, or infection, hence the patient's history along with other signs and parameters must always be taken into consideration during assessment. *Bradycardia* may be associated with respiratory insufficiency (hypoxia and hypercapnia), especially in the drowsy patient. *Hypotension* is a late sign of shock as BP is maintained by autonomic responses until decompensation occurs. *Acute hypertension* may be caused by untreated pain, thyroid toxicity, drug overdose, or autonomic dysreflexia in spinal injuries patients, and should be treated using appropriate medications. Centrally measured *capillary refill time* (see below), urine output (≥0.5–1 mg/kg/hour), and colour of central membranes (e.g. lips) are useful indicators of adequate tissue perfusion; peripheral temperature, colour, and capillary refill (e.g. of nailbeds) may be adversely affected by ambient temperature and hypothermia. Severe hypothermia (≤32°C) may also induce cardiac arrhythmias.

*Capillary refill time*: measurement of tissue perfusion achieved by pressing thumb on patient's sternum or forehead for 5 seconds; blanched skin should reperfuse in the well-hydrated patient within 2 seconds.

*Disability*

Assess patient's level of consciousness and pupil reactions to light (pupils equal and reactive to light). Immediate assessment of consciousness is best achieved using AVPU scale (patient is Alert, patient responds to Voice, patient responds to Pain, patient is Unresponsive), but a thorough neurological assessment requires repeated use of the Glasgow Coma Scale (GCS). An alert patient would normally be assessed as GCS 15; any patient with a GCS of 8 or below (corresponding with P on the AVPU scale) is classed as comatose and assumed incapable of protecting their own airway. Urgent endotracheal intubation should be considered in such cases.

*Exposure*

Perform systematic examination of patient's body, removing wet clothes as necessary to prevent unnecessary cooling, but ensuring maintenance of dignity as far as practicable. Signs such as bleeding from orifices, distended abdomen, possible fractures, surgical wounds, lacerations, and bruising should all be noted as part of the *secondary survey*, along with a detailed history and case note examination when planning further care.

## Other considerations

*Legal*

It is not always possible, or even ethically appropriate, to try and gain informed consent from critically ill or injured patients.

- Under English common law, healthcare professionals working in what they perceive to be the patient's best interests under such circumstances would not normally be required to gain formal consent.
- A possible exception to this might be the presence of a valid *advance directive* ('living will') in which the patient has documented their refusal to consent to certain treatments in specified circumstances.
- 'Do not attempt cardiopulmonary resuscitation' (*DNACPR*) orders are signed and *regularly updated* by the consultant or GP in charge of that patient's care, and are based on a considered decision that any attempt at resuscitation of that patient would not lead to prolonging his or her life at an acceptable quality (futility of treatment).
- This decision is taken by the senior clinician, but good practice recommends that the views of the patient, or relatives, should be sought before the decision is made.
- Unless lasting power of attorney (LPA) has been appointed under the Mental Capacity Act 2005, no person may give or withhold consent to treatment on behalf of another adult.

*Professional and ethical*

While it may seem obvious, it is always worth remembering that the experience of life-threatening illness or injury may cause intense emotional distress in patients and their relatives, as well as to staff, and the behaviour of healthcare practitioners at such times frequently leaves a lasting impression.

For this reason, it is particularly important to ensure that all communications are clear and unambiguous and that the team behaves in a calm and professional manner at all times, and that the rights and sensibilities of the patient and relatives are respected, as far as is practicable under the circumstances.

## Box 25.1 Types of shock

*Hypovolaemic shock*

Arises from loss of circulating volume caused by dehydration (e.g. through poor fluid balance, diarrhoea, vomiting, etc.), burns, or haemorrhage. Characterized by cool, clammy peripheries, pallor, and fast, thready pulses. Hypotension is a *late sign!*

Treatment of dehydration is by fluid and electrolyte replacement. Immediate fluid replacement in severe burns cases is calculated according to formulae, such as Muir and Barclay: [weight (kg) × %burn]/2 = mL colloid IV fluid (e.g. Gelofusine®) per time period (4 hours, 4 hours, 4 hours, 6 hours, 6 hours, 12 hours).

Haemorrhage is treated with oxygenation (to optimize remaining $O_2$ carrying capacity), application of direct pressure (tamponade) where possible, moderate fluid and blood product replacement with urgent surgical intervention where required; the use of tourniquets is discouraged in most cases and rapid, large volume infusions and transfusions are now viewed as being potentially counter-productive in the treatment of haemorrhage, especially following trauma.[3]

*Distributive shock*

Circulating volume is lost into the interstitial tissues through the capillary beds, as in anaphylactic and septic shock. Anaphylactic shock is characterized by a rapid decrease in BP, tachycardia, dyspnoea, wheezing, skin rash, etc. Recommended treatment of severe anaphylaxis involves removal of the offending allergen (e.g. blood transfusion), administration of IM adrenaline 0.5 mg (1:1000 solution) repeated at 5-minute intervals as required, the administration of crystalloid IV fluids if severe hypotension is present, and also IV antihistamines. Advanced airway management may also be required if oedema of the upper airway and bronchospasm are present.

Sepsis is characterized by a steady decrease in BP, tachycardia, tachypnoea, and hypo- or hyperthermia. Septic shock is a complex and potentially grave condition often requiring large volume fluid infusion and multiorgan support in a level 3 critical care facility (ICU).

*Cardiogenic shock*

This results from failure of the heart (due to arrhythmias or other dysfunction) to provide sufficient output to perfuse the tissues adequately. Characterized by decreasing BP, dyspnoea, raised CVP, and cool peripheries. The underlying heart condition should be treated urgently and IV fluids should only be given with extreme caution.

*Obstructive shock*

This results from physical obstruction to the circulation, as in PE, tension pneumothorax, or cardiac tamponade. Successful treatment involves identification of and removal of the cause of the obstruction. In cases of tension pneumothorax this may be relatively simple (◆ see 'Needle decompression', p. 747). Cardiac tamponade can occur as a result of trauma or ventricular rupture, and can be diagnosed by ultrasound and clinical signs such as muffled heart signs. Treatment by needle pericardiocentesis or emergency thoracotomy can be effective, but it is not always possible to achieve decompression and repair promptly, and a poor outcome is common.

# References

1. National Institute for Health and Care Excellence (2020). National Early Warning Score systems that alert to deteriorating adult patients in hospital. Medtech innovation briefing [MIB205]. Available at: ℘ https://www.nice.org.uk/guidance/mib205

2. Royal College of Physicians (2017). National Early Warning Score (NEWS) 2: standardising the assessment of acute illness severity in the NHS. Available at: ℘ https://www.rcplondon.ac.uk/projects/outputs/national-early-warning-score-news-2

3. Tran A, Yates J, Lau A, et al. (2018). Permissive hypotension versus conventional resuscitation strategies in adult trauma patients with hemorrhagic shock: a systematic review and meta-analysis of randomized controlled trials. Journal of Trauma and Acute Care Surgery, 84(5):802–808.

# Further reading

Craig A, Hatfield A (2020). The complete recovery room book (6th ed). Oxford: Oxford University Press.

Department of Health (2016). Mental Capacity Act 2016 (Northern Ireland). Available at: ℘ https://www.health-ni.gov.uk/mca

Freedman R, Herbert L, O'Donnell A, et al. (eds) (2022). Oxford handbook of anaesthesia (5th ed). Oxford: Oxford University Press.

Legislation.gov.uk (2005). Mental Capacity Act 2005. Available at: ℘ https://www.legislation.gov.uk/ukpga/2005/9/contents

National Institute for Health and Care Excellence (2020). Perioperative care in adults. NICE guideline [NG180]. Available at: ℘ https://www.nice.org.uk/guidance/ng180

O'Driscoll BR, Howard LS, Earis J, et al. (2017). BTS guideline for oxygen use in adults in healthcare and emergency settings. Thorax, 72(Suppl 1):ii1-ii90.

Pollard B, Kitchen G (eds) (2017). Handbook of clinical anaesthesia (4th ed). London: CRC Press.

Resuscitation Council (UK) (2021). Advanced life support provider manual (8th ed). London: Resuscitation Council (UK).

Resuscitation Council (UK) (2021). European paediatric life support provider manual (5th ed). London: Resuscitation Council (UK).

Royal College of Anaesthetists (2020). Chapter 5: guidelines for the provision of emergency anaesthesia. London: Royal College of Anaesthetists.

Smith G, Allan A, Gordon PAL, et al. (2012). ALERT™: acute life-threatening events, recognition and treatment (3rd ed). Portsmouth: Portsmouth Hospitals NHS Trust.

# Advanced resuscitation measures

- Basic life support (BLS) should only be interrupted to allow for checking of the ECG rhythm and defibrillation during resuscitation for cardiac arrest.
- The patient's airway and breathing should be maintained using appropriate airway adjuncts and manual ventilation, as described previously. Endotracheal intubation should only be attempted by those with suitable training and experience. Supraglottic airways (e.g. LMA, i-gel®) are recommended for use otherwise.
- Once the patient's airway has been satisfactory secured with either an ETT or supraglottic airway, chest compressions can be delivered continuously.
- IV or intraosseous access should be established promptly to facilitate the administration of drugs and IV fluids.

### Shockable rhythms: defibrillation

- Defibrillation is the internationally recognized treatment for cardiac arrest when the presenting rhythms are either pulseless ventricular tachycardia (VT) or ventricular fibrillation (VF),[1] and should be delivered as soon as the equipment becomes available.
- Safety is paramount when defibrillators are used, as they deliver potentially lethal electrical charges, so these must only be used by *suitably trained personnel*.
- Successful defibrillation requires sufficient electric current to pass through the heart to depolarize the myocardium, thereby terminating uncoordinated activity (fibrillation) and allowing the heart's natural pacemaker to instigate a normal, perfusing rhythm.
- Most defibrillators found in the operating department are of the manual variety and require the operator to analyse the patient's rhythm, then set and deliver the appropriate output charge.
- Automated external defibrillators are becoming increasingly common in wards and public access areas.
- Current guidelines recommend the delivery of a single, maximum power shock in VF/pulseless VT arrests, followed by 2 minutes of CPR, the cycle then being repeated as necessary with *10 mL (1 mg) 1:10,000 adrenaline (IV)* being administered before the *third shock*. It is also recommended that the antiarrhythmic drug *amiodarone* should be used in prolonged (refractory), shockable cardiac arrest rhythms after the third shock has been delivered.[2]

### Non-shockable rhythms

If the presenting rhythm is non-shockable, that is, pulseless electrical activity (PEA) or asystole:

- *10 mL (1 mg) 1:10,000 adrenaline* should be administered immediately and repeated every 3–5 minutes as necessary.
- BLS should be performed continuously until either the patient shows signs of life or all of the potentially reversible causes of cardiac arrest have been considered and treated.

## Potentially reversible causes

### Hypoxia
Ensure adequate and effective ventilation with high-flow $O_2$.

### Hypovolaemia
Establish IV access and administer 250–500 mL bolus of 0.9% sodium chloride or Hartmann's solution ('fluid challenge') and seek surgical opinion if haemorrhage is suspected.

### Hyper/hypokalaemia
Following biochemical testing, correct with potassium supplement (hypo) or insulin/dextrose infusion for potassium abnormality, or replacement of calcium or magnesium salts as necessary. Electrolyte and hydrogen ion (acid–base) levels can be measured swiftly in electronic blood-gas analysers. Blood glucose levels should also be measured and treated if necessary.

### Hypothermia
Rare in hospital inpatients but common in patients brought into the ED by ambulance (especially cases of trauma, overdose, drowning, etc.). If moderate or severe hypothermia present (<35°C), warm air blankets, warmed ventilator gases, and IV fluids should be employed to gradually rewarm the victim. In severe hypothermia, administration of drugs and defibrillation should be deferred following the initial attempts until a more normal temperature is achieved.

### Tension pneumothorax
Characterized by asymmetrical chest movement, hyper-resonance, and absent breath sounds on affected side together with symptoms of shock; must be treated by urgent needle decompression of the affected side (insertion of wide-bore cannula above third rib in midclavicular line) followed by chest drain insertion.

### Tamponade
Suspect in cases of penetrating chest trauma; treat with needle pericardiocentesis or emergency thoracotomy.

### Toxicity
Reactions to or overdose of therapeutic agents must be excluded or treated as required; in cases of poisoning, supportive treatment (CPR, ventilation) should be employed—contact with toxins centre (TOXBASE)[3] may be required to identify suitable antidote once agent identified.

### Thromboembolic
High index of suspicion of PE in surgical cases complicated by contraindication of thrombolysis following major surgery, haemorrhagic strokes, etc.

---

The potentially reversible causes of cardiac arrest should also be considered in cases of prolonged VF/pulseless VT cardiac arrest.

Following successful resuscitation, the patient's care should include the following:
- Continuing ventilatory support to maintain targeted $O_2$ saturation and acid–base balance.
- Capnography.
- Diagnostic 12-lead ECG and continuous three-lead rhythm strip monitoring.
- BP monitoring with inotropic support as necessary.
- Biochemical monitoring of electrolytes, cardiac enzymes, blood gases, etc.
- X-ray imaging of chest.
- The induction of mild hypothermia following resuscitation may demonstrate improved neurological outcomes.
- Following successful return of spontaneous circulation, the patient may be referred for *reperfusion therapy*—coronary artery stenting or thrombolysis.

## References

1. European Resuscitation Council (2021) Adult advanced life support. Available at: https://www. cprguidelines.eu/assets/guidelines/European-Resuscitation-Council-Guidelines-2021-Ad.pdf
2. Resuscitation Council (UK) (2021). Advanced life support providers manual (8th ed). London: Resuscitation Council (UK).
3. TOXBASE. Homepage. Available at: ✍ https://www.toxbase.org

## Further reading

Soar J, Nolan JP, Böttiger BW, et al. (2015). European Resuscitation Council Guidelines for Resuscitation 2015: Section 3. Adult advanced life support. Resuscitation, 95:100–147.

# Cardiac arrest in adults

Cardiac arrest can be defined as the failure of the heart to perfuse the body's tissues, especially those essential to life. In those patients who have suffered cardiac arrest and for whom resuscitation is indicated, *BLS* must be initiated and the cardiac arrest team called *immediately*.

### Basic life support—on finding a collapsed patient

- Ensure personal safety.
- Try to rouse patient by calling or gently shaking; if unresponsive call for help and commence **ABCDE** assessment:
  - **A**: open patient's mouth and check for possible cause of obstruction; perform head tilt/chin lift or, if patient is edentulous or neck trauma is suspected, jaw thrust manoeuvre.
  - **B**: look, listen, and feel for breathing (up to 10 seconds); if not breathing send for cardiac arrest team immediately. Where signs of life are present, support respiration until skilled help arrives. NB: 'mouth-to-mouth' expired air resuscitation is not recommended: self-inflating bag/valve/mask assemblies and pocket masks are both more hygienic and more effective.
  - **C**: assess for circulation (carotid pulse) or signs of life (coughing, purposeful movement, etc.); if none present, commence CPR—cycles of 30 chest compressions of the middle to lower half of victim's sternum (approx. one-third depth of chest) at a rate of 100 per minute, followed by two ventilations (using high-flow $O_2$, self-inflating resuscitator bag and mask or pocket mask, plus oropharyngeal airway if available). If the patient is intubated or secured by a well-fitting LMA, compressions should be continuous.

Attach cardiac monitor or adhesive defibrillator pads when available and initiate defibrillation as appropriate.

The ECG rhythms associated with cardiac arrest are as follows:
- *Pulseless VT* (broad complex rhythm with a rate >100 bpm; Fig. 25.1) or
- *VF* (uncoordinated, coarse or fine, 'bizarre' waveform with no recognizable complexes; Fig. 25.2).
- VF and pulseless VT are classified as the '*shockable*' rhythms.
- *PEA*—electrical activity of the heart might otherwise:
  - Be compatible with life but no effective pulse (cardiac output) is present) or
  - *Asystole* (normally a shallow wavy line on the ECG indicating an absence of electrical activity).
- PEA and asystole are classed as '*non-shockable*'. Correct identification of the rhythm is essential to guide subsequent resuscitation efforts.

In out-of-hospital settings, the majority of adult cardiac arrests are due to primary cardiac events (usually 'heart attacks'—MIs), and the presenting rhythm is, initially, pulseless VT or VF. These rhythms respond well to *early defibrillation* and CPR, and it has been suggested that for every minute defibrillation is delayed, the mortality rate increases by 7–10%.[1]

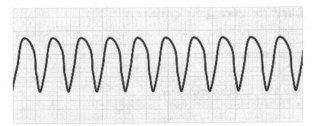

**Fig. 25.1** Ventricular tachycardia.

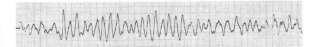

**Fig. 25.2** Ventricular fibrillation.

Reproduced from Myerson S, Choudhury P, and Mitchell A, Emergencies in Cardiology, 2005, with permission from Oxford University Press: Oxford.

In hospital settings the incidence of VF/VT arrests is decreased (<25%), as this figure includes patients admitted for non-cardiac conditions. The majority of patients who arrest in hospitals therefore present with PEA or asystole, and their survival rate is often considerably less, however, and in such cases it is particularly important to treat the *potentially reversible causes* (4Hs and 4Ts; ➲ see Advanced resuscitation measures, p. 746) while performing CPR and administering *10 mL (1 mg) 1:10,000 adrenaline (IV)* every 3–5 minutes.

## Reference

1. Resuscitation Council (UK) (2021). Advanced life support providers manual (8th ed). London: Resuscitation Council (UK).

## Further reading

Perkins G, Brace-McDonnell S (2015). The UK Out of Hospital Cardiac Arrest Outcome (OHCAO) project. Warwick: The OHCAO Project Group. Available at: ℬ http://bmjopen.bmj.com/content/5/10/e008736

# Cardiac arrest in children

Cardiorespiratory arrest in children is rarely due to a primary cardiac event, as in adults, but more usually secondary to *hypoxia* or *hypovolaemia*. Trauma and infection are common causes of hypovolaemia and airway obstruction, while choking is a common occurrence in young children (Box 25.2).

> **Box 25.2 Choking in children**
> - If <1 year old (or small toddler): if coughing is ineffective place child prone on lap with head supported in downwards position and deliver up to five sharp blows with the heel of hand between shoulder blades, followed by sharp compressions with two fingers to lower half of sternum, repeat cycle until foreign body displaced or child loses consciousness, in which event BLS protocol should be followed.
> - In the larger child, encourage coughing and deliver up to five slaps between shoulder blades followed by up to five abdominal thrusts (stand/kneel behind child and place clenched fist between xiphisternum and umbilicus, grasp fist with other hand and pull sharply inwards and upwards).
> - Repeat cycle if ineffective or proceed to BLS if child loses consciousness.

Paediatric physiology readily compensates for respiratory and circulatory failure, so signs such as decreased level of consciousness, bradypnoea, bradycardia, and hypotension indicate that the child is in extremis. It is imperative therefore that clinical signs indicating serious illness in children are recognized and treated promptly to prevent further deterioration. See Box 25.3.

## Signs of serious illness

- **A**: noisy (inspiratory stridor, expiratory wheeze) or silent breathing indicates partial or complete airway obstruction.
- **B**: tachypnoea, bradypnoea (late sign), decreased level of consciousness, increased effort of breathing including grunting, intercostal/subcostal/sternal recession, use of accessory muscles (neck and abdominal muscles, nasal flaring), asymmetrical breathing. NB: young children are diaphragmatic breathers so care is necessary to differentiate normal abdominal movement from obstructive 'see-saw' respiration.
- **C**: tachycardia, hypotension (late sign), bradycardia, pale or mottled skin, cool peripheries, central capillary refill time >2 seconds.

## Advanced airway management

- Endotracheal intubation of seriously ill young children requires great skill to avoid damaging an easily compromised airway and is consequently best left to experienced paediatricians or anaesthetists.
- The formula 'Age in years/4 + 4' is used when sizing ETT IDs for children, but experience suggests that at least one tube size either side of the resulting figure should be at hand when intubating children.

### Box 25.3 Basic life support—on finding a collapsed child

- Ensure safety.
- Gently stimulate.
- Shout for help if no response from child.

**A**: place head in neutral position (<1 year old) or head tilt (older children), open airway with chin lift or jaw thrust; check for foreign bodies or excessive secretions and remove if possible; NB: do not 'finger sweep'. Administer high-flow $O_2$.

**B**: look, listen, and feel for breathing (10 seconds). If absent or inadequate, give five rescue breaths using appropriate size self-inflating bag and mask attached to high-flow $O_2$ where available (use oropharyngeal airways as required); each breath should be delivered slowly (1–1.5 seconds) to avoid gastric distension and diaphragmatic splinting. If adequate respiration present, place child in recovery position.

**C**: check for central pulse (brachial <1 year old, otherwise carotid or femoral) or signs of life (coughing, purposeful movement, etc.); if pulse absent or <60/min commence CPR (ratio 2 breaths (see above) to 15 chest compressions (approx. one-third depth of chest, <1 year old two fingers to middle of sternum, 1–8 years old one hand on mid to lower half of sternum, two hands if larger child). Attach cardiac monitor when available to identify rhythm.

## Calculating child weights

- If the weight of a child is not known, measuring systems that indicate drug dosages and ETT sizes etc. based on the child's height are commercially available (e.g. Broselow system).
- In the absence of these, the following formula is recommended:
  - <1 year old: birth weight (full term) = 3.5 kg, weight at 6 months = 7 kg, weight at 1 year old =10 kg.
  - >1 year old = (age in years + 4) × 2 kg.

## Venous access

- Prompt and reliable venous access is a vital component in the successful resuscitation of children; venous cannulation should be attempted no more than three times in seriously ill children, after which the *intraosseous* route is recommended.
- This involves the insertion of a specialized. needle into the marrow cavity of a long bone, usually medial and inferior to the tibial tubercle (avoiding growth plate).
- This route is effective for both drug and fluid administration, which are most effectively administered using a syringe and three-way tap.

## Fluid resuscitation

- Boluses of 20 mL/kg of warmed 0.9% saline or Hartmann's IV solutions should be administered to the shocked child.
- The normal circulating volume for a child is in the region of 80 mL/kg, so after the second bolus of crystalloid fluids the use of blood products should be considered as should endotracheal intubation and controlled ventilation to counteract the risks of any pulmonary oedema resulting from fluid replacement.

- Children are also at serious risk from *hypoglycaemia*, so bedside glucose monitoring should be conducted regularly and treatment with boluses of 2 mL/kg of 10% glucose solution initiated as necessary.

### Adrenaline

- During CPR, the dosage of adrenaline is calculated as 10 mcg/kg or *0.1 mL/kg of 1:10,000* solution by the IV or intraosseous route every 3–5 minutes as required.

### Defibrillation

- If a rhythm of VF or pulseless VT is identified, defibrillator shocks should be administered by a *suitably trained* practitioner once every 2 minutes as required.
- The defibrillator power setting for children is calculated using the formula 4 J/kg.

### Further reading

Resuscitation Council (UK) (2021). European paediatric advanced life support providers manual (5th ed). London: Resuscitation Council (UK).

Skellett S, Maconochie I, Bingham R, et al. (2021). Paediatric advanced life support guidelines. Available at: ℜ https://www.resus.org.uk/library/2021-resuscitation-guidelines/paediatric-advanced-life-support-guidelines

# Sepsis

Sepsis is a life-threatening condition whereby the organs and tissues of the body are damaged in a dysregulated response to infection. In sepsis, disorder of inflammatory and coagulation pathways results in vasodilation and vessel leakage causing hypoperfusion and cell damage.

When somebody presents with any indication of infection, *always question* 'Could this be sepsis?'[1]

The disorder occurs when there is an abnormal response to invading pathogens including bacteria, fungi, and viruses with the most common sites of infection being the lungs, abdomen, and pelvis.

Sepsis can develop in previously healthy individuals of any age throughout the perioperative period; however, those with weakened immune systems are at particular risk. Risk factors include:
- Young children
- Older adults
- People with impaired immune systems (such as those receiving treatment for cancer or long-term users of steroids)
- People with indwelling catheters or devices (such as central lines, arterial lines, etc.)
- Patients with open wounds or impaired skin integrity
- Pregnant/postpartum women (particularly those who have comorbidities)
- Neonates (especially preterm or where there has been previous infection in other pregnancies, e.g. group B streptococci).

Sepsis can result in a prolonged critical care admission for those affected and failure to recognize and treat promptly can result in disability and death. Early identification and treatment is therefore essential. Signs and symptoms can be both specific and non-specific (Table 25.1) so alongside clinical observations, it is important to look out for indicators such as:
- The patient complaining of being 'extremely unwell', or feeling like they are 'going to die'
- They might also show signs of confusion and disorientation
- Younger children might present as being uninterested in anything or not responding to social cues. Babies could appear floppy with overall decreased activity.

Families and carers are also crucial as they might notice changes in behaviour which could be significant

A structured approach should be undertaken towards assessment and tools such as the National Early Warning Score (NEWS) and Paediatric Early Warning Score (PEWS) utilized for early identification of sepsis.

If sepsis is suspected, immediate referral should be made to the senior clinical decision maker.

**Table 25.1** Presentation of sepsis

| A | Audible abnormalities, accessory muscle use |
|---|---|
| B | Tachypnoea |
| | Breathlessness |
| | Low O₂ saturations |
| | Cyanosis |
| C | Tachycardia |
| | Hypotension |
| | Decreased urine output, decreased capillary refill time |
| | Cold to touch |
| | *Please note that patients may have a high or low temperature* |
| D | Confusion |
| | Feeling faint |
| | Disorientation, loss of consciousness |
| E | Rash |
| | Discoloured skin |

In terms of treatment, guidelines produced by the Surviving Sepsis Campaign are widely accepted and implementation of the 'Sepsis Six', within the first hour following recognition is recommended. This bundle is associated with improved outcomes and consists of the following:

1. Administer high-flow $O_2$. Target $O_2$ saturations >94%.
2. Take blood cultures.
3. Administer broad-spectrum IV antibiotics.
4. Commence fluid resuscitation.
5. Check lactate level.
6. Monitor hourly urine.

Patients should be monitored closely if not continuously.

Individuals who do not respond to initial interventions might require admission to critical care for organ support and more invasive monitoring, therefore referral should be made urgently.

> *Remember*, early identification and treatment of sepsis is essential to improving patient outcomes.

## Reference

1. UK Sepsis Trust. Homepage. Available at: ℘ https://sepsistrust.org/

## Further reading

National Institute for Health and Care Excellence (2020). National Early Warning Score systems that alert to deteriorating adult patients in hospital. Medtech innovation briefing [MIB205]. Available at: ℘ https://www.nice.org.uk/guidance/mib205

National Institute for Health and Care Excellence (2020). Sepsis. Quality standard [QS161]. Available at: ℘ https://www.nice.org.uk/guidance/qs161

Rhodes A, Evans LE, Alhazzani W, et al. (2017). Surviving Sepsis Campaign: international guidelines for management of sepsis and septic shock. Intensive Care Medicine, 43(3):304–377.

Royal College of Anaesthetists (2020). Chapter 5: guidelines for the provision of emergency anaesthesia. London: Royal College of Anaesthetists.

Surviving Sepsis Campaign (2016). International guidelines for management of sepsis and septic shock. Available at: ℘ http://www.survivingsepsis.org/Guidelines/Pages/default.aspx

# The deteriorating surgical patient

- When caring for a surgical patient, the practitioner must always be aware of the fact they could deteriorate during the perioperative phase.
- The fact that patients' primary immune defence (i.e. their skin) is breached in the vast majority of procedures predisposes them to developing infection, and also the need to cut through blood vessels means that bleeding is a reality in surgical practice.
- Although the majority of surgical procedures are conducted following careful assessment and planning in the preoperative phase, this does not guarantee a problem-free surgical journey; rather, it reduces the risk of complications. Indeed, emergency surgery carries a greater risk of complications, but the lifesaving nature of those operations outweighs the risk.
- This means the practitioner must be ever vigilant of changes in patient behaviours or physiological parameters, which could signify deterioration.

## Patient behaviours

Due to physiological compensatory mechanisms, patients will not always show overt signs of deterioration until those compensation mechanisms begin to fail. However, there may be subtle changes in their behaviour which could prompt the practitioner to systematically asses the patient. Some of these could be:
- Being quiet and withdrawn
- Reduced mobility (not influenced by surgical procedure or effects of anaesthetic)
- Delirium (indicating compromised cerebral perfusion)
- Complaining of increased intensity of pain
- Concern voiced by relatives.

This list is not exhaustive, but offers some areas of consideration. Essentially, if the practitioner feels concerned about a patient, a systematic assessment must be carried out in order to inform the escalation of care process.

## Risks of deterioration

Due to the multifactorial nature of surgery, there are many issues that place a particular patient at risk of deterioration; however, there are common risk factors which must be considered including:
- Advancing age
- Emergency surgery
- Presence of comorbidities.

## Causes of deterioration

The practitioner must adopt the same level of vigilance when caring for any perioperative patient as there are multiple causes of deterioration:
- Anaphylaxis due to anaesthetic drugs.
- Failure to ventilate, failure to intubate.
- Airway compromise due to opiates or incomplete reversal of muscle relaxant.
- Hypoxia.
- Sepsis.
- Multiorgan failure.
- Advanced disease.

- Cardiac failure.
- Respiratory failure.
- Bleeding.
- PE.

Whatever the cause of deterioration, the patient must always be monitored using a systematic approach to assessment, namely **ABCDE**.

## Airway

- Airway assessment begins with listening to airway sounds. Snoring indicates a partially obstructed airway, while a silent airway indicates complete obstruction.
- The airway must also be inspected for any obstructions, such as bodily fluids, displaced teeth, or soft tissue swelling.
- Any fluid should be carefully suctioned with a Yankauer sucker.
- Stridor indicates laryngeal obstruction and will quickly lead to significant hypoxia; relieving the obstruction will require expert help, which should be summoned immediately.
- The healthcare practitioner should take immediate action in cases of airway compromise.
- The airway should be opened using head tilt, chin lift (only jaw thrust in cervical spine injury), and assess for effectiveness of this manoeuvre.
- If successful, breathing should improve and normal breath sounds heard.
- Airway compromise of any cause and severity is a medical emergency and expert help should be summoned immediately.

## Breathing

- Initial assessment involves visualizing the patient's breathing effort and potential use of accessory muscles.
- Any increased work in breathing indicates respiratory distress.
- The respiratory rate should be counted (normal range 12–20 breaths/min), and the rhythm and depth of breathing also assessed.
- The chest should be inspected for bilateral chest rise, unilateral chest rise could indicate a pneumothorax.
- Effectiveness of breathing should be assessed by observing for any signs of peripheral or central cyanosis.
- This can be assessed in dark-skinned patients by checking the colour of their gums.
- Pulse oximetry is useful in assessing $O_2$ saturations at the bedside, with saturations >96% considered normal, 88–92% in chronic respiratory disease.
- Placing the patient in a semi-recumbent position may improve breathing, in doing so be cautious of a decrease in BP.
- Hypoxia of any cause is a risk to life and causes vital organ damage so the registered practitioner should correct hypoxia by giving $O_2$, the approach being reoxygenate at high flow then titrate down to maintain target $O_2$ saturations.
- $O_2$ should be prescribed at the time if a prescriber is present, or prescribed retrospectively if it was clearly clinically indicated.

### Circulation

- BP measurements should be taken to assess circulatory effectiveness; this should be done manually particularly in cases of atrial fibrillation.
- Low systolic BP indicates hypovolaemia or heart failure; diastolic BP indicates vascular resistance, so decreases suggests vasodilation seen in anaphylaxis or sepsis, with increased diastolic BP indicating vasoconstriction associated with hypovolaemia.
- Pulse should be taken manually so the practitioner can assess the rate and quality of the pulse.
- Tachycardia (pulse >100 bpm) indicates circulatory compensation.
- Thready rapid pulse indicates hypovolaemia, while a bounding rapid pulse indicates sepsis.
- In both cases the patient will need fluid resuscitation in accordance with local policies.
- Any changes in the pulse should be noted and reported, for instance, new-onset irregularity.
- The practitioner should also be vigilant for bradycardia (<60 bpm) as this can occur when an airway device is causing excessive vagal stimulation (e.g. LMA, ETT).
- It may be appropriate to continually monitor the patient with a three-lead ECG, as abdominal surgery and some anaesthetic drugs can give rise to arrhythmias.
- While ECG interpretation requires specialist knowledge and experience, practitioners in the surgical environment should be able to identify deviations from normal sinus rhythm or any changes from baseline.
- Peripheral temperature should be assessed by feeling the patient's hands and feet: cold peripheries indicate vasodilation, while warm peripheries will be observed in normally or in sepsis.
- Capillary refill time should be assessed by pressing an index finger on the sternum or forehead for 5 seconds—normally the area should reperfuse in <2 seconds. Any prolongation suggests poor perfusion and circulatory compromise.
- Urine output should be monitored, as poor renal perfusion due to circulatory compromise can result in reduced urine output. Urine output >30 mL/kg/hour is acceptable.

### Disability

- The patient's neurological function should be assessed using AVPU at the very least.
- Patients who have suffered a recent neurological event should be assessed using the GCS.
- Any recent-onset confusion should be considered as delirium which indicates compromised cerebral perfusion.
- The patient's pupils should be assessed using a pen torch for reaction to light:
  - The reaction should be a brisk pupillary constriction.
  - Recent administration of atropine will cause pupil dilation, while opiates will result in pupil constriction.
  - Any changes or lack of pupillary reaction should be reported immediately to the surgical team.
- Blood glucose should also be checked as fasting regimens will of course have an effect, more so in diabetic patients. Normal blood glucose concentration is 4–8 mmol/L.

## Exposure

- The patient's temperature should be taken; hypothermia can occur where inadequate patient warming was undertaken in theatre or when the patient requires fluid resuscitation. In either case, the patient should be warmed using warming blankets.
- Hyperthermia is highly suggestive of MH, in which case the practitioner should escalate care and follow the MH algorithm.
- This aspect of the assessment also requires a head-to-toe inspection to ascertain the possible cause of the deterioration.
- When exposing the patient, the practitioner should be mindful of maintaining the patient's body temperature and dignity.
- Surgical wounds should be visualized for any bleeding, and areas of distension should be noted and reported.
- Surgical drains should be inspected for any changes in the volume or nature of fluid drained.
- The patient's skin should be assessed for rashes, which could indicate an anaphylactic reaction.
- The patient's calves should be inspected for any swelling or redness associated with DVT, which often leads to PE.

## Post initial assessment

- This assessment should take 3–4 minutes and any areas of concern should prompt the practitioner to escalate case using the SBAR tool.
- Findings should also be clearly documented so that trends in the patient's condition can be assessed.
- It should also be borne in mind that younger patients will compensate for prolonged periods of time, therefore any signs of physiological compensation should cause concern.
- Once this is done, the practitioner should reassess the patient, still following the ABCDE approach, as the patient could deteriorate further.
- Regular reassessment will enable the practitioner to take prompt action should the patient's condition change.

## Further reading

Findlay G, Shotton H, Kelly K, et al. (2012). Time to intervene? London: National Confidential Enquiry into Patient Outcome and Death.

Herring N, Patterson DJ (2018). Levick's an introduction to cardiovascular physiology (6th ed). London: CRC Press.

National Institute for Health and Care Excellence (2020). National Early Warning Score systems that alert to deteriorating adult patients in hospital. Medtech innovation briefing [MIB205]. Available at: ℬ https://www.nice.org.uk/guidance/mib205

National Institute for Health and Care Excellence (2020). Sepsis. Quality standard [QS161]. Available at: ℬ https://www.nice.org.uk/guidance/qs161

O'Driscoll BR, Howard LS, Earis J, et al. (2017). BTS guideline for oxygen use in adults in healthcare and emergency settings. Thorax, 72(Suppl 1):ii1-ii90.

Resuscitation Council (UK) (2021). Advanced life support providers manual (8th ed). London: Resuscitation Council (UK).

Pollard B, Kitchen G (eds) (2017). Handbook of clinical anaesthesia (4th ed). London: CRC Press.

Robertson LC, Al-Haddad M (2013). Recognizing the critically ill patient. Anaesthesia and Intensive Care Medicine, 14(1):11–14.

Robson W, Daniels R (2013). Diagnosis and management of sepsis in adults. Nurse Prescribing, 11(2):76–82.

# Levels of consciousness

- Consciousness depends on a patient's arousability and awareness.
- Loss of consciousness can last for several minutes to more long term depending on the cause.
- Causes of unconsciousness are numerous and may dictate the length of the coma period.
- It is imperative to determine the cause of the coma so that appropriate treatment can be provided.
- Alterations in level of consciousness vary from slight to severe changes, indicating the degree of brain dysfunction.
- Previous or pre-existing conditions should be noted when assessing level of consciousness (e.g. hemiplegia, deafness, muteness).

Deteriorating levels of consciousness or unconsciousness can be classed into the categories identified in Table 25.2.

**Table 25.2** Deteriorating levels of consciousness or unconsciousness

| Poisons or drugs | Vascular causes |
|---|---|
| • Alcohol | • Post-cardiac arrest |
| • Overdose of solvents | • Haemorrhage |
| • GA | • Anaphylaxis |
| • Heavy metals, e.g. lead poisoning | • Infection |
| • Gases, e.g. carbon monoxide | • Septicaemia |
| • Prescribed/non-prescribed medications | • Viruses, e.g. HIV |
| Neurological disorders | Metabolic disorders |
| • Epilepsy | • Hypoxia |
| • Head injury | • Renal failure |
| • Pre-eclampsia | • Hepatic encephalopathy |
| • Hypoglycaemia | Other causes |
| • Hyperglycaemia | • Dehydration |
| • Meningitis | • Arrhythmias |
| • Encephalitis | • Hyperventilation |
| • Hydrocephalus | |
| • Stroke/transient ischaemic attack | |
| • Syncope | |

Assessment of vital signs is essential to monitor a patient's condition and should include pulse, BP, respiratory rate, temperature, $O_2$ saturation, and level of consciousness. Changes in vital signs may indicate:
- Shock
- Haemorrhage
- Electrolyte imbalance
- Raised ICP.

## Raised intracranial pressure

Signs of raised ICP that must be reported to an anaesthetist and neurosurgeon (Box 25.4) include:
- Rapid increase in BP
- Deterioration of level of consciousness
- Deterioration in responsiveness to speech or commands
- Changes in respiratory rate or breathing pattern
- Dilated pupil that indicates pressure on the ocular motor nerve and/or transtentorial herniation of the brain
- Decreased movement and muscle power down one side of the body.

---

**Box 25.4  Guide to raised intracranial pressure**
- ↑ BP.
- ↓ pulse.
- ↓ respiration.
- Potential small ↑ in temperature.
- Pupillary size and response changes (unilateral/bilateral).
- ↓ level of consciousness (lowering of score on GCS assessment).
- A change of one or more points on the GCS should be reported.

---

## Clinical events/complications associated with unconsciousness

The unconsciousness patient is subject to many clinical events/complications:
- Respiratory failure may develop shortly after the patient becomes unconscious.
- Pneumonia is common in patients receiving mechanical ventilation or in those who cannot maintain and clear their airway.
- Renal and GI reduced function.
- Pressure ulcers may become infected and therefore become a source of sepsis.

## Further reading

Association of Anaesthetists of Great Britain and Ireland (2019). Safe transfer of the brain-injured patient – trauma and stroke. Available at: ℘ http://dx.doi.org/10.1111/anae.14866

Craig A, Hatfield A (2020). The complete recovery room book (6th ed). Oxford: Oxford University Press.

Freedman R, Herbert L, O'Donnell A, et al. (eds) (2022). Oxford handbook of anaesthesia (5th ed). Oxford: Oxford University Press.

National Institute for Health and Care Excellence (2019). Hypertension in adults: diagnosis and management. NICE guideline [NG136]. Available at: ℘ https://www.nice.org.uk/guidance/NG136

Glasgow Coma Scale at 40 (2014). The new approach to Glasgow Coma Scale assessment. Available at: ℘ https://www.youtube.com/watch?v=v6qpEQxJQO4&ab_channel=GCSat40

National Institute for Health and Care Excellence (2019). Stroke and transient ischaemic attacks in over 16s: diagnosis and initial management. NICE guideline [NG128]. Available at: ℘ https://www.nice.org.uk/guidance/NG128

National Institute for Health and Care Excellence (2019). Suspected neurological conditions: recognition and referral. NICE guideline [NG127]. Available at: ℘ https://www.nice.org.uk/guidance/ng127

National Institute for Health and Care Excellence (2020). National Early Warning Score systems that alert to deteriorating adult patients in hospital. Medtech innovation briefing [MIB205]. Available at: ℛ https://www.nice.org.uk/guidance/mib205

National Institute for Health and Care Excellence (2020). Sepsis. Quality standard [QS161]. Available at: ℛ https://www.nice.org.uk/guidance/qs161

Peate I, MacLeod J (eds) (2020). Pudner's nursing the surgical patient (4th ed). Oxford: Elsevier.

Royal College of Anaesthetists (2020). Chapter 5: guidelines for the provision of emergency anaesthesia. London: Royal College of Anaesthetists.

Royal College of Anaesthetists (2021). Chapter 14: guidelines for the provision of neuro-anaesthetic services. London: Royal College of Anaesthetists.

# Assessing levels of consciousness

The assessment of level of consciousness involves three phases:
- *Eye opening* indicates that arousal mechanisms in the brain are active.
- *Evaluation of verbal response* may be orientated, confused, incomprehensible, or absent.
- *Evaluation of motor response* is used to assess brain function.

## Glasgow Coma Scale

See Table 25.3.

The GCS was first developed by the Institute of Neurological Sciences in Glasgow and was originally used to assess head injury. It is also used to assess conscious state during the postoperative period. Assessment of consciousness is as follows:
- Awake: alert, conscious, eyes open.
- Drowsy: eyes are shut except when spoken to; patient will cooperate on request.
- Rousable: the patient opens his/her eyes and also responds to stimulus.
- Coma: the patient does not respond to stimulus.

> The highest score in each category indicates a fully alert patient while the lowest score represents a patient who is unconscious and unresponsive. Any change of one or more points on the GCS should be reported immediately.

**Table 25.3** New Glasgow Coma Scale

|  |  | Score |
| --- | --- | --- |
| **Eye opening** | Spontaneous | 4 |
|  | To sound | 3 |
|  | To pressure | 2 |
|  | None | 1 |
|  | Non-testable | NT |
| **Verbal response** | Orientated | 5 |
|  | Confused | 4 |
|  | Words | 3 |
|  | Sounds | 2 |
|  | None | 1 |
|  | Non-testable | NT |
| **Motor response** | Obeys commands | 6 |
|  | Localizing | 5 |
|  | Normal flexion | 4 |
|  | Abnormal flexion | 3 |
|  | Extension | 2 |
|  | None | 1 |
|  | Non-testable | NT |
| **GCS maximum score 15; GCS minimum score 3** | | |

*Note: the lower the score, the more deeply unconscious the patient is. Patients presenting with a GCS score of <8 are in danger of a compromised airway.*

*Glasgow Coma Scale at 40*: 'The new approach to Glasgow Coma Scale assessment'[1]—this video provides a practical demonstration of how to use the GCS assessment accurately.

## AVPU scoring system

The AVPU is a simplified scale used to rapidly grade a patient's level of consciousness, responsiveness, or mental status. It is usually used during pre-hospital care and emergency rooms.[2]

- The AVPU scale is a system used to measure and record a person's level of consciousness.
- The AVPU scale has only four possible outcomes for recording.
- The patient is assessed from best (A) to worst (U) to avoid unnecessary tests on conscious (Table 25.4).
- It is a simplified GCS, which assesses a patient response in relation to:
  - Eyes
  - Voice
  - Motor skills.
- The AVPU scale should be assessed using the three identifiable traits listed above, identifying the best response of each.
- The scale is generally used as a first aid mechanism and may be followed with a more extensive assessment using the GCS.

Note that the AVPU scale is not suitable for long-term neurological use.

**Table 25.4** The AVPU scale

| A | **Alert** | Patient is fully responsive and lucid |
| | | Patient answers questions |
| V | **Voice** | Patient is responsive to voice |
| | | Patient may be drowsy with eyes closed |
| | | Patient may not speak coherently |
| P | **Pain** | Patient is not alert and does not respond to voice |
| | | Patient may respond to painful stimulus, e.g. shaking the shoulders or pinching an ear lobe |
| U | **Unresponsive** | Patient is unresponsive to any of the above |
| | | Patient is unconscious |

## References

1. Glasgow Coma Scale at 40 (2014). The new approach to Glasgow Coma Scale assessment. Available at: ℘ https://www.youtube.com/watch?v=v6qpEQxJQO4&ab_channel=GCSat40
2. Romanelli D, Farrell MW (2020). AVPU score. Available at: ℘ https://www.ncbi.nlm.nih.gov/books/NBK538431/

## Further reading

Craig A, Hatfield A (2020). The complete recovery room book (6th ed). Oxford: Oxford University Press.

Freedman R, Herbert L, O'Donnell A, et al. (eds) (2022). Oxford handbook of anaesthesia (5th ed). Oxford: Oxford University Press.

National Institute for Health and Care Excellence (2019). Recommendations. In: Head injury: assessment and early management. Clinical guideline [CG176]. Available at: https://www.nice.org.uk/guidance/cg176/chapter/1-recommendations

National Institute for Health and Care Excellence (2020). National Early Warning Score systems that alert to deteriorating adult patients in hospital. Medtech innovation briefing [MIB205]. Available at: https://www.nice.org.uk/guidance/mib205

National Institute for Health and Care Excellence (2020). Observations of patients with head injury in hospital. Available at: https://pathways.nice.org.uk/pathways/head-injury/observations-of-patients-with-head-injury-in-hospital

Reith FCM, Van den Brande R, Synnot A, et al. (2016). The reliability of the Glasgow Coma Scale: a systematic review. Intensive Care Medicine, 42(1):3–15.

Royal College of Physicians and Surgeons of Glasgow (2015). The Glasgow structured approach to assessment of the Glasgow coma scale. Glasgow: Royal College of Physicians and Surgeons of Glasgow.

# Death in the operating theatre

## Unexpected death

- This happens much less than might be thought even in emergency surgery; however, when patients do die in the operating theatre, it can be especially upsetting for those staff present.
- Whether death on the table was expected or occurred when least expected, the perioperative team are likely to be affected to some extent.
- Consideration should be given to providing support for staff who witness it and are involved with a deceased patient in the perioperative environment.
- It is particularly important to support junior and unqualified staff who may not have witnessed such an event previously.
- Post-event debriefing may be beneficial.
- A referral to the appropriate support services may also be considered for some staff who may be more affected by an unexpected death in the operating theatre.
- Offer relatives the best support possible. The bereaved relatives may wish to view the body and their wishes to do so must be respected. This will include respect of the patient and their family's religion which must be taken into consideration as certain faiths require the dead body to be treated in a certain way. The local policy should provide guidance on this matter.
- Relatives should be advised to contact the relevant NHS trust/health board officer who supports bereavement.
- Hospitals should have DNACPR guidance and documentation that complies with national requirements.[1]

## Expected death

- The medical and nursing teams must ensure that the patient and the patient's family/next of kin have been made aware of the patient's condition and that death is expected. This must be clearly documented within the patient's medical records.
- Deaths in certain circumstances must be referred to the coroner and may require a postmortem.
- A coroner is an independent judge who investigates unnatural or violent deaths, where the cause of death is unknown, or because the death took place in prison, police custody, or a type of state detention.[2] They are appointed by a local authority but remain independent judicial office holders. The coroner's role is to find out who died and how, when, and where they died.[3] A death should be reported to the coroner when:
  - Cause of death is unknown
  - Death occurred in hospital or another state detention centre
  - Death occurred as a result of anaesthesia or a surgical procedure
  - Death occurred within 24 hours of admission to hospital
  - Death may be caused by a medical procedure or treatment
  - Death may be caused by violence or trauma (intentional or otherwise)
  - Death may be caused by poisoning
  - Death may be caused by self-harm
  - Death may be caused by neglect
  - Death occurred in police custody or prison.

## Brainstem death

- This occurs when a patient has irreversibly lost the capacity for consciousness and breathing; this implies loss of brainstem function.
- A ventilator keeps the patient's heart beating and $O_2$ circulating through their bloodstream.
- A patient is confirmed as being dead when their brainstem function is permanently lost.
- Brain death can occur when the blood and/or $O_2$ supply to the brain is stopped. This could be caused by, for example, cardiac arrest, MI, stroke, brain haemorrhage, brain tumour or a head injury.
- Organ donation can only be instigated when a patient who has been diagnosed as brainstem dead and who has previously given consent (either themselves or by their relatives) to donate their organs to another person.
- Despite the predicable nature of this death, it may still be upsetting for certain members of staff as already described.
- In these situations, the transplant coordinator may be utilized to provide support for staff who might require it.
- Many cultures/religions do not support transplantation or organ donation.

> Patients who require surgical procedures with DNACPR decisions in place should have senior members of the anaesthetic and surgical team review the condition of the patient and the DNACPR status. Where feasible, a discussion should take place with the patient and/or their next of kin and it may be appropriate to suspend components of a DNACPR decision, for example, intubation, to allow surgery to safely proceed.[1]

## Care of the deceased

The body should be removed from the operating theatre to a place where the family can view it in some privacy, for example, the recovery room. It should also minimize the impact on other patients being treated in the theatre complex. The following is a guide as practitioners are required to follow local policy.

- The closed wound should be dressed to prevent leakage.
- Drains, IV cannulas, arterial and CVP lines, ETTs, and catheters should be secured and closed with a spigot where appropriate.
- Last offices should be carried out with respect and dignity.
- The body should be dressed in a shroud and placed in a body bag and labelled in accordance with local policy and the required documentation completed.
- Arrangements must then be made to transfer the body to the mortuary and be accompanied by a member of the operating theatre team.

## Requirements for people of different religious faiths

- Patients come from a diverse range of religious and cultural backgrounds and it is essential that awareness of faiths is recognized when caring for a deceased patient in theatre.
- Although not exhaustive, Box 25.5 outlines a few religions requirements that perioperative staff should observe when caring for a deceased patient.

## Box 25.5 Religious requirements for deceased patients

*Christianity*
*Cultural and/or religious requirements*
- Clergy may attend to say prayers and to support relatives.

*Last offices*
- No specific requirements.

*Postmortem/transplantation/organ donation*
- No objections.

*Burial or cremation requirements*
- No preference.

*Roman Catholic*
*Cultural and/or religious requirements*
- Priest requested to recite prayers for the dying and then prayers for the dead.

*Last offices*
- No specific requirements.
- A crucifix or rosary may accompany the patient's body.

*Postmortem/transplantation/organ donation*
- No objections.

*Burial or cremation requirements*
- No preference.

*Buddhism*
*Cultural and/or religious requirements*
- No specific rituals but a state of quiet and calm is required.
- A monk may be called to say prayers.
- Body to remain in one place for up to 7 days for the rebirth to take place but recognized this is not possible in a healthcare setting.

*Last offices*
- Delay last office for 4 hours to allow for prayers.
- Treated with care and respect.
- Do not wash the body unless essential.
- Body should be wrapped in a plain white sheet.

*Postmortem/transplantation/organ donation*
- No objections but some may prefer their bodies to be buried or cremated whole.

*Burial or cremation requirements*
- Cremation is preferable.

*Hinduism*
*Cultural and/or religious requirements*
- Last rites include tying a thread around the neck or wrist to bless the dying person, sprinkling holy water from the River Ganges on them, placing a sacred Tulsi leaf in their mouth if possible.

*Last offices*
- Close family members usually wash the body. They may be distressed if a non-Hindu touches the body so gloves should be worn.
- The body must be touched only by staff of the same sex.
- The eldest son must participate regardless of age.

*Postmortem/transplantation/organ donation*
- Only if necessary. Organs must be returned to the body if a postmortem occurs.

*Burial or cremation requirements*
- Cremation within 24 hours of death for arranged by the eldest son.
- Children <5 years are usually buried.

### Judaism
*Cultural and/or religious requirements*
- Orthodox Jews don't permit the touching or moving of a dying person. Following death, the Rabbi will be requested to perform last rites.

*Last offices*
- The family may wish to wash the body.
- Essential procedures can be performed by healthcare staff:
  - Close eyes and mouth.
  - All catheters and drains and fluid in them must be left as are considered part of the body.
  - Open wounds must be covered.
  - The body must be laid flat with hands open and arms parallel to the body.
  - Cover the body with a plain white sheet with the feet facing the door.
  - If death occurred during surgery check with the Rabbi and family if clothing that has blood on them should also be kept by the family for burial.

*Postmortem/transplantation/organ donation*
- Only if legally required.
- Organ donation is not permitted.

*Burial or cremation requirements*
- Burial but cremation is permitted for non-orthodox Jews.

### Jehovah's Witness
*Cultural and/or religious requirements*
- No specific rituals or requirements to observe.

*Last offices*
- No specific requirements.

*Postmortem/transplantation/organ donation*
- No specific requirements.

*Burial or cremation requirements*
- No preference.

### Islam

*Cultural and/or religious requirements*
- The Koran is recited until the point of death.

*Last offices*
- The body should be pointing East facing Mecca.
- Only wash the body, using gloves if relatives are absent.
- The body must be touched only by staff of the same sex.
- Close the eyes and bandage the lower jaw so the mouth doesn't open.
- Flex the joints of the arms and legs to stop them becoming rigid. The body should be wrapped in a Caffan. If there isn't one available, a white sheet will do. Maintaining modesty is essential.

*Postmortem/transplantation/organ donation*
- Postmortems are considered acceptable only if required by law.

*Burial or cremation requirements*
- Burial occurs as soon as possible after death.

### Sikhism

*Cultural and/or religious requirements*
- Prior to the death, comfort may be derived from reciting verses from the holy book.

*Last offices*
- The relatives may wish to prepare the body but this shouldn't be assumed.
- Observe guidance of the five Ks: Kesh, Kangha, Kara, Kirpan, Kaccha.
- The body must be touched only by staff of the same sex.

*Postmortem/transplantation/organ donation*
- No objections.

*Burial or cremation requirements*
- Cremation for adults.
- Burial for children.

## References

1. Royal College of Anaesthetists (2020). Chapter 5: guidelines for the provision of emergency anaesthesia. London: Royal College of Anaesthetists.
2. Bass S, Cowman S (2016). Anaesthetist's guide to the Coroner's Court in England and Wales. BJA Education, 16(4):130–133.
3. Ministry of Justice (2020). Guide to coroner services. London: HMSO.

## Further reading

Association of Anaesthetists of Great Britain and Ireland (2004). Catastrophes in anaesthetic practice – dealing with the aftermath. London: Association of Anaesthetists of Great Britain and Ireland.

Choudry M, Latif A, Warburton KG (2018). An overview of the spiritual importances of end-of-life care among the five major faiths of the United Kingdom. Clinical Medicine, 18(1):23–31.

Craig A, Hatfield A (2020). The complete recovery room book (6th ed). Oxford: Oxford University Press.

Freedman R, Herbert L, O'Donnell A, et al. (eds) (2022). Oxford handbook of anaesthesia (5th ed). Oxford: Oxford University Press.

Jithoo S, Sommerville TE (2017). Death on the table: anaesthetic registrars' experiences of perioperative death. Southern African Journal of Anaesthesia and Analgesia, 23(1):1–5.

Meara JG, Leather AJM, Farmer PE (2019). Making all deaths after surgery count. Lancet, 393(10191):2587.

# Surgical emergencies

The following topics discuss the presentation, anaesthesia, and surgical requirements, and postoperative care for a range of surgical emergencies.

# Ruptured abdominal aortic aneurysm repair

This is arguably the operation about which novice practitioners who work in departments that undertake emergency surgery feel most anxious about. It should be remembered that a patient with a ruptured (leaking) aneurysm will almost certainly be admitted via the ED and would not often be brought straight to the operating theatre.

## Presentation

- An abdominal aortic aneurysm (AAA) is defined as an increase in the diameter of the aorta by 50%, and is usually regarded as a diameter >3 cm.
- There is a higher incidence of AAA in elderly men with a ratio of 1:4 men to women.
- The mortality rate for an emergency repair of AAA is >50%.

## Anaesthesia management

- IV access urgently.
- Patient is usually anaesthetized in theatre using RSI.
- Close patient monitoring is essential during the perioperative period.
- Invasive monitoring including arterial BP, and triple-lumen CVP ± cardiac output if necessary.
- Attention to temperature regulation is vital during long surgical procedures.
- Hypertension, coughing, and straining should be avoided as this may precipitate further bleeding.
- Warm fluids and blood if possible.
- IV Hartmann's is a balanced solution and will help to prevent metabolic acidosis.
- Close monitoring of fluid balance is essential.
- Surgery can proceed once endotracheal intubation is confirmed.
- Ensure availability of intensive care bed.

## Surgical requirements

- General laparotomy set, arterial clamp set, two suction sets, large self-retaining abdominal retractor, selection of aortic grafts and sutures.
- To minimize the risk of the aneurysm further rupturing, the patient may be brought straight into the operating theatre and the IV access secured, CVP, arterial line and urinary catheter inserted, and the skin prepped and the patient draped prior to the administration of the GA.
- It will be necessary to explain carefully to the patient what is to happen to them as they are likely to be extremely anxious.

- Any accompanying relatives or friends must also be cared for and provided with the appropriate information, and this may fall to the perioperative staff since the medical staff may not have the opportunity to undertake this until after the procedure.

## Surgical approach

- The surgical approach is via a routine laparotomy and the intestines mobilized and pushed out of the way.
- The posterior peritoneum is incised to expose the aorta.
- In a ruptured AAA, the aorta must be cross-clamped as soon as possible.
- Patients are then heparinized as bleeding is not controlled until the cross-clamp is on.
- Once this has occurred then there is time and opportunity to take stock and continue to stabilize the patient before proceeding to repairing the aorta.
- Once the aorta is clamped, the aneurysm is then incised and repaired using a graft which is anastomosed using the vascular sutures.
- The clamp is then removed and the abdomen closed in the normal way.

## Postoperative management

- Most patients will transfer to critical care post surgery.
- Some can develop abdominal compartment syndrome after open surgical repair of a ruptured AAA.[1]

## Reference

1. National Institute for Health and Care Excellence (2020). Abdominal aortic aneurysm: diagnosis and management. Available at: ℘ https://www.nice.org.uk/guidance/ng156

## Further reading

Association of Anaesthetists of Great Britain and Ireland (2004). Catastrophes in anaesthetic practice – dealing with the aftermath. London: Association of Anaesthetists of Great Britain and Ireland.
Association of Anaesthetists of Great Britain and Ireland (2019). Checklist for draw-over anaesthetic equipment. Available at: ℘ http://dx.doi.org/10.21466/g.CFDAE2.2019
Craig A, Hatfield A (2020). The complete recovery room book (6th ed). Oxford: Oxford University Press.
Freedman R, Herbert L, O'Donnell A, et al. (eds) (2022). Oxford handbook of anaesthesia (5th ed). Oxford: Oxford University Press.
Peate I, MacLeod J (eds) (2020). Pudner's nursing the surgical patient (4th ed). Oxford: Elsevier.

# Appendicectomy

## Presentation

The patient will be admitted with central lower abdominal pain which may then move to the right lower quadrant and the patient may present with vomiting, anorexia, and low-grade pyrexia. Acute appendicitis is more common in children than in adults and the abdominal pain may be due to:

- Urinary tract infection
- Non-specific abdominal pain
- Pelvic inflammatory disease
- Renal colic
- Ectopic pregnancy
- Constipation
- Diagnosis of acute appendicitis is largely a clinical one and 10–20% of appendixes removed are normal.

## Anaesthesia management

- GA with RSI and muscle relaxation.
- Patient monitoring should include:
  - BP
  - ECG
  - Capnography
  - $SpO_2$
  - Temperature
  - IV fluid therapy.
- Analgesia can include:
  - NSAIDS administered PR if consent provided.
  - Local infiltration to wound site or right inguinal nerve block.
- Patient should be extubated awake in left lateral position.

## Main requirements

- Laparotomy or a minor intestinal tray.
- Suction.
- Abdominal lavage.
- Absorbable sutures 2/0 for purse string and 3/0 or 2/0 for closure of the muscle layer and then the desired skin closure.

## Operation

- The operation may be carried out as either an open procedure or laparoscopically.
- For the open procedure a transversely oblique incision (Lanz incision) is made in the right lower abdomen.
- A culture swab may also be taken.
- Care should be taken not to reuse instruments that have been in contact with the mucosal side of the bowel or the infected appendix.
- A washout using normal saline may be performed and the appendix is sent for pathological examination.

## Postoperative management

➔ See postoperative emergency care, p. 802.

# Further reading

Association of Anaesthetists of Great Britain and Ireland (2004). Catastrophes in anaesthetic practice – dealing with the aftermath. London: Association of Anaesthetists of Great Britain and Ireland.

Association of Anaesthetists of Great Britain and Ireland (2019). Checklist for draw-over anaesthetic equipment. Available at: ℜ http://dx.doi.org/10.21466/g.CFDAE2.2019

Craig A, Hatfield A (2020). The complete recovery room book (6th ed). Oxford: Oxford University Press.

Freedman R, Herbert L, O'Donnell A, et al. (eds) (2022). Oxford handbook of anaesthesia (5th ed). Oxford: Oxford University Press.

National Institute for Health and Care Excellence (2020). Appendicitis. Available at: ℜ https://cks.nice.org.uk/topics/appendicitis/

Peate I, MacLeod J (eds) (2020). Pudner's nursing the surgical patient (4th ed). Oxford: Elsevier.

Royal College of Surgeons of England (2014). Good surgical practice. Available at: ℜ https://www.rcseng.ac.uk/standards-and-research/gsp/

# Splenectomy

## Presentation

- The usual reason for removing the spleen is because of blunt trauma; often occurs along with lower rib fractures.
- The spleen can sometimes be damaged inadvertently during other abdominal operations.
- The patient may have lost blood and may be hypovolaemic and apart from the usual IV access is likely to require, CVP, and arterial lines.
- Fluid replacement with crystalloid, colloid fluid, or cross-matched blood may be required.

## Main requirements

Laparotomy tray, intestinal tray, arterial clamp set, abdominal closure sutures and ties for ligation (surgeon's preference), suction, and cell salvage equipment (optional).

## Surgical procedure

- The normal approach is by a midline incision.
- The surgeon will explore the surrounding area and the abdominal contents.
- Having identified and mobilized the spleen, the splenic artery and vein are identified, clamped and ligated, and then severed.
- Due to internal bleeding, it may prove necessary to evacuate clots from the abdomen so a large bowl will be required to receive these.
- The abdominal cavity may be irrigated with warm saline prior to the routine abdominal closure.

> Patients without a functioning spleen are at risk of overwhelming infection including pneumonia, sepsis, and meningitis.

## Postoperative management

→ See postoperative emergency care, p. 802.
The patient is likely to require a HDU or ITU bed postoperatively.

## Further reading

Association of Anaesthetists of Great Britain and Ireland (2004). Catastrophes in anaesthetic practice – dealing with the aftermath. London: Association of Anaesthetists of Great Britain and Ireland.

Association of Anaesthetists of Great Britain and Ireland (2019). Checklist for draw-over anaesthetic equipment. Available at: ℘ http://dx.doi.org/10.21466/g.CFDAE2.2019

Craig A, Hatfield A (2020). The complete recovery room book (6th ed). Oxford: Oxford University Press.

Freedman R, Herbert L, O'Donnell A, et al. (eds) (2022). Oxford handbook of anaesthesia (5th ed). Oxford: Oxford University Press.

Peate I, MacLeod J (eds) (2020). Pudner's nursing the surgical patient (4th ed). Oxford: Elsevier.

Royal College of Surgeons of England (2014). Good surgical practice. Available at: ℘ https://www.rcseng.ac.uk/standards-and-research/gsp/

# Bowel obstruction

## Small bowel

Small bowel obstructions account for approximately 5% of surgical admissions and in the UK the commonest causes are:
- Adhesions
- Strangulated hernia
- Malignancy
- Volvulus.

In the newborn, intestinal obstruction is the commonest GI surgical emergency intervention.

### Presentation

The patient may present with:
- Colicky abdominal pain
- Vomiting
- Abdominal distension
- Constipation.

### Anaesthesia management

- The patient is likely to require fluid resuscitation, arterial and CVP lines, and anaesthetic preparation for a major procedure supported with neuraxial blockade for postoperative analgesia.
- GA with RSI.
- Close patient monitoring is essential during the perioperative period.
- Attention to temperature regulation is vital during long surgical procedures.
- Warm fluids and blood if possible.
- Close monitoring of fluid balance is essential.

### Main requirements

- Laparotomy (or paediatric) tray, intestinal set, suction, intestinal surgical anastomosis set, normal saline for abdominal lavage, and abdominal closure and skin closing sutures or clips.
- Gloves and gowns (as per local procedure) for surgical team to change into following bowel resection.

### Surgical procedure

- The repair of the intestinal obstruction may include:
  - The division of an intestinal band
  - Release of an intestinal hernia
  - Resection of the bowel with anastomosis or creation of a stoma
  - Untwisting of a volvulus.
- A 'clean and dirty' or bowel technique should be utilized and instruments used while the bowel is opened not used during the abdominal closure.
- In many units the 'clean' period is following abdominal lavage where gloves and gowns are changed.

## Large bowel

- Large bowel obstruction is usually caused by a tumour with most patients being >70 years old.

- The risk of obstruction is greater in left-sided lesions and patients tend to present at a more advanced stage with 15% presenting with obstruction; patient may require fluid resuscitation and should be prepared.

*Presentation*
- Caecal tumours present with small bowel obstruction and the symptoms include:
  - Colicky abdominal pain
  - Early vomiting
  - Constipation
  - Variable extent of constipation.
- Left-sided tumours present with large bowel obstruction and symptoms include:
  - Change in bowel habit
  - Constipation
  - Abdominal distention
  - Early vomiting.
- The patient is likely to require fluid resuscitation, arterial and CVP lines, and anaesthetic preparation for a major procedure.

*Main requirements*
- Laparotomy tray, intestinal set, suction, intestinal surgical anastomosis set, stoma sutures, normal saline for abdominal lavage, and linear cutter stapler.
- Gloves and gowns (as per local procedure) for surgical team to change into following resection, and abdominal closure and skin closing sutures or clips.

---

Stenting or emergency surgery for those presenting with acute left-sided large bowel obstruction should be offered if potentially curative treatment is not suitable.[1]

---

*Surgical procedure*
A full laparotomy is carried out and the liver palpated for metastases and the colon inspected for tumour. Depending on the location of the tumour mass one of the following procedures may be carried out.
- Right hemicolectomy (right-sided lesions).
- Extended right hemicolectomy (transverse colon lesions).
- Various operations for left-sided lesions such as:

*Three-stage procedure*
- Defunctioning colostomy.
- Resection and anastomosis.
- Closure of colostomy.

*Two-stage procedure*
- Hartmann's procedure.
- Closure of colostomy.

*One-stage procedure*
- Resection and primary anastomosis (no colostomy).

*Postoperative management*
→ See postoperative emergency care, p. 802.

The patient is likely to require a HDU or ITU bed postoperatively.

## Reference

1. National Institute for Health and Care Excellence (2020). Colorectal cancer. Available at: ℬ https://www.nice.org.uk/guidance/qs20

## Further reading

Association of Anaesthetists of Great Britain and Ireland (2004). Catastrophes in anaesthetic practice – dealing with the aftermath. London: Association of Anaesthetists of Great Britain and Ireland.

Association of Anaesthetists of Great Britain and Ireland (2019). Checklist for draw-over anaesthetic equipment. Available at: ℬ http://dx.doi.org/10.21466/g.CFDAE2.2019

Craig A, Hatfield A (2020). The complete recovery room book (6th ed). Oxford: Oxford University Press.

Freedman R, Herbert L, O'Donnell A, et al. (eds) (2022). Oxford handbook of anaesthesia (5th ed). Oxford: Oxford University Press.

Peate I, MacLeod J (eds) (2020). Pudner's nursing the surgical patient (4th ed). Oxford: Elsevier.

Royal College of Anaesthetists (2020). Chapter 5: guidelines for the provision of emergency anaesthesia. London: Royal College of Anaesthetists.

Royal College of Surgeons of England (2014). Good surgical practice. Available at: ℬ https://www.rcseng.ac.uk/standards-and-research/gsp/

# Gastrointestinal bleed

## Presentation

Upper GI bleeding may be caused by:
- Peptic ulcer
- Gastric erosions
- Oesophageal or gastric varices
- Mallory–Weiss tear (caused by violent vomiting)
- Gastric neoplasia.

> Prophylactic antibiotic therapy should be considered in patients presenting with suspected or confirmed variceal bleeding.[1]

Patients will be likely to present with haematemesis and will require an early endoscopy to determine the site of the bleeding. There are several endoscopic therapies that can be utilized to stop the bleeding:
- Laser photocoagulation.
- Bipolar electrocautery.
- Heat probes.
- Adrenaline or sclerosant injection.

Should endoscopic therapy prove unsuccessful or there is recurrent bleeding, the patient will require a surgical intervention. The chosen operation is performed via a laparotomy.

## Anaesthesia management

- The patient may require fluid resuscitation, arterial and CVP lines, and anaesthetic preparation for a major procedure.
- GA with RSI.
- Close patient monitoring is essential during the perioperative period.
- Attention to temperature regulation is vital during long surgical procedures.
- Warm fluids and blood if possible.
- Close monitoring of fluid balance is essential.

## Main requirements

- Laparotomy tray.
- Intestinal set.
- Suction.
- Intestinal surgical anastomosis set.
- Anastomosis or under-sewing sutures.
- Normal saline for abdominal lavage.
- Abdominal closure and skin closing sutures or clips.
- A 'clean and dirty' technique should be utilized when the stomach or duodenum is open.
- NG or feeding tube.

## Surgical procedure

- For a duodenal ulcer, a gastroduodenostomy with the ulcer under-sewn with a 2/0 absorbable suture.
- For a gastric ulcer, a local resection or total or partial gastrectomy.

## Postoperative management

➔ See postoperative emergency care, p. 802.

The patient is likely to require a HDU or ITU bed postoperatively.

## Reference

1. National Institute for Health and Care Excellence (2016). Acute upper gastrointestinal bleeding in over 16s: management. Clinical guideline [CG141]. Available at: ℜ https://www.nice.org.uk/guidance/cg141

## Further reading

Association of Anaesthetists of Great Britain and Ireland (2004). Catastrophes in anaesthetic practice – dealing with the aftermath. London: Association of Anaesthetists of Great Britain and Ireland.

Association of Anaesthetists of Great Britain and Ireland (2019). Checklist for draw-over anaesthetic equipment. Available at: ℜ http://dx.doi.org/10.21466/g.CFDAE2.2019

Craig A, Hatfield A (2020). The complete recovery room book (6th ed). Oxford: Oxford University Press.

Freedman R, Herbert L, O'Donnell A, et al. (eds) (2022). Oxford handbook of anaesthesia (5th ed). Oxford: Oxford University Press.

Peate I, MacLeod J (eds) (2020). Pudner's nursing the surgical patient (4th ed). Oxford: Elsevier.

Royal College of Surgeons of England (2014). Good surgical practice. Available at: ℜ https://www.rcseng.ac.uk/standards-and-research/gsp/

# Obstetric emergencies

Emergency obstetric surgery can include:
- Caesarean section
- Vaginal delivery
- Removal of retained products of conception.

Caesarean section is generally performed for the benefit of the mother, fetus, or both (Box 25.6). Although caesarean section was traditionally classified as elective surgery, this procedure is now classified into four grades:
- Immediate threat to the life of the mother or fetus.
- Maternal or fetal compromise but not immediately life-threatening.
- No maternal or fetal compromise but early delivery required.
- Elective delivery to suit the mother and maternity team.

---

**Box 25.6 Indications for caesarean section**
- Previous caesarean section.
- Maternal exhaustion.
- Multiple pregnancy.
- Malposition.
- Pre-existing maternal disease.
- Placenta praevia.
- Placental abruption.
- Cord prolapse.
- Obstructed labour.
- Fetal compromise.

---

Anaesthetic management of obstetric surgery and the choice of anaesthetic technique are dependent on a number of factors:
- Degree of urgency.
- Anticipated obstetric complications.
- Anaesthetic history or anticipated anaesthetic complications.
- Whether an epidural catheter is *in situ*.
- To a lesser degree, anaesthetist's and patient's choice.

An obstetric early warning system has been recommended to improve timely recognition, management, and early referral of women who have or are developing a critical illness.[1] The early warning systems modified for maternity patients should include:
- Respiratory rate
- $O_2$ saturation
- Heart rate
- Systolic BP
- Diastolic BP
- Temperature
- Urine output
- Level of consciousness.

---

Maternity services should implement NICE[2] guidance on the recognition and response to acute illness in adults in hospital.

The AAGBI[3] and RCoA[1] make recommendations regarding obstetric services that include the following:
- A duty anaesthetist should be immediately available for the obstetric delivery suite 24 hours per day.
- A nominated consultant should be in charge of obstetric anaesthesia.
- There should be a clear line of communication from the duty anaesthetist to the supervising consultant at all times.
- Increasing workload in the modern obstetric unit requires an increase in anaesthetic staffing above currently accepted levels.
- When obstetric units are small, or workload is sporadic, that provision of the basic minimum staffing levels is not cost-effective, consideration should be given to amalgamation with other local units.
- Women should have antenatal access to information about the availability and provision of all types of analgesia and anaesthesia.
- An agreed system whereby the anaesthetist is given sufficient advance notice of all potential high-risk patients should be in place.
- Where a 24-hour epidural service is offered, the time from the anaesthetist being informed about an epidural until being able to attend the mother should not normally exceed 30 minutes, and must be within 1 hour except in exceptional circumstances.
- Provision should be made for those who cover the delivery suite on-call, but do not have regular sessions there, to spend time in the delivery suite in a supernumerary capacity with one of the regular obstetric anaesthetic consultants.
- Separate staffing and resources should be allocated to elective caesarean section lists to prevent delays due to emergency procedures and provision of regional analgesia in labour.
- The anaesthetic assistant must have no other conflicting duties, must be trained to a recognized national standard, and must work regularly in the obstetric unit.
- The training undergone by staff in the maternity recovery unit and the facilities provided must be to the same standard as for general recovery facilities.
- Appropriate facilities should be available for the antenatal and peripartum management of the sick obstetric patient.

The AAGBI[3] and RCoA[1] also make a list of recommended protocols that should be readily available in all obstetric departments including:
- Conditions requiring antenatal referral to the anaesthetist
- Management of major haemorrhage, pre-eclampsia, and eclampsia
- Management of failed/difficult intubation
- Management of regional anaesthesia, high regional block, and hypotension during regional block
- Management of accidental dural puncture and post-dural puncture headache
- Admission and discharge criteria from/to the HDU
- Management of regional techniques in patients on thromboprophylaxis
- Antacid prophylaxis for labour and delivery
- Oral intake during labour
- Resuscitation of the pregnant patient.

## Postoperative management

- ⮕ See postoperative emergency care, p. 802.
- The Modified Early Obstetric Warning Score (MEOWS) chart should be initiated in recovery by the recovery practitioner prior to transfer to midwifery care. The last set of observations taken in recovery should be recorded on both the theatre care and the MEOWS chart.
- Critical care units should have a named lead for maternal critical care to act as the liaison between critical care and obstetric services.[1]

## References

1. Royal College of Anaesthetists (2018). Care of the critically ill woman in childbirth; enhanced maternal care. Available at: ⅊ https://www.rcoa.ac.uk/sites/default/files/documents/2020-06/EMC-Guidelines2018.pdf
2. National Institute for Health and Care Excellence (2020). National Early Warning Score systems that alert to deteriorating adult patients in hospital. Medtech innovation briefing [MIB205]. Available at: ⅊ https://www.nice.org.uk/guidance/mib205
3. Association of Anaesthetists for Great Britain and Ireland (2013). Obstetric anaesthetic services. London: Association of Anaesthetists of Great Britain and Ireland.

## Further reading

Association of Anaesthetists of Great Britain and Ireland (2004). Catastrophes in anaesthetic practice – dealing with the aftermath. London: Association of Anaesthetists of Great Britain and Ireland.

Association of Anaesthetists of Great Britain and Ireland (2019). Checklist for draw-over anaesthetic equipment. Available at: ⅊ http://dx.doi.org/10.21466/g.CFDAE2.2019

Association of Anaesthetists of Great Britain and Ireland (2020). Safety guideline: neurological monitoring associated with obstetric neuraxial block. Available at: ⅊ https://doi.org/10.1111/anae.14993

Craig A, Hatfield A (2020). The complete recovery room book (6th ed). Oxford: Oxford University Press.

Freedman R, Herbert L, O'Donnell A, et al. (eds) (2022). Oxford handbook of anaesthesia (5th ed). Oxford: Oxford University Press.

Friedman AM, Campbell ML, Kline CR, et al. (2018). Implementing obstetric early warning systems. American Journal of Perinatology, 8(2):79–84.

National Institute for Health and Care Excellence (2019). Caesarean section. Clinical guideline [CG132]. Available at: ⅊ https://www.nice.org.uk/guidance/cg132

Peate I, MacLeod J (eds) (2020). Pudner's nursing the surgical patient (4th ed). Oxford: Elsevier.

Royal College of Anaesthetists (2020). Chapter 9: guidelines for the provision of anaesthesia services for an obstetric population. London: Royal College of Anaesthetists.

Royal College of Surgeons of England (2014). Good surgical practice. Available at: ⅊ https://www.rcseng.ac.uk/standards-and-research/gsp/

# Gynaecology emergencies

Emergency gynaecology surgery can include:
- Suspected ectopic pregnancy
- Ruptured ectopic pregnancy
- Evacuation of retained products of conception (ERCP)
- Incision and drainage of Bartholin's abscess (although this is sometimes performed at ward level).

## Ectopic pregnancy

- Ectopic or tubal pregnancy can be managed surgically or medically and this management should be tailored to the clinical condition and future fertility requirements of the woman.
- The Royal College of Obstetricians and Gynaecologists (RCOG)[1] advises that laparoscopic approach as opposed to an open approach to the surgical management of ectopic pregnancy, is preferable in a patient who is haemodynamically stable.
- Surgical procedures undertaken laparoscopically are often associated with decreased operation times, reduced blood loss, and lower analgesic requirements.
- If a patient is haemodynamically unstable, a laparotomy is the preferred method of management of ectopic pregnancy.
- IM methotrexate is advocated for medical management of ectopic pregnancy although surgical laparoscopy is often used to confirm its presence. Methotrexate should only be offered on a first visit when there is a definitive diagnosis of an ectopic pregnancy, and a viable intrauterine pregnancy has been excluded.[2]
- The RCOG advises against medical management of ectopic pregnancy if hypovolaemic shock is suspected.[1]
- Offer anti-D rhesus prophylaxis at a dose of 250 IU (50 mcg) to all rhesus-negative women who have a surgical procedure to manage an ectopic pregnancy or a miscarriage.[2]

## Early pregnancy loss

- Early pregnancy loss is defined by the RCOG as a loss within the first 12 completed weeks of pregnancy.[1]
- Early pregnancy loss can be managed surgically or medically.
- Surgical ERPC for early pregnancy loss used to be the main treatment for patients due to possible risks that include haemorrhage and infection.
- Treatment is now available on an outpatient basis.
- If a patient presents with excessive bleeding, unstable vital signs, or retained, infected tissue, then surgical evacuation via suction curettage is considered the treatment of choice.
- Complications of ERPC can include perforated uterus, haemorrhage, intra-abdominal trauma, intrauterine adhesions, and cervical tears.
- Medical management of early pregnancy loss involves the use of prostaglandin drugs but vaginal bleeding can occur for up to 3 weeks following miscarriage.
- Prophylactic antibiotic therapy should be administered according to individual need.

- The RCOG recommends that anti-D immunoglobulin should only be given for threatened miscarriage at <12 weeks of gestation when bleeding is heavy or associated with pain.[1] The RCOG states it is not required for complete miscarriage at <12 weeks of gestation when there has been no formal intervention to evacuate the uterus.[1]

## Anaesthetic management

- The majority of gynaecology patients presenting for emergency surgery are fit. Anaesthetic management of gynaecology surgery and the choice of anaesthetic technique are dependent on a number of factors: degree of urgency; anticipated complications; anaesthetic history or anticipated anaesthetic complications; and to a lesser degree, anaesthetists' and patients' choice.
- All professionals should be sensitive to the needs of patients as some may require considerable psychological support.
- Prophylactic antiemetic therapy should be considered as nausea and vomiting can be problematic postoperatively.
- Vagal stimulation can occur intraoperatively when dilating the cervix or during laparoscopic procedures.
- Attention to temperature regulation is vital during long surgical procedures.
- Intubation with ranitidine premedication is recommended where there are symptoms of reflux.
- RSI is advocated for ectopic pregnancy.

## Postoperative management

➔ See postoperative emergency care, p. 802.

## References

1. Royal College of Obstetricians and Gynaecologists (2016). Diagnosis and management of ectopic pregnancy (Green-top Guideline No. 21). Available at: ℅ https://www.rcog.org.uk/en/guidelines-research-services/guidelines/gtg21/
2. National Institute for Health and Care Excellence (2019). Ectopic pregnancy and miscarriage: diagnosis and initial management. Available at: ℅ https://www.nice.org.uk/guidance/NG126

## Further reading

Craig A, Hatfield A (2020). The complete recovery room book (6th ed). Oxford: Oxford University Press.

Freedman R, Herbert L, O'Donnell A, et al. (eds) (2022). Oxford handbook of anaesthesia (5th ed). Oxford: Oxford University Press.

National Institute for Health and Care Excellence (2020). National Early Warning Score systems that alert to deteriorating adult patients in hospital. Medtech innovation briefing [MIB205]. Available at: ℅ https://www.nice.org.uk/guidance/mib205

Peate I, MacLeod J (eds) (2020). Pudner's nursing the surgical patient (4th ed). Oxford: Elsevier.

Royal College of Anaesthetists (2020). Chapter 5: guidelines for the provision of emergency anaesthesia. London: Royal College of Anaesthetists.

# Ear, nose, and throat emergencies

ENT surgery is a speciality that is performed in most UK hospitals and, compared with many specialities, has relatively few emergency cases. This can make it more difficult for practitioners to maintain their skill level. It is therefore advisable that practitioners spend some time familiarizing themselves with elective ENT procedures and noting the whereabouts of instruments and equipment. Emergency ENT procedures include:

- Endoscopy for removal of foreign bodies in the airway or oesophagus
- Tracheostomy
- Mastoidectomy
- Treatment for epistaxis.

An airway emergency, including any lesion causing upper airway compromise, is potentially life-threatening in both adults and children. Stridor, acute epiglottitis, inhaled foreign body, and bleeding tonsils, all require a prompt, methodical approach.[1]

It is not uncommon for children to require a laryngoscopy for the removal of foreign bodies such as coins or small toys from their cricopharyngeus which may have been placed in the mouth by the child themselves.

- Once confirmed by an X-ray, and if it is not possible to reach the object with the child conscious, a GA will be required so that a rigid laryngoscopy can be performed and a grasping forceps used to grab the object.
- This can sometimes be carried out by the anaesthetist.
- If appropriate, the object can be cleaned and returned to the family in a suitable container as a reminder for the future.
- In adults, it is more likely that the foreign body will be in the oesophagus, sometimes ingested when intoxicated, and is often a food bolus that is caught at the aortic indentation or diaphragm.
- A rigid oesophagoscopy is performed under a GA and the foreign body removed or occasionally advanced into the stomach.

Tracheostomy may be performed to relieve an upper airway obstruction or to replace an ETT for a mechanically ventilated patient. Requirements include:

- Tracheostomy set.
- Selection of appropriately sized tracheostomy tubes
- Syringe to inflate tracheostomy tube cuff
- Suction and suction catheter
- Cotton tape to secure tracheostomy tube.

Mastoidectomy is occasionally performed as an emergency in the presence of a mastoid abscess. The condition is painful but not life-threatening and the operation is carried in the same way as the elective procedure.

Epistaxis can sometimes require a surgical intervention if the haemorrhage cannot be stemmed. Surgical techniques include:

- The insertion of a nasal balloon or posterior nasal pack
- Electrocautery to the affected area
- Ligation of maxillary and anterior ethmoidal artery.

## Anaesthesia management

Consideration should be given to identifying anaesthetists with advanced airway experience to support colleagues providing care to patients with complex airway emergencies.

## Postoperative management

➲ See postoperative emergency care, p. 802.

## Reference

1. Makepeace J, Patel A (2014). Ear, nose and throat emergencies. Anaesthesia and Intensive Care Medicine, 15(5):235–237.

## Further reading

Craig A, Hatfield A (2020). The complete recovery room book (6th ed). Oxford: Oxford University Press.

Freedman R, Herbert L, O'Donnell A, et al. (eds) (2022). Oxford handbook of anaesthesia (5th ed). Oxford: Oxford University Press.

Peate I, MacLeod J (eds) (2020). Pudner's nursing the surgical patient (4th ed). Oxford: Elsevier.

Royal College of Anaesthetists (2020). Chapter 12: guidelines for the provision of anaesthesia services for ENT, oral maxillofacial and dental surgery. London: Royal College of Anaesthetists.

Royal College of Surgeons of England (2014). Good surgical practice. Available at: ℜ https://www.rcseng.ac.uk/standards-and-research/gsp/

# Ophthalmology emergencies

## Retinal detachment

- Retinal detachment is a rare but serious and sight-threatening event.
- Not all cases of retinal detachment require urgent surgery but a delay in treatment should be avoided.
- The preservation of the macula anatomy is the most pressing indication for out-of-hours retinal detachment surgery.
- A retinal detachment usually happens naturally and occurs when the retina becomes separated from the underlying tissue. This may be caused by a hole or tear in the retina which allows fluid to get underneath, weakening the attachment of the retina which then becomes detached.
- Without treatment, this condition can lead to blindness in the affected eye.

Retinal detachment is one of the most common eye emergencies in the UK, with an annual incidence of about 10–15 per 100,000 people.[1]

Symptoms are not generally painful but can include a shadow or curtain spreading across the vision of one eye, bright flashes of light, and/or showers of dark spots called floaters. Those at a higher risk of developing a retinal detachment include people who are or have:

- Short-sighted
- Previous cataract surgery
- A recent severe direct blow to the eye
- Ocular tumours
- Diabetic eye disease
- Some are familial but these are rare.

Complications are rare and very rarely blindness can occur. Possible complications during the operation can include:

- Bleeding inside the eye.
- The surgery producing more holes in the retina.

Much of the ophthalmic surgical population is elderly and frail, and guidelines on perioperative care of elderly patients should be followed.[2]

## Anaesthetic management

- Many cases of primary retinal detachment can be managed with LA.
- Ophthalmic surgery is often required for ocular manifestations of systemic disease and there is a relatively high incidence of patients with uncommon medical conditions.
- GA should be considered if a patient cannot lie flat and still for up to 1 hour.
- A laryngeal mask is recommended unless contraindicated.
- Administration of glycopyrronium can reduce salivary function and avoid pooling behind an LMA.
- Sub-Tenon's block complements GA and improves intraoperative stability and reduces postoperative pain.

## Anaesthetic factors increasing intraocular pressure

- Laryngoscopy.
- Suxamethonium.
- Large volumes of LA drugs.
- External compression of the globe by tightly applied face mask.

The following should be considered emergency surgery, especially when outside of normal working hours:

- The eye condition
- ASA grade
- Age of patients
- The RCoA[2] advises that all ophthalmic theatre nurses, anaesthetic nurses, and ODPs must have up-to-date BLS training and ophthalmic nurses should be trained in cardiopulmonary resuscitation:
  - 'There must be a robust procedure for checking the laterality of the eye to be operated on prior to LA block. This should include the eye being marked by the responsible surgical team prior to admission to the surgical suite.
  - On arrival in the anaesthetic room the consent form must be checked. This must be done by the anaesthetist or surgeon performing the block and an ODP or theatre nurse. The patient must be asked to confirm on which eye they expect to have the operation.'

## Postoperative management

⊃ See postoperative emergency care, p. 802.

## References

1. National Institute for Health and Care Excellence (2019). Retinal detachment. Available at: ℗ https://cks.nice.org.uk/topics/retinal-detachment/
2. Royal College of Anaesthetists (2020). Chapter 13: guidelines for the provision of ophthalmic anaesthesia services. London: Royal College of Anaesthetists.

## Further reading

Craig A, Hatfield A (2020). The complete recovery room book (6th ed). Oxford: Oxford University Press.
Freedman R, Herbert L, O'Donnell A, et al. (eds) (2022). Oxford handbook of anaesthesia (5th ed). Oxford: Oxford University Press.
Peate I, MacLeod J (eds) (2020). Pudner's nursing the surgical patient (4th ed). Oxford: Elsevier.
Royal College of Anaesthetists (2020). Chapter 10: guidelines for the provision of paediatric anaesthesia services. London: Royal College of Anaesthetists.
Royal College of Ophthalmologists (2010). Management of acute retinal detachment. Available at: ℗ www.rcophth.ac.uk/docs/profstands/ophthalmic-services/ManagementRetinalDetachment.pdf
Royal College of Surgeons of England (2014). Good surgical practice. Available at: ℗ https://www.rcseng.ac.uk/standards-and-research/gsp/

# Orthopaedic trauma emergencies

- Trauma is an injury to the body caused by the application of external energy be it direct or indirect.
- The type and amount of energy exerted will result in a variety of injuries.
- The severity of the injuries is influenced by the violence of the impact.
- Trauma and fractures are not the same; however, the majority of trauma surgery is related to damage of bones, muscles, and joints.

The aim of fracture treatment is to preserve and restore function and normal anatomical position, with function being the priority.

## Principles of fracture treatment

Summarized as the 5 Rs:
- Resuscitation: shock, blood loss, pain.
- Reduction: realignment of the bone.
- Restriction: plaster cast, traction, open reduction/internal fixation, external fixation.
- Restoration.
- Rehabilitation.

## Diagnosis of fracture

*Look*
- Deformity: may not always be obvious.
- Bruising at site of injury.
- Impaired function.
- Swelling.
- Wounds
- Compare one side with the other.
- Colour of limb.

*Listen*
- History—what was the nature of the injury? The magnitude of the forces involved and the direction of the forces?

*Feel*
- Pain at site of injury.
- Tenderness.
- Crepitus.
- Is the limb warm? Check corresponding limb.
- Check for movement and sensation.
- Check for pulse.

## Investigations

- Radiological examination of the injured part, including the joint above and below; should be X-rayed in two views.
- CT scan.
- MRI scan.

## Management of fractures

See Fig. 25.3.
- Non-operative or operative techniques.
- Enhanced communication strategies.

## Anaesthetic management

- Airway management with cervical spine control.
- GA is usually advocated for major trauma patients with RSI.
- Blood loss may be extensive so monitor carefully.
- Recognition and management of major bleeding and coagulopathy strategies.
- Care should be taken when moving, handling, and transferring trauma patients.
- Patients should be positioned carefully with appropriate protection and padding of pressure areas.
- IV antibiotics prophylactically.
- Invasive monitoring may be necessary for patient with cardiovascular system disease.
- ICP monitoring with head injury patients.
- Urinary catheter for long procedures with observation of hourly urine output to assess renal perfusion and function.

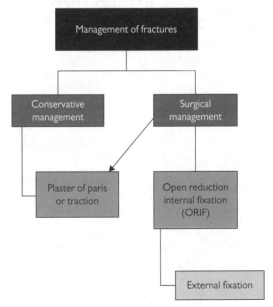

**Fig. 25.3** Management of fractures.

- A tourniquet is used to reduce bleeding but may be contraindicated due to fracture site.
- Intraoperative cell salvage and drain salvage may be considered.
- Patients should be actively warmed intraoperatively.
- Patients with limb fractures are at risk of fat embolism.
- Pain management.
- Management of skeletal muscle spasm.
- Management of stress response.
- Management of thromboembolic complications.

## Postoperative management

➔ See postoperative emergency care, p. 802.

## Further reading

Craig A, Hatfield A (2020). The complete recovery room book (6th ed). Oxford: Oxford University Press.

Freedman R, Herbert L, O'Donnell A, et al. (eds) (2022). Oxford handbook of anaesthesia (5th ed). Oxford: Oxford University Press.

Griffiths R, Brooks D (2022). Orthopaedic surgery. In: Freedman R, Herbert L, O'Donnell A, et al. (eds) Oxford handbook of anaesthesia (5th ed). Oxford: Oxford University Press.

National Institute for Health and Care Excellence (2019). Retinal detachment. Available at: ℰ https://cks.nice.org.uk/topics/retinal-detachment/

Peate I, MacLeod J (eds) (2020). Pudner's nursing the surgical patient (4th ed). Oxford: Elsevier.

Royal College of Anaesthetists (2020). Chapter 16: guidelines for the provision of anaesthesia services for trauma and orthopaedic surgery London: Royal College of Anaesthetists.

Royal College of Surgeons of England (2014). Good surgical practice. Available at: ℰ https://www.rcseng.ac.uk/standards-and-research/gsp/

# Postoperative emergencies

Postoperative emergencies are uncommon but emergency situations can occur spontaneously and can mostly be prevented. Emergency situations can be classified into two groups: *anaesthetic-related emergencies* (Box 25.7) and *general emergencies* (Box 25.8). These emergencies are specific to anaesthesia and post-anaesthetic care.

## Management of postoperative emergencies

Irrespective of the emergency, a universally methodical approach should be adopted by the practitioner. The **ABCDE** (primary survey) approach is an effective method in which to achieve this:

**A**: airway.
**B**: breathing.
**C**: circulation.
**D**: disability.
**E**: exposure.

### Airway

The airway is the priority in any emergency. The absence of a patent airway can lead to a quick death without intervention. The airway should be inspected, suctioned (if necessary), and appropriate adjuncts and techniques used to preserve its patency, such as oropharyngeal airways, jaw thrust/chin lift.

### Breathing and ventilation

The patient's chest rise/fall and pattern of breathing should be observed. Use of accessory muscles, bilateral or unilateral rise/fall, evidence of pain on inspiration/expiration, breath-holding, and alternative breathing patterns, such as Kussmaul's and Cheyne–Stokes should be noted.

$Sp/SaO_2$ levels should be observed and measured alongside peripheral/central perfusion (capillary refill, ashen/cyanosed appearance).

### Circulation

BP and circulating blood volume should be noted. The mean arterial pressure is a principal indicator of organ perfusion and should be kept at >60 mmHg; any decrease below this can lead to renal, coronary artery, and brain tissue ischaemia. Malignant increases or decreases in BP are concerning and require prompt treatment; these are often signs of an underlying cause, such as hypovolaemia. Heart rate should be observed in conjunction with BP, as both are interrelated. Tachycardias/bradycardias often correspond to a decreased and an increased BP, respectively. Compensatory mechanisms, such as this, are a principal indicator of shock. Rhythm should be analysed and any major abnormalities should be investigated further with a 12-lead ECG. VTs are an example and require prompt anaesthetic input. An unmanaged VT can quickly lead to cardiac arrest.

Fluid balance and urine output can be used as additional markers. Oliguria and anuria in postoperative patients can be initial signs of complication. Urine output should always be >1 mL/kg/hour (this calculation is negated when patients are administered diuretics).

*Disability (neurological assessment)*

Neurological status should be assessed. The use of an assessment tool such as the GCS is of significant benefit here. Consciousness level, responsiveness and coherence, sensory/motor weaknesses, visual acuity, and pupil reaction are all methods which can be used to assess and diagnose deficit. Neurological deficit can be expected with some types of surgery (neurosurgery) and preoperative status should always be noted (dementia, psychiatric disorders).

*Exposure (everything else)*

This part of the assessment should cover 'everything else'. Full exposure of the patient should occur: inspection of the wound site and surrounding tissue, palpation of the abdomen, and attention paid to 'additionals', such as temperature and blood sugar, can assist the practitioner with diagnosis.

Always turn the patient as haemorrhage can occur in a site which is non-evident while a patient is supine.

Patient dignity must be fully observed during this part of the assessment.

---

**Box 25.7 Anaesthetic-related emergencies**

- Atelectasis
- Compartment syndrome
- Delayed emergence and inadequate reversal
- Dehiscence
- DIC
- Hypoxaemia
- Laryngospasm
- MH suxamethonium apnoea
- Stridor
- Thyroid storm
- Upper airway obstruction

---

**Box 25.8 General emergencies**

- Allergy and anaphylaxis
- Arrhythmias
- Cardiac arrest
- Cardiac tamponade
- Chest pain
- Convulsions
- Extravasation
- Malignant hypo/hypertension
- MI
- Metabolic disturbances
- PE
- Pneumothorax
- Respiratory arrest
- Seizures
- Sepsis
- Severe hypo/hyperglycaemia
- Shock (normovolaemic/hypovolaemic)
- Sinus tachycardia
- Status epilepticus
- Supraventricular tachycardia
- Tension pneumothorax
- VT

## Further reading

Craig A, Hatfield A (2020). The complete recovery room book (6th ed). Oxford: Oxford University Press.

Freedman R, Herbert L, O'Donnell A, et al. (eds) (2022). Oxford handbook of anaesthesia (5th ed). Oxford: Oxford University Press.

National Institute for Health and Care Excellence (2020). National Early Warning Score systems that alert to deteriorating adult patients in hospital. Medtech innovation briefing [MIB205]. Available at: ℜ https://www.nice.org.uk/guidance/mib205

National Institute for Health and Care Excellence (2020). Perioperative care in adults. NICE guideline [NG180]. Available at: ℜ https://www.nice.org.uk/guidance/ng180

Peate I, MacLeod J (eds) (2020). Pudner's nursing the surgical patient (4th ed). Oxford: Elsevier.

Resuscitation Council (UK) (2021). Advanced life support providers manual (8th ed). London: Resuscitation Council (UK).

Resuscitation Council (UK) (2021). European paediatric life support provider manual (5th ed). London: Resuscitation Council (UK).

Royal College of Anaesthetists (2019). Chapter 4: guidelines for the provision of postoperative care. London: Royal College of Anaesthetists.

Royal College of Physicians (2017). National Early Warning Score (NEWS) 2: standardising the assessment of acute illness severity in the NHS. Available at: ℜ https://www.rcplondon.ac.uk/projects/outputs/national-early-warning-score-news-2

Smith G, Allan A, Gordon PAL, et al. (2012). ALERT™: acute life-threatening events, recognition and treatment (3rd ed). Portsmouth: Portsmouth Hospitals NHS Trust.

Tran A, Yates J, Lau A, et al. (2018). Permissive hypotension versus conventional resuscitation strategies in adult trauma patients with hemorrhagic shock: A systematic review and meta-analysis of randomized controlled trials. Journal of Trauma and Acute Care Surgery, 84(5):802–808.

# Cardiovascular emergencies

Cardiovascular disorders of the body can be classified as either complications or events. Cardiovascular complications describe minor–major conditions which are caused by homeostatic imbalance, such as hypotension and tachycardia. Cardiovascular events are conditions which arise as a result of these complications.

### Risk factors

The predominant risk factors for the development of cardiovascular complications/events postoperatively are identified in ➲ Chapter 5, as those with cardiac disease may be at higher risk of developing these cardiovascular complications. However, the risks can also include:

- Smoking
- Altered electrolyte physiology preoperatively
- Emergency surgery
- Regional anaesthetic technique.

### Cardiovascular complications

- Hypotension or hypertension.
- Arrhythmias.
- Sudden bradycardia or tachycardia.
- Chest pain.
- Cardiovascular events
- Hypovolaemia.
- Myocardial infarction (ST elevation MI).
- Cardiac tamponade.
- Cardiac rupture.
- Cardiac ischaemia.
- Cardiogenic shock.
- PE.
- Cardiac arrest.

### Contributors to cardiac arrest in the recovery room

Cardiac arrest is very rare in the recovery room and is always precipitated by one or more of the complications and/or events described here. Cardiac arrest protocols according to local policy should be followed.

- *Arrhythmias* are common in the recovery room as many patients undergoing surgical intervention have altered cardiac function and status. Five-lead monitoring should be used. Recognition of arrhythmia is not always easy. A 12-lead ECG should always be performed in any patient with an altered monitored rhythm. Patients who have previous cardiac surgery, MI, and ischaemia could have an altered ECG wave.
- *Hyper/hypokalaemia and metabolic disorders*: an increase or decrease in serum potassium is the most common metabolic cause of cardiac arrest. However, severe electrolyte disturbance can also cause arrest. Notable examples are hypoglycaemia, hypocalcaemia, and acidaemia. Correction of the abnormal value is the principal aim in such arrests.
- *Hypovolaemia*: severe intra/postoperative haemorrhage can result in arrest due to reduced circulatory blood volume. GI bleeding, dehiscence, and DIC are notable causes.

- *Thromboembolic/mechanical obstruction*: PE and MI are the most common causes of thromboembolic arrests. Surgical specialty can furthermore impact the risk of infarction—vascular and cardiac surgery being principal examples. Treatment of such arrests can be complicated and most are preventable if the signs of cardiac ischaemia (cardiac chest pain and radiation, ECG changes, shortness of breath) are recognized. Mechanical obstruction causing hypoxia could relate to ventilation and $O_2$ delivery system so a system check is warranted.
- *Tension pneumothorax*: the progressive deterioration of a simple pneumothorax can lead to a tension pneumothorax. In such cases, the gradual build-up of escaped air/pressure increases mediastinal pressure, which leads to tracheal deviation and cardiac compression. Upon diagnosis of such an arrest, a needle thoracocentesis and insertion of a chest drain can quickly alleviate the compression.
- *Cardiac tamponade*: tamponade acts in a similar manner to tension pneumothorax. It is caused by a large pericardial effusion (build-up of fluid in the pericardium) and causes arrest via excessive myocardial compression. Tamponade is largely caused by penetrating chest injuries, cardiac surgery, infarct, and sepsis (pericarditis). The immediate management of such an arrest is a pericardiocentesis. Further surgery is often required at a later stage once the patient has been stabilized, to repair the rupture.
- *Toxic/therapeutic disturbances*: arrests due to toxicity and therapeutic disturbances can either be attributed to septic shock, poisoning, or drug overdose.

## Post-resuscitation care

This should be multidisciplinary and focus on returning adequate organ perfusion through improving cardiopulmonary function. This is further discussed in ➔ Chapter 5.

## Further reading

Craig A, Hatfield A (2020). The complete recovery room book (6th ed). Oxford: Oxford University Press.

Freedman R, Herbert L, O'Donnell A, et al. (eds) (2022). Oxford handbook of anaesthesia (5th ed). Oxford: Oxford University Press.

National Institute for Health and Care Excellence (2020). National Early Warning Score systems that alert to deteriorating adult patients in hospital. Medtech innovation briefing [MIB205]. Available at: ⅌ https://www.nice.org.uk/guidance/mib205

National Institute for Health and Care Excellence (2020). Perioperative care in adults. NICE guideline [NG180]. Available at: ⅌ https://www.nice.org.uk/guidance/ng180

Parekh K, Shimabukuro D (2018). Cardiopulmonary resuscitation. In: Pardo M, Miller R (eds) Basics of anaesthesia (7th ed). Philadelphia, PA: Elsevier.

Ramrakha P, Hill J. (2012). Oxford handbook of cardiology (2nd ed). Oxford: Oxford University Press.

Resuscitation Council (UK) (2021). Advanced life support providers manual (8th ed). London: Resuscitation Council (UK).

Resuscitation Council (UK) (2021). European paediatric life support provider manual (5th ed). London: Resuscitation Council (UK).

Royal College of Anaesthetists (2019). Chapter 4: guidelines for the provision of postoperative care. London: Royal College of Anaesthetists.

Royal College of Anaesthetists (2020). Chapter 18: guidelines for the provision of anaesthesia services for cardiac and thoracic procedures. London: Royal College of Anaesthetists.

Royal College of Physicians (2017). National Early Warning Score (NEWS) 2: standardising the assessment of acute illness severity in the NHS. Available at: ⅌ https://www.rcplondon.ac.uk/projects/outputs/national-early-warning-score-news-2

Smith G, Allan A, Gordon PAL, et al. (2012). ALERT™: acute life-threatening events, recognition and treatment (3rd ed). Portsmouth: Portsmouth Hospitals NHS Trust.

# Respiratory emergencies

Respiratory disorders are common within the post-anaesthetic setting. An incidence of between 1% and 30% is suggested, depending upon the complication and its severity. They can occur as a direct result of the surgery or anaesthesia and are the most common cause of life-threatening incidents in the recovery room. Respiratory disorders can be classified as being either airway or breathing in nature and an early diagnosis and resolve of the cause can prevent further deterioration and death.

## Airway

Airway compromise is the principal cause of all respiratory complications. In most instances, compromise is due to airway obstruction, which can arise from either the upper (nose/lips to bronchus) or lower bronchioles to alveoli part of the airway. Airway sounds emitted by the patient are usually the first indicators of obstruction. Stridor and snoring are indicative of upper airway obstruction while wheezing and excessive coughing denote the presence of obstruction in the bronchioles and lower airway.

### Stridor

Stridor is always a medical emergency and presents as a 'crowing' noise, which is most often caused by partial airway obstruction in the larynx. Stridor can occur on inspiration or expiration; postoperatively, inspiratory stridor is most common, occurring as a result of laryngospasm. The management of stridor should follow a systematic approach:

- Open and inspect the airway by use of jaw thrust or chin lift manoeuvres.
- If airway difficult to visualize, use laryngoscope.
- Clear the airway of any secretions or foreign bodies via suction.
- Administer 100% $O_2$ via high concentration non-rebreather mask.

*If these methods do not improve the patient's condition*

- Call for assistance.
- Insert an oropharyngeal/nasopharyngeal airway (if patient is not fully conscious).
- Fully extend jaw (not possible with confirmed/?cervical spine fracture).
- Hand-ventilate airway using bag and mask, ensure that the seal between the airway and mask is effective—the aim of hand ventilation is the application of positive pressure.

*In worst case scenarios, if the above measures have failed*

- Suxamethonium and an induction agent (e.g. propofol should be readily available in cases of stridor).
- Administer a small bolus dose of suxamethonium or propofol.
- Prepare for emergency endotracheal intubation and/or cricothyroidotomy.

*Wheezing and bronchospasm*

Wheezing is a principal sign of bronchial irritation, inflammation, and/or oedema and predominantly indicates bronchospasm. The risk of a patient developing a bronchospasm postoperatively is greatly affected by their preoperative respiratory physiology. Increased incidence in asthmatics, smokers, and patients with COPD.

Wheezing is an initial sign of complication and should never be ignored, it is often accompanied by:
- Dyspnoea and tachypnoea
- Decrease in BP
- Paradoxical ('see-saw') breathing
- Cyanosis.

When bronchospasm is detected, it should be managed with high-flow $O_2$ (100%) administered via a non-rebreather mask. The patient should be closely monitored and if the wheeze persists, the anaesthetist consulted. Reassurance is often beneficial if the patient is conscious. A continuous wheeze can indicate allergy, aspiration, or pulmonary oedema.

## Breathing

Several conditions directly influencing the respiratory drive can cause postoperative complication. These include:
- Suxamethonium apnoea
- Respiratory paralysis (inadequate reversal of neuromuscular blockade)
- Hypoventilation
- Aspiration pneumonitis (➔ see Chapter 11).

## Hypoxia

- The eventual consequence of any airway/breathing event is hypoxia and the principal function of the recovery room is to prevent its occurrence.
- Cyanosis is an intermediary sign; peripheral cyanosis usually indicates a $SpO_2$ of <85%.
- Hypoxia can cause death quickly and subtly and the most effective treatment is prompt recognition.
- Patients who develop cyanosis should be given 100% $O_2$ via a non-rebreather mask.
- Airway patency and efficiency of breathing should then be assessed.
- Once the cause of hypoxia is ascertained, appropriate methods should be taken to correct it.
- If left untreated, hypoxia leads to cardiac arrest.

## Risk factors

Several factors increase the risk of developing airway/breathing events postoperatively, these are:
- Age: ≤1 year or ≥60 years
- Obesity: 120 kg+ in men/100 kg+ in women
- ASA grading: increased grading = increased risk
- Pre-existing illness and lifestyle: COPD, renal disease
- Cardiovascular disease, diabetes mellitus, smoker
- Type of surgery; thoracic and abdominal surgery increase the risk of postoperative respiratory complications.

## Further reading

Craig A, Hatfield A (2020). The complete recovery room book (6th ed). Oxford: Oxford University Press.

Freedman R, Herbert L, O'Donnell A, et al. (eds) (2022). Oxford handbook of anaesthesia (5th ed). Oxford: Oxford University Press.

National Institute for Health and Care Excellence (2020). Asthma: diagnosis, management and chronic asthma management. NICE guideline [NG80]. Available at: ℅ https://www.nice.org.uk/guidance/ng80

National Institute for Health and Care Excellence (2020). Perioperative care in adults. NICE guideline [NG180]. Available at: ℅ https://www.nice.org.uk/guidance/ng180

Pollard B, Kitchen G (eds) (2017). Handbook of clinical anaesthesia (4th ed). London: CRC Press.

Royal College of Anaesthetists (2020). Chapter 18: guidelines for the provision of anaesthesia services for cardiac and thoracic procedures. London: Royal College of Anaesthetists.

Royal College of Anaesthetists (2019). Chapter 4: guidelines for the provision of postoperative care. London: Royal College of Anaesthetists.

Royal College of Physicians (2017). National Early Warning Score (NEWS) 2: standardising the assessment of acute illness severity in the NHS. Available at: ℅ https://www.rcplondon.ac.uk/projects/outputs/national-early-warning-score-news-2

Smith G, Allan A, Gordon PAL, et al. (2012). ALERT™: acute life-threatening events, recognition and treatment (3rd ed). Portsmouth: Portsmouth Hospitals NHS Trust.

# Neurosurgery

Neurosurgical emergencies often progress rapidly hence emergency management is essential to minimize further neurological damage. The brain can be injured in many ways, the most common being through direct traumatic brain injury.

In the Western world, the most common mechanisms of these injuries are road traffic collisions, falls from height, and assaults.

- Ischaemic injury through embolic stroke or haemorrhagic injury from ruptured vascular malformations (e.g. cerebral aneurysms) are also common causes of neurosurgical emergencies.
- Acute hydrocephalus (excessive fluid on the brain) and infection problems (e.g. abscesses) are other conditions where prompt intervention is required.
- Similarly, acute spinal injuries can be traumatic, compressive, and infective.

## Patient assessment

- Patients requiring emergency neurosurgical procedures will normally be transferred to a specialist regional centre for their treatment; and then to a specialist neurosurgical unit.
- Initial assessment of the patient's vital signs and GCS score is vital.
- The GCS provides a practical method for assessment of impairment of conscious level in response to defined stimuli. It also aids staff to communicate about the level of consciousness of patients with a neurosurgical condition. This includes pupil size and reactivity, limb movements, respiratory rate, heart rate, BP, temperature, and blood $O_2$ saturation; this score is out of 15. All are documented and checked hourly, or until stable.
- IV access should be established, fluids and pain relief should be prescribed and administered.
- Complete blood tests and any imaging should be performed.
- Visual assessment of how the patient appears at the time of observation also requires documenting.
- Development of severe or increasing headache or persisting vomiting, or new or evolving neurological symptoms or signs such as pupil inequality or asymmetry of limb or facial movement.
- To reduce inter-observer variability and unnecessary referrals, a second member of staff should confirm deterioration before involving the supervising doctor. This should be carried out immediately. An immediate CT scan should be considered, and the patient's clinical condition reassessed and managed appropriately.
- If a patient deteriorates by >3 points on their GCS score an ITU referral is required with possibly an ITU admission.

*Emergency operations can be carried out for*

- Intracranial haematoma.
- Subarachnoid haemorrhage.
- Hydrocephalus.

*Types of intracranial haematomas*
- Extradural.
- Subdural.

Extradural haematoma can be the result of a low-velocity injury and the patient may experience:
- A transient loss of consciousness that can rapidly recover
- A period of lucidity
- Rapid deterioration in their level of consciousness
- Increase in BP and decrease in heart rate
- Limb weakness.
- Dilatation of pupils.

The treatment of choice will be to carry out an emergency decompression operation, such as burr holes (Fig. 25.4), to evacuate the clot and reduce the ICP.

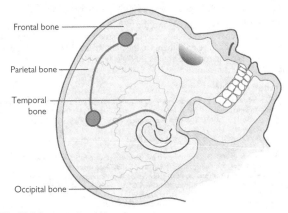

Frontal bone

Parietal bone

Temporal bone

Occipital bone

**Fig. 25.4** Emergency burr holes.

Adapted with permission from Gardiner M and Borley N (2009). *Training in Surgery*, Oxford University Press, Oxford.

Subdural haematoma can be a complication of a high-velocity injury and the patient will usually:
- Be unconscious from the time of injury
- Exhibit a deteriorating level of consciousness.

The patient will require a decompressive craniotomy. Causes of subarachnoid haemorrhage may be:
- Intracranial aneurysm
- Arteriovenous malformation
- Hypertension
- Idiopathic.

Common symptoms include:
- Sudden-onset severe headache
- Nausea
- Photophobia
- Vomiting
- Neck stiffness.

If the patient is fit enough, they may undergo a craniotomy to clip the aneurysm at its neck while maintaining the blood flow in the native vessel. The timing of surgical intervention is controversial with some cases being delayed for 10 days after the initial haemorrhage. Early surgery may be associated with reduced mortality and no increased morbidity.

Hydrocephalus is a condition in which there is an increase in CSF in the cranial cavity. This may be due to:
- Excessive production
- Inadequate absorption
- An obstruction that impedes flow through the ventricular system.

The surgical treatment may involve the insertion of a ventriculoperitoneal (VP) shunt where a catheter is placed in the lateral ventricle, connected via a valve and a long tunnelled catheter to the peritoneum. The valve is located under the scalp and can be compressed digitally to flush CSF from the ventricle to the peritoneum.

## Further reading

Association of Anaesthetists of Great Britain and Ireland (2019). Safe transfer of the brain-injured patient – trauma and stroke. Available at: ℘ http://dx.doi.org/10.1111/anae.14866

Craig A, Hatfield A (2020). The complete recovery room book (6th ed). Oxford: Oxford University Press.

Freedman R, Herbert L, O'Donnell A, et al. (eds) (2022). Oxford handbook of anaesthesia (5th ed). Oxford: Oxford University Press.

Glasgow Coma Scale at 40 (2014). The new approach to Glasgow Coma Scale assessment. Available at: ℘ https://www.youtube.com/watch?v=v6qpEQxJQO4&ab_channel=GCSat40

National Institute for Health and Care Excellence (2019). Recommendations. In: Head injury: assessment and early management. Clinical guideline [CG176]. Available at: ℘ "https://www.nice.org.uk/guidance/cg176/chapter/1-recommendations

National Institute for Health and Care Excellence (2019). Suspected neurological conditions: recognition and referral. Available at: https://www.nice.org.uk/guidance/ng127

National Institute for Health and Care Excellence (2020). National Early Warning Score systems that alert to deteriorating adult patients in hospital. Medtech innovation briefing [MIB205]. Available at: ℘ https://www.nice.org.uk/guidance/mib205

Pollard B, Kitchen G (eds) (2017). Handbook of clinical anaesthesia (4th ed). London: CRC Press.

Royal College of Anaesthetists (2020). Chapter 14: guidelines for the provision of neuro-anaesthetic services. London: Royal College of Anaesthetists.

Royal College of Physicians (2017). National Early Warning Score (NEWS) 2: standardising the assessment of acute illness severity in the NHS. Available at: ℘ https://www.rcplondon.ac.uk/projects/outputs/national-early-warning-score-news-2

Smith G, Allan A, Gordon PAL, et al. (2012). ALERT™: acute life-threatening events, recognition and treatment (3rd ed). Portsmouth: Portsmouth Hospitals NHS Trust.

# Seizure/convulsion management

A *seizure* can be defined as a sudden and uncontrollable discharge of electricity in the brain.

A *convulsion* is the abnormal motor response that occurs during a seizure.

Seizures can occur as a result of epilepsy or as a result of an underlying pathology, such as CNS imbalance. Epilepsy is a common condition that affects approximately 1 in 103 people. It is usually diagnosed in childhood and in people aged >65 years, but it can affect anyone. It may be hard to tell if someone is having a seizure, as some seizures only cause a person to have vacant episodes. These may go unnoticed. Specific symptoms depend on which part of the brain is involved. Irrespective of their cause, seizures should always be managed similarly—the maintenance of the airway taking precedence.

## Types of seizure

There are several types of seizure that a patient can endure. These can be broadly categorized as generalized, partial, and complex partial seizures.
- Generalized seizures summarize the traditional 'fit'. These describe tonic–clonic (grand mal) convulsions, myoclonic (brief arm contractions), and clonic seizures (rhythmic symmetrical movements of the arms, neck, and face).
- Partial seizures (also known as focal seizures) are usually non-motor and involve sensory, autonomic, and/or higher conscious impairment.
- Complex partial seizures involve loss of consciousness, spatial awareness, and memory.

Seizures can progress from one type to another. For example, complex partial seizures commonly develop into generalized seizures. The predominant causes of seizures in the recovery room are identified in Table 25.5.

**Table 25.5** Causes of seizures in recovery

| | |
|---|---|
| A patient with epilepsy who has not taken his/her medication or is undiagnosed | *Most common* |
| Adverse reaction to anaesthetic agents | |
| Neurosurgery | |
| Hyperpyrexia and sepsis | |
| Hypoglycaemia | |
| Hypoxia | |
| Fluid overload | |
| Hypocalcaemia | |
| Norpethidine toxicity (pethidine overdose) | *Least common* |

*Adverse reaction to anaesthetic agents*
- With the exception of epilepsy, this is one of the most common reasons for postoperative seizures.
- Methohexitone, propofol, enflurane, and LAs are agents which can directly stimulate convulsions.
- Abrupt withdrawal of alcohol (in alcoholics), benzodiazepines, and antiparkinsonians can also indirectly stimulate seizures.

> All neurosurgical patients are at an increased risk of postoperative seizure, this may be attributed to the surgery or the patient's medical history (which indicates the need for surgery).

*Hyperpyrexia, sepsis, and febrile convulsions*
- Hyperpyrexia (high fever) refers to a core temperature >40°C.
- As the body's temperature begins to exceed this, its thermoregulatory cooling mechanisms begin to fail.
- A core temperature of 41°C+ can stimulate seizures and cellular decay in the brain.
- The body's consumption for $O_2$ will increase by 15% for every degree Celsius above 37°C, therefore hyperpyrexic patients should always be administered high-flow $O_2$.
- This can prevent and delay the onset of hyperpyrexic seizures.

In children aged up to 6 years, seizures can occur once their core temperature reaches 39°C.
- In such instances, these seizures are referred to as febrile convulsions and are characterized by a rapid increase in core temperature.
- Febrile convulsions should be therapeutically managed by the administration of rectal diazepam (while the child is convulsing) and an antipyretic, such as paracetamol (if not administered prior to convulsion).

In adults, sepsis is the most common cause of hyperpyrexia and the nature and type of operation can influence the risk of its development (e.g. ruptured appendixes, external trauma, surgery involving the meninges).

*Hypoglycaemia*
- A blood glucose level of <2 mmol/L can result in a hypoglycaemic seizure.
- This type of seizure should be managed according to local policy and alongside an infusion of 50% glucose until the blood glucose level reaches between 5.5 and 11 mmol/L.

## Management

The prevention of seizure is always the best form of management. A proactive approach, such as ensuring the epileptic patient is administered his/her anticonvulsant, maintenance of blood glucose level via sliding scale of insulin, and cooling of a patient before he/she becomes hyperpyrexic, can prevent a potential crisis from occurring.

When managing a convulsing patient reactively, a systematic approach should be adopted:

- Immediately check the pulse—if pulse absent, treat as cardiac arrest.
- Call for assistance and request the emergency trolley.
- Open the airway and support using jaw thrust/chin lift.
- Have suction available.
- Administer high-flow $O_2$ via non-rebreather mask, monitor breathing.
- Protect the patient, raise cot sides on bed/trolley and support with padding or pillows, and place patient in the recovery position.
- Monitor the seizure, note the time of onset, and record the duration of convulsion.
- Ascertain cause of seizure: check blood sugar level, $SpO_2$, temperature, and medical/drug history.

## Pharmacological management

- Most seizures will last no more than 3–5 minutes. Pharmacological management should be considered if the seizure exceeds this duration.
- The first-line treatment of postoperative seizures is benzodiazepines:
  - IV or IM lorazepam (0.1 mg/kg, administered over 2 minutes) or diazepam (0.15–0.2 mg/kg, administered over 5 minutes) should be used if the patient has IV access.
  - PR diazepam can be administered (0.5 mg/kg) if the patient does not have IV access.
- Second-line treatments (if the seizure has not resolved following administration of first-line agents) patients can be given a loading dose IV of most commonly, phenytoin, dose 20 mg/kg (maximum per dose 2 g) or levetiracetam.
- Seizures that continue for 30 minutes or more is a condition known as status epilepticus. It can occur with all types of seizures, but with tonic–clonic seizures it represents a medical emergency requiring immediate treatment. In such instances, the patient should be re-intubated, ventilated, and transferred to intensive care.

## Further reading

Association of Anaesthetists of Great Britain and Ireland (2019). Safe transfer of the brain-injured patient – trauma and stroke. Available at: ℘ http://dx.doi.org/10.1111/anae.14866

Craig A, Hatfield A (2020). The complete recovery room book (6th ed). Oxford: Oxford University Press.

Glasgow Coma Scale at 40 (2014). The new approach to Glasgow Coma Scale assessment. Available at: ℘ https://www.youtube.com/watch?v=v6qpEQxJQO4&ab_channel=GCSat40

Joint Formulary Committee (2022). British national formulary. Available at: ℘ https://bnf.nice.org.uk/

Joint Formulary Committee (2022). British national formulary for children. Available at: ℘ https://bnfc.nice.org.uk/

National Institute for Health and Care Excellence (2019). Recommendations. In: Head injury: assessment and early management. Clinical guideline [CG176]. Available at: ℘ https://www.nice.org.uk/guidance/cg176/chapter/1-recommendations

National Institute for Health and Care Excellence (2019). Suspected neurological conditions: recognition and referral. NICE guideline [NG127]. Available at: ℘ https://www.nice.org.uk/guidance/ng127

National Institute for Health and Care Excellence (2020). Epilepsies: diagnosis and management. Clinical guideline [CG137]. Available at: ℘ https://www.nice.org.uk/guidance/cg137

National Institute for Health and Care Excellence (2020). National Early Warning Score systems that alert to deteriorating adult patients in hospital. Medtech innovation briefing [MIB205]. Available at: ℘ https://www.nice.org.uk/guidance/mib205

Pollard B, Kitchen G (eds) (2017). Handbook of clinical anaesthesia (4th ed). London: CRC Press.

Royal College of Anaesthetists (2020). Chapter 14: guidelines for the provision of neuro-anaesthetic services. London: Royal College of Anaesthetists.

Royal College of Physicians (2017). National Early Warning Score (NEWS) 2: standardising the assessment of acute illness severity in the NHS. Available at: &#8518; https://www.rcplondon.ac.uk/projects/outputs/national-early-warning-score-news-2

Smith G, Allan A, Gordon PAL, et al. (2012). ALERT™: acute life-threatening events, recognition and treatment (3rd ed). Portsmouth: Portsmouth Hospitals NHS Trust.

# Index

Notes: Tables, figures and boxes are indicated by an italic *t*, *f* or *b* following the page/paragraph number.